Physical Activity and Health

Physical Activity and Health explains clearly, systematically and in detail the relationship between physical activity, health and disease, and examines the role of exercise in the prevention and management of a wide range of important conditions.

Now in a fully updated and expanded third edition, this is the most complete and engaging textbook on the subject. It offers a balanced examination of the latest evidence linking levels of physical activity with the risk of mortality, cardiovascular diseases, diabetes, obesity, cancer, osteoporosis and dementia. Designed to help the reader evaluate the quality of the evidence, the book includes an invaluable discussion of common study designs and the inherent difficulties of measuring physical activity. It examines the evidence in relation to child and adolescent health, older adults, hazards of exercise, sedentary behaviour, public health policy and, in a new chapter, mental health, and an epilogue considers the emerging evidence regarding the significance of physical activity and COVID-19.

Containing chapter summaries, study tasks, guides to supplementary reading, a glossary of key terms and an abundance of figures and tables, *Physical Activity and Health* is an essential course text, and important reading for undergraduate, masters and postgraduate research students of sport and exercise science, public health, physical therapy, medicine and nursing.

This third edition is supported by an updated companion website featuring self-test questions, PowerPoint slides, learning activities and website links.

David J. Stensel is Professor of Exercise Metabolism and Associate Dean for Research in the School of Sport, Exercise and Health Sciences at Loughborough University, UK. He is also the Lifestyle Theme Lead for the National Institute for Health Research (NIHR) Leicester Biomedical Research Centre and Editor-in-Chief for the *International Journal of Obesity*.

Adrianne E. Hardman is Emeritus Professor of Human Exercise Metabolism at Loughborough University, UK. She has over 30 years' experience in university teaching and research, has published widely, given invited lectures in many countries, and has contributed to the development of guidelines on physical activity in the UK and in North America.

Jason M.R. Gill is Professor of Cardiometabolic Health at the University of Glasgow, UK. He leads an active multidisciplinary research group investigating the effects of physical activity and wider lifestyle on the prevention and management of vascular and metabolic diseases. He is also Director of his university's MSc in Sport and Exercise Science and Medicine.

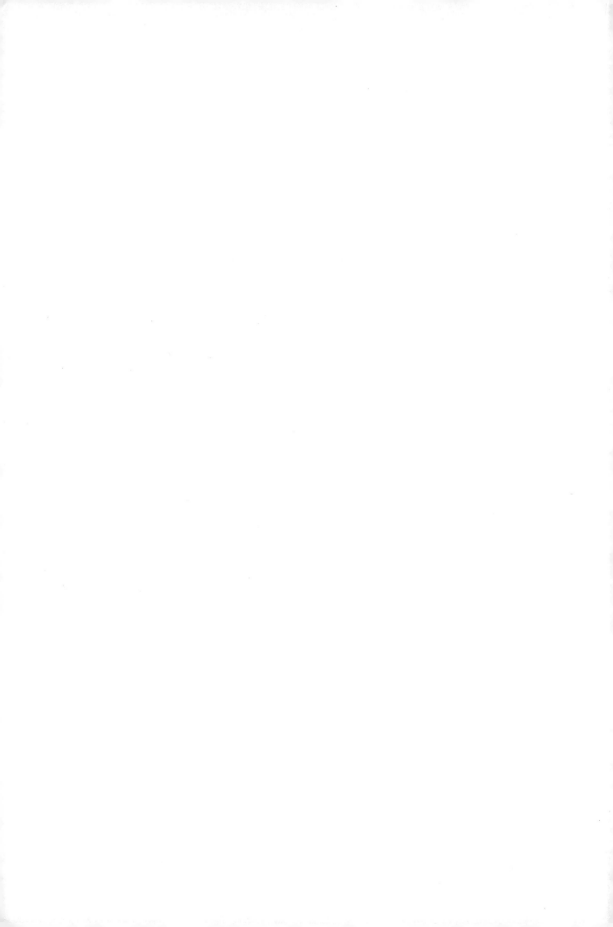

Physical Activity and Health
The Evidence Explained

Third edition

Edited by
David J. Stensel, Adrianne E. Hardman
and Jason M.R. Gill

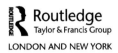
Routledge
Taylor & Francis Group

LONDON AND NEW YORK

Third edition published 2022
by Routledge
2 Park Square, Milton Park, Abingdon, Oxon, OX14 4RN

and by Routledge
605 Third Avenue, New York, NY 10158

Routledge is an imprint of the Taylor & Francis Group, an informa business

First edition published by Routledge 2003
Second edition published by Routledge 2009

British Library Cataloguing-in-Publication Data
A catalogue record for this book is available from the British Library

Library of Congress Cataloging-in-Publication Data
Names: Stensel, David J., 1964- editor. | Hardman, Adrianne E., 1944-
editor. | Gill, Jason M. R., editor.
Title: Physical activity and health : the evidence explained / David J.
Stensel, Adrianne E. Hardman, and Jason M.R. Gill.
Description: Third edition. | Abingdon, Oxon ; New York, NY :
Routledge, 2021. | Revised edition of: Physical activity and health /
Adrianne E. Hardman and David J. Stensel. 2nd ed. 2009. | Includes
bibliographical references and index. |
Identifiers: LCCN 2020055921 | ISBN 9780415632959 (hardback) |
ISBN 9780415632966 (paperback) | ISBN 9780203095270 (ebook)
Subjects: LCSH: Exercise therapy. | Exercise—Health aspects. | Health
risk assessment. | Epidemiology. | Medicine—Research—Evaluation.
Classification: LCC RM725 .H337 2021 | DDC 615.8/2—dc23
LC record available at https://lccn.loc.gov/2020055921

ISBN: 978-0-415-63295-9 (hbk)
ISBN: 978-0-415-63296-6 (pbk)
ISBN: 978-0-203-09527-0 (ebk)

Typeset in Adobe Garamond Pro
by codeMantra

Access the companion website: www.routledge.com/cw/stensel

Contents

5 Type 2 diabetes

JASON M.R. GILL

6 Obesity

JAMES A. KING

Figures

Tables

Boxes

Contributors

Katherine Brooke-Wavell is Senior Lecturer in Human Biology at the School of Sport, Exercise and Health Sciences, Loughborough University, UK.

Stephen F. Burns is Associate Professor in the Department of Physical Education and Sports Science at the National Institute of Education, Nanyang Technological University, Singapore.

Kevin Deighton is Health Economist and Statistician at Delta Hat, Nottingham, UK.

James A. King is Senior Lecturer in Exercise Physiology at the School of Sport, Exercise and Health Sciences, Loughborough University, UK.

Fehmidah Munir is Reader in Health Psychology at the School of Sport, Exercise and Health Sciences, Loughborough University, UK.

Marie H. Murphy is Professor, Dean of Postgraduate Research and Director of the Ulster Doctoral College, Ulster University, Northern Ireland.

Clare Stevinson is Senior Lecturer in Behavioural Aspects of Physical Activity and Health at the School of Sport, Exercise and Health Sciences, Loughborough University, UK.

Alice E. Thackray is Senior Research Associate in Exercise Metabolism at the School of Sport, Exercise and Health Sciences, Loughborough University, UK.

Foreword

THIRD EDITION

The forewords to the first and second editions of this text were written by Professor Jeremy N. Morris, a pioneer of the epidemiology of physical activity and coronary heart disease. We were, and remain, proud that someone of his unique stature in the field chose to endorse our book. Sadly, Professor Morris died in October 2009, only months after the publication of the second edition. It seemed inappropriate to include a new foreword to this third edition; instead, Professor Morris's valued contributions to the earlier editions are reprinted here.

Foreword

SECOND EDITION

I am delighted to welcome this second updated edition that seeks to report and interpret the international study effort. This could not be more timely. It appears that at long last our government is serious about its responsibility to promote physical activity as essential for the health of the nation. Mounting concern over children's obesity, treated here in model new theoretical and practical chapters, may have triggered the shift in policy. Newcomers to physical activity and health can be expected, including many newly involved in public approaches. They will be seeking instruction, understanding and guidance – and will find a splendid resource in this distinguished text.

Jerry N. Morris, January 2009

Foreword

FIRST EDITION

It is a privilege and pleasure to welcome this fine work by a leading investigator and her colleague, both of them experienced teachers in the famous school at Loughborough. The text meets the needs of countless students of physical activity and health now to be found in university sports sciences, clinical medicine, epidemiology and in the social domain, from transport planning to the fitness industry. Many of these students, like myself, have not had systematic teaching in the physiology of exercise. Yet, we are constantly meeting its concepts and observations that are plainly fundamental to understanding and to application. Until now, there hasn't been a book to meet our needs. Two features, moreover, characterise their contribution: throughout, the nature and quality of the evidence are clearly described, and the collective – the population – aspects as well as the individual and personal are emphasised.

Our field today presents some remarkable features. In the half-century since the Second World War, there has been an explosion of research and thinking on the needs for, and benefits of, physical activity/exercise across the lifespan and bodily systems. This knowledge is widely not being applied in practice. In consequence there is an epochal waste of human potential for health, functional capacities, wellbeing. This the authors document and illuminate.

Three of today's major associated issues may be cited. First, the pandemic of obesity in the developed and, increasingly, the developing world. The scientific consensus now is that physical inactivity bears much and possibly most of the responsibility. The authors devote two chapters to the issue, giving us a lucid straightforward description plus a highly instructive account of the metabolic, insulin resistance, syndrome, a seminal concept that public health has not yet begun to take on board. The characteristic 'modern epidemic' of coronary heart disease is dealt with again in two chapters. These are typically helpful in elucidating the roles of physical activity and physical fitness and in distinguishing disease and risk factors for disease. A third instance is the welfare of old people. When history comes to be written, society's failure to apply modern knowledge of normal ageing processes, in particular the loss of muscle, and the remedial possibilities, is likely to shame us. Scientific evidence in randomised controlled trials is impeccable. And yet, one of the great gifts of physiology to public health is massively ignored. There cannot be any excuse for any in health care with such a convincing demonstration now so readily available in this book.

We are, the generality of us, the first generation in history to require little, often scarcely any, physical activity in our everyday lives. We have therefore deliberately to introduce this ourselves, and commonly in an unhelpful environment. Many readers will be seeking one way and another to serve in this field. They will find much support in this splendid book. It is surely a tract for the times. *Bon voyage*!

Jerry N. Morris
Public and Environmental Health Research Unit
London School of Hygiene and Tropical Medicine

Preface

It has been 12 years since the second edition of this textbook was published. During this time there has been a huge increase in the volume of literature published across many areas. This is due in part to the continuation of several trends which were identified in previous editions. Rates of obesity and type 2 diabetes have continued to climb worldwide, in children and adolescents as well as in adults, and in low- and middle-income countries as well as in high-income countries. Another trend highlighted in previous editions – the ageing of the population – has continued, increasing the prevalence of many chronic diseases, notably cancer, dementia and type 2 diabetes. Collectively, these trends bring a renewed sense of urgency to research into the potential of physical activity to prevent disease and facilitate healthy ageing.

A notable development has been increased attention on the potential adverse consequences of high levels of sedentary behaviour, and whether this is independent of overall physical activity levels. Quantification of the dose–response relationships between physical activity and sedentary behaviour with adverse health outcomes has been facilitated by the increased utilisation of accelerometers and inclinometers for measuring not just physical activity but also body posture (standing, sitting, lying down). This has enhanced the accuracy and detail with which physical activity and sedentary behaviour profiles can be characterised. Moreover, the past decade has seen greater use of imaging techniques, including dual energy X-ray absorptiometry and magnetic resonance imaging. This has strengthened knowledge and understanding of the effects of physical activity not only on muscle, bone, fat and body composition but also on the structure of organs including the heart, the liver and the brain, all of which may be influenced by regular physical activity.

Another important development has been the increased use of systematic reviews and meta-analyses to collate and summarise research evidence. These ensure that all available data are captured when addressing specific research questions and thus provide a more objective and comprehensive assessment of the literature. In addition, new large epidemiological cohorts, such as the UK Biobank, have enabled the contributions of genetic predisposition and environmental exposure (including physical activity) to the development of disease to be captured. Such developments have enhanced understanding of the association between physical activity/sedentary behaviour and a variety of chronic diseases which have contributed to revised public health recommendations for physical activity in the US in 2018 and the UK in 2019. These guidelines and other issues central to public health are addressed in the final chapter of this book.

It would be remiss of us not to mention the worldwide pandemic of COVID-19 which erupted during the writing of this book and which is discussed in our Epilogue. Its effects have been particularly pernicious among older adults, those with chronic disease and those who are obese. Thus COVID-19, an infectious disease, has brought to the fore concerns about lifestyle behaviours, including physical activity, and their contribution to disease prevention/alleviation and the maintenance of individual and public health.

In producing the third edition of this textbook, David and Adrianne decided to move to an edited book and enlisted a valued co-editor, Professor Jason Gill, as well as a distinguished group of contributors each of whom brought a fresh perspective to the issues addressed in the book, whilst at the same time ensuring a continuity of the style adopted in previous editions.

Acknowledgements

We are indebted to all contributors for devoting time to this project. Thanks go, in particular, to Dr Alice Thackray who not only wrote a key chapter but also assisted with the formatting and preparation of the final manuscript. Her attention to detail was exemplary. David thanks his wife, Para, and his daughters, Chandini and Rohini, for their continued support and patience, particularly when holidays were used for book writing! Adrianne is grateful to her late husband, Peter, for his understanding of her commitment to this text over many years. Jason is grateful to Adrianne and David for including him in this exciting and important project, and to Christine and Freya for their understanding and forbearance on the many occasions when writing spilled over into family time. Finally, the editors extend warm and wholehearted thanks to Simon Whitmore and Rebecca Connor of Routledge for their unwavering support and enthusiasm during the preparation of this book.

Part I
Assessing the evidence

1 Introduction

David J. Stensel

EARLY OBSERVATIONS

Physical activity and physical fitness have been linked with health and longevity since ancient times. The earliest records of organised exercise used for health promotion are found in China, around 2500 BC. However, it was the Greek physicians of the fifth and early fourth centuries BC who established a tradition of maintaining positive health through 'regimen' – the combination of correct eating and exercise. Hippocrates (c. 460–370 BC), often called the Father of Modern Medicine, wrote:

all parts of the body which have a function, if used in moderation and exercised in labours in which each is accustomed, become thereby healthy, well-developed and age more slowly, but if unused and left idle they become liable to disease, defective in growth and age quickly.

(Hippocrates 1967)

Modern-day exercise research began after the Second World War in the context of post-war aspirations to build a better world. Public health was changing to focus on chronic, non-communicable diseases and the modification of individual behaviour. Whilst Doll and Hill worked on the links between smoking and lung cancer, Professor Jeremy Morris and his colleagues set out to test the hypothesis that deaths from coronary heart disease (CHD) were less common among men engaged in physically active work than among those in sedentary jobs. In seminal papers published in 1953, they reported that conductors working on London's double-decker buses who climbed around 600 stairs per working day experienced less than half the incidence of heart attacks as the sedentary drivers who sat for 90% of their shift (Morris et al. 1953) (Figure 1.1).

Subsequent studies by Morris and others, in particular Morris's close friend Ralph Paffenbarger in the United States (US), confirmed that the postponement of cardio-vascular disease through exercise represents a cause-and-effect relationship. For their contribution, Morris and Paffenbarger were, in 1996, jointly awarded the first International Olympic Medal and Prize for research in exercise sciences.

In the 70 years since Morris's early papers, research into the influence of physical activity on health has burgeoned. This book is not a comprehensive account of this literature; rather it is an attempt to illustrate its extent, strengths and weaknesses, and to help students understand the process of evaluation of evidence. Our emphasis will be on topics that comprise major public health issues. But first, it is necessary to 'paint a picture' of some relevant features of today's societies.

Figure 1.1 A London double-decker bus in the 1950s. Jeremy Morris and colleagues compared the incidence of heart attack in sedentary drivers with that in physically active conductors.

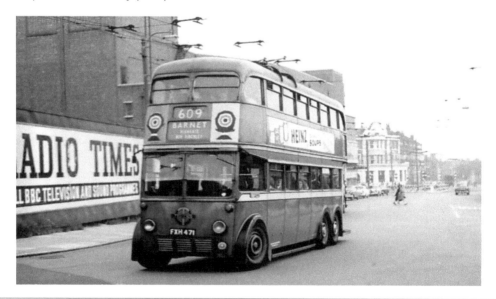

MODERN TRENDS

Over the past century or so the predominant diseases afflicting society in most countries have changed from those transmitted through infection (pneumonia, influenza, tuberculosis, diphtheria) to those that are influenced to some extent by lifestyle, e.g. heart disease, cancer, stroke and diabetes (Jones et al. 2012) (Figure 1.2). Of course, there is a genetic element to these diseases (i.e. some people have a greater genetic predisposition to these conditions than others) but three modern trends are exacerbating the prevalence of these lifestyle-related diseases. These are physical inactivity, obesity and the ageing of the population. Before examining physical inactivity, we will briefly survey trends in obesity and ageing.

According to research, published in *The Lancet* in 2014, more than 2.1 billion (approximately 30%) of the world's population are overweight or obese (Ng et al. 2014) (Figure 1.3). Since 1980 the proportion of adults with a body mass index (BMI) of 25 kg m^{-2} or greater has increased from 29% to 37% in men and from 30% to 38% in women. In adults, estimated obesity prevalence exceeds 50% in some countries

Figure 1.2 Top ten causes of death in the United States: 1900 versus 2010.

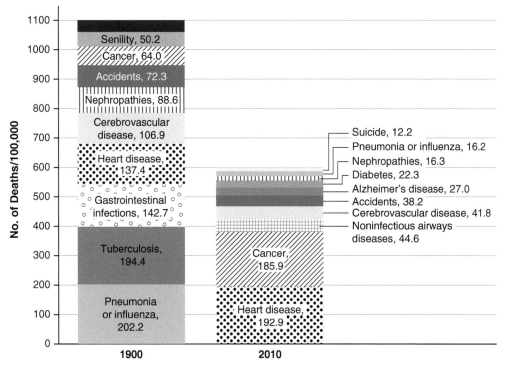

Source: Data are from the Centers for Disease Control and Prevention. Figure reprinted from the *New England Journal of Medicine*, Jones, D.S., et al., 'The burden of disease and the changing task of medicine', 366: 2333–8. Copyright © 2012 Massachusetts Medical Society. Reprinted with permission from Massachusetts Medical Society.

Figure 1.3 Prevalence of overweight and obesity and obesity alone, by age and sex, 2013.

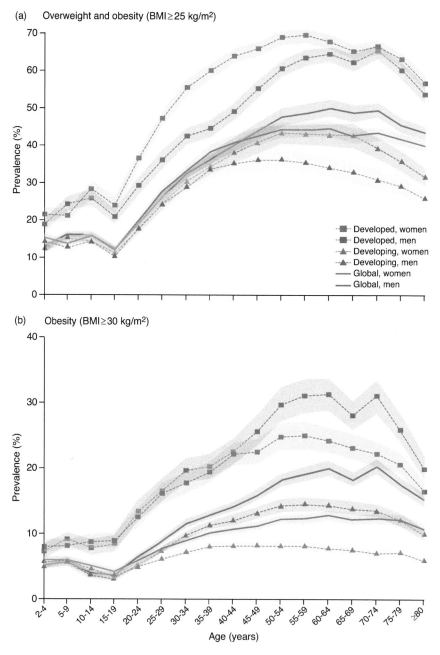

Source: Reprinted from *The Lancet*, 384: 766–81, Ng, M. et al., 'Global, regional, and national prevalence of overweight and obesity in children and adults during 1980–2013: a systematic analysis for the Global Burden of Disease Study 2013', page 769, copyright © 2014, with permission from Elsevier.

Note: Data are displayed for countries classed as developed and developing separately as well as combined (global). Shaded areas represent 95% uncertainty intervals. BMI: body mass index.

(e.g. more than 50% of men in Tonga and more than 50% of women in Kuwait are estimated to be obese). The prevalence of overweight and obesity has also increased in children and adolescents. In 2013, 24% of boys and 23% of girls in developed countries were either overweight or obese while in developing countries approximately 13% of both boys and girls were overweight or obese. This represents a 47% increase in the worldwide prevalence of overweight and obesity for children since 1980. While there are some signs that the increase in adult obesity prevalence is slowing in developed countries this does not appear to be the case in developing countries. Perhaps more ominous is the observation that there are no national success stories in the struggle to control obesity prevalence over the last three decades (Ng et al. 2014).

A recent report on adult obesity prevalence in the US (employing data from the Behavioural Risk Factor Surveillance System Survey) estimates that by 2030 nearly one in two American adults will be obese (BMI $\geq$ 30 kg m^{-2}) and the prevalence of obesity is projected to be higher than 50% in 29 US states. Nearly one in four US adults are predicted to be *severely* obese (BMI $\geq$ 35 kg m^{-2}) by 2030 and this is predicted to become the most common BMI category among women (27.6%), non-Hispanic black adults (31.7%) and low-income adults (31.7%) in the US (Ward et al. 2019) (Figure 1.4).

Consistent with findings from the US, data from the Health Survey for England suggest that 67% of men and 60% of women in England were overweight or obese in 2018. This includes 26% of men and 29% of women in England who were obese (BMI $\geq$ 30 kg m^{-2}) and 2% of men and 4% of women who were *morbidly* obese (BMI $\geq$ 40 kg m^{-2}). Data from this survey also revealed that 34% of men and 48% of women had a very high waist circumference measurement (>102 cm in men; >88 cm in women), indicating central obesity and placing them at elevated risk of chronic disease (Health Survey for England, 2018 courtesy of the National Centre for Social Research (NatCen) and the Department of Epidemiology and Public Health, University College London, 2019). The Health Survey for England 2018 also reports that 28% of children aged 2 to 15 are overweight or obese, of whom 15% are obese. The National Child Measurement Programme (2019) reports that nearly 10% of children are categorised as obese when starting school, i.e. in reception year (aged 4 to 5 years). As noted by the former chief medical officer for England, Professor Dame Sally Davies, childhood obesity disproportionately affects those living in the most deprived areas and has 'profound impacts on the health and life chances of children' (Davies 2019).

The reason there is such concern about obesity is because it is a risk factor for a variety of diseases including cancer, chronic kidney disease, diabetes, hypertension and cardiovascular disease. This will be discussed in greater detail in the coming chapters, but one example here is useful to illustrate the implications of the unrelenting rise in obesity prevalence in recent decades. The disease most closely associated with obesity is type 2 diabetes. In 2008, the global age-standardised adult diabetes prevalence was 9.8% in men and 9.2% in women (up from 8.3% and 7.5% in 1980). Although this includes type 1 diabetes as well as type 2 diabetes, type 2 diabetes accounts for most cases. The estimated number of people with diabetes in 2008 worldwide was 347 million (up from 153 million in 1980). The region with the highest prevalence of diabetes in 2008 was Oceania where 15.5% of men and 15.9% of women had diabetes. Other regions with high diabetes prevalence include South Asia, Latin America and the Caribbean, central Asia, North Africa and the Middle East (Danaei et al. 2011).

Figure 1.4 Estimated prevalence of overall obesity (Panel A) and severe obesity (Panel B) among adults in each state in the United States, from 1990 through 2030.

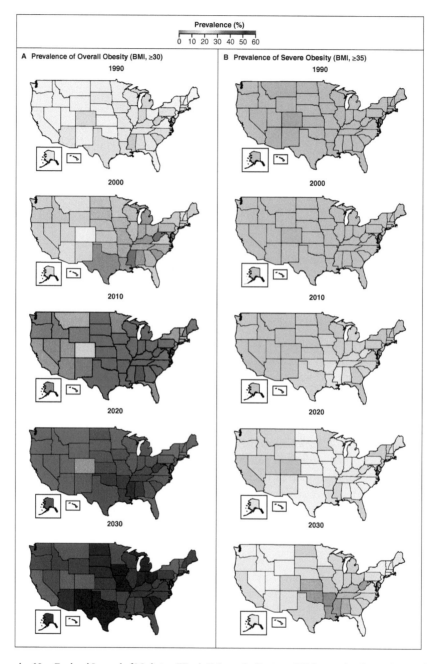

Source: From the *New England Journal of Medicine*, Ward, Z.J., et al., 'Projected U.S. state-level prevalence of adult obesity and severe obesity', 381: 2440–50. Copyright © 2019 Massachusetts Medical Society. Reprinted with permission from Massachusetts Medical Society.
Note: Overall obesity includes the BMI (body mass index) categories of moderate obesity (BMI 30 to < 35 kg m^{-2}) and severe obesity (BMI ≥ 35 kg m^{-2}).

Among major developed countries, the US has one of the highest rates of diabetes. Between 1980 and 2010 the number of diagnosed diabetes cases increased from 5.6 million to 20.9 million, representing 2.5% and 6.9% of the population respectively (Figure 1.5). Approximately 27% of 65-year-old Americans have diabetes and the American Diabetes Association estimated that the cost of the disease in the US was US$174 billion in 2007. If current trends continue, diabetes prevalence could reach 30% in the US by 2050 (Polonsky 2012). In the United Kingdom (UK), 3.8 million people are living with a diagnosis of diabetes and 90% of these have type 2 diabetes. One in ten people over 40 years of age has diabetes in the UK, and it is estimated that an additional 1 million people in the UK have undiagnosed type 2 diabetes. The total number of people living with diabetes (diagnosed and undiagnosed) in the UK is projected to increase to 5.5 million by 2030 (Diabetes UK 2019). Until relatively recently this type of diabetes was considered an adult disease. In England, the first cases among children were reported in 2000. There are now over 100 diagnoses in children in England every year and over 700 children are living with diabetes (Davies 2019). In the US approximately one in five adolescents and one in four young adults have pre-diabetes and the prevalence of this condition is higher in adolescents and young adults who are obese (Andes et al. 2020).

Although a rising obesity prevalence worldwide is one reason for the increased rates of diabetes globally, another important factor is the ageing of the population. Data presented by Christensen and colleagues (2009) for various developed nations (England and Wales, France, Germany, Japan, Sweden and the US) shows that in 1850 average life expectancy was less than 50 years. This increased to around 85 years by 2010 (Figure 1.6). Christensen and colleagues (2009) contend that if the pace of increase in life expectancy continues through the twenty-first century as it has over the past two centuries then most (i.e. >50%) babies born since 2000 in France, Germany, Italy, the UK, the US, Canada, Japan and other countries with long life expectancies will celebrate their 100th birthdays. These increases in life expectancy have been driven by improvements in infant and childhood survival and improved prevention/treatment of infectious diseases together with reductions in old-age mortality in more recent years.

The result is population ageing whereby there is a shift in the percentage of older adults within the population. In Germany, for example, only one person in ten was aged 65 or older in the 1950s. This figure has now nearly doubled, and the proportion of octogenarians, nonagenarians and centenarians has more than tripled. This shift in ageing demographics in Germany is nicely demonstrated using population pyramids (Figure 1.7) and is typical of the pattern seen in many countries. Christensen and colleagues (2009) note that in the past life was typically considered to comprise three stages, childhood, adulthood and old age, whereas now old age has evolved into two segments, a third age (young old) and a fourth age (oldest old). The ageing of a population has enormous social and economic implications, including an increase in age-related diseases and an increased number of frail elderly people. One indicator of such challenges is the old-age dependency ratio which is calculated by dividing the number of people at retirement ages (>65 years) with the number of people at working ages (15 to 64 years). There were about 15 to 16 retired people for every 100 people of working age in Germany in 1956. Fifty years later, there were 29 people aged older than 65 years for every 100 people aged 15 to 64 years and this figure is predicted to

Figure 1.5 Number of persons and percentages of the population with diagnosed diabetes in the United States, 1980–2010.

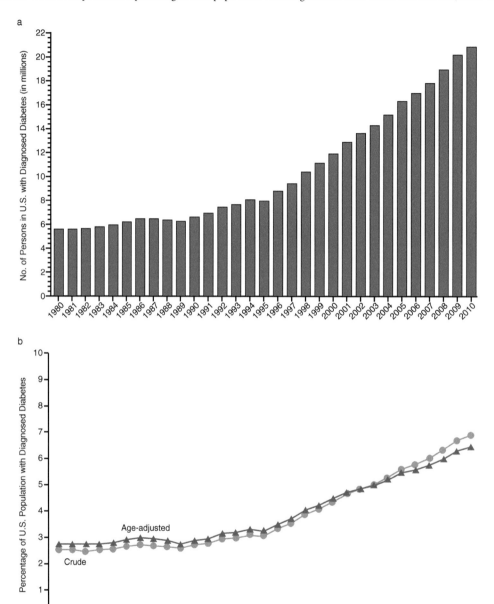

Source: Data are from the Centers for Disease Control and Prevention. Figures reprinted from the *New England Journal of Medicine*, Polonsky, K.S., 'The past 200 years in diabetes', 367: 1332–40. Copyright © 2012 Massachusetts Medical Society. Reprinted with permission from Massachusetts Medical Society.

Note: Panel a shows the number of cases of diagnosed diabetes between 1980 and 2010 among US adults 18 to 79 years of age. During this period, the number increased from 5.6 million to 20.9 million. Panel b shows the crude and age-adjusted percentages of the US population with diagnosed diabetes for this same period.

Figure 1.6 Life expectancy for women in selected countries from 1840 to 2007.

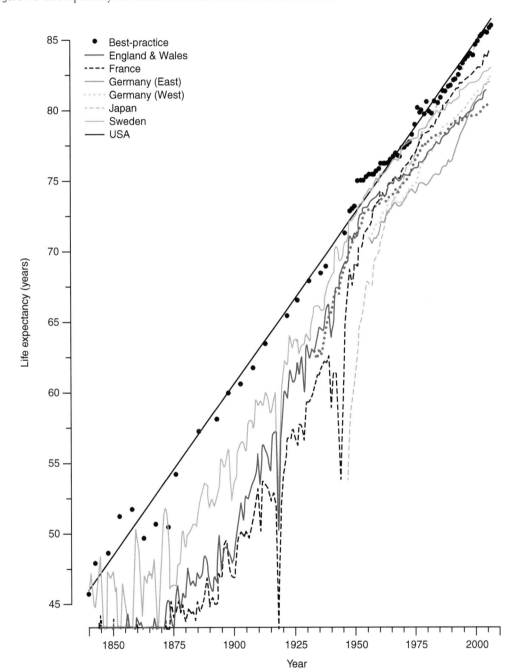

Source: Reprinted from *The Lancet*, 374: 1196–208, Christensen, K. et al., 'Ageing populations: the challenges ahead', page 1198, copyright © 2009, with permission from Elsevier.
Note: Best practice life expectancy refers to the highest value recorded in a national population. The solid black line displays the linear regression trend with a slope of 0.24 per year.

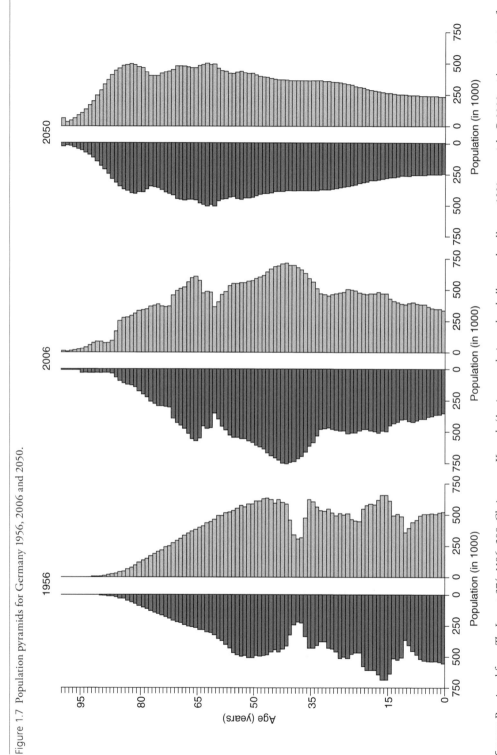

Figure 1.7 Population pyramids for Germany 1956, 2006 and 2050.

Source: Reprinted from *The Lancet*, 374: 1196–208, Christensen, K. et al., 'Ageing populations: the challenges ahead', page 1201, copyright © 2009, with permission from Elsevier.
Note: Horizontal bars are proportional to number of men (blue) and women (grey).

increase to around 60 by 2060 (Christensen et al. 2009). A similar pattern is expected to occur in most if not all developed nations in the coming years. Although these gains in life expectancy are a remarkable accomplishment, they also bring great challenges for society. Indeed, 'widespread concern exists that exceptional longevity has grim results both for individuals and for societies' (Christensen et al. 2009). The outbreak of coronavirus (COVID-19) in 2019–2020 demonstrates the legitimacy of this concern. At the time of writing, COVID-19 has afflicted over 145 million people worldwide and has been responsible for around 3.0 million deaths (Johns Hopkins University 2021). Most deaths have been in older adults with pre-existing medical conditions (Office of National Statistics 2020) and the disease has placed an unprecedented strain on healthcare systems around the world.

One of the conditions most closely associated with ageing is dementia; indeed age is the strongest risk factor for dementia. In 2015 the global prevalence of dementia was estimated to be over 46 million and this number is predicted to increase to over 130 million by 2050. The estimated global cost of dementia is close to a trillion US dollars (World Alzheimer Report 2015). Ahmadi-Abhari and colleagues (2017) assessed dementia trends in England and Wales and concluded that although the age-specific incidence of dementia has decreased in recent years the overall prevalence of dementia is rising and the number of people with dementia is likely to increase by 57% from 2016 to 2040 with more than 1.2 million people living with dementia in England and Wales by 2040. This increase is mainly driven by improved life expectancy i.e. the ageing of the population (Figure 1.8).

About 80% of the general public are concerned about developing dementia at some stage in their lives and one in four people think that there is nothing they can do to prevent it (World Alzheimer Report 2019). Yet research conducted by Norton and colleagues (2014) suggests that up to one in three cases of Alzheimer's disease (a major form of dementia) could be prevented by paying attention to seven major modifiable risk factors. These are: diabetes, mid-life hypertension, mid-life obesity, physical inactivity, depression, smoking and low educational attainment. Norton and colleagues (2014) estimate that, of these seven risk factors, the largest proportion of cases of Alzheimer's disease in the US, Europe and the UK may be attributed to physical inactivity. The role of physical activity in preventing dementia is supported by the findings of Sallis and colleagues (2016) who estimate that physical inactivity accounts for about 3.8% of dementia cases worldwide. Sallis and colleagues (2016) also estimate that nearly 300,000 cases of dementia could be avoided annually if all people were adequately active, and this figure is increasing as the global population ages.

This brief overview of modern trends has emphasised the rising prevalence of obesity over many decades and the resulting impact on chronic disease risk particularly, though not exclusively, type 2 diabetes. The ageing of the population has also been emphasised and whilst this may be considered an achievement for society its accompanying challenges have been highlighted. Physical activity has much to offer all sections of society to counteract the risks of chronic disease associated with obesity and ageing and this will be explored in the coming chapters. The next section of this chapter will examine current levels of physical activity/inactivity in the UK and globally.

Figure 1.8 Age-specific estimated number of cases of dementia 2010–40 in men and women in England and Wales.

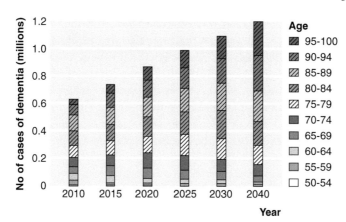

PREVALENCE OF PHYSICAL ACTIVITY/INACTIVITY WORLDWIDE

Governments and other agencies monitor health behaviours, including physical activity, to inform public health policy and to review the progress of interventions that aim to change behaviours. Many countries survey only leisure-time physical activity because this type of activity is assumed to be the most amenable to interventions and because energy expended in occupational and household work has declined significantly in recent decades. Evidence from one study indicates that mean daily energy expenditure due to work-related physical activity has dropped by more than 100 kcal since 1960 in both women and men in the US (Church et al. 2011) (Figure 1.9). Another study examining household management energy expenditure in women observed a 42% decrease in energy expenditure in non-employed women and a 30% decrease in energy expenditure in employed women in the US between 1965 and 2010. These decreases were estimated to be equivalent to decrements of 2518 kcal week^{-1} (360 kcal day^{-1}) in non-employed women and 923 kcal week^{-1} (132 kcal day^{-1}) in employed women (Archer et al. 2013) (Figure 1.10). The assessment methods used to monitor physical activity in populations unfortunately are varied and although there is increasing use of accelerometers to assess physical activity levels many assessments still rely on questionnaires.

There are two frequently used approaches to presenting data on population physical activity levels: one is to report the proportion of individuals in a specified age/sex group who are judged to be inactive; the other is to report the proportion of individuals meeting the criteria that identify the minimal 'dose' of activity needed for health benefits. The former approach has been more common in recent years. Figure 1.11 shows the percentage of adults in selected European countries who report that they never or seldom exercise or play sport. In the UK, the figure is 54% which is lower than the European average

Figure 1.9 Occupational METs and energy expenditure for US adults between 1960 and 2010.

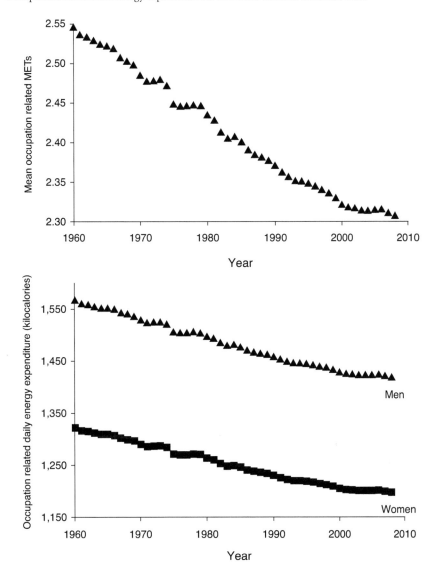

Note: The upper panel displays the mean occupation related METs since 1960 and the lower panel presents the mean occupational daily energy expenditure in men and women since 1960. MET: metabolic equivalent of task.

of 59%. Based on these data Bulgaria is the least active country with 87% of survey participants reporting that they seldom or never exercise or play sport. These data need to be interpreted with caution, however. In answer to another question about taking part in extended periods of walking on four or more days of the week 77% of Bulgarian adults

Figure 1.10 Household management energy expenditure per week between 1965 and 2010 in US women aged 19 to 64 years.

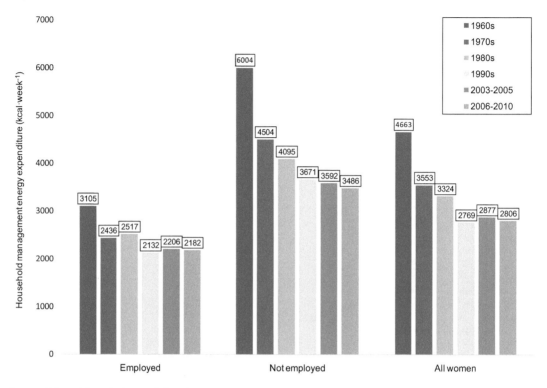

Source: Adapted from Archer et al. (2013).
Note: Household management energy expenditure was calculated using body weights from national surveys and metabolic equivalents.

met this criterion – the highest of any country surveyed (British Heart Foundation 2015). This clearly highlights the difficulties inherent in assessing and interpreting physical activity behaviour and in making cross-country comparisons.

At the time of the 2012 London Olympics the prevalence of physical inactivity worldwide was estimated to be 31% among adults (Hallal et al. 2012). By the time of the Rio Olympics in 2016 although more countries were monitoring and promoting physical activity, population physical activity levels had not increased (Sallis et al. 2016). Two features of the data on physical activity are common to most countries: the rapid decline with increasing age; and higher levels of inactivity in women than in men. For example, the data from Figure 1.12 show that in Northern Ireland, whereas 23% of men and 40% of women aged 19 to 24 did not meet physical activity recommendations, these figures increase to 86% and 92%, respectively, in the 75+ age group. Activity levels within countries also vary considerably with racial/ethnic group. In the UK, adults of Bangladeshi or Pakistani origin are the least active, and in the US, there is concern at the low levels of activity among Hispanics. In developing countries, a decline in physical activity appears to follow in the wake of economic growth, so the

Figure 1.11 Percentage of adults reporting that they never or seldom exercise or play sport, EU 2013.

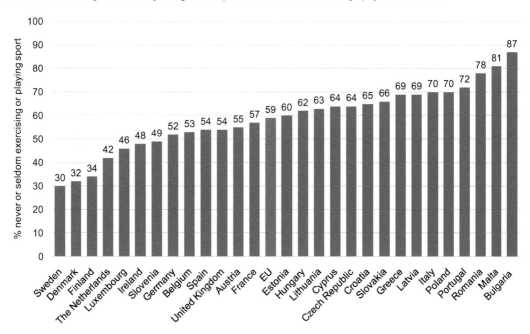

Source: British Heart Foundation (2015).
Note: Question asked: how often do you exercise or play sport?

Figure 1.12 Percentage of adults not meeting physical activity recommendations in England, Scotland, Wales and Northern Ireland.

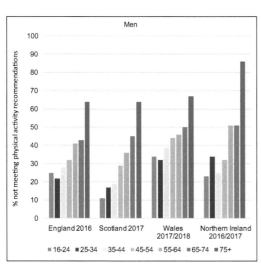
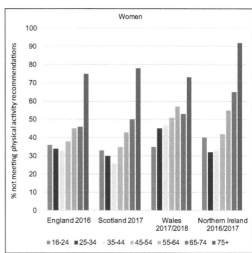

Source: British Heart Foundation (2019).
Note: Guidelines are for at least 150 minutes of moderate or 75 minutes of vigorous physical activity per week or an equivalent combination.

prevalence of inactivity worldwide may be expected to rise as the economies of these countries progress.

Exposure to physical inactivity is also an issue for children and adolescents. One recent report used data from 298 school-based surveys from 146 countries to assess the worldwide prevalence of insufficient physical activity levels in 1.6 million students aged 11 to 17 years. Insufficient physical activity was defined as not meeting the World Health Organization's recommendations on physical activity for health (i.e. not achieving 60 minutes of daily physical activity of moderate-to-vigorous intensity). This report revealed that 81% of students aged 11 to 17 years were insufficiently active (77.6% of boys and 84.7% of girls). There was no clear pattern according to country income group: insufficient activity prevalence in 2016 was 84.9% in low-income countries, 79.3% in lower-middle-income countries, 83.9% in upper-middle-income countries and 79.4% in high-income countries. The authors of this report concluded that most adolescents do not meet current physical activity guidelines and called for urgent policies and programmes to increase physical activity in adolescents (Guthold et al. 2020).

SEDENTARY BEHAVIOUR

Sedentary behaviour refers to activities in which energy expenditure is very low and sitting or lying is the dominant mode of posture. Since the second edition of this book (published in 2009) there has been a huge increase in research directed specifically at sedentary behaviour as distinct from physical activity. Evidence now suggests that even those who meet physical activity guidelines may be at increased risk of chronic disease if they spend long periods of time engaged in sedentary behaviours. This has been confirmed in recent systematic reviews examining outcomes for total mortality (Ekelund et al. 2019b) as well as cardiovascular disease and cancer mortality (Ekelund et al. 2019a). Moreover, a recent report from the 2018 Physical Activity Guidelines Advisory Committee in the US concluded there is strong evidence that high amounts of sedentary behaviour increase the risk for all-cause and cardiovascular disease mortality as well as the development of cardiovascular disease and type 2 diabetes. The report also observed moderate evidence that sedentary behaviour is associated with endometrial, colon and lung cancer (Katzmarzyk et al. 2019).

According to the British Heart Foundation (2017) the average woman and man in the UK spends the equivalent of 74 and 78 days respectively each year sitting with much of this time spent watching television – almost 30 hours per week for the average adult. A meta-analysis of 16 studies involving 1 million men and women observed that watching television for 3 hours or more per day was associated with increased mortality regardless of physical activity level in all but the most active quartile of the study population (Ekelund et al. 2016). Another study using a prevalence-based approach to estimate the impact of sedentary behaviour on mortality rates concluded that life expectancy in the US would be 2.00 years longer if adults reduced their time spent sitting to less than 3 hours each day and 1.38 years longer if they reduced television viewing to less than 2 hours each day (Katzmarzyk and Lee 2012). Unfortunately, an analysis of trends in sedentary behaviour in the US involving nearly 52,000 individuals enrolled in the National Health and Nutrition Examination Survey (NHANES) indicates that

Figure 1.13 Total sitting time in US adolescents and adults, 2007–2008 through to 2015–2016.

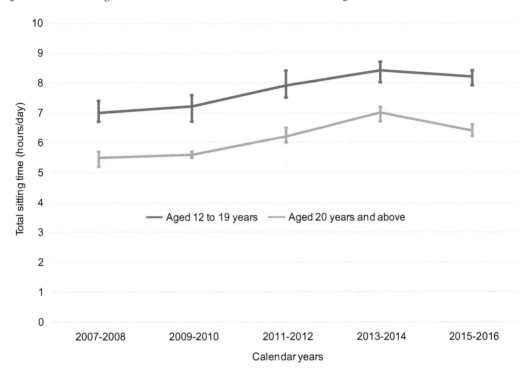

Source: Yang et al. (2019).
Note: Data are from the National Health and Nutrition Examination Survey (NHANES).

total sitting time has increased among US adolescents and adults in recent years (Yang et al. 2019) (Figure 1.13).

Evidence linking sedentary behaviour with disease and mortality risk and data showing high levels of sedentary behaviour across many sections of society have led to calls for strategies aimed specifically at reducing sedentary behaviour. To be successful such strategies will likely need to involve multiple environmental settings including work, school, home and local neighbourhoods as well as the provision of enhanced opportunities for active transport (Owen et al. 2014). With this in mind guidelines have recently been established for 'the sedentary office' where workers are recommended to accumulate two hours/day of standing and light activity (light walking) during working hours initially, progressing over time to a total accumulation of four hours/day (Buckley et al. 2015).

Exactly how sedentary behaviour (as distinct from physical activity) increases disease risk is a subject for ongoing research (Owen et al. 2010). One theory proposed by Hamilton and colleagues (2007) focuses on the enzyme lipoprotein lipase (LPL) which facilitates triglyceride clearance from the blood and increases production of high-density lipoprotein cholesterol (which is associated with a reduced risk of cardiovascular disease). Hamilton and colleagues (2007) demonstrate that reduced skeletal muscle contraction through sedentary activity leads to suppression of skeletal muscle LPL activity, compromising triglyceride clearance. They also observe that experimentally reducing normal spontaneous standing and ambulatory time has a much greater effect on LPL regulation than adding vigorous exercise training on top of the normal level of non-exercise activity. Skeletal muscle inactivity may also reduce blood glucose uptake thereby increasing the risk of type 2 diabetes. These mechanisms will be explored further in the coming chapters.

THERAPEUTIC POTENTIAL OF PHYSICAL ACTIVITY

In view of the high levels of physical inactivity and sedentary behaviour outlined in previous sections, physical activity is hugely underutilised by individuals and societies as a strategy for maintaining health and avoiding chronic disease. Research presented in later chapters of this book will show there is ample evidence supporting the benefits of exercise for body composition, skeletal health and metabolic health and hence a reduced risk of various chronic diseases including cardiovascular disease, cancer, type 2 diabetes and osteoporosis as well as enhanced longevity and benefits for mental health. These benefits apply to children, adults and older adults (i.e. they apply across the lifespan). Lee and colleagues (2012) estimate that worldwide, physical inactivity causes 6% of the burden from CHD, 7% of type 2 diabetes, 10% of breast cancer, 10% of colon cancer and 9% of premature mortality (Figure 1.14). Based on this analysis more than 5.3 million of the 57 million deaths that occurred worldwide in 2008 were due to physical inactivity (Lee et al. 2012).

Very recent evidence from a prospective multi-cohort study, including 12 European studies and 116,043 participants, suggests that physical activity is one of four key healthy lifestyle behaviours (together with non-smoking, maintenance of a BMI <25 $kg\,m^{-2}$ and moderate alcohol consumption) that can increase the number of years lived free from chronic disease. In this study, those with the best lifestyle scores lived for over nine years longer without developing chronic disease than those with the worst lifestyle scores (Nyberg et al. 2020). Despite such findings the prevalence of healthy lifestyle behaviours is low, even among those who have been afflicted by chronic disease, with some evidence that the situation is worse in low-income than high-income countries (Teo et al. 2013). Yet the benefits of exercise are not restricted to those at elevated risk of developing disease. One observational study has shown that even among individuals who are judged to be at low risk of CHD (based on the Framingham Risk Score) those who exhibit high levels of physical fitness (presumably due to higher physical activity levels) are at lower risk of CHD than their less fit counterparts (Barlow et al. 2012).

In view of the volume of evidence supporting the health benefits of physical activity combined with the high levels of physical inactivity and sedentary behaviour across many sections of society, there have been calls for more concerted efforts to prescribe exercise in primary care. Kahn and colleagues (2011) recommend that general practitioners begin by administering physical activity questionnaires and adopting brief counselling approaches as well as avoiding 'the knee jerk reaction of prescribing "preventive" drugs as a first response to diseases of inactivity' (Kahn et al. 2011). This latter point is pertinent considering the findings of a meta-analysis of randomised controlled

Figure 1.14 Estimates of the prevalence of physical inactivity, relative risks and population attributable fractions for coronary heart disease, type 2 diabetes, breast cancer, colon cancer and all-cause mortality associated with physical inactivity.

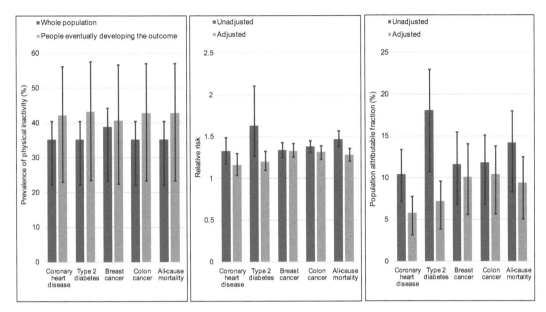

Source: Lee et al. (2012).
Note: Prevalence of physical inactivity values are overall median with the range of medians for WHO regions shown by the vertical black bars. Vertical black bars for relative risk are 95% confidence intervals. Population-attributable fraction values are overall median with the range of medians for WHO regions shown by the vertical black bars. Adjusted relative risk and population-attributable fraction values are adjusted for potential confounders. Breast cancer data are for women only.

trials showing that exercise and many drug interventions are often similar in terms of their mortality benefits in the secondary prevention of CHD, rehabilitation after stroke, treatment of heart failure and prevention of diabetes (Naci and Ioannidis 2013). Kahn and colleagues (2012) suggest that exercise might also be considered as a fifth vital sign (in addition to body temperature, blood pressure, heart rate and respiratory rate) and should be recorded in patients' electronic medical records while Yancey and colleagues (2013) note that being sedentary is a 'way of life' for many health professionals and call for medical professionals to lead the way in adopting and promoting physical activity.

COSTS OF PHYSICAL INACTIVITY

Knowing the financial costs of physical inactivity is important for policy makers so that they can make informed decisions about the allocation of funds to address the issue. A review paper by Pratt and colleagues (2014) identified 11 studies from six highly developed countries which have assessed national-level health-care costs of physical inactivity. Despite using a variety of methods, the findings of these 11 studies are quite consistent in estimating that 1–2.6% of total health-care costs are due to physical inactivity.

More recently, Ding and colleagues (2016) quantified the economic burden of physical inactivity at a global level using national physical activity prevalence data from 142 countries, representing 93% of the world's population. They assessed direct health-care costs, productivity losses and disability adjusted life years (DALYs: the sum of years of potential life lost due to premature mortality and the years of productive life lost due to disability). In calculating these costs, they considered five major non-communicable diseases related to physical inactivity: CHD, stroke, type 2 diabetes, breast cancer and colon cancer. They 'conservatively' estimated that physical inactivity cost health-care systems international $ (INT$) 53.8 billion worldwide in 2013 plus an additional INT$13.7 billion in productivity losses giving a total economic cost of INT$67.5 billion. They also estimated that physical inactivity was responsible for 13.4 million DALYs worldwide. While high-income countries suffered a larger proportion of the economic burden, low- and middle-income countries suffered a larger proportion of the disease burden related to physical inactivity.

Another cost-based analysis was conducted at the time of the 2012 London Olympics to estimate the potential effect of increased walking and cycling in urban England and Wales on costs to the National Health Service (NHS) for several diseases associated with physical inactivity. This analysis suggested that within 20 years, reductions in the prevalence of type 2 diabetes, dementia, ischaemic heart disease, cerebrovascular disease and cancer if there were to be increased physical activity would lead to savings of roughly UK £17 billion (in 2010 prices) for the NHS, after adjustment for an increased risk of road traffic injuries (Jarrett et al. 2012). (Note: road traffic and other potential hazards of exercise are discussed in Chapter 13.) Not surprisingly such costs have prompted widespread calls for increased promotion and scaling up of physical activity interventions worldwide (Reis et al. 2016) and this topic is addressed further in Chapter 14 ('Public Health').

DEFINITIONS OF KEY TERMS

Before concluding this chapter, it is helpful to briefly define some of the key terms used throughout this book. Surprisingly, defining common, everyday terms such as exercise, health and disease can be challenging and controversial. In previous editions of this book we wrote that disease is relatively easy to define, either according to aetiology (e.g. tuberculosis is caused by a bacterium, *Mycobacterium tuberculosis*) or in terms of symptoms (e.g. the term asthma describes a disease characterised by fits of laboured breathing). While this remains true in many cases, there is ongoing debate about whether obesity should be classified as a disease (Wilding et al. 2019) and the distinction between disease and disease risk factors is sometimes blurred as is the distinction between normal ageing and disease (Mellor and Merali 2019). The reader wanting greater clarity on the diseases examined in this book may refer to the WHO's International Classification of Disease catalogue which is now in its 11th edition (WHO 2018).

Defining health can also be problematic. Is health merely the 'other side of the coin', that is, the absence of disease? Somehow this fails to capture the essence of our everyday use of the term health as encapsulated in phrases such as 'picture of health' and 'rude health'. Something wider is needed. The most ambitious definition is that proposed by the WHO in 1948: 'Health is a state of complete physical, mental and social well-being and not merely the absence of disease or infirmity.' However, this definition has been criticised because it is unachievable for many, it would leave most people classed as unhealthy most of the time and it has unintentionally contributed to the medicalisation of society (Godlee 2011). In view of this Huber and colleagues (2011) propose a new definition of health as 'the ability to adapt and self-manage' in the face of social, physical and emotional challenges. In the context of this book both definitions may be considered helpful – the former definition is an aspiration for some people while the latter definition is relevant to many if not most people. Physical activity contributes more to health than just helping to prevent disease and it enables people to maintain productive and fulfilling lives while coping with disease.

Finally – a note on our use of the terms 'physical activity', 'exercise', 'sedentary behaviour' and 'physical inactivity'. As in previous editions we have adopted the definitions of physical activity and exercise proposed by Howley (2001). Thus, physical activity is 'any bodily movement produced by contraction of skeletal muscle that substantially increases energy expenditure'. Hence the title of this book is broad – *physical activity and health*. Exercise (or exercise training) is defined as 'a subcategory of leisure-time physical activity in which planned, structured and repetitive bodily movements are performed to improve or maintain one or more components of physical fitness'. However, the distinction between physical activity and exercise is sometimes neither helpful nor necessary, so there are occasions in the text where these terms are used more loosely. With respect to the terms 'sedentary behaviour' and 'physical inactivity' we are guided by the Sedentary Behaviour Research Network (Sedentary Behaviour Research Network 2012; Tremblay et al. 2017) which defines sedentary behaviour as 'any waking behaviour characterised by an energy expenditure ≤ 1.5 METs while in a sitting or reclining posture'. In contrast, the term 'inactive' describes those who are performing insufficient amounts of moderate-to-vigorous physical activity (i.e. not meeting specified physical activity guidelines).

SUMMARY

- The modern history of exercise science began after the Second World War, when epidemiologists began the scientific study of the role of exercise in protection against heart disease.
- An epidemic of obesity in adults and children is leading to an increase in obesity-related diseases – most notably type 2 diabetes.
- Improvements in life expectancy for both men and women mean that the total number of older people worldwide is increasing, changing the age structure of populations. This means more age-related disease and an increased number of frail elderly people.
- Many adults and children around the world are insufficiently active to benefit their health, placing them at increased risk of developing chronic disease.
- A decline in physical activity appears to follow in the wake of economic growth, so that the prevalence of inactivity worldwide may be expected to rise as the economies of developing countries progress.

- High levels of sedentary behaviour are associated with an increased risk of disease independently from physical activity levels. Many adults and children exhibit high levels of sedentary behaviour.
- The therapeutic potential of physical activity is underutilised across the globe and this has detrimental economic and social consequences.

STUDY TASKS

1 Why do the figures describing the prevalence of overweight and obesity in children and adolescents give rise to so much concern?

2 In your opinion, what factors can be invoked to explain the low levels of physical activity in children and adolescents?

3 Do some research to find out what the latest overweight and obesity statistics are for children, adolescents, and adults in your country.

4 Why is the age structure of the population of a country such as Germany (Figure 1.7) expected to change so much in the decades to come? What are the implications of this change for public health policy?

5 Access the papers by Church and colleagues (2011) and Archer and colleagues (2013) and briefly summarise the methods employed to calculate the data displayed in Figures 1.9 and 1.10, respectively.

6 Examine the data in all three panels of Figure 1.14 and explain as fully as possible what the data are showing.

7 Do some research to find out what the latest physical activity/inactivity statistics are for your country.

FURTHER READING

British Heart Foundation. (2015) Physical activity statistics 2015 [online], available at: https://www.bhf.org.uk/informationsupport/publications/statistics/physical-activity-statistics-2015 (accessed 16 April 2020).

British Heart Foundation. (2019) Heart and circulatory disease statistics 2019 [online], available at: https://www.bhf.org.uk/what-we-do/our-research/heart-statistics/heart-statistics-publications/cardiovascular-disease-statistics-2019 (accessed 15 April 2020).

Christensen, K., Doblhammer, G., Rau, R. and Vaupel, J.W. (2009) Ageing populations: the challenges ahead. *The Lancet* 374: 1196–208.

Davies, S.C. (2019) Time to solve childhood obesity. Department of Health and Social Care [online], available at: https://assets.publishing.service.gov.uk/government/uploads/system/uploads/attachment_data/file/837907/cmo-special-report-childhood-obesity-october-2019.pdf (accessed 13 April 2020).

Hamilton, M.T., Hamilton, D.G. and Zderic, T.W. (2007) Role of low energy expenditure and sitting in obesity, metabolic syndrome, type 2 diabetes, and cardiovascular disease. *Diabetes* 56: 2655–67.

Jones, D.S., Podolsky, S.H. and Greene, J.A. (2012) The burden of disease and the changing task of medicine. *New England Journal of Medicine* 366: 2333–8.

Owen, N., Healy, G.N., Matthews, C.E. and Dunstan, D. (2010) Too much sitting: the population health science of sedentary behaviour. *Exercise and Sport Sciences Reviews* 38: 105–13.

REFERENCES

Ahmadi-Abhari, S., Guzman-Castillo, M., Bandosz, P., Shipley, M.J., Muniz-Terrera, G., Singh-Manoux, A. et al. (2017) Temporal trend in dementia incidence since 2002 and projections for prevalence in England and Wales to 2040: modelling study. *British Medical Journal* 358: j2856. doi: 10.1136/bmj.j2856.

Andes, L.J., Cheng, Y.J., Rilke, D.B., Gregg, E.W. and Imperatorin, G. (2020) Prevalence of pre-diabetes among adolescents and young adults in the United States, 2005–2016. *Journal of the American Medical Association Pediatrics* 174: e194498. doi: 10.1001/jamapediatrics.2019.4498.

Archer E., Shook, R.P., Thomas, D.M., Church, T.S., Katzmarzyk, P.T., Hébert, J.R. et al. (2013) 45-year trends in women's use of time and household management energy expenditure. *PLoS One* 8: e56620. doi: 10.1371/journal.pone.0056620.

Barlow, C.E., DeFina, L.F., Radford, N.B., Berry, J.D., Cooper, K.H., Haskell, W.L. et al. (2012) Cardiorespiratory fitness and long-term survival in 'low-risk' adults. *Journal of the American Heart Association* 1:e001354. doi: 10.1161/JAHA.112.001354.

British Heart Foundation. (2015) Physical activity statistics 2015 [online], available at: https://www.bhf.org.uk/informationsupport/publications/statistics/physical-activity-statistics-2015 (accessed 16 April 2020).

British Heart Foundation. (2017) Physical activity and sedentary behaviour report [online], available at: https://www.bhf.org.uk/informationsupport/publications/statistics/physical-inactivity-report-2017 (accessed 15 April 2020).

British Heart Foundation (2019) Heart and circulatory disease statistics 2019 [online], available at: https://www.bhf.org.uk/what-we-do/our-research/heart-statistics/heart-statistics-publications/cardiovascular-disease-statistics-2019 (accessed 15 April 2020).

Buckley, J.P., Hedge, A., Yates, T., Copeland, R.J., Loosemore, M., Hamer, M. et al. (2015) The sedentary office: an expert statement on the growing case for change towards better health and productivity. *British Journal of Sports Medicine* 49: 1357–62.

Christensen, K., Doblhammer, G., Rau, R. and Vaupel, J.W. (2009) Ageing populations: the challenges ahead. *The Lancet* 374: 1196–208.

Church, T.S., Thomas, D.M., Tudor-Locke, C., Katzmarzyk, P.T., Earnest, C.P., Rodarte, R.Q. et al. (2011) Trends over 5 decades in U.S. occupation-related physical activity and their associations with obesity. *PLoS One* 6: e19657. doi: 10.1371/journal.pone.0019657.

Danaei, G., Finucane, M.M., Lu, Y., Singh, G.M., Cowan, M.J., Paciorek, C.J., et al. on behalf of the Global Burden of Metabolic Risk Factors of Chronic Diseases Collaborating Group (Blood Glucose). (2011) National, regional, and global trends in fasting plasma glucose and diabetes prevalence since 1980: systematic analysis of health examination surveys and epidemiological studies with 370 country-years and 2.7 million participants. *The Lancet* 378: 31–40.

Davies, S.C. (2019) Time to solve childhood obesity. Department of Health and Social Care [online], available at: https://assets.publishing.service.gov.uk/government/uploads/system/uploads/attachment_data/file/837907/cmo-special-report-childhood-obesity-october-2019.pdf (accessed 13 April 2020).

Diabetes UK. (2019) Facts and stats update [online], available at: https://www.diabetes.org.uk/about_us/news/new-stats-people-living-with-diabetes (accessed 13 April 2020).

Ding, D., Lawson, K.D., Kolbe-Alexander, T.L., Finkelstein, E.A., Katzmarzyk, P.T., van Mechelen, W. and Pratt, M. for the Lancet Physical Activity Series 2 Executive Committee. (2016) The economic burden of physical inactivity: a global analysis of major non-communicable diseases. *The Lancet* 388: 1311–24.

Ekelund, U., Brown, W.J., Steene-Johannessen, J., Fagerland, M.W., Owen, N., Powell, K.E. et al. (2019a) Do the associations of sedentary behaviour with cardiovascular disease mortality and cancer mortality differ by physical activity level? A systematic review and harmonised meta-analysis of data from 850 060 participants. *British Journal of Sports Medicine* 53: 886–94.

Ekelund, U., Steene-Johannessen, J., Brown, W.J., Fagerland, M.W., Owen, N., Powell, K.E. et al. for the Lancet Physical Activity Series 2 Executive Committee and the Lancet Sedentary Behaviour Working Group. (2016) Does physical activity attenuate, or even eliminate, the detrimental association of sitting time with mortality? A harmonised meta-analysis of data from more than 1 million men and women. *The Lancet* 388: 1302–10.

Ekelund, U., Tarp, J., Steene-Johannessen, J., Hansen, B.H., Jefferis, B., Fagerland, M.W. et al. (2019b) Dose–response associations between accelerometry measured physical activity and sedentary time and all-cause mortality: systematic review and harmonised meta-analysis. *British Medical Journal* 366: l4570. doi: 10.1136/bmj.l4570.

Godlee, F. (2011) What is health? *British Medical Journal* 343: d4817. doi: 10.1136/bmj.d4817.

Guthold, R., Stevens, G.A., Riley, L.M. and Bull, F.C. (2020) Global trends in insufficient physical activity among adolescents: a pooled analysis of 298 population-based surveys with 1.6 million participants. *The Lancet Child and Adolescent Health* 4: 23–35.

Hallal, P.C., Andersen, L.B., Bull, F.C., Guthold, R., Haskell, W. and Ekelund, U. for the Lancet Physical Activity Series Working Group. (2012) Global physical activity levels: surveillance progress, pitfalls, and prospects. *The Lancet* 380: 247–57.

Hamilton, M.T., Hamilton, D.G. and Zderic, T.W. (2007) Role of low energy expenditure and sitting in obesity, metabolic syndrome, type 2 diabetes, and cardiovascular disease. *Diabetes* 56: 2655–67.

Hippocrates (1967) *Hippocrates* (trans. W.H.S. Jones). Cambridge, MA: Harvard University Press.

Howley, E.T. (2001) Type of activity: resistance, aerobic and leisure versus occupational physical activity. *Medicine and Science in Sports and Exercise* 33: S364–9.

Huber, M., Knottnerus, J.A., Green, L., van der Horst, H., Jadad, A.R., Kromhout, D. et al. (2011) How should we define health? *British Medical Journal* 343: d4163. doi: 10.1136/bmj.d4163.

Jarrett, J., Woodcock, J., Griffiths, U.K., Chalabi, Z., Edwards, P., Roberts, I. and Haines, A. (2012) Effect of increasing active travel in urban England and Wales on costs to the National Health Service. *The Lancet* 379: 2198–205.

Johns Hopkins University (2021) Coronavirus Resource Centre [online], available at: https://coronavirus.jhu.edu/map.html (accessed 24 February 2021).

Jones, D.S., Podolsky, S.H. and Greene, J.A. (2012) The burden of disease and the changing task of medicine. *New England Journal of Medicine* 366: 2333–8.

Kahn, K.M., Thompson, A.M., Blair, S.N., Sallis, J.F., Powell, K.E., Bull, F.C. and Bauman, A.E. (2012) Sport and exercise as contributors to the health of nations. *The Lancet* 380: 59–64.

Kahn, K.M., Weiler, R. and Blair, S.N. (2011) Prescribing exercise in primary care. *British Medical Journal* 343: d4141. doi: 10.1136/bmj.d4141.

Katzmarzyk, P.T. and Lee, I.-M. (2012) Sedentary behaviour and life expectancy in the USA: a cause-deleted life table analysis. *British Medical Journal Open* 2: e000828. doi: 10.1136/bmjopen-2012–000828.

Katzmarzyk, P.T., Powell, K.E., Jakicic, J.M., Troiano, R.P., Piercy, K. and Tennant, B. for the 2018 Physical Activity Guidelines Advisory Committee. (2019) Sedentary behaviour and health:

update from the 2018 physical activity guidelines committee. *Medicine and Science in Sports and Exercise* 51: 1227–41.

Lee, I.-M., Shiroma, E.J., Lobelo, F., Puska, P., Blair, S.N. and Katzmarzyk, P.T., for the Lancet Physical Activity Series Working Group. (2012) Effect of physical inactivity on major non-communicable diseases worldwide: an analysis of burden of disease and life expectancy. *The Lancet* 380: 219–29.

Mellor, D. and Merali, S. (2019) What exactly is disease? *The Conversation*, 24 July [online], available at: https://theconversation.com/what-exactly-is-a-disease-120622 (accessed 18 April 2020).

Morris, J.N., Heady, J.A., Raffle, P.A.B., Parks, J.W. and Roberts, C.G. (1953) Coronary heart disease and physical activity of work. *The Lancet* 262: 1053–7.

Naci, H. and Ioannidis, J.P.A. (2013) Comparative effectiveness of exercise and drug interventions on mortality outcomes: metaepidemiological study. *British Medical Journal* 347:f5577. doi: 10.1136/bmj.f5577.

National Centre for Social Research (NatCen), University College London, Department of Epidemiology and Public Health. (2019) Health Survey for England, 2018 [online], available at: http://digital.nhs.uk/pubs/hse2018 (accessed 13 April 2020).

National Child Measurement Programme (2019) England 2018/19 School Year [online]: available at: https://digital.nhs.uk/data-and-information/publications/statistical/national-child-measurement-programme/2018-19-school-year (accessed 13 April 2020).

Ng, M., Fleming, T., Robinson, M., Thomson, B., Graetz, N., Margono, C. et al. (2014) Global, regional, and national prevalence of overweight and obesity in children and adults during 1980–2013: a systematic analysis for the Global Burden of Disease Study 2013. *The Lancet* 384: 766–81.

Norton, S., Matthews, F.E., Barnes, D.E., Yaffe, K. and Brayne, C. (2014) Potential for primary prevention of Alzheimer's disease: an analysis of population-based data. *The Lancet Neurology* 13: 788–94.

Nyberg, S.T., Singh-Manoux, A., Pentti, J., Madsen, I.E.H., Sabia, S., Alfredsson, L. et al. (2020) Association of healthy lifestyle with years lived without major chronic diseases. *Journal of the American Medical Association Internal Medicine*. 180: 760–8. doi: 10.1001/jamainternmed.2020.0618.

Office for National Statistics (2020) Deaths involving COVID-19, England and Wales: deaths occurring in March 2020 [online], available at: https://www.ons.gov.uk/peoplepopulationandcommunity/birthsdeathsandmarriages/deaths/bulletins/deathsinvolvingcovid19englandandwales/deathsoccurringinmarch2020 (accessed 17 April 2020).

Owen, N., Healy, G.N., Matthews, C.E. and Dunstan, D. (2010) Too much sitting: the population health science of sedentary behaviour. *Exercise and Sport Sciences Reviews* 38: 105–13.

Owen, N., Salmon, J., Koohsari, M.J., Turrell, G. and Giles-Corti, B. (2014) Sedentary behaviour and health: mapping environmental and social contexts to underpin chronic disease prevention. *British Journal of Sports Medicine* 48: 174–7.

Polonsky, K.S. (2012) The past 200 years in diabetes. *New England Journal of Medicine* 367: 1332–40.

Pratt, M., Norris, J., Lobelo, F., Roux, L. and Wang, G. (2014) The cost of physical inactivity: moving into the 21st century. *British Journal of Sports Medicine* 48: 171–3.

Reis, R.S., Salvo, D., Ogilvie, D., Lambert, E.V., Goenka, S. and Brownson R.C., for the Lancet Physical Activity Series 2 Executive Committee. (2016) Scaling up physical activity interventions worldwide: stepping up to larger and smarter approaches to get people moving. *The Lancet* 388: 1337–48.

Sallis, J.F., Bull, F., Guthold, R., Heath, G.W., Inoue, S., Kelly, P. et al., for the Lancet Physical Activity Series 2 Executive Committee. (2016) Progress in physical activity over the Olympic quadrennium. *The Lancet* 388: 1325–36.

Sedentary Behaviour Research Network (2012) Standardised use of the terms "sedentary" and "sedentary behaviours". *Applied Physiology, Nutrition and Metabolism* 37: 540–2.

Teo, K., Lear, S., Islam, S., Mony, P., Dehghan, M., Li, W. et al., on behalf of the PURE Investigators. (2013) Prevalence of a healthy lifestyle among individuals with cardiovascular disease in high-, middle- and low-income countries. The Prospective Urban Rural Epidemiology (PURE) Study. *Journal of the American Medical Association* 309: 1613–21.

Tremblay, M.S., Aubert, S., Barnes, J.D., Saunders, T.J., Carson, V., Latimer-Cheung, A.E. et al., on behalf of SBRN Terminology Consensus Project Participants. (2017) Sedentary Behavior Research Network (SBRN) – Terminology consensus project, process, and outcome. *International Journal of Behavioral Nutrition and Physical Activity* 14: 75. doi: 10.1186/s12966-017-0525-8.

Ward, Z.J., Bleich, S.N., Cradock, A.L., Barrett, J.L., Giles, C.M., Flax, C. et al. (2019) Projected U.S. state-level prevalence of adult obesity and severe obesity. *New England Journal of Medicine* 381: 2440–50.

Wilding, J.P.H., Mooney, V. and Pile, R. (2019) Should obesity be recognised as a disease? *British Medical Journal* 366: l4258. doi: 10.1136/bmj.l4258.

World Alzheimer Report. (2015) The global impact of dementia: an analysis of prevalence, incidence, costs and trends. *Alzheimer's Disease International* [online], available at: https://www.alz.co.uk/research/world-report-2015 (accessed 14 April 2020).

World Alzheimer Report. (2019) Attitudes to dementia. *Alzheimer's Disease International* [online], available at: https://www.alz.co.uk/research/world-report-2019 (accessed on 14 April 2020).

World Health Organization. (2018) *International Classification of Diseases* [online], available at: https://icd.who.int/browse11/l-m/en (accessed 18 April 2020).

Yancey, A.K., Sallis, R.E. and Bastani, R. (2013) Changing physical activity participation for the medical profession. *Journal of the American Medical Association* 309: 141–2.

Yang, L., Cao, C., Kantor, E.D., Nguyen, L.H., Zheng, X., Park, Y. et al. (2019) Trends in sedentary behaviour among the US population, 2001–2016. *Journal of the American Medical Association* 321: 1587–97.

2 The nature of the evidence

Jason M.R. Gill

INTRODUCTION

There are several forms of evidence available to help evaluate the effects of physical activity (or fitness, or strength, or sedentary behaviour – see Chapter 1 for definitions of these related concepts) on health and the mechanisms responsible for these effects. These lines of evidence are complementary: it is important to consider the different evidence types together to obtain a clear overall picture of both *what* the effects of physical activity on health are, and *how* and *why* they occur. Each type of evidence has inherent strengths and limitations. It is important to recognise these constraints and to be able to identify research that has been well conducted. Good research generally requires a plausible hypothesis, a robust study design, and data that are collected and interpreted with adequate allowance for potential sources of error.

Research can be broadly divided into two categories: observational and experimental. In observational studies researchers allow nature to take its course and merely collect information about one or more groups of participants. The simplest observational studies are merely descriptive, but most go beyond this by analysing relationships between health status and other variables. In experimental studies researchers intervene to affect what happens to one or more of the groups.

OBSERVATIONAL RESEARCH

Much of the evidence on the relationship between physical activity and health comes from the field of epidemiology. This has been defined by the World Health Organization (WHO) as 'the study of the distribution and determinants of health-related states or events in specified populations, and the application of this study to control of health problems' (Porta 2008). The use of the phrase 'health-related states or events' (rather than the older term 'disease frequency') reflects the fact that our concept of health now includes aspects of positive health – for example, a good quality of life – and not only the absence of disease. For simplicity, the term 'health-related outcome' will be used in this text to include both disease and other health-related states or events. Health-related outcomes may be defined simply, for example as 'disease present' or 'disease absent', or graded, for example 'normal weight', 'overweight' or 'obese'. Epidemiological research can be observational or experimental, but in the physical activity and health field, most epidemiological studies have been observational. The main types of observational epidemiological study are summarised in Table 2.1.

Case reports or case series describe the experience of a single patient or group of patients with a similar diagnosis. Such studies usually report an unusual feature and may lead to the formulation of a new hypothesis. Few studies on physical activity or fitness are of this form, but one example is the autopsy study of Clarence DeMar, a runner who had participated in over 1,000 distance races, including 100 marathons; the diameter of his coronary arteries was estimated to be two or three times the normal diameter, leading to conjecture that years of running training might lead the arteries to adapt to the larger demand for blood flow (Currens and White 1961).

In ecological studies (sometimes called correlational studies), the characteristics of entire populations are used to describe the frequency of a health-related outcome in

Table 2.1 Types of epidemiological study.		
CATEGORY	TYPE OF STUDY	UNIT OF STUDY
Observational		
Descriptive studies	Case reports of case series	Individuals
Analytical studies	Correlational (Ecological)	Populations
	Cross-sectional surveys	Individuals
	Case-control studies	Individuals
	Cohort studies	Individuals
Experimental	Randomised controlled trials	Individuals

Source: Adapted from Beaglehole et al. (1993).

relation to some factor/s relevant to the research question or hypothesis. A classic example of a correlational study is the Seven Countries Study where rates of mortality from coronary heart disease (CHD) between populations were highly correlated with the median plasma cholesterol concentrations in the different populations (Keys 1980) (Figure 2.1). While these data demonstrate an association at the population level, they cannot be used to infer a link between cholesterol and CHD at the individual level. A more recent physical activity-related example of an ecological study is a report examining the relationship between trends in occupation-related physical activity and population body weight in the United States over the past five decades (Church et al. 2011). Using employment data from the Bureau of Labor statistics, the authors estimated that daily occupation-related physical activity declined by over 100 kcal from the early 1960s to early 2000s. They then used computational energy balance models to predict how much this energy expenditure change would be expected to change population body weight over this period and compared this with the actual population body weight trend. The model matched the real trend well and the authors concluded that reductions in occupational activity could account for a substantial portion of the increase in mean population body weight over this period. However, it is important to recognise that the authors of this report made a number of assumptions when undertaking this analysis and not all researchers agree with this interpretation. Other data suggest that changes in dietary intake may play a more important role. The influence of physical activity and diet on obesity will be covered in more depth in Chapter 6.

Cross-sectional surveys describe the prevalence of a health-related outcome in representative samples and relate this to personal or demographic characteristics. For example, surveys from nationally representative population samples from a number of different countries (such as the Canada Fitness Survey, the Health Survey for England, and the National Health and Nutrition Examination Survey in the United States) have shown associations between levels of physical activity and indices of health status or risk of disease. This concept is illustrated in Figure 2.2. Although cross-sectional surveys can potentially be very large and provide results quickly, they have the inherent problem that they cannot explain the direction of any relationship observed. For example, if an inverse relationship between level of physical activity and obesity was observed, it would not be possible to determine whether physical activity helped to

Figure 2.1 Relationship between the median serum cholesterol concentration and ten-year mortality from CHD in 16 cohorts of men in the Seven Countries Study.

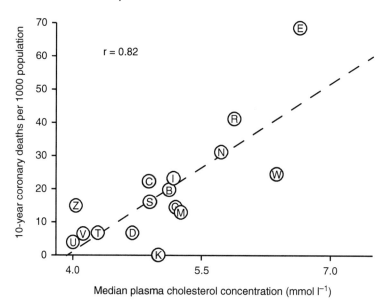

Notes: B = Belgrade (Yugoslavia, now Serbia); C = Crevalcore (Italy); D = Dalmatia (Yugoslavia, now Croatia); E = East Finland; G = Corfa; I = Italian railroad; K = Crete; M – Montegiorgio (Italy); N = Zutphen (the Netherlands); R = American railroad; S = Slavonia (Yugoslavia, now Croatia); T = Tanushimaru (Japan); U = Ushibuka (Japan); V = Velika Krsna (Yugoslavia, now Serbia); W = West Finland; Z = Zrenjanin (Yugoslavia, now Serbia).

protect against obesity or if those who were obese chose to be less physically active. This is a key limitation which needs to be taken into consideration whenever cross-sectional study data are interpreted. Observing trends over time in serial cross-sectional surveys can provide a means of evaluating population-based interventions.

In a case-control study (also called a retrospective study), the occurrence of a possible cause is compared between people known to have a disease (the cases) and a reference group who do not have the disease (the controls). The investigators look back from the disease to a possible cause, seeking associations with exposure to the factors of interest. The most difficult aspect of this design is the selection of controls because this can introduce bias (systematic error). However, case-control studies offer a way to identify adequate numbers of patients even when the outcome under study is relatively rare. Many studies of physical activity and the risk of specific cancers are therefore of this type.

Cohort studies, sometimes called follow-up studies, are conceptually simple. They begin with a group of people who are free of disease (or other health-related outcome) and determine their exposure to a suspected risk factor. Subgroups are defined on the basis of exposure to the risk factor. For a study of physical (in)activity, subgroups might comprise individuals engaging in low, moderate or high levels of physical activity. Participants are then followed for a period of time, usually a number of years, so that

Figure 2.2 Cross-sectional survey study design.

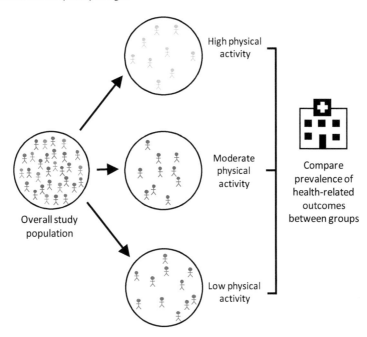

the occurrence of the specified outcome can be compared between the subgroups. In contrast to case-control studies, a range of outcomes can be studied. The concept of the cohort study is illustrated in Figure 2.3.

There have been a number of large cohort studies which have studied the effects of physical activity, fitness or sedentary behaviour on a variety of health-related outcomes. For example, the Nurses' Health Study – which began in 1976 with over 100,000 American nurses aged 35 to 55 on entry, and was expanded in 1989 with a further 116,000 women aged 25–42 recruited to the Nurses' Health Study II cohort (a further Nurses' Health Study III cohort started recruitment in 2010) – has investigated the association between physical activity, or sedentary behaviour, on risk of future cardio-vascular disease, diabetes, obesity, several site-specific cancers, depression, cognitive function, psoriasis, inflammatory bowel syndrome, hip fractures, and even infertility and hearing loss. The Aerobics Center Longitudinal Study, based in Texas in the United States, is perhaps the best-known prospective cohort study which has evaluated the effects of cardiorespiratory fitness on future incidence of a range of health-related outcomes. Such studies are expensive, but represent the strongest study design for an observational study, with a lower potential for reverse causality influencing the outcomes (i.e. presence of disease leading to lower physical activity or fitness) than case-control or cross-sectional study designs. Risk of reverse causality is not completely eliminated by a cohort study, as presence of undiagnosed disease at baseline could conceivably influence physical activity or fitness, but this can be minimised by long follow-up periods and, where possible, undertaking landmark analyses where adverse health-related outcomes occurring in the first year or more after baseline measurement are excluded from the analysis.

Figure 2.3 Cohort study design.

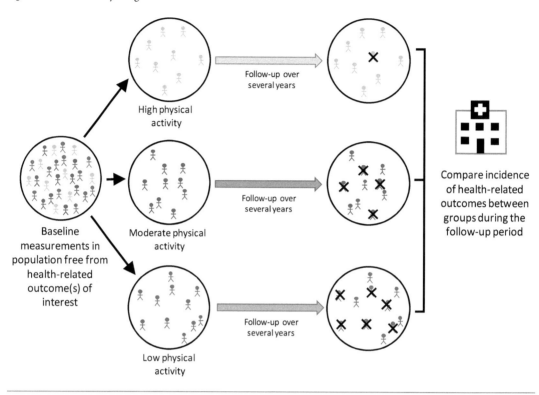

Cohort studies also provide the potential to address more complex issues, such as gene–environment interactions. For example, a publication using data from the Nurses' Health Study and Health Professionals Follow-up Study found that high levels of physical activity in leisure time attenuated, and high levels of television watching (often used as a proxy measure of sedentary behaviour) accentuated, the effects of a genetic predisposition to obesity on body mass index (Qi et al. 2012).

MEASURES OF HEALTH-RELATED OUTCOMES IN EPIDEMIOLOGICAL STUDIES

Measures of the occurrence of health-related outcomes are basic tools of epidemiology. They permit comparison of the frequency of the outcome(s) of interest between populations, as well as among individuals, with and without exposure to a particular risk factor. A number of measures are in common usage, giving different types of information. All require correct definition of the population at risk. For instance, sports injuries only occur among people who play sport, so the population at risk are sports players.

Prevalence and incidence are the measures most commonly used. Prevalence quantifies the proportion of individuals in a population that exhibits the outcome of interest at a specified time. For example, in the 2010 Scottish Health Survey, the prevalence of

Scottish women undertaking sufficient physical activity to meet current physical activity recommendations was 33%. Prevalence is helpful in assessing the need for health care or preventive strategies. The formula for calculating prevalence (P) is:

P = Number of people with the health-related outcome at a specified time / Number of people in the population at risk at the specified time

Incidence quantifies the number of new occurrences of an outcome that develop during a specified time interval in the population at risk of experiencing the event during this period. The most accurate is the person–time incidence rate (I), calculated as:

I = Number of people who develop the health-related outcome in a specified period / Sum of the periods of time for which each person in the population is at risk

The denominator is the best available measure of the total time for which individuals are free of the outcome in question. Each person in the study population contributes one person-year for each year of observation before the outcome develops or that person is lost to follow-up. Figure 2.4 illustrates this schematically, based on a study of five participants over a five-year observation period.

The commonest outcome measures are rates of morbidity (illness) and mortality (death). Because the age structure of a population affects both rates, these are often reported as age-specific or age-adjusted rates. This is essential when older people are more likely to become ill, as is the case, for instance, for CHD or stroke. Measures of health status may also encompass some measure of the quality of life – for example, life expectancy free from disability, quality-adjusted life years or disability-adjusted life years lost.

Figure 2.4 Calculation of person–time incidence rate.

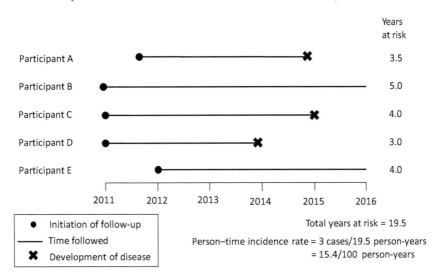

Source: Adapted from Hennekens and Buring (1987).

Comparisons of disease occurrence between exposed and unexposed groups, for example smokers versus non-smokers, or people with high and low levels of physical activity, are essential tools in epidemiology. Measures used include risk difference, relative risk, odds ratio and hazard ratio. An explanation of these terms is provided in Box 2.1. When interpreting epidemiological data, it is important to appreciate the difference between absolute and relative risk. Increasing incidence from one in a million to two in a million, or from 250,000 in a million to 500,000 in a million, both represent a doubling of relative risk. However, in the former case the absolute risk is trivial and in the latter it is huge. Thus, relative risk statistics can be difficult to interpret in the absence of absolute risks or prevalence data.

BOX 2.1 KEY MEASURES OF RISK IN EPIDEMIOLOGY.

Risk difference	Also called excess risk. The absolute difference in rates of occurrence between individuals who have and have not been exposed to the factor of interest. For example, if incidence of stroke is 17.7 events per 100,000 person-years in non-smokers and 49.6 events per 100,000 person-years in smokers, the risk difference in strokes between smokers and non-smokers is 31.9 events (49.6 minus 17.7) per 100,000 person-years.
Relative risk	Also called risk ratio. The risk of occurrence in the exposed group divided by the risk of occurrence in the unexposed. In the example above, the relative risk of stroke in smokers compared with non-smokers would be 2.8 (49.6/17.7). In other words, smokers are 2.8 times as likely to have a stroke as non-smokers.
Odds ratio	Used to measure the association between an exposure and a health-related outcome in case-control and cross-sectional studies. It is very similar to the relative risk, particularly if the outcome is relatively rare (occurring in less than ~10% of the unexposed group).
Hazard ratio	A hazard is the rate at which an outcome (e.g. morbidity or mortality) occurs. Thus, the hazard ratio compares the rates at which outcomes occur between groups over time. Hazard ratios are calculated using a relatively complex statistical technique called survival analysis and can be interpreted as the relative risk averaged over time.

When dealing with exposures that are associated with a decreased risk of disease – as is often the case for physical activity – researchers sometimes take the unexposed group (the inactive group) as the reference category. The relative risk in the group exposed to physical activity is thus less than 1. Box 2.2 illustrates both approaches.

Survival analyses, resulting in the calculation of hazard ratios (see Box 2.1), are increasingly being used in epidemiological research. These analyses are often presented using Kaplan–Meier (or survival) curves, which show cumulative probability of either developing, or remaining free of (i.e. surviving), an outcome over time. Figure 2.5 shows a Kaplan–Meier curve for the probability of remaining free from all-cause mortality according to level of fitness in 1,263 men with type 2 diabetes from the Aerobics Center Longitudinal Study over an average follow-up period of 12 years (14,777 person-years of observation). Over this period, 180 men died, and the rate of mortality

---

BOX 2.2 COMPARISONS OF DISEASE OCCURRENCE.

Table 2.2 Vigorous sports and incidence of coronary heart disease in male civil servants.

EPISODES OF VIGOROUS SPORT IN PREVIOUS FOUR WEEKS, REPORTED IN 1976	CORONARY HEART DISEASE CASES	PERSON-YEARS	AGE STANDARDISED RATE* (CASES PER 1000 PERSON-YEARS)
None (reference group)	413	72,282	5.8
1–3	37	7,786	4.5
8–12+	7	3,349	2.1

Source: Adapted from Morris et al. (1990).

Note: * Rates are slightly different from values obtained from calculations based on data in columns 2 and 3 because of adjustment for age.

In Table 2.2, the absolute difference in CHD between men reporting no vigorous sports and those reporting between 8 and ≥12 episodes is (5.8 – 2.1), that is 3.7 cases per 1,000 person-years. This gives no indication of the strength of the association, however, which is estimated by calculating the relative risk. Relative risk can be expressed in two ways:

1 Taking men reporting no vigorous sport as the reference group, the relative risk in men reporting between 8 and ≥12 episodes is (2.1/5.8), or 0.36. Thus, men who were the most active in vigorous sport had a risk of developing CHD that was around one-third of that experienced by the least active men in such sports.
2 Taking men with the highest level of participation in vigorous sports as the reference group, the relative risk of not engaging in these is (5.8/2.1), or 2.76. Thus, men who did not engage in vigorous sport were more than two-and-a-half times as likely to develop CHD as those with the highest level of participation in such sport.

---

was 2.1 times higher in unfit compared with fit men; in other words, unfit men had a hazard ratio for mortality of 2.1.

For public health policy, it is informative to estimate the incidence of a disease (or other health outcome) in a population that can be attributed to exposure to a particular risk factor. This measure is the population-attributable risk. It reflects not only the strength of the risk associated with an exposure (information vital for assessment of the risk to an individual) but also its prevalence. Population-attributable risk estimates can therefore help to determine which exposures have the most relevance to the health of a community. For example, the relative risk of developing lung cancer in smokers is high (14 in a classic study of British doctors). Nevertheless, if only 1% of the population smoke, the population-attributable risk is low; on the other hand, if 30% of people smoke, then the population-attributable risk is high and this behaviour represents a considerable public health burden that justifies investment in strategies to reduce its prevalence. A second example, based on World Health Organization data comparing the global burden of smoking and physical inactivity, is shown

Figure 2.5 Kaplan–Meier plot showing probability of remaining free from all-cause mortality amongst 1,263 men with type 2 diabetes in the Aerobic Center Longitudinal Study. Solid line represents fit participants and dashed line represents unfit participants.

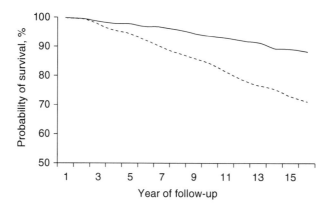

Source: From *Annals of Internal Medicine*, Wei, M., et al., 'Low cardiorespiratory fitness and physical inactivity as predictors of mortality in men with type 2 diabetes', 132: 605–11. Copyright © 2000 American College of Physicians. All Rights Reserved. Reprinted with the permission of American College of Physicians, Inc.

Table 2.3 Global burden on mortality of smoking and physical inactivity.

RISK FACTOR	HAZARD RATIO FOR ALL-CAUSE MORTALITY	PREVALENCE OF RISK FACTOR (% OF POPULATION)	POPULATION ATTRIBUTABLE RISK (%)	GLOBAL DEATHS PER YEAR
Smoking	1.57	26	8.7	5.1 million
Physical inactivity	1.28	35	9.0	5.3 million

Source: Adapted from Wen and Wu (2012).

in Table 2.3. Although the hazard ratio of death associated with smoking is higher than that associated with physical inactivity, the estimates of population-attributable risk for these two exposures, and number of global deaths attributed to these two risk factors are similar because the prevalence of physical inactivity is much higher than the prevalence of smoking.

EXPERIMENTAL RESEARCH

Observational studies have limited ability to identify a causal link between an exposure and an outcome, as there is potential for observational findings to be influenced by bias and confounding (these concepts will be discussed further), but often lead to the generation of hypotheses that can be tested experimentally. Experimental studies (often called intervention studies), in which researchers intervene to change a variable in one

Figure 2.6 Randomised controlled trial study design.

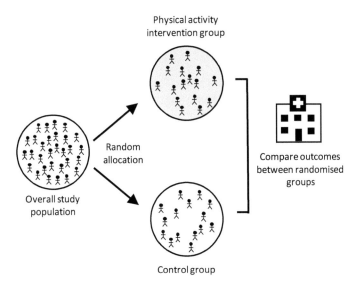

or more groups and then measure the effect on the outcome of interest, can reduce these sources of error.

The 'gold-standard' study design for establishing a causal relationship between an exposure variable (e.g. physical activity) and a disease or health outcome is the randomised controlled trial (RCT). In an RCT, participants are assigned to one or more intervention groups or a control group in a random manner. This ensures that differences between groups in the outcomes at the end of the study are due to the imposed intervention rather than other inherent differences between the groups. Figure 2.6 illustrates this concept.

There are relatively few RCTs considering the effect of physical activity on disease outcomes, and those that do exist have all evaluated specific populations who are at high risk of developing the disease in question. This contrasts with the body of observational data on physical activity and health or disease outcomes, where samples from the general population have generally been studied. This is because the relatively low rate of disease 'events' in the general (healthy) population means that an RCT would need to be unfeasibly long (over many decades) and large (with many thousands of participants) for an effect of an intervention to be detected. The Finnish Diabetes Prevention Study is an example of one RCT that has been undertaken. In this study, 522 patients with impaired glucose tolerance (a pre-diabetic condition that substantially increases risk of developing type 2 diabetes) were randomly assigned to lifestyle intervention (comprising increased physical activity and dietary modification) or control groups, with incidence of diabetes over a follow-up period of up to six years as the primary study outcome. Lifestyle intervention reduced incident diabetes by 58% compared with the control group (Tuomilehto et al. 2001). However, in 'lifestyle' interventions, which include changes to both physical activity and diet and often lead to weight loss, it can be difficult to ascertain the specific contribution of increased physical activity (i.e. independent of dietary changes and weight loss) on the study outcome measures. An RCT examining the effects of an intervention on a disease outcome, such as the Finnish Diabetes Prevention study, is an experimental epidemiological study, and the outcome measures are assessed in the same way as the observational epidemiological studies described above.

OUTCOME MEASURES IN EXPERIMENTAL STUDIES

In physical activity research, it is often difficult to undertake experiments to test the effect of physical activity on a disease outcome directly. Thus, many experimental studies in the field of physical activity and health consider the effects of a physical activity intervention on risk factors (or biomarkers) for the disease of interest. For example, an experimental study might investigate whether a particular type of physical activity intervention reduces blood pressure, which is an important causal risk factor for cardiovascular disease (Figure 2.7). From this, we can infer that physical activity is likely to also reduce risk of cardiovascular disease. Studies of this nature also provide information about the mechanisms by which physical activity might reduce cardiovascular disease risk, in this instance through its effects in reducing blood pressure.

Laboratory-based experimental studies can go beyond looking at risk markers to examine the mechanisms in more detail. Taking the blood pressure example above, an experimental study might investigate how exercise influences factors which determine blood pressure, for example looking at how physical activity might improve the ability of blood vessels to relax. This may involve investigation of how exercise influences concentrations in the blood of molecules that influence blood vessel relaxation or may involve examination of small muscle or fat samples collected from a biopsy. In some instances, it can be helpful to use animal models to examine the mechanisms by which

Figure 2.7 Using RCT data on effects of physical activity on a risk factor together with established data on causal link between the risk factor and the disease outcome to infer a causal link between physical activity and the disease outcome.

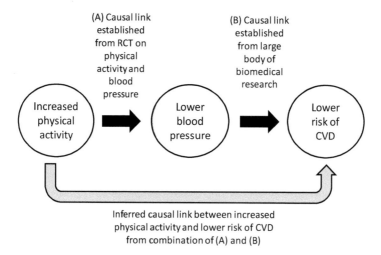

physical activity, fitness or sedentary behaviour influences health-related outcomes in more detail than is possible in a study of humans. For example, a group of researchers has experimentally bred rats with high and low levels of cardiorespiratory fitness to examine the mechanisms by which fitness influences a number of health-related variables such as cardiac function and energy metabolism in muscle (Koch et al. 2012). Another group of investigators used an experimental model where rats' hind limbs were held above the ground (and therefore not subject to any weight bearing) by suspending them by their tails, to examine the effects of extreme inactivity on the activity of lipoprotein lipase (an enzyme responsible for clearing fat from the blood) within the muscles of the rats' hind limbs (Hamilton et al. 2007). While animal models enable examination of the mechanisms by which (in)activity or fitness influence health in more detail than would be possible in studies of humans, species differences in physiology and metabolism mean that care is sometimes needed in translating the findings of these experiments to humans.

TYPES OF EXPERIMENTAL STUDY DESIGN

The RCT design described above, where control and intervention groups are studied in parallel and differences in a binary health or disease outcome measure between the groups are assessed (e.g. developing or remaining free from diabetes), is an example of a parallel study design. A parallel study design can also be used to evaluate the effects of an intervention on health-related variables of a continuous nature. For example, a study investigating the effects of exercise training on weight loss might randomly assign individuals to a 12-week exercise programme or control group (who just undergo their normal activities for the study duration), and then compare the difference in change in weight from the start to the end of the study in the two groups. Random assignment of participants to groups in an intervention generates the highest degree of confidence in the findings and provides strong internal validity, reducing the likelihood that the findings are influenced by chance, bias or confounding. Without randomisation, there is potential for the introduction of bias. For example, given the choice, 'couch potatoes' will typically choose to be controls, whereas those who are already fit and active will happily volunteer to be exercisers. If not controlled for by randomisation, such underlying differences can lead to differences in the variables of interest between the groups that confound the study findings.

Another type of study design is the cross-over, or repeated measures, design where each participant acts as their own control. For example, if researchers wished to study the effects of a single exercise session on bone metabolism, each participant would be studied twice, once after no exercise and once after an exercise session. The within-participant changes between the conditions would then be compared. In such experiments it is best practice to randomly allocate the order of testing. If all participants were to do the exercise trial first, there is the potential for the findings to be confounded by order-of-testing effects. These effects might derive from, for example, the environment (hot weather during the first trials, followed by a cold snap), but more often relate to changes in the participants themselves. Participants' anxiety levels decrease with repeated trials, resulting in changes to physiological and metabolic responses.

A third type of experimental study design is a before–after study, where the effect of an intervention on a health-related variable is evaluated without a parallel control group. For example, a study might compare blood glucose values in newly diagnosed type 2 diabetes patients before and after a three-month walking intervention programme. This is a much weaker experiment design than the parallel or cross-over designs described above because without a control group there is a risk of confounding from systematic effects unrelated to the intervention. In the example here, it is possible that effects of diabetes medications, dietary changes during the intervention period, or an order-of-testing effect, might also have influenced glucose values. Thus, the observed effects on blood glucose would have been the effects of the walking intervention as well as any effects of medications, diet or testing order. Thus, without a control group, the effects of an intervention are often overestimated.

Figure 2.8 illustrates parallel, cross-over and before–after study designs. Here the simplest forms of parallel and cross-over studies are shown, with the effects of only one intervention being compared to a control condition. However, it is possible to extend either of these designs to study multiple intervention groups; for example, a parallel study might randomly assign participants to control, moderate intensity exercise and vigorous intensity exercise intervention arms and the differences between these three conditions would be compared.

Figure 2.8 Types of experimental study design.

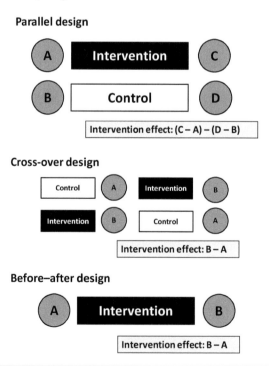

ERROR: NATURE, SOURCES AND IMPLICATIONS

Evaluation of the validity of the findings of a study depends on the extent to which these could also be explained by chance, bias or confounding. A critical appreciation of the literature on exercise and health requires an understanding of all three sources of error. First, however, it is essential to make the distinction between precision and accuracy, both essential features of measurement. Figure 2.9 depicts these important concepts. Briefly, data are accurate if they are close to the true values and precise if the same measurement, when repeated, consistently yields similar values. Good data have to be both accurate and precise (Figure 2.9, top left); neither is sufficient alone (Box 2.3).

Random error is due to chance and leads to imprecision in measurement. It derives from several sources, including: individual biological variation; sampling error (as the study group(s) are a sample from a larger population); and measurement error. These errors cannot be eliminated, but they can be reduced by making individual measurements as precise as possible and by increasing the size of the study. In the laboratory, precision is achieved by calibration of instruments, by making careful measurements and by increasing the number of measurements. Precise measurements are often impossible in epidemiology because it is difficult to measure physical activity, sedentary behaviour, or fitness (this is addressed below) and, often, health outcomes. This imprecision may be compensated by studying a large sample which increases statistical power (see below).

Bias is error in research design or collection of data that produces results which differ in a systematic manner from the true values. It can take many forms, but the most important are selection bias and measurement bias. Selection bias arises when the characteristics of people selected to participate in a study differ systematically from those of people who are not selected. In an experimental study, selection bias may influence the subsequent generalisability of findings, but not its validity. In observational studies, where associations between a putative risk factor and a health outcome are sought, selection bias threatens the validity of a study. For example, if people are asked to participate in a study of physical activity, responders are likely to differ in their exercise habits from non-responders. An investigator can also introduce bias (knowingly or unknowingly) by including people who appear more (or less) receptive to the notion that physical activity improves health rather than other potential participants. Another source of selection bias is the 'healthy worker effect'; people in employment have to be healthy enough to do their job, whereas those who are ill or disabled may often be excluded.

Systematic error in measurements is an issue in both experimental and observational studies. For example, in a large multi-centre study, one clinical biochemistry laboratory may consistently measure plasma cholesterol concentrations lower than another. This bias can be evaluated if each laboratory participating in a study analyses a portion of a 'pooled' serum sample and a correction factor is applied. Other sources of bias are more difficult to deal with. One of the most important relates to measurements that rely on human memory (e.g. consumption of coffee or of foods high in fat or, of course, participation in physical activities) and these are common in epidemiology. For example, underweight individuals tend to over-report food intake on questionnaires, while obese

BOX 2.3 ACCURACY AND PRECISION.

- If an individual's $\dot{V}O_2$max is measured on four occasions during one week and recorded as 25 ml kg^{-1} min^{-1}, 35 ml kg^{-1} min^{-1}, 15 ml kg^{-1} min^{-1} and 42 ml kg^{-1} min^{-1}, the measurements have low precision; they are so different that no meaningful interpretation can be placed on them – even if the average of these values is close to the true value (Figure 2.9, bottom left).
- On the other hand, repeated measurements of 34 ml kg^{-1} min^{-1}, 32 ml kg^{-1} min^{-1}, 33 ml kg^{-1} min^{-1} and 33 ml kg^{-1} min^{-1} indicate high precision, but are inaccurate if the person's *true* $\dot{V}O_2$max is 19 ml kg^{-1} min^{-1} (Figure 2.9, top right). This is important because the average value recorded (33 ml kg^{-1} min^{-1}) suggests that brisk walking at 4.5 METs would be very light exercise for this person (<50% $\dot{V}O_2$max), whereas it would actually be very vigorous (>80% $\dot{V}O_2$max).
- Only if repeated values are close to each other (high precision) and cluster around the true value (high accuracy), can we have confidence in the data.

Figure 2.9 Schematic representation of accuracy and precision in measurement.

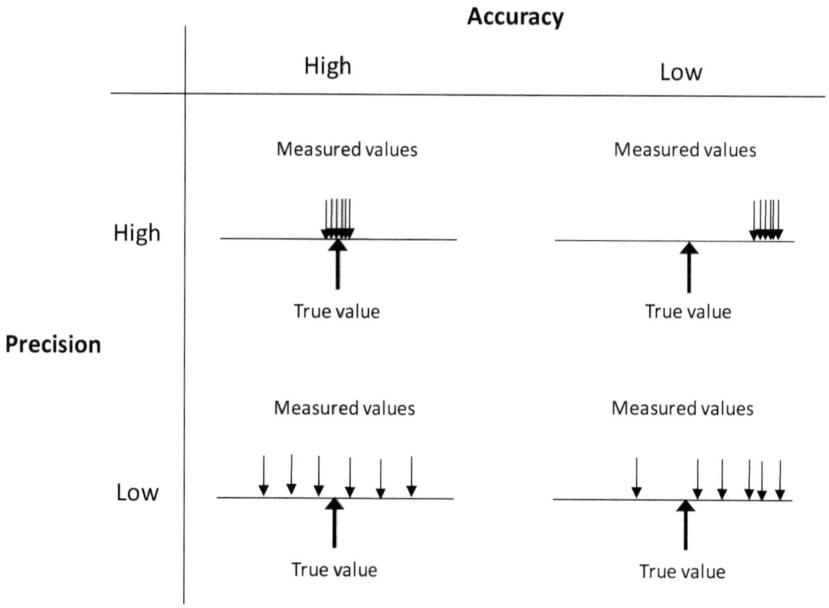

Source: Adapted from Beaglehole et al. (1993).

participants under-report it. This error is called recall bias and is particularly important in case-control studies when individuals recently diagnosed with a disease tend to recall their past exposures with greater accuracy than controls, especially if it is widely known that the risk factor under study may be associated with that disease.

Bias is not confined to individual studies but may be evident in the literature as a whole. For example, there is a tendency for editors of journals to accept research papers reporting 'positive' findings (where the research hypothesis is supported) more readily than those who report 'negative' findings. This tendency for publication bias is compounded by the fact that researchers are less likely to submit studies with negative findings for publication.

As explained early in this chapter, an epidemiological study seeks to identify an association between exposure to a designated causal (or risk) factor and a health-related outcome. Often, however, a third factor is associated both with the exposure being studied and the outcome being studied. If this third factor is unequally distributed between the exposure subgroups, it may confuse the findings. This problem is called confounding. It can even create the appearance of a cause-and-effect relationship that does not exist. Randomisation is the best way to control the problem of confounding factors in intervention trials. In case-control and cohort studies, the problem is most commonly addressed at the analysis stage by statistical modelling to estimate the strength of associations, while controlling simultaneously for confounding variables. An example of confounding can be seen in a paper published from the US National Health and Nutrition Examination Survey, in which an inverse relationship between energy intake and cardiovascular disease mortality rate was observed – in other words those with the *highest* energy intakes had the *lowest* incidence of cardiovascular disease mortality (Fang et al. 2003) (Figure 2.10). This is not a biologically plausible causal relationship and thus the association is likely to be mediated by confounding factors. Indeed, once the data were statistically adjusted for the confounding effects of physical activity and body mass index, the initial inverse association between energy intake and cardiovascular disease mortality was no longer evident. However, this analytical approach cannot alter the fundamental quality of the data and it is not possible to statistically adjust for all sources of confounding. Thus, in observational studies, residual confounding will inevitably introduce biases that cannot be controlled statistically.

Figure 2.10 Cardiovascular disease mortality rates (per 1,000 person-years) adjusted for age and ethnicity, by tertile of dietary caloric intake, in men and women in the National Health and Nutrition Examination Survey I Epidemiologic Follow-up Study.

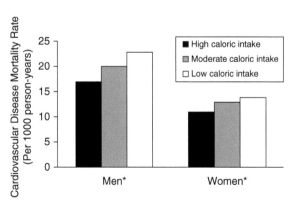

Source: Reprinted from the *American Journal of Preventive Medicine*, 25: 283–9, Fang, J. et al., 'Exercise, body mass index, caloric intake, and cardiovascular mortality', page 286, copyright © 2003, with permission from Elsevier.
Note: * Significant difference between groups, p < 0.01.

Another potential form of systematic error in observational studies is reverse causality. For example having cardiovascular disease may lead to a reduction in physical activity, so in cross-sectional studies, there is potential that an inverse relationship between physical activity and disease status could conceivably be influenced by cardiovascular disease leading to a reduction in physical activity. This effect can also be seen to some extent in cohort studies as some people may have low levels of physical activity at baseline because they are already in the early stages of having a disease that influences physical activity levels. This effect can be minimised by undertaking landmark analyses which remove data from individuals who experience a disease event soon (e.g. within a year or two years) after the baseline measurements.

STATISTICAL ANALYSIS OF DATA

Researchers use hypothesis testing to evaluate the degree to which chance variation may account for the results by calculating either the significance value (p-value) or a confidence interval. Their hypothesis is accepted or rejected on the basis of these statistical tests. The p-value describes the probability that the result may be due to chance alone. In medical research, investigators conventionally adopt a critical p-value (α) of 0.05. This means that the probability of obtaining the observed association (or difference) is less than 5% (or 1 in 20) if the null hypothesis was in fact true. In other words, the researcher is reasonably certain that the observed data are 'unusual' enough to rule out the null hypothesis. Two types of error are associated with this decision: to reject the null hypothesis when it is true (type I or α error), and to accept the null hypothesis when it is false (type II or β error). The probability of making a type I error is the level of significance of a statistical test.

The probability of rejecting the null hypothesis when it is in fact false and should be rejected is known as its power. This reflects the potential of a study to detect an important effect. ('Important' has to be defined by the investigators, often on the basis of what is judged to be clinically meaningful.) Statistical power is affected by three factors: the size of the difference between groups, the number of participants and the variability of the factor being measured (error variance). Thus, larger group sizes enable smaller differences to be detected between groups, and high variability in the factor of interest (due to large variability within the group and/or low precision of measurement) reduces power to detect small differences. In epidemiological studies, it is possible to obtain sufficient statistical power to detect effects with imprecise measures because sample sizes are typically large. In laboratory studies, where variability in measurement is low and intervention effects can be large, it is possible to have sufficient power with relatively small sample sizes. Researchers can perform power calculations before embarking on an investigation to determine how large a sample is needed to detect statistically significant effects.

The p-value in itself does not provide information about the importance of the difference between groups. For example, with a large sample and low error variance, it is possible for very small differences between groups, that may be clinically or biologically unimportant, to be detected. To understand how important a difference is, investigators need to consider the magnitude of the effect. This can be expressed in absolute terms – for example, an exercise intervention resulted in 3 kg greater weight loss than control; or in percentage terms – for example, a training programme led to a 10% increase in maximal oxygen uptake. An increasingly common approach is to calculate a standardised effect size such as the Cohen's *d* effect size, which is calculated by dividing the difference in mean values by the standard deviation. Whether a given effect size can be considered large or small is often dependent on the context, but as a rule of thumb, Cohen's *d* effect size values of 0.2, 0.5 and 0.8 are typically considered as 'small', 'medium' and 'large', respectively. Odds ratios, relative risks and hazard ratios described earlier in this chapter are other examples of standardised effect sizes.

Confidence intervals are being increasingly used to assess differences between groups. They provide the range within which the true magnitude of the effect lies, with a certain level of assurance. Conventionally 95% confidence intervals are used, so the confidence limits contain the true value for the variable of interest 95% of the time. For example, in the UK Biobank cohort, cycling to work was associated with a hazard ratio for all-cause mortality of 0.59, compared with non-active commuting (Celis-Morales et al. 2017). The 95% confidence interval for this hazard ratio was 0.42–0.83, so we can be assured that, if the study were repeated 20 times on different samples, on 19 occasions the relative risk would lie between 0.42 and 0.83. This value did not cross 1.00, so lower relative risk would be considered significant at the $p < 0.05$ level. Thus, the confidence interval gives both a measure of effect size and statistical significance in a single statistic. Increasing sample size or reducing error variance reduces the width of confidence interval but does not (systematically) change the effect size.

PHYSICAL ACTIVITY, SEDENTARY BEHAVIOUR, CARDIORESPIRATORY FITNESS AND STRENGTH: CONCEPTS AND INTER-RELATIONSHIPS

Physical activity is defined as bodily movement produced by skeletal muscles that substantially increases energy expenditure. Over the course of a day, humans can engage in a range of physical activities that cover a range of intensities, from light activities of daily living to very high intensity exercise. The most appropriate approach to quantify these complex behaviours depends on the nature of the research question and study outcome being addressed. For example, in a study of the potential effects of physical activity on body weight, the most appropriate measure might be total activity energy expenditure, whereas for studies evaluating effects on cardiovascular disease risk, details about intensity, type, duration and frequency of physical activity are likely to be of importance. Often, researchers are interested in quantifying time spent engaged in moderate and vigorous physical activities, which are sometimes grouped together as moderate-to-vigorous physical activity (MVPA; i.e. all activity of at least moderate intensity). Moderate and vigorous intensities can be defined either in terms relative to the individual – such as perceived effort level, or percentages of maximum heart rate or maximal oxygen uptake ($\dot{V}O_2max$) – or in terms of absolute values. A common approach in epidemiological research and public health guidance is to characterise activity intensities using metabolic equivalents (METs), which measures intensity in multiples of the resting metabolic rate (assumed to correspond to an oxygen uptake of 3.5 ml kg^{-1} min^{-1}). Using this approach, activities of 3 to 6 MET intensity are typically classed as moderate intensity, with >6 MET activities being classed as vigorous. Multiplying time spent in physical activities by the MET score can be used to provide a summary measure of volume of physical activity (expressed in MET-hours or MET-minutes). For example, if a woman did two hours of high-impact aerobic dance (intensity 7 METs) each week, as well as three hours of brisk walking at 4 METs, her total physical activity could be described as $[(2 \times 7) + (3 \times 4)] = 26$ MET-hour week^{-1}.

Historically, the term **sedentary** has been used to define individuals who engaged in low levels of physical activity. However, in recent times, the terminology has shifted, with 'inactive' becoming the preferred term to describe such individuals, and the term 'sedentary behaviour' being used to characterise low energy expenditure activities (<1.5 METs) in a seated or reclining position (Tremblay et al. 2017). Accordingly, MVPA and sedentary behaviour are independent factors and it is possible for an individual to be both highly physically active and highly sedentary; for example, if they run for an hour per day, but spend the rest of the day sitting down. Light intensity activity (typically classed as 1.5 to 3 METs) has historically received relatively limited attention in physical activity for health epidemiology, partly due to difficulties in capturing it well using self-report questionnaires, but, increasingly, researchers are adopting more integrated approaches to capture physical activity behaviours across the entire intensity spectrum encompassing sedentary, light, moderate and vigorous activities.

Cardiorespiratory fitness is a physiological trait defined as the ability of the cardiovascular and respiratory systems to supply oxygen to working muscles during sustained physical activity. It is typically assessed by measuring $\dot{V}O_2$max, either directly or indirectly. Higher levels physical activity generally leads to higher fitness levels, with vigorous activity influencing fitness to a greater extent than moderate or light intensity activity. However, it is estimated that up to half of the variance in fitness (and the extent to which fitness improves in response to exercise training) can be explained by

Figure 2.11 Inter-relationships between activity behaviours, genetics, cardiorespiratory fitness and muscular strength.

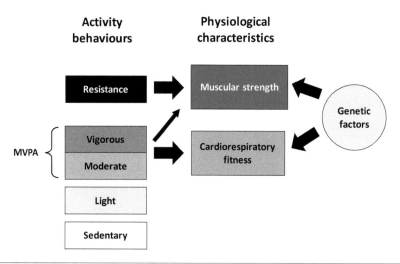

heritable factors (Bouchard et al. 1998; Bouchard 2012). Thus, it is possible to have a high level of fitness and be physically inactive, or to have a low level of fitness despite being physically active, depending on an individual's genetic make-up.

A further class of physical activity is resistance exercise which involves muscles contracting against an external resistance, for example weights, which has the effect of increasing muscle size and strength. However, like cardiorespiratory fitness, muscular strength also has a large genetic component (Silventoinen et al. 2008). Figure 2.11 shows the inter-relationships between activity behaviours, genetics, cardiorespiratory fitness and muscular strength.

MEASUREMENT OF PHYSICAL ACTIVITY, SEDENTARY BEHAVIOUR, CARDIORESPIRATORY FITNESS AND STRENGTH

In the early years of research into physical activity and health, job classification was a useful tool. For example, the classic study by Morris and co-workers compared the incidence of CHD in London postmen who delivered mail on foot or by bicycle (a physically active group) with that in colleagues who sorted the mail (designated as less active) (Morris et al. 1953). Occupational tasks have sometimes been classified using 'on-the-job' measurements of oxygen uptake as in Paffenbarger's study of San Francisco longshoremen (dockworkers) in the 1970s (Paffenbarger and Hale 1975). However, as the physical demands of so many occupations decreased, leisure-time physical activity became the dominant component of total activity. This has most commonly been measured using a questionnaire or diary (in 'real time' or retrospectively). In addition, self-reported indices of sedentary behaviour, such as hours spent watching television, provide useful information. Approaches that are increasingly adopted as technology progresses include monitoring physical activity using wearable monitors, such as pedometers or accelerometers, and measurement of total energy expenditure using the doubly labelled water technique.

Self-report questionnaires

Questionnaires of self-reported physical activity behaviours are inexpensive and easy to administer which makes them particularly suitable for studies of large populations. They can be self-administered either on paper or, increasingly, using computer-based online forms; or completed during a telephone or face-to-face interview with an investigator. A wide range of questionnaires for the assessment of physical activity and sedentary behaviour are available. The simplest of these classify people as active or inactive, based on two or three questions. More detailed questionnaires ask a range of questions about time spent engaged in activities of different intensities and the context in which these activities occur (e.g. leisure time, occupational, transport). Sedentary behaviour is often assessed by asking questions about time spent sitting down, or time engaged in subcategories of sitting such as television watching, screen-time (i.e. television watching and computer use) or driving. Questionnaires may ask questions about recent physical activity or sedentary behaviours (for example in the past week or month), usual physical activity/sedentary behaviours, or lifetime exposures. Asking about recent activity improves recall and avoids difficulties in interpretation about what constitutes 'usual', but the validity of the data is limited by the extent to which the period sampled reflects an individual's usual behaviour.

There has long been a need for a standardised approach to obtaining data on self-reported physical activity levels to facilitate international comparisons and global surveillance. To this end the International Physical Activity Questionnaire (IPAQ) has now been developed in both long and short forms. Details are available at https://sites. google.com/site/theipaq/. Its reliability and validity are 'at least as good as other established self-reports', even in diverse settings (Craig et al. 2003).

The precision (repeatability) of questionnaires, assessed by test–retest correlation coefficients, is high (at an interval of one month this mostly exceeds 0.75). It is, however, best for high-intensity leisure-time activities and much poorer for those of moderate and light intensity. Several approaches have been used for questionnaire validation including: detailed interview by a trained interviewer; use of a motion detector, usually an accelerometer; and assessment of cardiorespiratory fitness. Questionnaire measures correlate relatively poorly with accelerometer recordings or with measurements of total energy expenditure obtained by the doubly labelled water method. Figure 2.12 shows the relationship between MVPA assessed using the IPAQ and physical activity assessed objectively using an accelerometer in one study, indicating both the modest correlation between the two physical activity measures and the systematic overestimation of MVPA by the questionnaire (Celis-Morales et al. 2012). The relationships between questionnaire scores of physical activity and fitness

Figure 2.12 Relationship between accelerometer-derived and IPAQ-reported MVPA in 317 adults.

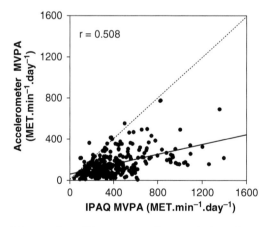

Source: Reprinted with no modifications from 'Objective vs. self-reported physical activity and sedentary time: effects of measurement method on relationships with risk biomarkers', Celis-Morales, C.A. et al., *PLoS One*, 2012, 7: e36345. Article distributed under the terms of the Creative Commons Attribution 4.0 International (CC BY) Licence (http:// creativecommons.org/licenses/by/4.0/).
Note: Solid line represents the linear regression line; dotted line represents the line of equality, y = x; r is the Pearson correlation coefficient.

also tend to be modest (typical correlation coefficients 0.3–0.5); this is likely to reflect both the genetic influence on fitness and the imprecision involved in measuring physical activity by questionnaire.

The relative inaccuracy of questionnaire-based assessment of physical activity acts to attenuate any apparent relationship between physical activity and a health-related outcome (i.e. bias towards a null effect). This phenomenon is called regression dilution bias, and thus in epidemiological studies, the observed relationships between questionnaire-assessed physical activity and health outcomes are likely to be underestimates of the true effect. Figure 2.13 illustrates this effect in a cross-sectional study of physical activity level (determined by quartile of MVPA) and plasma triglyceride concentrations. When MVPA quartile was assessed by accelerometer, a clear dose–response effect was observed with higher level physical activity associated with lower triglyceride concentrations. However, this dose–response relationship is less evident when MVPA quartile was assessed using the IPAQ (Celis-Morales et al. 2012).

Despite their shortcomings, questionnaires can provide important information about the context of physical activity and sedentary behaviours that objective measures do not. This information can be particularly helpful in the design of interventions to increase physical activity or reduce sedentary behaviour. Thus, questionnaire-based and objective measures of physical activity and sedentary behaviour provide complementary information and a number of recent studies have used both measurement approaches in parallel.

Figure 2.13 Triglyceride concentrations by quartile of MVPA for accelerometer-derived and IPAQ-reported physical activity measures in 317 adults.

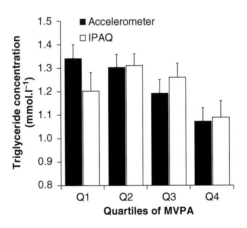

Source: Reprinted with no modifications from 'Objective vs. self-reported physical activity and sedentary time: effects of measurement method on relationships with risk biomarkers', Celis-Morales, C.A. et al., *PLoS One*, 2012, 7: e36345. Article distributed under the terms of the Creative Commons Attribution 4.0 International (CC BY) Licence (http://creativecommons.org/licenses/by/4.0/).
Note: The trend for triglyceride concentration by MVPA quartile was statistically significant for the accelerometer ($p = 0.022$), but not the IPAQ ($p = 0.139$), activity measure.

Measures of physical activity and sedentary behaviour which do not rely on self-report

Pedometers and accelerometers are wearable sensors that provide objective real-time measurement of activity behaviours. Pedometers are usually worn on the hip and count steps either using a horizontal, spring-suspended lever arm that bounces with vertical motion during walking or running or using a piezoelectric (electricity resulting from mechanical stress) sensor that measures accelerations in the vertical plane. Pedometers do not capture intensity of activity and data are typically reported as steps per day.

Accelerometers are small, minimally intrusive, devices that use piezoelectric or solid-state sensors to measure bodily accelerations. Both uniaxial (measuring accelerations in a single, usually vertical, plane) and triaxial accelerometers (measuring accelerations in all three planes) are available. The latter theoretically allow for more comprehensive assessment of body movement, although in practice often only vertical accelerations are used in data analysis. Accelerometers are typically worn (on the hip, wrist, thigh, upper arm or ankle) during waking hours, for at least four days (often seven days) to provide a reliable measure of usual physical activity and sedentary behaviour, but some devices are worn 24 hours per day. Computer software is used to convert raw acceleration outputs (often called 'counts') into meaningful indicators of physical activity such as time spent in different intensity domains or energy expenditure. This requires prior validation of accelerometer outputs over a range of activities against measures such as direct observation or oxygen uptake (or against doubly labelled water measures for total energy expenditure). Commonly used analytical approaches include the use of thresholds of acceleration counts (known as cut-points) to define periods of sedentary, light, moderate and vigorous intensities; and the use of regression-based models to estimate energy expenditure. Some devices (particularly those positioned on the thigh) can determine body posture as well as dynamic accelerations and can therefore classify periods of sitting or lying down, standing and stepping. This permits more accurate determination of sedentary behaviour than devices classifying sedentary time simply on the basis of low acceleration counts. In validation studies, moderate to high correlations are generally observed between accelerometer counts and oxygen uptake or physical activity energy expenditure (typical correlation coefficients 0.5–0.9). There are also devices that combine accelerometry with other technologies such as heart-rate monitoring that may enhance the ability accurately to determine energy expenditure. Devices using Global Positioning Systems (GPS) are being developed that have the potential to help provide context about where activities are taking place, and some researchers have started to use smartphones (which have inbuilt accelerometers and other sensors) to monitor physical activity. Development of new technologies, and of more sophisticated methods to analyse the data generated, is progressing rapidly and readers wishing to consider these methodological issues further will find the series of papers 'Objective measurement of physical activity: best practices and future directions' a valuable resource (*Medicine and Science in Sports and Exercise* 2012; 44 (Suppl. 1S): S1–89).

The use of accelerometry in research is increasing exponentially, and over the past decade a number of large-scale population-based studies, such as the US National Health and Nutrition Examination Survey, the Australian AusDiab study and the UK

Biobank, have used accelerometers to objectively measure physical activity and sedentary behaviour.

Doubly labelled water

This non-intrusive method is regarded as the gold standard for measuring total energy expenditure in free-living situations. A brief description of the principle and procedures involved are given in Box 2.4. It provides a more accurate measure of total energy expenditure than either questionnaires or accelerometers, but it is expensive and cannot distinguish different rates of energy expenditure. Doubly labelled water is often used in combination with a measure of resting metabolic rate (either determined from a resting expired air sample via indirect calorimetry, or estimated from a regression equation) to provide an index called the 'physical activity level', which is the ratio of total energy expenditure to resting metabolic rate.

BOX 2.4 MEASUREMENT OF ENERGY EXPENDITURE USING DOUBLY LABELLED WATER.

The principle is as follows:

- Participants drink water containing stable (non-radioactive) isotopes of hydrogen ^{2}H, or deuterium) and oxygen (^{18}O, or oxygen-18).
- The isotopes distribute throughout all body fluids.
- ^{2}H leaves the body as water ($^{2}H_2O$) in urine, sweat, and vapour from breathing.
- ^{18}O leaves the body as both water ($H_2^{18}O$) and carbon dioxide ($C^{18}O_2$).
- The difference between the rates of loss of ^{18}O and ^{2}H enables carbon dioxide production to the estimated.
- Oxygen consumption is calculated from carbon dioxide production.
- Energy expenditure is calculated using stoichiometry.

Measurement of cardiorespiratory fitness

The gold-standard measure of cardiorespiratory fitness is direct measurement of $\dot{V}O_2max$, during an incremental exercise test on a treadmill or cycle ergometer. In the Aerobics Center Longitudinal Study, time to 'volitional fatigue' during an incremental treadmill test has been used as a surrogate measure of $\dot{V}O_2max$ (Blair et al. 1989). The validity of this method derives from the strong, essentially linear, relationship between $\dot{V}O_2max$ and treadmill test performance. Maximal oxygen uptake can also be estimated outside of the laboratory using an incremental shuttle running protocol to volitional fatigue (e.g. bleep test) or from time taken to complete an endurance run (e.g. 1.5-mile-run test). Often, because of practical and ethical constraints fitness is assessed using a submaximal test. Maximal oxygen uptake can be estimated from the heart rate response to submaximal cycling, treadmill or stepping exercise (with or without direct measurement of oxygen uptake). Alternatively, the heart rate at a given work rate may be adopted as a marker. In field settings, maximal oxygen uptake can be estimated using regression equations from time taken to walk a given distance and the heart rate achieved (e.g. the UKK (Urho Kaleka Kekkonen) 2 km walk test or the Rockport walking test). In clinical research, in older or physically impaired individuals, tests such as the shuttle walking test or 6-minute-walk test are commonly used. These can be conducted in a physiotherapy department or even in a hospital corridor and are appropriate and safe for various patient groups. As with measures of physical activity, each approach has its strengths and limitations. Indirect measures are less accurate but can permit larger numbers to be studied. Maximal testing improves accuracy but often has to be restricted to apparently healthy people.

Measurement of strength

Strength has been less commonly measured than cardiorespiratory fitness in epidemiological research, and unlike cardiorespiratory fitness, there is no single gold-standard measure. In laboratory-based studies, measures of maximal voluntary isokinetic (constant speed) or isometric (static) strength of major groups can be assessed using a dynamometer. Alternatively, one-repetition-maximum (1RM), the maximum amount of weight that can be lifted for a single repetition, can be assessed. In large-scale studies outside of the laboratory, grip strength (assessed using a hand-grip dynamometer), which correlates reasonably well with other measures of limb muscle strength (Bohannon et al. 2012), is often used as a measure of muscular strength. Other approaches to assess muscular strength outside of the laboratory include functional measures such as maximal push-up capacity (Yang et al. 2019), or the sit-to-stand test, which assesses time taken to repeatedly stand up and sit down again on a chair for a set number of repetitions (usually five or ten), or number of repetitions completed in a set period of time (usually 30 seconds) (Bohannon et al. 2010).

SUMMARISING THE EVIDENCE BASE: SYSTEMATIC REVIEWS AND META-ANALYSIS

Individual studies are subject to error and can lack generalisability, thus a single study is rarely sufficient to permit firm conclusions to be drawn. Indeed, it is not unusual for different studies on a similar topic to give different, and potentially contradictory, findings. It is therefore important for researchers to review and summarise the totality of evidence before drawing any firm conclusions. Review papers summarise and provide an overview of a research topic and provide very useful background reading, particularly for those who are unfamiliar with the field. However, like individual studies, review papers can be subject to bias, for example if the author does not rigorously search for all of the relevant evidence or even selectively cites studies to support their personal beliefs. Systematic reviews attempt to overcome these shortcomings by addressing a defined research question (for example, 'Is fitness level associated with risk of type 2 diabetes?') using an explicit and comprehensive search strategy to identify relevant literature; using defined inclusion and exclusion criteria for inclusion of studies within the review; evaluating the methodological quality of studies against consistent standards; and drawing clear conclusions based on the evidence. Identifying all of the relevant literature can be difficult and typically requires searching more than one database. For example, searching MEDLINE and PubMed will typically only identify 70–80% of the relevant literature. One of the most comprehensive systematic reviews on physical activity and health outcomes is the systematic review of evidence for Canada's physical activity guidelines for adults, which was published in 2010 (Warburton et al. 2010).

Some systematic reviews include a meta-analysis. This is a statistical approach to combine results from multiple studies to provide a quantitative estimation of the overall magnitude of effect with a measure of the uncertainty around the effect size. The overall magnitude in a meta-analysis is not a simple average of the effect size in each study; larger studies, with more precise effect size estimates, receive greater weighting. Thus, a meta-analysis including studies with sample sizes of 10, 40, 100 and 250 participants, would be equivalent to a single study of 400 participants, but the weighting of the largest study to the overall effect would (assuming similar measurement errors across the studies) have 25 times the weighting of the smallest study in the calculation of the overall effect size. The increased overall sample size in a meta-analysis compared to the individual studies increases the precision of the effect size estimate and increases the power to detect small, but clinically important effects. Results of meta-analyses are typically presented in a forest plot (Box 2.5, Figure 2.14). It is important to recognise that a meta-analysis can only reflect results that have been published, and publication bias (caused by studies showing no effect being less likely to be published) can inflate the estimate of the overall effect size.

BOX 2.5 FOREST PLOTS.

Forest plots provide a graphical representation of the results of a meta-analysis. Figure 2.14 shows a forest plot for a meta-analysis of eight RCTs investigating the effects of pedometer-based interventions for weight loss in overweight and obese adults with type 2 diabetes. Each study is represented by a rectangle (box) indicating the mean difference in weight loss between the intervention and control study arms. Boxes to the left of the solid vertical line indicate greater weight loss with the intervention; boxes to the right of the line indicate greater weight loss in the control group. The horizontal lines, or 'whiskers' going through each box, indicate the 95% confidence interval (95% CI) for each study. If these whiskers cross the solid vertical line indicating no difference, there was no significant effect of the intervention in the study. In this instance, all individual studies, except Andrews et al., showed no significant effect of the intervention on weight loss. The size of the box indicates the weighting of the study to the overall results (the weighting is also shown in the right-hand column). Larger, more powerful studies, with more precise estimates of the effect size have larger weighting. Here, the study by Andrews et al., which had 494 participants, had a much larger weighting in the meta-analysis than any of the other studies, which ranged in size from 39 to 92 participants. The WMD (weighted mean difference) column numerically shows the mean difference and 95% CIs illustrated graphically by the box and whiskers. The overall effect of the intervention across all studies is illustrated by the diamond at the bottom, with the width of the diamond representing 95% CI of the overall estimate. In this case, the overall effect was a modest (0.65 kg), but statistically significant (as the 95% CI does not cross 0), greater weight loss in the intervention groups. Finally, the 'I^2' statistic provides a measure of heterogeneity. When this is low (<50%),

Figure 2.14 Forest plot showing results of a meta-analysis of eight studies investigating the effects of pedometer-based interventions for weight loss in overweight and obese adults with type 2 diabetes.

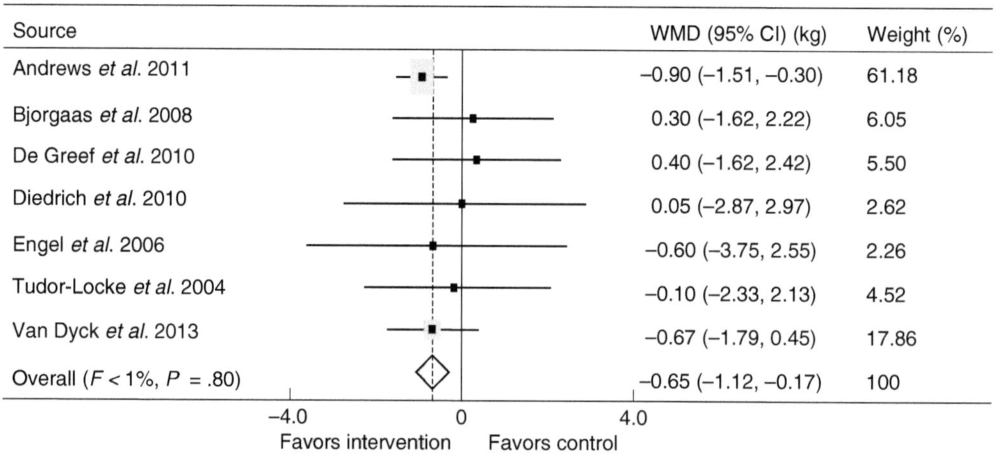

Source: Reprinted from 'Pedometer intervention and weight loss in overweight and obese adults with Type 2 diabetes: a meta-analysis', Cai, X. et al., *Diabetic Medicine* 33: 1035–44: doi 10.1111/dme.13104, with permission from John Wiley and Sons. Copyright © 2016 The Authors.

as it is in this case, it indicates that the results are similar between studies (data are homogeneous) which increases the likelihood that the results are conclusive. A high level of heterogeneity indicates that the effect size differed meaningfully between studies reduces and leads to lower confidence in the overall effect size estimate.

Establishing causality

This is an important issue because the designation of a risk factor as 'causal' is the starting point for initiating disease prevention programmes based on reducing exposure to the risk factor.

Observational epidemiological studies and experimental studies in the form of clinical trials and laboratory studies investigating mechanisms all contribute evidence on physical activity and health. Assessment of the strength of this evidence involves consideration of each type of research. As noted in the previous section, large RCTs of physical activity with disease endpoints are difficult to undertake and studies of this nature have been limited. Epidemiological research in this area is therefore largely observational and, because of bias and confounding, a rather blunt tool. Indeed, these two sources of error have been described as 'a plague upon the house of epidemiology' (Taubes 1995). How, then, does the research community assess whether physical inactivity (or low fitness or high levels of sedentary behaviour) is a causal factor for a particular health outcome? (In considering the diseases which are big public health problems in the twenty-first century, for example heart disease, diabetes and osteoporosis, it is appropriate to talk about 'causal factors', rather than a single cause.)

Several criteria for causal significance in epidemiological studies have been proposed, and these are summarised in Box 2.6. One of the most important criteria is the strength of the association between the causal factor and the outcome. Some authorities take the view that no single epidemiological study is persuasive by itself unless the relative risk of exposure is three or more. If this were the only criterion, very few studies would indicate that physical inactivity and low fitness are causal factors for important health-related outcomes.

BOX 2.6 CRITERIA USED TO ASSESS WHETHER EPIDEMIOLOGICAL EVIDENCE IS SUFFICIENT TO CONCLUDE THAT A RISK FACTOR IS CAUSAL.

- Appropriately sequenced – does the measure of level of physical activity (or fitness) precede the onset of disease?
- Plausibility – is the association consistent with other knowledge (mechanisms of action; animal studies)?
- Consistency – are the findings consistent in different populations?
- Strength – what is the strength of the association between physical activity/fitness and the effect, i.e. what is the relative risk?
- Dose–response – are increasing levels of physical activity or fitness associated with greater effect?
- Reversibility – is becoming less active or fit associated with a loss of benefit?
- Strong study design – are findings based on strong study designs? (The randomised controlled trial is the 'gold standard'.)

Source: Adapted from Hill (1965).

However, judgements on causality need also to take other aspects of the evidence into account. Two requirements must be satisfied before a causal claim is accepted: empirical demonstration of an association and a proposed underlying explanatory mechanism. Thus, associations reported in epidemiological studies must be shown to be concordant with biologically plausible mechanisms. In this way, evidence from experimental laboratory-based studies complements and extends that from epidemiology. The former demonstrate mechanisms but cannot show links with disease endpoints: the latter can establish links with morbidity and mortality but cannot by themselves establish causality. Reaching a conclusion on whether or not physical inactivity and/or low fitness may be causal factors in specific health outcomes therefore involves making judgements based on multiple lines of evidence.

Frameworks for grading the strength of research evidence are now widely used, particularly among medical researchers. A number of different approaches to describe 'levels of evidence' have been described and, while these differ in detail, they generally rank RCTs above observational studies, with 'expert opinion' and anecdotal experience being ranked at the bottom. Systematic reviews and meta-analyses of RCTs are often placed at the top of the evidence hierarchy. In physical activity research, where the evidence base comprises substantial observational data and a more limited body of data from RCTs, this can present challenges for interpreting the strength of the evidence base. While RCTs minimise selection bias, observational studies can facilitate larger samples in diverse populations and settings, longer follow-up periods and assessment of 'hard' health outcomes (such as incidence of CVD or mortality). Thus, RCT and observational data are often complementary and when findings are consistent across study types, the strength of the evidence is enhanced. Box 2.7 shows two slightly different approaches to grade strength of evidence which were used for the American College of Sports Medicine Position Stand on Exercise and Physical Activity for Older Adults (Chodzko-Zajko et al. 2009), and for the systematic review of evidence for Canada's Physical Activity Guidelines for Adults (Warburton et al. 2010).

BOX 2.7 EXAMPLES OF APPROACHES USED TO EVALUATE STRENGTH OF RESEARCH EVIDENCE IN PHYSICAL ACTIVITY AND HEALTH.

Criteria used to evaluate strength of evidence in the American College of Sports Medicine Position Stand on Exercise and Physical Activity for Older Adults.

EVIDENCE LEVEL	EVIDENCE LEVEL DESCRIPTION
Evidence Level A	Overwhelming evidence from randomised controlled trials and/or observational studies, which provides a consistent pattern of findings on the basis of substantial data.
Evidence Level B	Strong evidence from a combination of randomised controlled trials and/or observational studies but with some studies showing results that are inconsistent with the overall conclusion.
Evidence Level C	Generally positive or suggestive evidence from a smaller number of observational studies and/or uncontrolled or non-randomised trials.
Evidence Level D	Panel consensus judgement that the strength of the evidence is insufficient to place it in categories A through C.

Source: Reprinted with permission from Wolters Kluwer Health, Inc.: Chodzko-Zajko, W.J. et al. (2009) 'American College of Sports Medicine position stand: exercise and physical activity for older adults', *Medicine and Science in Sports and Exercise*, 41: 1510–30. Available at: https://doi.org/10.1249/MSS.0b013e3181a0c95c.

Levels and grades of evidence used in the systematic review of evidence for Canada's Physical Activity Guidelines for Adults.

LEVEL OF EVIDENCE	CRITERIA
Level 1	Randomised controlled trials without important limitations
Level 2	• Randomised controlled trials with important limitations • Observational studies (non-randomised clinical trials or cohort studies) with overwhelming evidence
Level 3	Other observational studies (prospective cohort studies, case-control studies, case series)
Level 4	Inadequate or no data in population of interest Anecdotal evidence or clinical experience

GRADE OF EVIDENCE	CRITERIA
Grade A	Strong recommendation (action can apply to most individuals in most circumstances • Benefits clearly outweigh risks (or vice versa) • Evidence is at Levels 1, 2 or 3
Grade B	Weak recommendation (action may differ depending on individual's characteristics of other circumstances) • Unclear if benefits outweigh risks • Evidence is at Levels 1, 2 or 3
Grade C	Consensus recommendation (alternative actions may be equally reasonable) • Unclear if benefits outweigh risks • Evidence is at Levels 3 or 4

Source: Reprinted with no modifications from 'A systematic review of the evidence for Canada's Physical Activity Guidelines for Adults', Warburton, D.E. et al., *International Journal of Behavioral Nutrition and Physical Activity*, 2010, 7: 39. Article distributed under the terms of the Creative Commons Attribution 2.0 (CC BY) Licence (https://creativecommons.org/licenses/by/2.0/).

SUMMARY

- Epidemiology is the study of the distribution and determinants of health-related states or events in specified populations and the application of this study to control of health problems. It can identify risk factors but not, in itself, causality.
- Outcome measures include mortality and morbidity, but also indices of quality of life. An important measure of disease frequency is the person–time incidence rate. For example, heart attacks per 1,000 person-years. These are compared between groups, yielding a relative risk that estimates the strength of an association with the risk factor under study.
- Associations may reflect the true effect on an exposure, but may have an alternative explanation, i.e. chance, bias or confounding.
- While most epidemiological research on physical activity and health has focused on moderate-to-vigorous physical activity, physical activity behaviours exist across a continuum encompassing sedentary, light, moderate, vigorous activities as well as resistance exercise. Cardiorespiratory fitness and muscular strength are physiological characteristics which are related to the level and types of physical activity undertaken. However, both these traits also have a large genetic component.
- In epidemiological studies, physical activity levels have most often been measured by self-report questionnaire. This can lead to inaccuracies which decrease the strength of the observed associations with health outcomes, thus relationships between questionnaire-assessed physical activity and health outcomes are likely to be underestimates of the true relationship. Other, more objective (but more expensive) measures involve use of wearable motion sensors (pedometers and accelerometers) and the doubly labelled water technique.
- Experimental, or intervention, studies reduce the risk of bias and confounding present in observational studies. The gold-standard study design for establishing a

causal relationship is the randomised controlled trial (RCT). However, there are relatively few RCTs evaluating the effects of physical activity on disease outcomes. Laboratory-based studies can achieve excellent control and precision and indicate potential mechanisms. However, their outcome measures are removed from the clinical endpoints of morbidity and mortality.

- Individual studies are subject to error and different studies on a similar topic can provide different findings. It is therefore important to review all relevant studies before drawing firm conclusions. Here, systematic reviews and meta-analyses, which synthesise the available evidence and draw clear evidence-based conclusions to defined research questions, can be valuable tools.
- Establishing causality requires evidence from epidemiology for strong and consistent associations, as well as evidence for plausible mechanisms from laboratory-based studies. These types of evidence are complementary, and neither is sufficient alone. The totality of the evidence determines decisions as to causality.

STUDY TASKS

1 In epidemiology, what is considered the strongest study design and why? Discuss the reasons why this design would be extremely difficult to implement in the study of physical activity and risk of mortality amongst the general population.

2 What is confounding, and what is reverse causality? Explain steps that can be taken to minimise these in a cohort study investigating the association between cardiorespiratory fitness and risk of cardiovascular disease.

3 Discuss the strengths and limitations of using self-report questionnaires, accelerometers and doubly labelled water to measure physical activity in epidemiological research.

4 A study is aiming to investigate the acute effects of a single exercise session on mechanisms controlling blood pressure. What study design would you use and why? Would you use the same study design to investigate the effects of a 12-month exercise programme on blood pressure?

5 In the UK in 2017, the relative risk for mortality in HIV patients was 5.7 compared with the general population, and approximately 0.15% of the population was infected. Comment on the population-attributable risk for mortality from HIV versus physical inactivity in the UK, and the implications of these findings for (a) the individual; and (b) public health policy.

FURTHER READING

Bhopal, R. (2008) Concepts of epidemiology: integrating the ideas, theories, principles and methods of epidemiology. 2nd edn, Oxford: Oxford University Press.

Impellizzeri, F.M. and Bizzini M. (2012) Systematic review and meta-analysis: a primer. *International Journal of Sports Physical Therapy* 7: 493–503.

Lee, I.-M (ed) (2008) *Epidemiologic methods in physical activity studies*. New York: Oxford University Press.

Objective measurement of physical activity: best practices and future directions. (2012) *Medicine and Science in Sports and Exercise* 44(Suppl. 1S): S1–89.

Thomas, J.R., Nelson J.K. and Silverman, S.J. (2015) *Research methods in physical activity*. 7th edn, Champaign, IL: Human Kinetics.

REFERENCES

Beaglehole, R., Bonita, R. and Kjellström, T. (1993) *Basic epidemiology*. Geneva: World Health Organization.

Blair, S.N., Kohl, H.W., Paffenbarger, R.S., Clark, D.G., Cooper, K.H. and Gibbons, L.W. (1989) Physical fitness and all-cause mortality: a prospective study of healthy men and women. *Journal of the American Medical Association* 262: 2395–401.

Bohannon, R.W., Bubela, D.J., Magasi, S.R., Wang, Y.C. and Gershon, R.C. (2010) Sit-to-stand test: performance and determinants across the age-span. *Isokinetics and Exercise Science* 18: 235–40.

Bohannon, R.W., Magasi, S.R., Bubela, D.J., Wang, Y.C. and Gershon, R.C. (2012) Grip and knee extension muscle strength reflect a common construct among adults. *Muscle and Nerve* 46: 555–8.

Bouchard, C. (2012) Genomic predictors of trainability. *Experimental Physiology* 97: 347–52.

Bouchard, C., Daw, E.W., Rice, T., Perusse, L., Gagnon, J., Province, M.A. et al. (1998) Familial resemblance for VO_2max in the sedentary state: the HERITAGE family study. *Medicine and Science in Sports and Exercise* 30: 252–8.

Cai, X., Qiu, S.H., Yin, H., Sun, Z.L., Ju, C.P., Zügel, M. et al. (2016) Pedometer intervention and weight loss in overweight and obese adults with Type 2 diabetes: a meta-analysis. *Diabetic Medicine* 33: 1035–44.

Celis-Morales, C.A., Lyall, D.M., Welsh, P., Anderson, J., Steell, L., Guo, Y. et al. (2017) Association between active commuting and incident cardiovascular disease, cancer, and mortality: prospective cohort study. *British Medical Journal* 357: j1456. doi: 10.1136/bmj.j1456.

Celis-Morales, C.A., Perez-Bravo, F., Ibañez, L., Salas, C., Bailey, M.E. and Gill, J.M. (2012) Objective vs. self-reported physical activity and sedentary time: effects of measurement method on relationships with risk biomarkers. *PLoS One* 7: e36345. doi: 10.1371/journal.pone.0036345.

Chodzko-Zajko, W.J., Proctor, D.N., Fiatarone Singh, M.A., Minson, C.T., Nigg, C.R., Salem, G.J. and Skinner, J.S. (2009) American College of Sports Medicine position stand: exercise and physical activity for older adults. *Medicine and Science in Sports and Exercise* 41: 1510–30.

Church, T.S., Thomas, D.M., Tudor-Locke, C., Katzmarzyk, P.T., Earnest, C.P., Rodarte, R.Q. et al. (2011) Trends over 5 decades in U.S. occupation-related physical activity and their associations with obesity. *PLoS One* 6: e19657. doi: 10.1371/journal.pone.0019657.

Craig, C.L., Marshall, A.L., Sjöström, M., Bauman, A.E., Booth, M.L., Ainsworth, B.E. et al. (2003) International physical activity questionnaire: 12-country reliability and validity. *Medicine and Science in Sports and Exercise* 35: 1381–95.

Currens, J.H. and White, P.D. (1961) Half a century of running: clinical, physiologic and autopsy findings in the case of Clarence DeMar ("Mr. Marathon"). *New England Journal of Medicine* 265: 988–93.

Fang, J., Wylie-Rosett, J., Cohen, H.W., Kaplan, R.C. and Alderman, M.H. (2003) Exercise, body mass index, caloric intake, and cardiovascular mortality. *American Journal of Preventive Medicine* 25: 283–9.

Hamilton, M.T., Hamilton, D.G. and Zderic, T.W. (2007) Role of low energy expenditure and sitting in obesity, metabolic syndrome, type 2 diabetes, and cardiovascular disease. *Diabetes* 56: 2655–67.

Hennekens, C.H. and Buring, J.E. (1987) *Epidemiology in medicine.* Philadelphia: Lippincott, Williams and Wilkins.

Hill, A.B. (1965) The environment and disease: association or causation? *Proceedings of the Royal Society of Medicine* 58: 295–300.

Keys, A. (1980) *Seven countries: a multivariate analysis of death and coronary heart disease.* Cambridge, MA: Harvard University Press.

Koch, L.G., Britton, S.L. and Wisløff, U. (2012) A rat model system to study complex disease risks, fitness, aging, and longevity. *Trends in Cardiovascular Medicine* 22: 29–34.

Morris, J.N., Clayton, D.G., Everitt, M.G., Semmence, A.M. and Burgess, E.H. (1990) Exercise in leisure time: coronary attack and death rates. *British Heart Journal* 63: 325–34.

Morris, J.N., Heady, J.A., Raffle, P.A.B., Roberts, C.G. and Parks, J.W. (1953) Coronary-heart disease and physical activity of work. *The Lancet* 262: 1053–7, 1111–20.

Paffenbarger, R.S. and Hale, W.E. (1975) Work activity and coronary heart mortality. *The New England Journal of Medicine* 292: 545–50.

Porta, M. (2008) *Dictionary of Epidemiology.* 5th edn, Oxford: Oxford University Press for the International Epidemiological Association.

Qi, Q., Li, Y., Chomistek, A.K., Kang, J.H., Curhan, G.C., Pasquale, L.R. et al. (2012) Television watching, leisure time physical activity, and the genetic predisposition in relation to body mass index in women and men. *Circulation* 126: 1821–7.

Silventoinen, K., Magnusson, P.K., Tynelius, P., Kaprio, J. and Rasmussen, F. (2008) Heritability of body size and muscle strength in young adulthood: a study of one million Swedish men. *Genetic Epidemiology* 32: 341–9.

Taubes, G. (1995). Epidemiology faces its limits. *Science* 269: 164–9.

Tremblay, M.S., Aubert, S., Barnes, J.D., Saunders, T.J., Carson, V., Latimer-Cheung, A.E. et al. (2017) Sedentary Behavior Research Network (SBRN) – Terminology Consensus Project process and outcome. *International Journal of Behavioral Nutrition and Physical Activity* 14: 75. doi: 10.1186/s12966-017-0525-8.

Tuomilehto, J., Lindström, J., Eriksson, J.G., Valle, T.T., Hämäläinen, H., Ilanne-Parikka, P. et al. (2001) Prevention of type 2 diabetes mellitus by changes in lifestyle among subjects with impaired glucose tolerance. *New England Journal of Medicine* 344: 1343–50.

Warburton, D.E., Charlesworth, S., Ivey, A., Nettlefold, L. and Bredin, S.S. (2010) A systematic review of the evidence for Canada's physical activity guidelines for adults. *International Journal of Behavioral Nutrition and Physical Activity* 7: 39. doi: 10.1186/1479-5868-7-39.

Wei, M., Gibbons, L.W., Kampert, J.B., Nichaman, M.Z. and Blair, S.N. (2000) Low cardiorespiratory fitness and physical inactivity as predictors of mortality in men with type 2 diabetes. *Annals of Internal Medicine* 132: 605–11.

Wen, C.P. and Wu, X. (2012). Stressing harms of physical inactivity to promote exercise. *The Lancet* 380: 192–3.

Yang, J., Christophi, C.A., Farioli, A., Baur, D.M., Moffatt, S., Zollinger, T.W. and Kales, S.N. (2019) Association between push-up exercise capacity and future cardiovascular events among active adult men. *Journal of the American Medical Association Network Open* 2: e188341. doi: 10.1001/jamanetworkopen.2018.8341.

3 Physical activity and mortality

Jason M.R. Gill

INTRODUCTION

In this chapter, we will examine the evidence that high levels of physical activity, cardiorespiratory fitness and strength, and low levels of sedentary behaviour, reduce the risk of dying prematurely. The studies included in this chapter are those that have addressed all-cause mortality; that is, death from any cause. Studies that have examined the link between activity/fitness and specific causes of death such as cardiovascular disease (CVD) and cancer are covered elsewhere in the book (Chapters 4 and 8, respectively, for CVD and cancer). Moreover, the studies discussed in this chapter are predominantly epidemiological cohort studies which, on their own, cannot provide proof of cause and effect for reasons outlined in the previous chapter. Furthermore, these studies do not begin to answer the question, 'Why do active/fit people live longer than inactive/unfit people?' Answers to this question are provided in later chapters.

PHYSICAL ACTIVITY AND MORTALITY

Although there was some limited information linking physically active occupations to longevity in the eighteenth and nineteenth centuries, systematic study of the relationship between physical activity and longevity only began in the twentieth century. Initially, research focused on occupational activity and longevity. One such study was of US railroad industry employees. This study examined mortality rates over a two-year period (1955–6) and found lower rates among section men (classified as the most active group) compared with clerks (classified as the least active group) and switchmen (Taylor et al. 1962). However, there were limitations to these early studies. It was possible, for example, that the relationship between occupation and mortality risk was simply due to self-selection; that is, men who were in the process of developing chronic diseases (and therefore likely to die prematurely) might have chosen physically less demanding jobs. Also, other characteristics predictive of mortality, such as smoking, obesity and diet, were not accounted for. Moreover, leisure-time physical activity was not measured and thus there was no clear assessment of total physical activity. Nevertheless, such studies were the catalyst for future investigations with improved study designs.

In the latter half of the twentieth century, attention switched to leisure-time physical activity and the findings of several cohort studies were published from the 1980s onwards. The Harvard Alumni Health Study – a cohort study of men enrolled in Harvard College between 1916 and 1950 – was an early seminal investigation in this field. One publication from this study concerned the relationship between physical activity and all-cause mortality in 16,936 men aged 35–74 years at baseline (Paffenbarger et al. 1986). Baseline data, in which questionnaires were used to estimate the amount of energy expended in walking, stair climbing, sports and recreational activities, were collected either in 1962 or 1966. Follow-up was conducted 12–16 years later in 1978, by which time 1,413 alumni had died. The findings revealed an inverse dose–response relationship between physical activity and the risk of all-cause mortality. Death rates were 25–33% lower among alumni who reported expending 2,000 kcal per week (8,400 kJ per week) or more in weekly physical activity compared with those who reported expending less than this amount. These findings remained significant following control for smoking, hypertension, extremes or gains in body mass and early parental death. Moreover, the inverse association between activity and mortality risk held when findings were examined within different age bands (35–49, 50–59, 60–69 and 70–84 years).

The findings from the Harvard Alumni Health study were typical of those observed in other prospective cohort studies of physical activity and mortality. These findings are summarised in a meta-analysis of 80 studies involving a total of 1,338,143 participants (118,121 deaths) investigating the relationship between physical activity (assessed by self-reported questionnaire) and all-cause mortality (Samitz et al. 2011). In analyses adjusted for a range of confounding variables (including age, sex, cardiovascular risk factors, behavioural factors (such as smoking) and socio-economic variables), those reporting the highest amounts of total physical activity had a relative risk of all-cause mortality of 0.65 (95% confidence interval 0.60–0.71) compared with those reporting the lowest levels of total physical activity. In other words, the most physically active had a 35% reduction in mortality risk. Similar relationships were observed when context-specific physical activity levels (e.g. occupational, transport, leisure time) were assessed (Figure 3.1).

A dose–response relationship between amount of physical activity and mortality risk was observed, such that increasing amounts of reported physical activity were associated with increasing reductions in mortality risk. Both vigorous and moderate intensity

Figure 3.1 Relative risk of all-cause mortality associated with the highest compared with lowest levels of physical activity across different domains from a meta-analysis of 80 studies with over 1.3 million participants.

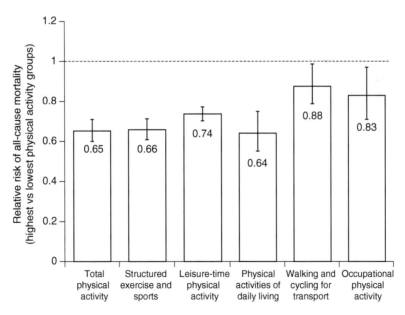

Source: Samitz et al. (2011).
Notes: Error bars represent 95% confidence intervals. Relative risks are from maximally adjusted statistical models (adjustments included age, sex, cardiovascular risk factors, behavioural and socio-economic variables).

Figure 3.2 Relative risk for all-cause mortality associated with undertaking 60, 150 and 300 minutes/week of physical activity of different intensities, compared with lowest levels of activity, in a meta-analysis from Samitz and colleagues.

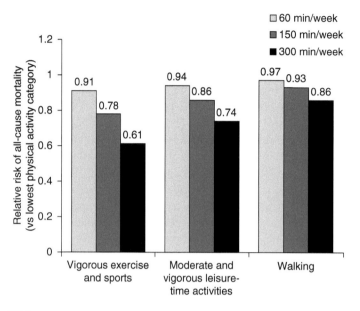

Source: Samitz et al. (2011).
Notes: Relative risks are from maximally adjusted statistical models (adjustments included age, sex, cardiovascular risk factors, behavioural and socio-economic variables).

physical activity were associated with lower mortality risk, but, minute-for-minute, engaging in vigorous exercise and sports was associated with greater reductions in all-cause mortality risk than engaging in walking or moderate intensity activity (Figure 3.2).

The studies included in the meta-analysis by Samitz and colleagues all used self-report questionnaires to assess physical activity and are therefore liable to error due to inadequate or inaccurate recall. As discussed in Chapter 2, this error would act to attenuate the apparent relationship between physical activity and mortality. Thus, the protective effect of physical activity on mortality risk observed in these studies is potentially greater than these observations suggest. In recent years, a growing body of studies have attempted to address this limitation by using more objective measurements of physical activity. The Health, Ageing and Body Composition (Health ABC) Study (Manini et al. 2006) used doubly labelled water (the gold-standard method) to assess energy expenditure over a two-week period in 302 'high-functioning' community-dwelling older adults aged 70–82 years. (Box 2.4 provides a brief description of the doubly labelled water method.) Participants (men and women) were divided into tertiles according to their free-living activity energy expenditure as follows: low, <521 kcal day^{-1} (2,188 kJ day^{-1}); middle, 521–770 kcal day^{-1} (2,188–3,234 kJ day^{-1}); high, >770 kcal day^{-1} (3,234 kJ day^{-1}). During an average 6.15 years of follow-up, 55 participants died, and a significant association was found between objectively measured

Figure 3.3 Association between free-living activity energy expenditure and all-cause mortality in the Health, Ageing and Body Composition (Health ABC) Study.

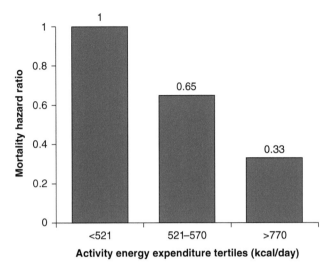

Source: Manini et al. (2006).
Notes: Free-living activity energy expenditure was assessed using doubly labelled water. The findings were adjusted for age, sex, race, study site, weight, height, percentage body mass, sleep duration, self-rated health, education, smoking status and history, CVD, lung disease, diabetes, hip or knee osteoarthritis, cancer and depression.

physical activity and risk of death. Death rates were two-thirds lower in the high physical activity group compared with the low physical activity group (Figure 3.3). This is a substantially larger mortality risk reduction than has been observed in studies that have assessed physical activity by self-report, which is consistent with the suggestion that questionnaire-based physical activity measurement leads to underestimation of potential benefit. Thus, the objective measurement of activity energy expenditure in the Health ABC study provides a novel and important contribution to this research field. One limitation of the doubly labelled water method is that it does not provide any information on intensity of physical activity, and thus the findings cannot be used to provide information about intensity of physical activity and mortality risk. In addition, the cost of the technique makes it unsuitable for use in very large studies.

The increasing use of accelerometry to objectively assess physical activity in large-scale population-based studies means that more robust estimates of the magnitude of the effect of physical activity on mortality risk are becoming increasingly available. In 2019, Ekelund and colleagues published a meta-analysis of prospective cohort studies that measured physical activity using accelerometry and assessed risk of all-cause mortality (Ekelund et al. 2019). Eight studies, including 36,383 participants (mean age 62.6 years), were included. Median follow-up was 5.8 years (range 3.0–14.5 years) and 2,149 deaths occurred over this period. The findings of this meta-analysis are shown in Figure 3.4. There are a number of important observations from this analysis. First, the study demonstrated that any physical activity, regardless of intensity, was associated with lower risk of mortality. Compared with individuals in the lowest quartile for

Figure 3.4 Association between accelerometer-measured total physical activity (left panel), moderate-to-vigorous physical activity (MVPA) (middle panel), light physical activity (right panel) and all-cause mortality in a meta-analysis from Ekelund and colleagues.

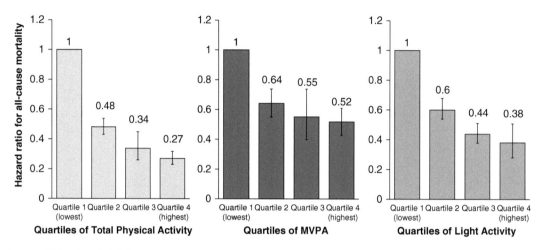

Source: Ekelund et al. (2019).
Notes: Error bars represent 95% confidence intervals. Hazard ratios were adjusted for age, sex, body mass index, socioeconomic position and accelerometer wear time. Analysis of MVPA also adjusted for sedentary time.

overall physical activity, those in the second, third and fourth quartiles, had 52%, 66% and 72% lower risks of mortality, respectively. This is a substantially larger magnitude of risk reduction with increasing levels of physical activity than observed in studies which assessed physical activity by self-report. Second, the relationship was not linear, with the largest benefits seen in moving from the first to second activity quartiles. Third, increasing levels of both MVPA and light physical activity were associated with lower mortality risk. The association between light physical activity and mortality risk had previously been poorly understood as this aspect of activity is difficult to measure using self-report questionnaires. Finally, the amounts of physical activity required to lower mortality risk appear to be substantially lower for accelerometer measured compared with self-reported physical activity. For example, in this meta-analysis, undertaking just ~5–6 minutes per day of MVPA was associated with a ~30% reduction in mortality risk, whereas ~20–40 minutes per day of self-reported physical activity is needed for a similar mortality risk reduction (Moore et al. 2012). In addition, maximal risk reduction occurred with ~20 minutes per day of accelerometer-measured MVPA, in comparison to the >60 minutes of self-reported MVPA required to observe maximal reductions in mortality risk (Moore et al. 2012). A recent analysis of 96,476 participants in UK Biobank, who had physical activity measured by accelerometer, similarly found the increasing levels of both MVPA and light activity were associated with lower risk of mortality over 3.1 years of follow-up, with a substantially steeper dose–response relationship for reduced risk with increasing activity than observed when physical activity is assessed by self-report (Strain et al. 2020). These new findings from studies where physical activity has been objectively measured by accelerometer has led to the observation by the author that, 'The benefits of physical activity may be greater, and the levels of physical activity at which they occur may be lower, than previously considered' (Gill 2020). However, it should be noted that the follow-up period in the studies that have measured physical activity by accelerometer are, to date, relatively short, which increases the potential contribution of reverse causality to the findings (i.e. presence of chronic disease at baseline leading to lower physical activity levels; see Chapter 2 for explanation). Longer-term follow-up over time in these and other studies using accelerometer-based physical activity measurement will help determine the extent to which this is likely to have influenced the magnitude of the mortality risk estimates, and enable more robust quantification of the strength of association between physical activity and mortality risk than has been possible to date.

The studies described above considered the association between aerobic physical activities (or physical activity energy expenditure) and risk of mortality. Fewer studies have investigated the association between muscle strengthening resistance exercise and mortality risk. One such report comes from the Women's Health Study in which 28,879 women (average age at baseline 62.2 years), who were free from CVD, cancer or diabetes at baseline, completed a physical activity questionnaire including questions on walking pace, flights of stairs climbed and time spent engaged in various leisure time activities including 'weight lifting/strength training' (Kamada et al. 2017). They were followed up for an average of 12.0 years (346,843 person-years of observation), during which 3055 participants died. In analyses adjusted for a range of confounding variables, including aerobic physical activity, there was a non-linear J-shaped relationship between weekly time spent in strength training and risk of mortality. Compared with women undertaking no strength training, those undertaking between 1–19, 20–59 and 60–149 minutes per week of strength training had between 19% and 29% lower risks of mortality, with hazard ratios of 0.73 (95% confidence interval 0.65–0.82), 0.71 (0.62–0.82) and 0.81 (0.67–0.97), respectively. However, women undertaking the highest amounts of strength training ($\geq$150 minutes/week) did not have a lower mortality risk (hazard ratio 1.10 (0.77–1.56)), although the confidence interval here was wide. Benefits of engaging in MVPA and strength training appeared to be additive. Compared with women undertaking no strength training and <150 minutes per week of MVPA; women undertaking $\geq$150 minutes per week of MVPA and no strength training had a hazard ratio for mortality of 0.71 (0.64–0.79); women undertaking any strength training and <150 minutes per week of MVPA had a hazard ratio of 0.74 (0.65–0.85); and women undertaking any strength training and $\geq$150 minutes per week of MVPA has a hazard ratio of 0.54 (0.57–0.61). The authors also conducted a landmark analysis excluding all deaths occurring within the first two years of follow-up, which did not materially alter the results, indicating that the findings are unlikely to have been substantially influenced by reverse causality. A further report based on data from the Health Survey for England and the Scottish Health Survey in 80,306 adults aged $\geq$30 years (mean follow-up 6.2 years, 736,463 person-years of observation, 5763 deaths), similarly reported lower risk of mortality amongst individuals undertaking strength-promoting exercise (Stamatakis et al. 2018). After exclusion of deaths occurring in the first two years of follow-up, participation in any strength exercise was associated with a hazard ratio for all-cause mortality of 0.77 (95% confidence interval 0.69–0.87), compared with no strength exercise participation, in analyses adjusted for a range of confounders including other forms of physical activity. Reports from other cohorts, including, for example, the US National Health and Nutritional Examination Survey (n = 8872, 6.7 years follow-up) (Dankel et al. 2016) and older adults participating in the US National Health Interview Survey (n = 30,162, 15 years follow-up) (Kraschnewski et al. 2016), have similarly reported lower mortality risk amongst those reporting participation in strength training. Thus, although the evidence base is less established than that for aerobic physical activity, there is an accumulating body of evidence that regular participation in muscle strengthening exercise is associated with lower mortality risk.

POPULATION-ATTRIBUTABLE RISK FOR MORTALITY ASSOCIATED WITH PHYSICAL INACTIVITY

In public health terms, it is important to quantity the population-attributable risk (see Chapter 2) for mortality associated with physical inactivity. A report in *The Lancet*, based on self-reported measures of physical activity, estimated the population-attributable risk-fraction mortality associated with physical inactivity, and the gains in population life-expectancy if physical inactivity was eliminated throughout the world (Lee et al. 2012). Data for selected countries are shown in Table 3.1. Worldwide, it was estimated that 9.4% of all deaths could be attributed to physical inactivity, and if everyone who was inactive, became active, it was estimated that worldwide life expectancy would increase by 0.68 years. (Of course, this estimate for change in life expectancy is at the population level and averages the effect on individual life expectancy in those who move from inactive to active across the whole population. The estimated difference in life expectancy between an active individual compared with an inactive individual is substantially greater than this, at approximately 1.5 to 4 years (Paffenbarger et al. 1986; Wen et al. 2011).) However, these population-level estimates are subject to substantial error as they depend on accurate data for the prevalence of physical inactivity, which were difficult to obtain outside of Europe and North America, and can vary depending on which instrument was used to measure physical activity (for example whether the questionnaire used only assessed leisure time physical activity, or also included occupational, transport and home-based activities). In addition, the relative risk for mortality associated with physical inactivity used in these estimates was based on questionnaire-based assessments of physical activity, which may underestimate the true mortality risk, as discussed in paragraphs above.

SEDENTARY BEHAVIOUR AND MORTALITY

Over the past decade there have been an increasing number of reports from prospective cohort studies investigating the relationship between sedentary behaviour and mortality. In these studies sedentary behaviour has been typically quantified by self-report of either total time spent sitting daily, or by self-report of time spent engaged in specific sedentary behaviours, such as television watching or driving, although, as with studies of physical activity and mortality, there is an emerging body of evidence which is using accelerometers to quantify sedentary behaviour more objectively.

Table 3.1 Estimated population attributable risk fraction associated with physical inactivity and estimated gains in life expectancy if physical inactivity was eliminated in selected countries.

COUNTRY	POPULATION ATTRIBUTABLE RISK FRACTION	GAINS IN POPULATION LIFE EXPECTANCY IF PHYSICAL INACTIVITY WAS ELIMINATED (YEARS)
Argentina	18.2%	1.39
Australia	10.1%	0.56
Bangladesh	1.3%	0.10
Brazil	13.2%	1.08
China	8.3%	0.61
France	8.7%	0.55
India	4.2%	0.34
Ireland	14.2%	0.87
Jamaica	12.8%	1.01
Japan	16.1%	0.91
Kenya	4.4%	0.37
Kuwait	17.2%	1.12
Malawi	2.7%	0.21
Netherlands	4.9%	0.29
South Africa	14.0%	1.26
Thailand	5.1%	0.41
Turkey	15.0%	1.06
United Kingdom	16.9%	1.07
USA	10.8%	0.78
Median Worldwide	**9.4%**	**0.68**

Source: Adapted from Lee et al. (2012).

Much of this work has been summarised in a recent meta-analysis, including 34 studies and over 1.3 million participants, which investigated the dose–response relationship between total sedentary behaviour and television viewing on a range of adverse health outcomes, including all-cause mortality (Patterson et al. 2018). In analyses adjusted for a range of confounders, including physical activity, each additional hour of total sedentary behaviour below a threshold of 8 hours per day was associated with a 1% increase in mortality risk, whereas every hour above 8 hours per day was associated with a 4% risk increase. Similarly, every hour of television viewing below 3.5 hours per day was associated with 3% increase in risk of mortality, whereas every additional hour beyond this was associated with a 6% increase in mortality risk. This is illustrated in Figure 3.5. There are two important observations here. First, the association between sedentary behaviour and mortality risk is not linear, with risk only increasing steeply for individuals who report sitting for more than about a third of the day (about half of all waking hours), or watch more than three to four hours of television per day. Second, the association between television viewing and risk of mortality is substantially stronger than the risk associated with overall sitting. This may reflect the clustering of other risk factors for mortality – including unhealthy dietary behaviours, lower socio-economic status, and poorer mental health – with high levels of television viewing and demonstrates that television viewing and sitting should not be considered synonymous when considering

Figure 3.5 Associations between total sedentary behaviour (top panel) and television viewing (bottom panel) and all-cause mortality in a meta-analysis from Patterson and colleagues.

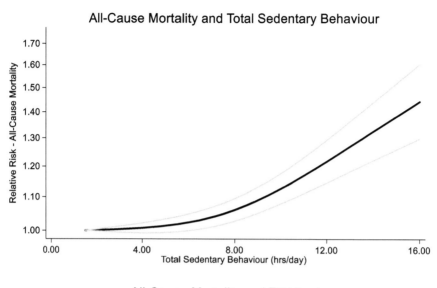

All-Cause Mortality and Total Sedentary Behaviour

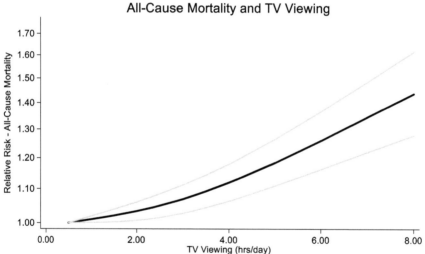

All-Cause Mortality and TV Viewing

Source: Reprinted with no modifications from 'Sedentary behaviour and risk of all-cause, cardiovascular and cancer mortality, and incident type 2 diabetes: a systematic review and dose response meta-analysis', Patterson, R. et al., *European Journal of Epidemiology*, 2018, 33: 811–29. Article distributed under the terms of the Creative Commons Attribution 4.0 International (CC BY) Licence (http://creativecommons.org/licenses/by/4.0/).
Notes: Grey lines represent 95% confidence intervals. Relative risks from models adjusted for all available confounders, including physical activity.

the relationship between sedentary behaviour and risk of adverse health outcomes (Stamatakis et al. 2019).

Recently, there has been increasing interest in whether the adverse association between high levels of sedentary behaviour and mortality risk could be offset by engaging in a sufficiently large amount of physical activity. Ekelund and colleagues undertook a meta-analysis including 13 studies and over a million participants investigating the association between reported daily sitting time and risk of mortality across quartiles of self-reported physical activity (Ekelund et al. 2016). This found that whilst sitting for more than 8 hours per day, compared with sitting less than 4 hours per day, was associated with a 27% higher risk of mortality (hazard ratio 1.27, 95% confidence interval 1.22–1.32) amongst those in the lowest quartile of physical activity (corresponding to ~5 minutes per day of moderate intensity physical activity), this association was substantially attenuated as levels of physical activity increased, such that for those in the highest quartile of physical activity (corresponding to at least 60–75 minutes per day of moderate intensity activity), there was no difference in the mortality risk between those sitting less than 4 hours and more than 8 hours per day (hazard ratio 1.04, 95% confidence interval 0.98–1.10). This is shown in Figure 3.6. Thus, it appears that risk of mortality associated with high levels of sitting can be mitigated by being sufficiently active, and that someone who is both highly sedentary and physically inactive could reduce the excess mortality risk associated with their high level of sitting by either sitting less, and/or by increasing their level of physical activity so that the mortality risk associated with their sitting is minimised.

Figure 3.6 Association between sitting time and all-cause mortality according to level of physical activity in a meta-analysis from Ekelund and colleagues.

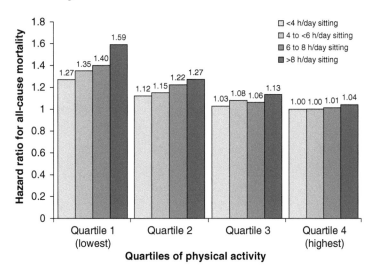

Source: Ekelund et al. (2016).
Notes: Reference category was highest quartile of physical activity and <4 h per day sitting. Upper boundary of physical activity quartile 1 was 2.5 MET-h week^{-1} (equivalent to ~5 minutes of moderate intensity physical activity per day); upper boundary of quartile 2 was 16 MET-h week^{-1} (~25–35 minutes of moderate intensity physical activity per day); upper boundary of quartile 3 was 30 MET-h week^{-1} (~50–65 minutes of moderate intensity physical activity per day); and lower boundary of quartile 4 was 35.5 MET-h week^{-1} (~60–75 minutes of moderate intensity physical activity per day). The findings were adjusted for all available covariates.

CARDIORESPIRATORY FITNESS AND MORTALITY

Cardiorespiratory fitness is a physiological trait which is influenced by both level of physical activity and genetic factors (see Chapter 2). In comparison to the questionnaire-based assessment of physical activity that has been commonly used in epidemiological studies, fitness can typically be measured more objectively (usually using either submaximal or maximal treadmill or cycle ergometer tests). Thus, the observed relationships between fitness and mortality are not subject to the regression dilution bias errors (see Chapter 2) that are present in most epidemiological studies of the relationship of physical activity and mortality.

One of the first studies to demonstrate an association between cardiorespiratory fitness and all-cause mortality risk was the Aerobics Center Longitudinal Study (Blair et al. 1989). In this study, a maximal treadmill exercise test was conducted in 10,224 men and 3,120 women, and time to exhaustion on this test was used to indicate fitness. The average period of follow-up was just over eight years, during which there were 240 deaths in men and 43 deaths in women.

Participants were classified into quintiles: quintile one contained those with the shortest treadmill times (lowest fitness); and quintile five contained those with the longest treadmill times (highest fitness). Those with the lowest fitness levels had the highest risk of death during follow-up. The lowest risk of death was seen in those with the highest fitness in men and in those in quintile four in women (Table 3.2). These trends remained after statistical adjustment for age, smoking habit, cholesterol level, systolic blood pressure, fasting blood glucose level, parental history of coronary heart disease (CHD) and follow-up interval. Blair and colleagues concluded that high levels

Table 3.2 Physical fitness (time to exhaustion on a treadmill test) was associated with a reduction in the risk of all-cause mortality in both men and women in the Aerobics Center Longitudinal Study.

FITNESS GROUP	PERSON-YEARS OF FOLLOW-UP	NO. OF DEATHS	AGE-ADJUSTED RATES PER 10,000 PERSON-YEARS	RELATIVE RISK
Men				
1 (low)	14,515	75	64.0	3.44
2	16,898	40	25.5	1.37
3	17,287	47	27.1	1.46
4	18,792	43	21.7	1.17
5 (high)	17,557	35	18.6	1.00
Women				
1 (low)	4,916	18	39.5	4.65
2	5,329	11	20.5	2.42
3	5,053	6	12.2	1.43
4	5,522	4	6.5	0.76
5 (high)	4,613	4	8.5	1.00

Source: Reproduced with permission from the *Journal of the American Medical Association.* 1989. 262(17): 2395–401. Copyright © (1989) American Medical Association. All rights reserved.

of physical fitness appear to delay all-cause mortality primarily due to lowered rates of CVD and cancer.

The results of the Aerobics Center Longitudinal Study are consistent with the findings of other studies investigating the relationship between cardiorespiratory fitness and mortality. A meta-analysis by Kodama and colleagues of 33 studies, including a total of 102,980 individuals found that compared with the reference category of high fitness (>10.8 METs in age- and sex-adjusted analysis; see Chapter 2 for an explanation of METs), the relative risk for all-cause mortality for intermediate (7.9–10.8 METs) and low (<7.9 METs) fitness was 1.13 (95% confidence interval 1.04–1.22) and 1.70 (95% confidence interval 1.51–1.92), respectively (Kodama et al. 2009) (Figure 3.7). Thus, in terms of mortality risk reduction, the greatest reduction in mortality risk was seen in moving from the low to intermediate fitness category. Based on these findings, the authors calculated that men aged 40, 50 and 60 years would need to achieve cardiorespiratory fitness levels of 9, 8 and 7 METs, respectively (7, 6 and 5 METs respectively, for women), to achieve substantial mortality risk reduction. Overall, each 1-MET increase in cardiorespiratory fitness (equivalent to a 1 km h^{-1} faster maximum intensity running speed) was associated with a 13% reduction in mortality risk.

In Kodama's meta-analysis, higher levels of fitness were consistently protective against mortality risk in subgroups aged both below and above 50 years of age; in people with both normal and abnormal exercise electrocardiograms (indicating presence of coronary heart disease); and in participants exhibiting less than three, or three or more cardiovascular disease risk factors. This final observation is important. A high

Figure 3.7 Association between cardiorespiratory fitness and all-cause mortality in a meta-analysis from Kodama and colleagues.

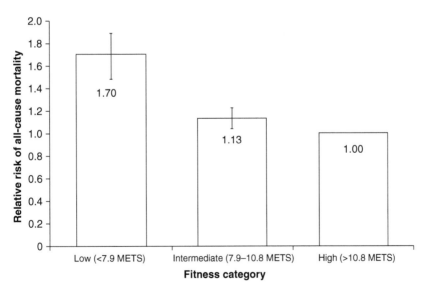

Source: Kodama et al. (2009).
Notes: Error bars represent 95% confidence intervals. Relative risks are adjusted for all available covariates.

level of fitness is associated with lower risk of mortality in people with a range of health conditions, including cardiovascular disease, diabetes and chronic obstructive lung disease (COPD) and in those exhibiting a range of risk factors for cardiovascular or metabolic disease. This is illustrated in a Californian study of 3,679 men with CVD and 2,534 men without CVD (Myers et al. 2002), who had cardiorespiratory fitness estimated from treadmill speed and incline achieved during a maximal exercise test, and were followed up for an average of 6.2 years, during which there were 1,256 deaths. Higher levels of fitness were associated with lower mortality risk in participants both with and without CVD at baseline (Figure 3.8), as well as in subgroups of participants who were at increased risk of death due to the presence of other risk factors, including a history of hypertension, COPD, diabetes, smoking, obesity and hypercholesterolaemia (Figure 3.9).

Two further recent studies on the relationship between cardiorespiratory fitness and mortality and fitness warrant particular mention. The first of these took advantage of the fact that Sweden has had mandatory military service for men over a century and that all men undergoing military service underwent a standardised incremental fitness test on a cycle ergometer, during which resistance was increased by 25 W m^{-1} until volitional fatigue, on enrolment at age ~18 years. Thus, Högström and colleagues were able to assess the relationship between fitness at age ~18 years (assessed as maximum

Figure 3.8 Exercise capacity (METs) was inversely related to the risk of death in Californian men with and without CVD.

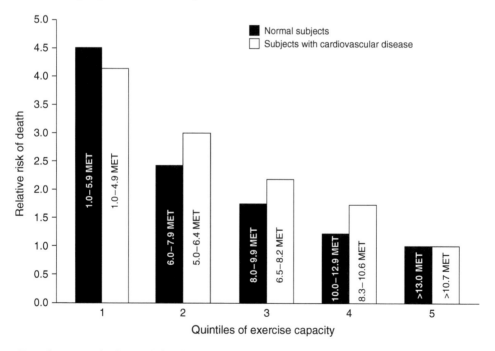

Source: From the *New England Journal of Medicine*, Myers, J., et al., 'Exercise capacity and mortality among men referred for exercise testing', 346: 793–801. Copyright © 2002 Massachusetts Medical Society. Reprinted with permission from Massachusetts Medical Society.

Figure 3.9 High exercise capacity was associated with a reduced risk of all-cause mortality even in the presence of established risk factors in a study of Californian men.

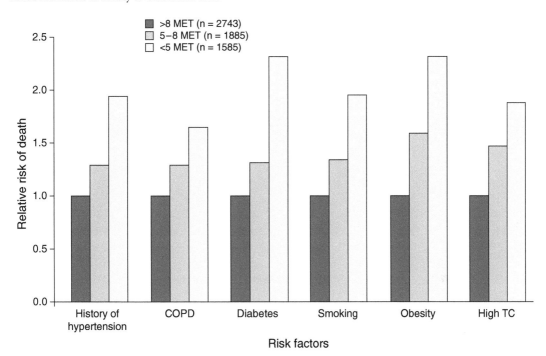

Source: From the *New England Journal of Medicine*, Myers, J., et al., 'Exercise capacity and mortality among men referred for exercise testing', 346: 793–801. Copyright © 2002 Massachusetts Medical Society. Reprinted with permission from Massachusetts Medical Society.
Notes: The figure shows age-adjusted relative risk of death from any cause in men with various risk factors classified according to exercise capacity in METs. COPD: chronic obstructive pulmonary disease. Obesity was defined as a BMI ≥ 30 kg m^{-2}. High TC: high total cholesterol i.e. ≥ 5.7 mmol l^{-1}.

power output achieved during the fitness test) and risk of mortality in 1,317,713 Swedish men who were conscripted between 1969 and 1996, making this the largest ever study investigating fitness and mortality risk (Högström et al. 2016). The men were followed up for a mean of 29 years, during which time 44,301 men died. After adjustment for confounding variables, higher levels of fitness were associated with lower risk of mortality in a dose-dependent manner, with those in the top 20% of the study population for fitness at age 18 years having a 31% lower risk of mortality over the follow-up period compared with those in the bottom 20% (Figure 3.10). A key difference between this study and other studies investigating the relationship between fitness and risk of mortality is that here fitness was measured in youth, rather than in middle-age. Fitness in youth was protective against risk of mortality, which contrasts with data about youthful physical activity and mortality risk, where high levels of physical activity in youth were not protective unless continued into later life (see section on 'Changes in physical activity and mortality' below and Chapter 4 for more details). This may be due to the fact that a large component of fitness is genetic, so

Figure 3.10 Association between cardiorespiratory fitness at age ~18 years and all-cause mortality in 1.3 million Swedish men.

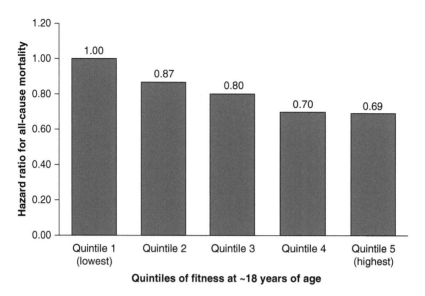

Source: Högström et al. (2016).
Notes: Quintiles of fitness determined by maximum power output achieved in an incremental cycle ergometer fitness test. Quintile 1: 100–228 W; Quintile 2: 229–254 W; Quintile 3: 255–283 W; Quintile 4: 284–320 W; Quintile 5: >321 W. The findings were adjusted for age, year of conscription, BMI, systolic and diastolic blood pressure, socio-economic variables 15 years after conscription, and common diagnoses at baseline.

that fitness levels in youth are likely to correlate quite strongly with fitness levels later life – in others words youthful fitness is likely to be a reasonably good proxy for fitness in middle-age – which is not necessary the case for physical activity.

The second paper, from the Copenhagen Male Study, investigated the association between cardiorespiratory fitness and longevity (Clausen et al. 2018). Here, 5,245 men aged 40–59 years at baseline, had cardiorespiratory fitness estimated from a submaximal cycle ergometer test, and were categorised as having fitness levels below the lower limit of normal (bottom 5% of population), low normal (between 6th and 50th centile), high normal (51st to 95th centile), or above the upper limit of normal (top 5%). The men were followed up for 46 years – the longest follow-up period to date for a study investigating the relationship between fitness and mortality – during which 4,700 (92%) of the men died. After statistical adjustment for age, BMI, self-reported physical activity, presence of diabetes, smoking, alcohol intake, systolic blood pressure and socio-economic status, being in the top 5% of the population for fitness was associated with 4.9 years longer life expectancy compared with the bottom 5%, and every 1 ml kg^{-1} min^{-1} increase in maximum oxygen uptake ($\dot{V}O_2$max) was associated with a 45-day increase in longevity. Importantly, the very long follow-up period enabled a robust assessment of the potential contribution of reverse causality to the findings, by repeating the analyses excluding all men who died within the first ten years of follow-up (n = 361). This landmark analysis had only had a modest effect on the life-expectancy

Table 3.3 Association between mid-life cardiorespiratory fitness and survival over 46 years of follow-up in the Copenhagen Male Study.

FITNESS CATEGORY	ALL PARTICIPANTS			EXCLUDING DEATHS WITHIN TEN YEARS		
	NUMBER OF PARTICIPANTS	NUMBER OF EVENTS (%)	ADDITIONAL YEARS OF SURVIVAL* (95% CI)	NUMBER OF PARTICIPANTS	NUMBER OF EVENTS (%)	ADDITIONAL YEARS OF SURVIVAL* (95% CI)
Below lower limit of normal (lowest 5% of population)	257	246 (96%)	0.0 (reference)	230	219 (95%)	0.0 (reference)
Low normal (6th to 50th centile)	2276	2095 (92%)	2.1 (0.7–3.4)	2107	1928 (92%)	1.8 (0.6–3.1)
High normal (51st to 95th centile)	2299	2107 (92%)	2.9 (1.5–4.2)	2147	1956 (91%)	2.6 (1.4–3.9)
Above upper limit of normal (highest 5% of population	256	234 (91%)	4.9 (3.1–6.7)	244	222 (91%)	4.3 (2.6–5.9)

* adjusted for age, body mass index, self-reported leisure-time physical activity, diabetes, smoking, alcohol, hypertension and socio-economic status.

Source: Reprinted from the *Journal of the American College of Cardiology*, 72: 987–95, Clausen, J.S. et al., 'Midlife cardiorespiratory fitness and the long-term risk of mortality: 46 years of follow up', page 993, copyright © 2018, with permission from Elsevier.

estimates, indicating a minimal contribution of reverse causation to the study findings. More details are shown in Table 3.3 and Figure 3.11.

The large body of observational data showing strong associations with cardiorespiratory fitness and risk of mortality is supported by evidence from animal models. To test the hypothesis that low capacity for oxidative metabolism, manifesting in low endurance exercise capacity (i.e. low cardiorespiratory fitness), was causally related to adverse health outcomes, Koch and colleagues undertook an innovative research programme in which they artificially selected rats on the basis of their aerobic capacity (Koch et al. 2012). Rats from a founder population performed incremental treadmill running tests to determine maximal endurance capacity, and then 'low capacity runners' and 'high capacity runners' were interbred for several generations. By generation 20, there was a 4.7-fold difference in running capacity between the low- and high-capacity running groups, with rats in the low-capacity group completing about 300 m on the treadmill test, and the high-capacity rats managing 1600 m before exhaustion. Life expectancy was 28% longer in the high-capacity rats (hazard ratio for mortality in the low compared with high-capacity rats was 5.7), and within both the high- and low-capacity strains $\dot{V}O_2$max was a strong predictor of lifespan. Thus, these data support the interpretation that the association between cardiorespiratory fitness and mortality risk observed in epidemiological data in humans is likely to be causal, as selectively breeding

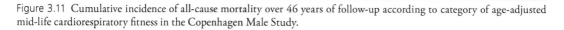

Figure 3.11 Cumulative incidence of all-cause mortality over 46 years of follow-up according to category of age-adjusted mid-life cardiorespiratory fitness in the Copenhagen Male Study.

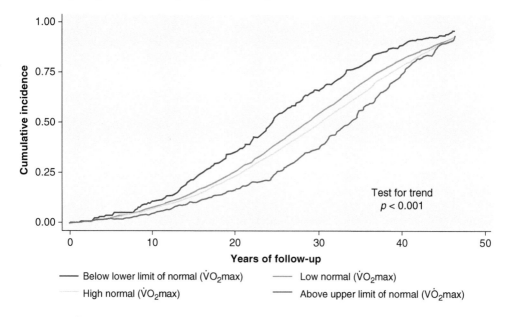

Source: Reprinted from the *Journal of the American College of Cardiology*, 72: 987–95, Clausen, J.S. et al., 'Midlife cardiorespiratory fitness and the long-term risk of mortality: 46 years of follow up', page 991, copyright © 2018, with permission from Elsevier.

Notes: Below lower limit of normal corresponded to age-adjusted fitness level in lowest 5% of population; Low normal corresponded to 6th to 50th centile for age-adjusted fitness; High normal corresponded to 51st to 95th centile; and Above upper limit of normal corresponded to the top 5%.

for the trait of cardiorespiratory fitness had a direct effect on risk of mortality and life expectancy (at least in rats).

The importance of (low) cardiorespiratory fitness as a risk factor for mortality has led to suggestions that fitness measurement should be a routine component of all clinical assessments (Kraus and Douglas 2005). However, one potential barrier to the widespread routine measurement of fitness in clinical practice is the need to undertake exercise tests on participants, which can be time-consuming and impractical in routine clinical settings. To address this, a non-exercise test to predict cardiorespiratory fitness using a regression equation based on age, sex, body mass index, resting heart rate and self-reported physical activity level has been developed, which had correlations of 0.72 to 0.80 with directly measured cardiorespiratory fitness in cross-validation studies (Jurca et al. 2005). This test has not yet been widely adopted but in a study of 32,319 adults drawn from the Health Survey for England and the Scottish Health Survey and followed up for a mean of 9 years (2165 deaths occurred during follow-up), the hazard ratio for all-cause mortality associated with a one standard deviation increase in cardiorespiratory fitness assessed using this non-exercise test was 0.85 (95% confidence interval 0.78–0.93) in men and 0.88 (95% confidence interval 0.80–0.98) in women, in analyses adjusted for a range of confounding factors (Stamatakis et al. 2013).

MUSCULAR STRENGTH AND MORTALITY

Like cardiovascular fitness, muscular strength is a physiological trait which is influenced by both physical activity (particularly resistance exercise) and genetic factors. In contrast with the wealth of studies examining the relationship between cardiorespiratory fitness and mortality, fewer studies have examined the relationship between muscular strength and mortality. A meta-analysis of 14 studies, mostly in older adults (>60 years at baseline), with a total of 53,476 participants, compared risk for mortality between the weakest and strongest, sex-specific quartiles for hand-grip strength, reporting a hazard ratio for low grip strength of 1.67 (95% confidence interval 1.45–1.93) in analyses adjusted for age, sex and body size, and a graded relationship between grip strength and mortality was apparent across strength quartiles (Cooper et al. 2010). Since publication of this meta-analysis, other larger studies with a wider age range of participants have reported similar findings. The Prospective Urban Rural Epidemiology (PURE) study, enrolled households with at least one member aged 35–70 years across 17 countries of varying socio-economic levels (Leong et al. 2015). 139,691 participants had hand-grip strength measured at baseline using a dynamometer and were followed up for a median of four years, during which time there were 3,379 deaths. In analyses adjusted for a range of confounding variables, grip strength was inversely associated with risk of mortality, with each 5 kg decrement in grip strength associated with a 16% increase in risk of all-cause mortality (i.e. hazard ratio of 1.16 (95% confidence interval 1.13 to 1.20) per 5 kg reduction in grip strength). In UK Biobank, 502,293 men and women aged 40–69 from the general UK population had hand-grip strength measured at baseline and were followed up for a mean of 7.1 years, during which 13,322 died (Celis-Morales et al. 2018). After statistical adjustment for a range of confounding variables, the hazard ratio for mortality per 5 kg reduction in grip strength was 1.20 (95% confidence interval 1.17 to 1.23) in women, and 1.16 (95% confidence interval 1.15 to 1.17) in men, a similar magnitude of association to that observed in the PURE study. A key observation in the UK Biobank study was that the addition of grip strength to an established mortality risk prediction score (which included age, sex, diabetes, body mass index, blood pressure and smoking) improved prediction of all-cause (and CVD) mortality, suggesting that measurement of grip strength might become a useful addition to routine risk screening in health-care settings.

Grip strength has been the most widely used measure of muscular strength in epidemiological studies of musculoskeletal fitness and mortality. However, a small number of studies have used other measures. For example, in a report of 8,116 people who were followed up for 13 years after participation in the 1981 Canada Fitness Survey found that the number of sit-ups performed in 60 seconds was associated with all-cause mortality, with a relative risk for being in the bottom compared to top quartile of 2.72 (95% confidence interval 1.56–4.64) for men and 2.26 (95% confidence interval 1.15–4.43) for women, in analyses adjusted for age, smoking, body mass and $\dot{V}O_2$max (Katzmarzyk and Craig 2002).

IS FITNESS OR PHYSICAL ACTIVITY MORE IMPORTANT FOR MORTALITY RISK?

In prospective cohort studies where measurements of both physical activity and cardiorespiratory fitness (or muscular strength) have been made, the strength of association with mortality is consistently greater for fitness or muscular strength than for physical activity (Blair et al. 2001; Celis-Morales et al. 2017). For example, in a report from UK Biobank, a one standard deviation decrease in physical activity was associated with a 5% higher risk of mortality, but one standard deviation decreases in cardiorespiratory fitness and grip strength were associated with 22% and 18% increases in mortality risk, respectively, after adjustment for a comprehensive range of confounding variables (Celis-Morales et al. 2017). This may be related to self-report measurement of physical activity diluting the strength of the apparent relationship with mortality but may also reflect the innate genetic contribution to fitness and strength which may influence mortality risk independently of physical activity.

Indeed, recent evidence from UK Biobank suggests that the association between physical activity and risk of mortality may differ according to level of cardiorespiratory fitness and grip strength (Celis-Morales et al. 2017). Here, 498,135 adults aged 40–69 years underwent baseline measurements including hand-grip strength and self-reported physical activity, and a subset of 67,702 participants underwent baseline measurements of cardiorespiratory fitness (based on a submaximal cycle ergometer test). They were followed up for a median of 4.9 years during which 8,591 participants died. Participants were stratified into age- and sex-specific tertiles (low, moderate and high) for grip strength and cardiorespiratory fitness and the association between physical activity and mortality was evaluated for participants in each strength and fitness category. In participants with low grip strength there was a strong association between physical activity and mortality risk, with a hazard ratio for mortality of 1.11 (95% confidence interval 1.09 to 1.14) per quintile decrease in physical activity level. Similarly, amongst those with low fitness, each quintile decrease in physical activity was associated with a hazard ratio for mortality of 1.13 (95% confidence interval 1.02 to 1.26). In contrast, the mortality hazard ratio per quintile decrease in physical activity was 1.04 (95% confidence interval 1.01 to 1.08) for those highest tertile for grip strength and 1.03 (95% confidence interval 0.91 to 1.16) for those in the highest tertile for cardiorespiratory fitness (Figure 3.12 and Figure 3.13). These data suggest that the mortality risk associated with a low level of physical activity is greatest in those with low levels of fitness and strength, and that those with high fitness and strength have relatively low risk of mortality, even when their physical activity levels are low. Thus, those with the lowest levels of strength and fitness may benefit most from interventions to increase physical activity, and physical activity may be less important for mortality risk in those with innately high levels of fitness and strength.

However, it is also clear that changes in physical activity can have profound effects on cardiorespiratory fitness (American College of Sports Medicine 1998). Thus, by increasing their level of physical activity individuals can potentially modify their mortality risk by altering their level of fitness, as well as via mechanisms which may be

Figure 3.12 Association between physical activity and all-cause mortality according to level of grip strength in the UK Biobank.

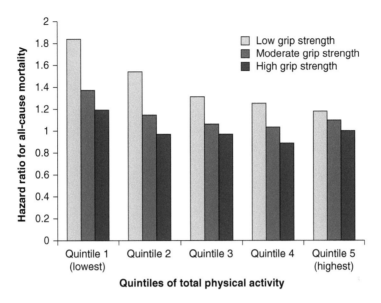

Source: Adapted from Celis-Morales et al. (2017).
Notes: Low, moderate and high grip strength refer to age- and sex-specific tertiles. Reference category was quintile 5 for physical activity and high grip strength. The findings were adjusted for age, sex, ethnicity, deprivation index, BMI, smoking status, total sedentary time, alcohol intake, depression, diabetes, hypertension, cancer diagnosis, stroke, angina, heart attack and long-standing illness.

independent of fitness level. Evidence to support this assertion is available in the form of studies that have examined changes in either activity or fitness to determine whether or not there is an associated change in all-cause mortality. This evidence is discussed in the section below.

CHANGES IN PHYSICAL ACTIVITY AND MORTALITY

The first major epidemiological study to examine changes in physical activity and risk of all-cause mortality was the Harvard Alumni Health Study (Paffenbarger et al. 1993). In this study, exercise habits were assessed via a questionnaire at baseline (either 1962 or 1966) and again in 1977 in 10,269 men aged 45–84 years in 1977. These men reported being free from life-threatening disease at both observation points. Follow-up was continued until 1985 during which time 476 men died. At each observation point individuals were grouped according to: (1) their weekly physical activity levels (<2,000 kcal per week (8.4 MJ per week) versus ≥2,000 kcal per week); and (2) their participation or lack of participation in 'moderately vigorous' sports activities (defined as those requiring an intensity ≥4.5 METs) such as swimming, tennis, squash, racquetball, handball, jogging

Figure 3.13 Association between physical activity and all-cause mortality according to level of cardiorespiratory fitness in the UK Biobank.

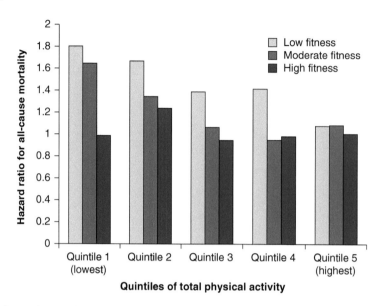

Source: Adapted from Celis-Morales et al. (2017).
Notes: Cardiorespiratory fitness determined from a submaximal cycle ergometer test. Low, moderate and high fitness refer to age- and sex-specific tertiles. Reference category was quintile 5 for physical activity and high fitness. The findings were adjusted for age, sex, ethnicity, deprivation index, BMI, smoking status, total sedentary time, alcohol intake, depression, diabetes, hypertension, cancer diagnosis, stroke, angina, heart attack and long-standing illness.

and running. The findings revealed that changes in exercise habits between observation points were associated with differences in mortality risk during follow-up. Specifically, there was a lower mortality rate in those who became more active and/or increased the intensity of their physical activity between observation points than in those who did not (Figure 3.14). Other studies have also examined the relationship between changes in physical activity and mortality risk. Reports from the British Regional Heart Study (Wannamethee et al. 1998), the Copenhagen City Heart Study (Schnohr et al. 2003), and the Baltimore Longitudinal Study of Aging (Talbot et al. 2007) have demonstrated that, amongst 'older' men, an increase in physical activity is associated with a decrease in mortality risk. The findings in studies of women are somewhat less clear-cut, but the Study of Osteoporotic Fractures (Gregg et al. 2003) reported that increasing physical activity was associated with a decrease, and reducing physical activity was associated with an increase, in all-cause mortality risk among older women. Thus, the available evidence is broadly supportive of the hypothesis that inactive people can lower their risk of dying prematurely by becoming more active, even in later life. The evidence also suggests that past activity alone is not protective and only continuing current physical activity reduces mortality risk: Figure 3.14 illustrates this observation for the Harvard Alumni Health Study cohort.

Figure 3.14 Increases in the amount and/or intensity of physical activity over time are associated with a lower risk of mortality in comparison with the risk in those who remain inactive amongst men in the Harvard Alumni Health Study.

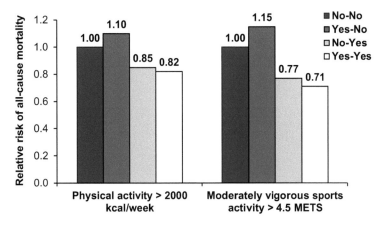

Source: Paffenbarger et al. (1993).
Notes: This study involved 10,269 men assessed in 1962 or 1966 and again in 1977, and followed up until 1985. The figure legend indicates group classifications; e.g. those in the 'No–No' group expended less than 2000 kcal week^{-1} (8.4 MJ week^{-1}) at both observation points.

CHANGES IN FITNESS AND MORTALITY

The largest study to investigate the relationship between change in cardiorespiratory fitness and all-cause mortality is the Aerobics Center Longitudinal Study. A report from this cohort evaluated mortality in 14,345 men who completed at least two maximal treadmill tests between 1974 and 2002 (Lee et al. 2011). The mean interval between treadmill tests was 6.3 years, and the mean follow-up duration after the final test was 11.4 years, during which time there were 914 deaths. Participants whose fitness levels changed by between –0.06 and +0.19 METs per year between the first and second treadmill tests were classified as having 'stable' fitness levels (n = 4,781), those whose fitness levels decreased by more than 0.06 METs per year were classified as losing fitness (n = 4,782), and those whose fitness levels increased by more than 0.19 METs per year were classified as gaining fitness (n = 4,782). In analyses adjusted for a range of confounding factors, including change in BMI, men who maintained fitness between the first and second tests had a 30% lower risk, and men who improved fitness had a 39% lower risk, of all-cause mortality, compared to men who lost fitness (Figure 3.15). Each 1-MET increase in fitness between tests was associated with 15% lower risk of all-cause mortality. These findings were consistent irrespective of fitness level at baseline. A smaller study of 1,428 healthy Norwegian men reported similar findings (Erikssen et al. 1998).

Thus, collectively, studies of changes in activity/fitness provide evidence that changes in activity habits have an influence on mortality risk, particularly if such

Figure 3.15 Association between changes in fitness and risk of all-cause mortality in the Aerobics Center Longitudinal Study.

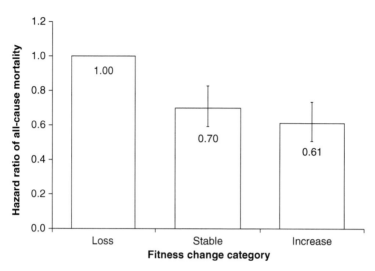

Source: Lee et al. (2011).
Notes: This study involved 14,345 men who completed two treadmill tests with a mean interval of 6.3 years and were followed up for a further 11.4 years. Participants were divided into tertiles for change in fitness between the two tests. Loss of fitness was a decrease in fitness of >0.06 METs between measurements; stable fitness was a change between −0.06 and +0.19 METs; and increase in fitness was an increase of >0.19 METs. Error bars represent 95% confidence intervals. The findings were adjusted for age, examination year, parental cardiovascular disease, baseline BMI, baseline maximal METs, smoking status, alcohol intake, physical activity, abnormal ECG, hypertension, diabetes, hypercholesterolaemia, change in BMI and number of clinic visits.

changes result in a change in cardiorespiratory fitness. These studies therefore suggest that human beings have an element of control over their own mortality. It is important to re-emphasise, however, that these studies are observational and are not proof of a cause-and-effect relationship. It is not always clear, for example, why individuals have changed their activity levels, nor is it clear to what extent overall physical activity levels can be sustainably changed over the long term.

PHYSICAL ACTIVITY, FITNESS, BODY COMPOSITION AND MORTALITY

Most of the studies discussed so far relate to initially 'healthy' individuals, although some studies have included 'healthy' and 'unhealthy' groups based on the presence or absence of disease at baseline. An issue that has been debated more recently is the extent to which physical activity and cardiorespiratory fitness influences mortality risk in obese individuals irrespective of any influence on body fatness.

A number of studies have attempted to determine whether a high level of physical activity is protective against the increased mortality risk associated with obesity. One report from the Nurses' Health Study, which followed up 116,564 female nurses for 24

Figure 3.16 Risk of mortality by level of physical activity and body mass index category in the Nurses' Health Study.

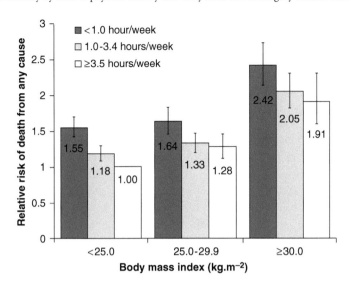

Source: Hu et al. (2004).
Notes: Reference category was physical activity ≥ 3.5 hours week^{-1} and BMI < 25 kg m^{-2}. The findings were adjusted for age, smoking status, parental history of coronary heart disease, menopausal status and hormone use. Error bars represent 95% confidence intervals.

years, during which time 10,282 deaths occurred, found that a high level of physical activity ameliorated, but did not eliminate, the excess mortality risk associated with obesity (Hu et al. 2004). Compared with women who were lean (BMI < 25 kg m^{-2}) and active (≥3.5 hours of physical activity per week), relative risk of death was 1.55 (95% confidence interval 1.42–1.70) for lean inactive (less than one hour of physical activity per week) women, 1.91 (95% confidence interval 1.60–2.30) for obese (BMI ≥ 30 kg m^{-2}) women who were active and 2.42 (95% confidence interval 2.14–2.73) for obese women who were inactive, in multivariate analyses adjusted for a range of confounders (Figure 3.16). Similar findings have been reported in a number of other large cohort studies of middle-aged and older men and women, including the American National Institutes of Health–AARP Diet and Health Study (n = 185,412, 10 years of follow-up) (Koster et al. 2009) and the Swedish National March Cohort (n = 40,729, 9.7 years of follow-up) (Bellocco et al. 2010). Overall, the weight of evidence suggests that low levels of physical activity and obesity are independent and additive risk factors for all-cause mortality.

Studies examining the relationship between cardiorespiratory fitness, obesity and mortality have produced slightly different findings from studies which considered physical activity. A meta-analysis evaluated the joint effects of BMI category and fitness on all-cause mortality in ten reports, including a total of 92,986 participants. Mean follow-up ranged from 7.7 to 16 years and there were 6,663 deaths across all studies (Barry et al. 2014). Nine of the ten studies classed normal weight as BMI < 25 kg m^{-2}, overweight as BMI 25 to 29.9 kg m^{-2} and obese as BMI ≥ 30 kg m^{-2}

(the other classified obesity as BMI $\geq$ 27.8 kg m^{-2}). Seven of the ten studies classified low fitness as having fitness in the lowest 20% of the population for their age group, with the remainder of the population classified as fit; the remaining three reports classified fitness using a study-specific threshold. The findings indicated that, compared with normal weight fit individuals, unfit individuals had approximately twice the risk of mortality, irrespective of BMI category. In contrast, fit overweight and obese individuals had similar mortality risk to fit and normal weight individuals (Figure 3.17). These findings suggest that risk of death was more dependent on fitness level than BMI. Thus, overweight or obese individuals who were fit did not have a greater risk of all-cause mortality, and the benefits of leanness are restricted to those who are fit. However, there are two important factors to take into account when interpreting these findings. Firstly, the distribution of low fitness is not even across BMI categories. For example, in one large report from the Aerobics Center Longitudinal Study included in the meta-analysis (n = 25,714), only 9% of normal weight men but 51% of obese men were classified as unfit (Wei et al. 1999). Thus, it is relatively uncommon for a person to be normal weight and unfit, but relatively common to be obese and unfit. Secondly, as fitness measured in terms of $\dot{V}O_2$max or METs is expressed according to bodyweight (i.e. in ml kg^{-1} min^{-1}), obesity and fitness are not entirely independent. Thus, while an unfit obese person could increase their fitness level by becoming more physically active in the absence of weight loss, they could also increase their fitness level by losing weight.

Figure 3.17 Risk of mortality by level of cardiorespiratory fitness and body mass index category in a meta-analysis by Barry and colleagues.

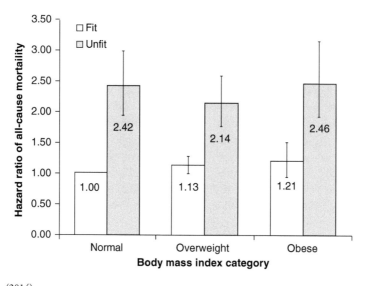

Source: Barry et al. (2014).
Notes: Unfit was defined as having fitness in the lowest 20% of the population for their age-group (seven out of ten included studies) and using study-specific thresholds in the other three studies. Reference category was fit with normal BMI (< 25 kg m^{-2}). Most studies classed overweight as a BMI 25–29.9 kg m^{-2}, and obese as a BMI $\geq$ 30 kg m^{-2}. Error bars represent 95% confidence intervals.

Thus, overall, the evidence indicates that physically active obese individuals have lower risk of mortality than inactive obese individuals, but that a high level of activity does not fully protect from the excess mortality risk associated with obesity. In contrast, a high level of physical fitness does appear to protect from the adverse effects of obesity on mortality risk. This difference may be related to the inaccuracies in self-report physical activity measures attenuating the apparent benefit (i.e. regression dilution bias), the innate genetic contribution to fitness influencing mortality risk independently of physical activity, or the fact that fitness and body weight are not completely independent. In any case, the data do indicate that overweight and obese individuals may gain benefit from increased physical activity, even in the absence of weight loss. However, it seems that to maximise benefit, obese persons would also need to increase their cardiorespiratory fitness level and/or lose weight. This might have implications for the optimal type of physical activity to undertake, as vigorous activity induces greater increases in fitness than activities of light and moderate intensity (American College of Sports Medicine 1998).

ARE RANDOMISED CONTROLLED TRIALS OF PHYSICAL ACTIVITY AND MORTALITY RISK POSSIBLE?

It is very difficult to undertake randomised controlled trials to investigate the effects of physical activity on risk of mortality because of the low absolute risk of mortality over a given time period for individuals in the general population. For example, the risk of dying within the next ten years for a healthy, normal weight, non-smoking but inactive woman in the UK aged 50–59 years is less than 3%, and for an equivalent man is ~7% (Kobayashi et al. 2017); thus a study will need to be extremely large (several thousand participants) and long (likely more than a decade) for sufficient deaths to occur to be able to establish whether increasing physical activity changes risk of mortality amongst the general population. Further complications include ensuring adherence to physical activity in the intervention group (and inactivity in the control group) for such a long period and drop-out. One way to address at least the first of these issues is to study older populations where the risk of mortality is higher. The Generation 100 Study is a randomised controlled trial with the primary aim of determining the effects of regular exercise training over a five-year period on overall mortality in Norwegian adults aged 70–76 years at baseline (a population in which the mortality rate is ~2% per year) (Stensvold et al. 2015). Between August 2012 and June 2013, the Generation 100 Study randomly assigned 1567 participants to exercise (n = 787) and control (n = 780) intervention arms. Within the exercise arm, 387 participants were randomised to moderate intensity exercise (50 minute sessions of continuous exercise at ~70% maximum heart rate, twice per week), and 400 were assigned to high-intensity exercise (40-minute sessions including 4 x 4 minute intervals at ~85–95% maximum heart rate, twice per week) to investigative whether intensity of exercise influenced outcomes. Analyses will be performed on both an *intention-to-treat* (i.e. data will be analysed according to the group participants were assigned to, irrespective of adherence to the intervention) and a *per protocol* (i.e. based on adherence to the intervention, including only those who completed at least 50% of the prescribed training sessions) basis, and follow-up is planned until the year 2035. At the time of writing, no outcome data from this trial have yet been published, but findings are eagerly awaited.

SOME FINAL THOUGHTS

This chapter has focused on the association between physical activity, sedentary behaviour, cardiorespiratory fitness and muscular strength on risk of mortality, providing evidence of lower risk of premature mortality and a modest increase in life-expectancy. However, it is important to recognise that there is much more to health than avoiding early death. Health is also about living without illness, having functional capacities to do things (what might be termed 'positive health') and feeling good (wellbeing). This is where physical activity possibly has the most to offer. In the chapters that follow, we will examine a wide variety of evidence to explain:

1 the aetiology of the major diseases and conditions that might be influenced by physical activity;
2 the associations between these diseases/conditions and physical activity/sedentary behaviour/fitness/strength; and
3 the mechanisms by which physical activity may enhance health.

SUMMARY

- Observational studies consistently show that physical activity is inversely associated with risk of mortality. This has been demonstrated for physical activity across a range of contexts (including occupational, transport and leisure time) and associations remain statistically significant after adjustment for a range of potential confounding factors.
- Both vigorous and moderate intensity physical activity are associated with lower mortality risk, but minute-for-minute, vigorous activity is associated with a greater risk reduction.
- Most studies have assessed physical activity using self-report questionnaires which are liable to errors due to inaccurate recall. These errors can lead to an underestimation of the true relationship between physical activity and mortality. Stronger relationships between physical activity and mortality have been observed in the limited number of studies which have used more objective measures of physical activity.
- There is an accumulating body of evidence that participation in muscle-strengthening exercise, as well as aerobic physical activity, is associated with lower risk of mortality.
- It has been estimated that almost 10% of deaths worldwide can be attributed to physical inactivity.
- Sedentary behaviour is associated with risk of mortality in a non-linear manner, with mortality risk increasing by ~4% per hour increase in daily sitting time beyond 8 hours. A stronger association with mortality is observed for television

viewing than overall sitting, which may reflect clustering of other risk factors for mortality with high levels of television viewing.

- Risks associated with high levels of sedentary behaviour differ according to level of physical activity and can be minimised by being sufficiently active.
- Both cardiorespiratory fitness and muscular strength (usually assessed using hand-grip strength) are inversely associated with risk of mortality. These associations are stronger than the association between physical activity and mortality risk and may reflect more accurate measurement and/or the genetic contribution to fitness and strength influencing risk independently of physical activity.
- Risks associated with physical inactivity appear to be greatest in those who also have low levels of fitness or strength.
- Changes in levels of physical activity or cardiorespiratory fitness are associated with changes in risk of mortality.
- Evidence suggests that obese individuals who are physically active have a lower risk of mortality than inactive obese individuals, but a high level of physical activity does not fully protect from the adverse effects of obesity on mortality risk. Obese individuals with a high level of cardiorespiratory fitness appear to have similar risk of mortality as fit normal weight adults. However, a high level of fitness is substantially less common in obese than normal weight individuals.
- The available evidence suggests that those with the highest levels of physical activity or cardiorespiratory fitness have approximately 1.5 to 4 years longer life expectancy than those with the lowest levels of activity/fitness.
- There are many plausible biological mechanisms to explain the associations between physical activity/sedentary behaviour/fitness/strength and all-cause mortality. These will be discussed in the chapters that follow and provide strong evidence for a cause-and-effect relationship.

STUDY TASKS

1 Describe in details the findings from one study on physical activity or sedentary behaviour and one study on cardiorespiratory fitness or muscular strength. State what is novel about each study and how the study has advanced knowledge and understanding.
2 Make a list, in order of importance, of all the possible confounding factors that may preclude cause-and-effect relationship between physical activity/sedentary behaviour/fitness/strength and all-cause mortality.
3 List the aspects of the evidence linking physical activity/sedentary behaviour/fitness/strength with all-cause mortality that are supportive of a cause-and-effect relationship.
4 The association of physical activity with risk of mortality appears to be less strong than the association of cardiorespiratory fitness and muscular strength with mortality risk. Why is this the case?
5 Discuss the evidence that risk of mortality associated with high levels of sitting may vary according to level of physical activity. What are the strengths and limitations of these data?

6 Discuss the strengths and limitations of studies examining changes in physical activity/fitness and risk of all-cause mortality.

7 Can being fit and physically active eliminate the excess risk of mortality associated with obesity? Provide a reasoned answer based on the available evidence.

8 How fit, strong and active does someone need to be to reduce risk of premature mortality? Justify your answer with reference to the research literature.

9 Write a 500-word description of a hypothetical study which will examine the relationships between physical activity, sedentary behaviour, cardiorespiratory fitness, and/or muscular strength and risk of all-cause mortality. What study design will you use? Which population will you study? What questions will this design allow you to answer? How will you assess physical activity/sedentary behaviour/fitness/strength? How will the findings advance knowledge? What will be the limitations of the study?

FURTHER READING

Barry, V.W., Baruth, M., Beets, M.W., Durstine, J.L., Liu, J. and Blair, S.N. (2014). Fitness vs. fatness on all-cause mortality: a meta-analysis. *Progress in Cardiovascular Diseases* 56: 382–90.

Celis-Morales, C.A., Lyall, D.M., Anderson, J., Iliodromiti, S., Fan, Y., Ntuk, U.E. et al. (2017) The association between physical activity and risk of mortality is modulated by grip strength and cardiorespiratory fitness: evidence from 498 135 UK-Biobank participants. *European Heart Journal* 38: 116–22.

Ekelund, U., Tarp, J., Steene-Johannessen, J., Hansen, B.H., Jefferis, B., Fagerland, M.W. et al. (2019) Dose–response associations between accelerometry measured physical activity and sedentary time and all-cause mortality: systematic review and harmonised meta-analysis. *British Medical Journal* 366: l4570. doi: 10.1136/bmj.l4570.

Gill, J.M.R. (2020) Linking volume and intensity of physical activity to mortality. *Nature Medicine* 26: 1332–4.

Hu, F.B., Willett, W.C., Li, T., Stampfer, M.J., Colditz, G.A. and Manson, J.E. (2004) Adiposity as compared with physical activity in predicting mortality among women. *New England Journal of Medicine* 351: 2694–703.

Kodama, S., Saito, K., Tanaka, S., Maki, M., Yachi, Y., Asumi, M. et al. (2009) Cardiorespiratory fitness as a quantitative predictor of all-cause mortality and cardiovascular events in healthy men and women: a meta-analysis. *Journal of the American Medical Association* 301: 2024–35.

Patterson, R., McNamara, E., Tainio, M., de Sá, T.H., Smith, A.D., Sharp, S.J. et al. (2018) Sedentary behaviour and risk of all-cause, cardiovascular and cancer mortality, and incident type 2 diabetes: a systematic review and dose response meta-analysis. *European Journal of Epidemiology* 33: 811–29.

Samitz, G., Egger, M. and Zwahlen, M. (2011) Domains of physical activity and all-cause mortality: systematic review and dose-response meta-analysis of cohort studies. *International Journal of Epidemiology* 40: 1382–400.

Stensvold, D., Viken, H., Rognmo, O., Skogvoll, E., Steinshamn, S., Vatten, L.J. et al. (2015) A randomised controlled study of the long-term effects of exercise training on mortality in elderly people: study protocol for the Generation 100 study. *British Medical Journal Open* 5: e007519. doi: 10.1136/bmjopen-2014–007519.

REFERENCES

American College of Sports Medicine. (1998) American College of Sports Medicine Position Stand. The recommended quantity and quality of exercise for developing and maintaining cardiorespiratory and muscular fitness, and flexibility in healthy adults. *Medicine and Science in Sports and Exercise* 30: 975–91.

Barry, V.W., Baruth, M., Beets, M.W., Durstine, J.L., Liu, J. and Blair, S.N. (2014) Fitness vs. fatness on all-cause mortality: a meta-analysis. *Progress in Cardiovascular Diseases* 56: 382–90.

Bellocco, R., Jia, C., Ye, W. and Lagerros, Y.T. (2010) Effects of physical activity, body mass index, waist-to-hip ratio and waist circumference on total mortality risk in the Swedish National March Cohort. *European Journal of Epidemiology* 25: 777–88.

Blair, S.N., Cheng, Y. and Holder, J.S. (2001) Is physical activity or physical fitness more important in defining health benefits? *Medicine and Science in Sports and Exercise* 33: S379–99.

Blair, S.N., Kohl, H.W., Paffenbarger, R.S., Clark, D.G., Cooper, K.H. and Gibbons, L.W. (1989) Physical fitness and all-cause mortality. A prospective study of healthy men and women. *Journal of the American Medical Association* 262: 2395–401.

Celis-Morales, C.A., Lyall, D.M., Anderson, J., Iliodromiti, S., Fan, Y., Ntuk, U.E. et al. (2017) The association between physical activity and risk of mortality is modulated by grip strength and cardiorespiratory fitness: evidence from 498 135 UK-Biobank participants. *European Heart Journal* 38: 116–22.

Celis-Morales, C.A., Welsh, P., Lyall, D.M., Steell, L., Petermann, F., Anderson, J. et al. (2018) Associations of grip strength with cardiovascular, respiratory, and cancer outcomes and all-cause mortality: prospective cohort study of half a million UK Biobank participants. *British Medical Journal* 361: k1651. doi: 10.1136/bmj.k1651.

Clausen, J., Marott, J.L., Holtermann, A., Gyntelberg, F. and Jensen, M.T. (2018) Midlife cardiorespiratory fitness and the long-term risk of mortality: 46 years of follow-up. *Journal of the American College of Cardiology* 72: 987–95.

Cooper, R., Kuh, D. and Hardy, R. (2010) Objectively measured physical capability levels and mortality: systematic review and meta-analysis. *British Medical Journal* 341: c4467. doi: 10.1136/bmj.c4467.

Dankel, S.J., Loenneke, J.P. and Loprinzi, P.D. (2016) Dose-dependent association between muscle-strengthening activities and all-cause mortality: prospective cohort study among a national sample of adults in the USA. *Archives of Cardiovascular Diseases* 109: 626–33.

Ekelund, U., Steene-Johannessen, J., Brown, W.J., Fagerland, M.W., Owen, N., Powell, K.E. et al. (2016) Does physical activity attenuate, or even eliminate, the detrimental association of sitting time with mortality? A harmonised meta-analysis of data from more than 1 million men and women. *The Lancet* 388: 1302–10.

Ekelund, U., Tarp, J., Steene-Johannessen, J., Hansen, B.H., Jefferis, B., Fagerland, M.W. et al. (2019) Dose–response associations between accelerometry measured physical activity and sedentary time and all-cause mortality: systematic review and harmonised meta-analysis. *British Medical Journal* 366: l4570. doi: 10.1136/bmj.l4570.

Erikssen, G., Liestøl, K., Bjørnholt, J., Thaulow, E., Sandvik, L. and Erikssen, J. (1998) Changes in physical fitness and changes in mortality. *The Lancet* 352: 759–62.

Gill, J.M.R. (2020) Linking volume and intensity of physical activity to mortality. *Nature Medicine* 26: 1332–4.

Gregg, E.W., Cauley, J.A., Stone, K., Thompson, T.J., Bauer, D.C., Cummings, S.R. and Ensrud, K.E. (2003) Relationship of changes in physical activity and mortality among older women. *Journal of the American Medical Association* 289: 2379–86.

Högström, G., Nordström, A. and Nordström, P. (2016) Aerobic fitness in late adolescence and the risk of early death: a prospective cohort study of 1.3 million Swedish men. *International Journal of Epidemiology* 45: 1159–68.

Hu, F.B., Willett, W.C., Li, T., Stampfer, M.J., Colditz, G.A. and Manson, J.E. (2004) Adiposity as compared with physical activity in predicting mortality among women. *New England Journal of Medicine* 351: 2694–703.

Jurca, R., Jackson, A.S., LaMonte, M.J., Morrow, J.R., Blair, S.N., Wareham, N.J., et al. (2005) Assessing cardiorespiratory fitness without performing exercise testing. *American Journal of Preventive Medicine* 29: 185–93.

Kamada, M., Shiroma, E.J., Buring, J.E., Miyachi, M. and Lee, I.-M. (2017) Strength training and all-cause, cardiovascular disease, and cancer mortality in older women: a cohort study. *Journal of the American Heart Association* 6: e007677. doi: 10.1161/JAHA.117.007677.

Katzmarzyk, P.T. and Craig, C.L. (2002) Musculoskeletal fitness and risk of mortality. *Medicine and Science in Sports and Exercise* 34: 740–4.

Kobayashi, L.C., Jackson, S.E., Lee, S.J., Wardle, J. and Steptoe, A. (2017) The development and validation of an index to predict 10-year mortality risk in a longitudinal cohort of older English adults. *Age and Ageing* 46: 427–32.

Koch, L.G., Britton, S.L. and Wisløff, U. (2012) A rat model system to study complex disease risks, fitness, aging, and longevity. *Trends in Cardiovascular Medicine* 22: 29–34.

Kodama, S., Saito, K., Tanaka, S., Maki, M., Yachi, Y., Asumi, M. et al. (2009) Cardiorespiratory fitness as a quantitative predictor of all-cause mortality and cardiovascular events in healthy men and women: a meta-analysis. *Journal of the American Medical Association* 301: 2024–35.

Koster, A., Harris, T.B., Moore, S.C., Schatzkin, A., Hollenbeck, A.R., van Eijk, J.T. and Leitzmann, M.F. (2009) Joint associations of adiposity and physical activity with mortality: the National Institutes of Health–AARP Diet and Health Study. *American Journal of Epidemiology* 169: 1344–51.

Kraschnewski, J.L., Sciamanna, C.N., Poger, J.M., Rovniak, L.S., Lehman, E.B., Cooper et al. (2016) Is strength training associated with mortality benefits? A 15 year cohort study of US older adults. *Preventive Medicine* 87: 121–7.

Kraus, W.E. and Douglas, P.S. (2005) Where does fitness fit in? *New England Journal of Medicine* 353: 517–19.

Lee, D.C., Sui, X., Artero, E.G., Lee, I.-M., Church, T.S., McAuley, P.A. et al. (2011) Long-term effects of changes in cardiorespiratory fitness and body mass index on all-cause and cardiovascular disease mortality in men: the Aerobics Center Longitudinal Study. *Circulation* 124: 2483–90.

Lee, I.-M., Shiroma, E.J., Lobelo, F., Puska, P., Blair, S.N. and Katzmarzyk, P.T. (2012) Effect of physical inactivity on major non-communicable diseases worldwide: an analysis of burden of disease and life expectancy. *The Lancet* 380: 219–29.

Leong, D.P., Teo, K.K., Rangarajan, S., Lopez-Jaramillo, P., Avezum, A., Orlandini, A. et al. (2015) Prognostic value of grip strength: findings from the Prospective Urban Rural Epidemiology (PURE) study. *The Lancet* 386: 266–73.

Manini, T.M., Everhart, J.E., Patel, K.V., Schoeller, D.A., Colbert, L.H., Visser, M. et al. (2006) Daily activity energy expenditure and mortality among older adults. *Journal of the American Medical Association* 296: 171–9.

Moore, S.C., Patel, A.V., Matthews, C.E., Berrington de, G.A., Park, Y., Katki, H.A. et al. (2012) Leisure time physical activity of moderate to vigorous intensity and mortality: a large pooled cohort analysis. *PLoS Medicine* 9: e1001335. doi: 10.1371/journal.pmed.1001335.

Myers, J., Prakash, M., Froelicher, V., Do, D., Partington, S. and Atwood, J.E. (2002) Exercise capacity and mortality among men referred for exercise testing. *New England Journal of Medicine* 346: 793–801.

Paffenbarger, R.S., Hyde, R.T., Wing, A.L. and Hsieh, C.C. (1986) Physical activity, all-cause mortality, and longevity of college alumni. *New England Journal of Medicine* 314: 605–13.

Paffenbarger, R.S., Hyde, R.T., Wing, A.L., Lee, I.-M., Jung, D.L. and Kampert, J.B. (1993) The association of changes in physical-activity level and other lifestyle characteristics with mortality among men. *New England Journal of Medicine* 328: 538–45.

Patterson, R., McNamara, E., Tainio, M., de Sá, T.H., Smith, A.D., Sharp, S.J. et al. (2018) Sedentary behaviour and risk of all-cause, cardiovascular and cancer mortality, and incident type 2 diabetes: a systematic review and dose response meta-analysis. *European Journal of Epidemiology* 33: 811–29.

Samitz, G., Egger, M. and Zwahlen, M. (2011) Domains of physical activity and all-cause mortality: systematic review and dose-response meta-analysis of cohort studies. *International Journal of Epidemiology* 40: 1382–400.

Schnohr, P., Scharling, H. and Jensen, J.S. (2003) Changes in leisure-time physical activity and risk of death: an observational study of 7,000 men and women. *American Journal of Epidemiology* 158: 639–44.

Stamatakis, E., Ekelund, U., Ding, D., Hamer, M., Bauman, A.E. and Lee, I.-M. (2019) Is the time right for quantitative public health guidelines on sitting? A narrative review of sedentary behaviour research paradigms and findings. *British Journal of Sports Medicine* 53: 377–82.

Stamatakis, E., Hamer, M., O'Donovan, G., Batty, G.D. and Kivimaki, M. (2013) A non-exercise testing method for estimating cardiorespiratory fitness: associations with all-cause and cardiovascular mortality in a pooled analysis of eight population-based cohorts. *European Heart Journal* 34: 750–8.

Stamatakis, E., Lee, I.-M., Bennie, J., Freeston, J., Hamer, M., O'Donovan, G. et al. (2018) Does strength-promoting exercise confer unique health benefits? A pooled analysis of data on 11 population cohorts with all-cause, cancer, and cardiovascular mortality endpoints. *American Journal of Epidemiology* 187: 1102–12.

Stensvold, D., Viken, H., Rognmo, O., Skogvoll, E., Steinshamn, S., Vatten, L.J. et al. (2015) A randomised controlled study of the long-term effects of exercise training on mortality in elderly people: study protocol for the Generation 100 study. *British Medical Journal Open* 5: e007519. doi: 10.1136/bmjopen-2014–007519.

Strain, T., Wijndaele, K., Dempsey, P.C., Sharp, S.J., Pearce, M., Jeon, J. et al. (2020) Wearable-device-measured physical activity and future health risk. *Nature Medicine* 26: 1385–91.

Talbot, L.A., Morrell, C.H., Fleg, J.L. and Metter, E.J. (2007) Changes in leisure time physical activity and risk of all-cause mortality in men and women: the Baltimore Longitudinal Study of Aging. *Preventive Medicine* 45: 169–76.

Taylor, H.L., Klepetar, E., Keys, A., Parlin, W., Blackburn, H. and Puchner, T. (1962) Death rates among physically active and sedentary employees of the railroad industry. *American Journal of Public Health and the Nation's Health* 52: 1697–707.

Wannamethee, S.G., Shaper, A.G. and Walker, M. (1998) Changes in physical activity, mortality, and incidence of coronary heart disease in older men. *The Lancet* 351: 1603–8.

Wei, M., Kampert, J.B., Barlow, C.E., Nichaman, M.Z., Gibbons, L.W., Paffenbarger, R.S. and Blair, S.N. (1999) Relationship between low cardiorespiratory fitness and mortality in normal-weight, overweight, and obese men. *Journal of the American Medical Association* 282: 1547–53.

Wen, C.P., Wai, J.P., Tsai, M.K., Yang, Y.C., Cheng, T.Y., Lee, M.C. et al. (2011) Minimum amount of physical activity for reduced mortality and extended life expectancy: a prospective cohort study. *The Lancet* 378: 1244–53.

Part II
Influence of physical activity on the risk of disease

4 Cardiovascular disease

Stephen F. Burns

INTRODUCTION

Cardiovascular diseases (CVDs), primarily coronary heart disease (CHD), accounted for over half the deaths in the United Kingdom in the early 1960s and 1970s. Cohort studies around that time discovered that this epidemic, which affected many Western countries, was largely due to environmental influences. One key environmental influence related to CHD occurrence is physical activity. In the previous chapter, evidence was presented that people who are physically active or fit are less likely to die over a defined period than those who are inactive and/or unfit. This chapter shows that one important reason for this is that individuals who are active and fit experience a lower incidence of CVD. More than 60 years after Professor Jeremy Morris's pioneering studies, the evidence that physical inactivity and low fitness are risk factors for CVD is compelling. This evidence will be presented in accordance with the principles set out in Chapter 2. First, however, it is important to clarify the term CVD.

WHAT IS CVD?

CVD is the name of a group of diseases of the heart and blood vessels (Box 4.1). The main disease endpoints for primary prevention that have been studied in relation to physical activity or fitness are CHD, stroke and hypertension. In CHD, myocardial blood flow is compromised because of progressive narrowing or sudden blocking of a coronary artery or arteries. When blood flow to the myocardium is impaired a heart attack occurs, either because a thrombus forms or because the artery goes into spasm. The extent of the myocardial damage depends on the site of the obstruction; if flow is interrupted to a large area, the attack is life-threatening because the heart no longer effectively pumps oxygenated blood around the body. A stroke causes neurological damage either because a blood vessel in the brain becomes blocked or because there is bleeding into the tissues of the brain from a ruptured vessel. Hypertension is the term for abnormally high arterial blood pressure which increases the work of the heart, damages the arterial wall and increases the possibility that a blood vessel in the brain will rupture. As a modifiable risk factor for CVD, evidence showing that physical activity can modify the occurrence of hypertension is presented in Chapter 7. There is less evidence for primary prevention of other types of CVD in relation to physical activity but they are included in Box 4.1 for completeness. The components of classification in Box 4.1 are not mutually exclusive. For example, heart failure is the principal manifestation of coronary atherosclerosis, heart attack, damaged valves or hypertension. For physical activity as a strategy for secondary prevention of CVD, endpoints have been examined for CHD, stroke and heart failure, along with appraising physical activity as a therapy for improving quality of life outcomes.

GLOBAL IMPACT OF CVD

It was estimated that worldwide there were 422.7 million cases of CVD in 2015. The prevalence ranged from <5,000 cases per 100,000 individuals in countries such as Australia, Greece, Ireland, Israel, Italy, Japan, New Zealand, Singapore and South Korea

---

BOX 4.1 CATEGORIES OF CVD.

- Cardiomyopathies: disorders that occur due to major structural abnormalities of the myocardium.
- Cerebrovascular disease (stroke): this can be due to the formation of a thrombus (blood clot), that is, a thromboembolytic or ischaemic stroke, or to a bleed into the brain, that is, a haemorrhagic stroke.
- CHD (ischaemic heart disease): this category includes angina and myocardial infarction (heart attack).
- Heart failure: the heart is unable to pump blood forward at a rate sufficient to meet the metabolic demands of the body, usually because of impaired left ventricular function.
- Hypertension (high blood pressure).
- Peripheral vascular disease: this is a narrowing of peripheral arteries which compromises blood flow. This most often affects the femoral artery, causing pain on walking.
- Rheumatic heart disease: the valves of the heart are damaged, impairing its capability to control the direction of blood flow.

---

to >9,000 cases per 100,000 in Iran, Madagascar, Mozambique, Morocco, Oman and Zambia. In the same year, CVD accounted for 17.9 million deaths and was the most common cause of death globally (Roth et al. 2017). In Europe, for example, nearly half of all deaths – 47% in women and 42% in men – were from CVD in 2012, primarily CHD and stroke. CHD is the most common cause of death in Europe and was responsible for 1.8 million deaths; stroke was the second most common cause, accounting for almost 1.1 million deaths (Nichols et al. 2012) (Figure 4.1).

Worldwide, age-standardised death rates from CVD vary greatly, with reported death rates from heart disease and stroke in 2008 as low as 29.2 and 21.7 deaths per 100,000 of the population in France and as high as 399.8 and 125.1 in Ukraine (World Health Organization 2011) (Figure 4.2). Trends over time vary substantially among countries. In the United Kingdom, for example, death rates from CHD in men aged <65 years fell from 137 per 100,000 of the population in 1981 to 33 per 100,000 in 2009. Conversely, in Belarus CHD mortality in men increased from 137 to 213 per 100,000 over the same period (Nichols et al. 2012). These strong temporal changes, within populations with presumably relatively stable gene pools, illustrate the important contribution from environmental factors, including physical activity, to the aetiology of CHD.

This chapter discusses the relationship between physical activity and fitness with CVD. The relationship of physical activity/fitness with CVD risk factors will be touched upon here but dealt with in detail in Chapter 7. Before examining these relationships, the process of atherosclerosis, which is by far the most important cause of CVD, and its complications will be discussed.

ATHEROSCLEROSIS

Atherosclerosis is a process which begins early in life and is considered by far the most important cause of CVD. In a landmark study published in 1953 pathologists

Figure 4.1 Proportion of deaths from coronary heart disease (CHD), stroke and other cardiovascular diseases (CVDs) in men and women in Europe.

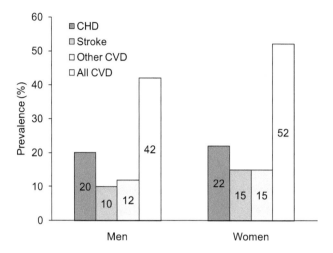

Source: Nichols et al. (2012).
Notes: Statistics are for the latest available year.

Figure 4.2 Age standardised death rates from ischaemic heart disease (IHD) and stroke per 100,000 population for selected countries in 2008.

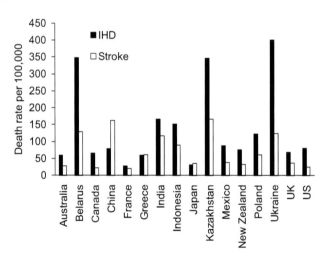

Source: World Health Organization (2011).
Notes: Observe the wide variation in rates.

conducting autopsies of US soldiers killed in action in the Korean War observed gross evidence of atherosclerotic plaques in 77% of the men, despite the fact that the average age was only 22 years (Enos et al. 1953). A subsequent report included autopsy data on young Japanese men (20–30 years old). Here, although lesions were found in 65% of cases, no plaques over 50% luminal narrowing – the threshold for clinical symptoms – were observed, whereas 20 such cases were found among the American men (Enos et al. 1955). Later autopsy reports of US soldiers who died in the Vietnam War found that most of these young men did not have severe atherosclerosis (McNamara et al. 1971). The reason for this discrepancy is unclear, but some evidence of atherosclerosis was found in all these reports, confirming that the disease begins early in life. More recent autopsy data from 2,876 individuals in the US aged 15 to 34 years who had died from external causes reinforces this notion. Fatty streaks and intimal lesions appeared in all the aortas examined and in more than half of the right coronary arteries of the youngest age group (aged 15–19 years) and these increased in prevalence and extent with age (oldest age group 30–34 years) irrespective of sex or race (Strong et al. 1999).

The pathological hallmarks of atherosclerosis are the fatty streak (the earliest visible lesions) and the fibrous plaque (advanced lesions that are the source of clinical symptoms). The mechanisms responsible for atherosclerosis are built on the 'response to injury' hypothesis proposed in the early 1970s. This states that the disease begins with an injury – a lesion – to the endothelium, the inner lining of the artery, which may be caused by numerous factors such as elevated or modified low-density lipoprotein (LDL), high blood pressure (hypertension), type 2 diabetes mellitus or smoking (for in-depth discussion of cardiovascular risk factors please see Chapter 7). The wall of normal muscular arteries consists of three layers: the intima (the most 'intimate' with the blood), the media (the middle layer) and the outer adventitia. The intima – the battleground of the atherosclerotic process – comprises a single layer of endothelial cells that rests on a bed of connective tissue.

Normal endothelial cells serve several critically important functions: they comprise a barrier restricting the passage of large molecules and cells; they resist thrombosis (the formation of blood clots) through releasing anti-clotting molecules and platelet inhibitors; they help regulate the blood flow to meet metabolic needs by secreting vasodilator substances; and they inhibit the proliferation and migration of smooth muscle cells. Endothelial injury or dysfunction in a lesion-prone area of the vasculature alters these normal functions. Leukocytes or platelets migrate and adhere to the site of injury, increasing the permeability of the endothelium itself. An inflammatory process begins, which, if not effective in controlling the offending agents, can continue unabated, stimulating proliferation of smooth muscle cells at the site and thickening the artery wall. In response, the artery may compensate by gradually dilating so that lumen size, and consequently blood flow, remains unaltered – a term called 'remodelling'. Over time, continued inflammation at the lesion causes white blood cells, called monocytes, to adhere and subsequently cross the endothelium where they become macrophages which engulf oxidised lipids, causing them to take on a 'foamy' appearance. These macrophages multiply within the lesion along with smooth muscle cells which proliferate and produce collagen and other molecules that further enlarge and increase the bulk of the lesion which may become covered by a fibrous cap covering the fat and cellular debris within and a fibrous plaque is formed. The artery may compensate for this increased deposition via dilation and the lesion intrudes into the lumen, compromising blood flow. Moreover, some lipid-laden macrophages within the lesion may emigrate back into the bloodstream. If this occurs at sites where blood flow is turbulent, such as where an artery branches or bifurcates, thrombi can form. The site of the lesion can also become calcified, reducing the artery's elasticity (Ross 1993, 1999).

Figure 4.3 Cross-sectional and longitudinal view of an artery that has undergone remodelling with the development of atheromatous plaque. The thin fibrous cap has ruptured and provoked the formation of a thrombus.

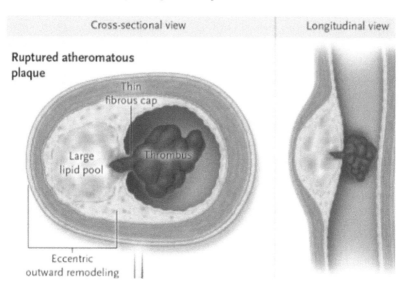

Source: From the *New England Journal of Medicine*, Libby, P., 'Mechanisms of acute coronary syndromes and their implications for therapy', 368: 2004–13. Copyright © 2013 Massachusetts Medical Society. Reprinted with permission from Massachusetts Medical Society.

The traditional view of this atherosclerotic process suggested that continued proliferation and deposition of smooth muscle cells within the plaque caused a marked stenosis (narrowing) of the arterial lumen leading to ischaemia and a myocardial infarction. However, clinical data have affirmed that invasive procedures which treat stenoses do not prevent future thrombotic events more effectively than non-invasive procedures (Boden et al. 2007; Hochman et al. 2006). Indeed, at least 12 randomised trials between 1987 and 2007 and involving >5,000 patients found no reduction in myocardial infarction attributable to angioplasty (a procedure to open up a blocked artery using a catheter) (Rothberg 2013). Current thinking and evidence focus instead on plaque rupture, exposing pro-thrombotic material from the core of the plaque to the blood, as the most common cause of fatal coronary syndromes (Figure 4.3). Studies examining the characteristics of plaques that have ruptured identify them as having thin fibrous caps (50 to 65 μm thick), large lipid cores, an abundance of inflammatory cells and punctuated calcification. An abundance of activated immune cells where the fibrous cap is thin produces the pro-inflammatory molecules and proteolytic enzymes. These disrupt and weaken the collagen matrix which provides the tensile strength to the cap jeopardising its integrity. Moreover, they can initiate thrombus formation by activating cells in the core of the plaque. This process can thus transform a stable plaque into a vulnerable, unstable one, prone to rupture, which subsequently induces a thrombus leading to an acute coronary syndrome (Hansson 2005; Libby 2013) (Figure 4.4). Indeed, one autopsy study found that a fibrous-cap thickness of 55 μm was the best indicator of plaques that cause fatal ruptures even though more than 30% were associated with a luminal stenosis of less than 75% and with few smooth muscle cells (Narula et al. 2013).

Figure 4.4 Cross-section of a coronary artery from a patient who died of a myocardial infarction.

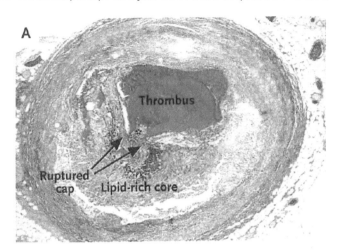

Source: From the *New England Journal of Medicine*, Hansson, G.K., 'Inflammation, atherosclerosis, and coronary artery disease', 352: 1685–95. Copyright © 2005 Massachusetts Medical Society. Reprinted with permission from Massachusetts Medical Society.
Note: There is an occlusive thrombus superimposed on a lipid-rich atherosclerotic plaque. The fibrous cap covering the lipid-rich core has ruptured (area between the arrows), exposing the thrombogenic core to the blood.

ATHEROSCLEROSIS – GENETIC AND ENVIRONMENTAL INFLUENCES

Many scientists assume that the widespread prevalence of atherosclerotic lesions at an early age is lifestyle related and driven by post-industrial and modern agricultural lifestyles and that reversal of such lifestyles could potentially prevent atherosclerosis or avoid its clinical manifestations. However, a unique examination of 137 mummies, from four different geographical regions and populations spanning more than 4,000 years analysed for the presence of calcified plaques challenges this hypothesis. Atherosclerosis was present in the aorta of 20% of the mummies and existed in 12% of carotid arteries and 4% of coronary arteries. Moreover, estimated age at the time of death correlated significantly with the existence of atherosclerosis. That these findings were in individuals with different genetic backgrounds and environmental exposures across disparate geographical regions and chronological cultures raises the possibility that atherosclerosis is not simply associated with modern living but suggests a more basic human predisposition to the disease (Thompson et al. 2013). Evidence from a study of human foetal aortas supports this with foetal plasma cholesterol levels correlating with maternal cholesterol levels and those foetal aortas from mothers with high cholesterol showing the presence of lesions which were greater in number and larger in size (Napoli et al. 1997).

Nevertheless, the role of the environment in atherosclerotic development cannot be downplayed. A recent study of 705 Tsimane, a Bolivian people who survive via a lifestyle of subsistence hunting, gathering, fishing and farming, showed that 85% were free from coronary artery calcium – a marker of atherosclerotic disease. Even in

Figure 4.5 Percentage of Tsimane with moderately increased coronary artery calcium (CAC) (score >100) compared with individuals in the US Multiethnic Study of Atherosclerosis (MESA) by age group.

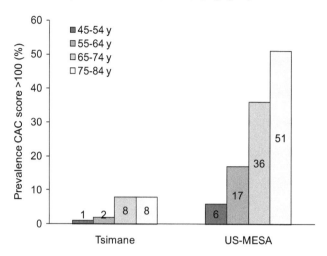

Source: Kaplan et al. (2017).

individuals aged 75 years or older, 65% were free of coronary artery calcium with only 8% of older individuals showing moderately increased levels. This compares with 51% of individuals from a multi-ethnic US cohort of the same age (Figure 4.5). Moreover, the prevalence of several coronary artery disease risk factors, including raised cholesterol, elevated blood glucose and high blood pressure, was low in all age groups among the Tsimane. In terms of lifestyle, Tsimane men and women spend 6–7 hours and 4–6 hours per day engaging in physical activity, respectively, and less than 10% of their daylight hours engaged in sedentary activities (Kaplan et al. 2017). Such observational evidence suggests that coronary atherosclerosis can be avoided with a lifetime of high physical activity coupled with a low number of coronary artery disease risk factors.

EPIDEMIOLOGY OF PHYSICAL ACTIVITY AND CHD

A historical context – the ground-breaking work of Jeremy Morris and Ralph Paffenbarger

That physical activity affords some protection against CHD was first discovered in studies of occupational activity. Professor Jeremy Morris and colleagues compared the incidence of heart attack in men in a variety of occupations. They found that drivers on London's double-decker buses were twice as likely to experience a heart attack or a 'sudden death' from a heart attack as the conductors who walked up and down stairs 11 days per fortnight for 50 weeks each year (Morris et al. 1953). Similarly, postmen, who spent much of their shift time walking, cycling and climbing stairs, had approximately half the incidence of mortality from heart disease as male telephone exchange workers who sat in chairs for most of their work time. Whilst these studies were seminal in establishing the hypothesis that physical activity through work offered protection from CHD and mortality, self-selection bias was a major weakness: did healthier and leaner men seek more physically active jobs? To account for some of this difference Morris and colleagues subsequently examined the trouser waist measurement of the uniforms issued to the London busmen as a crude proxy for central obesity (Chapter 6). Irrespective of the category of waist size – small or large – the death rates and likelihood of experiencing a CHD event in the conductors was about half that of the drivers (Heady et al. 1961). Thus, it seemed as if physical activity imparted some protection against coronary events irrespective of body fatness.

At a similar time to these studies of Morris and colleagues, Professor Ralph Paffenbarger and co-workers were investigating the work activity of 6,351 San Francisco dock workers (longshoremen) aged 35 to 75 years. The work of these longshoremen was classified as light, moderate or heavy according to measurements of oxygen uptake. Overall death rates from CHD of the dockworkers engaged in heavy activity was approximately half that of those in medium to light activity categories (Figure 4.6). Notably, the issue of selection bias was overcome as the dockworkers were assigned to their positions, at least upon initial entry into the industry (Paffenbarger and Hale 1975).

By the late 1960s heavy occupational work was declining in developed countries. Thus, it became clear that the populations of these countries would derive most of their activity from leisure-time pursuits. Two pioneering investigations on opposite sides of the Atlantic were instrumental in demonstrating that individuals could reduce their risks

Figure 4.6 Death rates from CHD in San Francisco dockworkers between 1951 and 1972, according to intensity of physical activity at work and age at death.

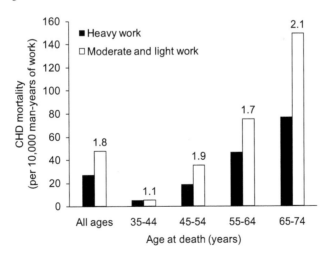

Source: Adapted from Paffenbarger and Hale (1975).
Notes: Open bars, moderate and light work at 6.3–20.9 kJ min^{-1} (1.5–5.0 kcal min^{-1}); dark bars heavy work at 21.8–31.4 kJ min^{-1} (5.1–7.5 kcal min^{-1}). Figures over bars show relative risk within each age band, with reference group as heavy work. Difference between heavy and moderate/light work significant for all ages ($P < 0.001$) and for men in all ten-year age bands ($P < 0.01$) except 35–44 years.

of CHD through leisure-time activity. The first of these studies recruited 16,936 men, aged 35 to 74 years, who graduated from Harvard University between 1916 and 1950 and collated information by questionnaire on their physical activity habits in 1962 or 1966. The alumni were followed until 1972 when records of fatal or non-fatal heart attacks were obtained. Several important observations emerged. Firstly, the risk of a heart attack was inversely related to total weekly estimates of energy expenditure in physical activity across all ages within an energy expenditure range of 2.1–8.4 MJ week^{-1} (<500–2000 kcal week^{-1}). Secondly, energy expenditure was not the only important exercise variable in mitigating risk. Strenuous but not light sports were associated with a significant decrease in heart attacks and the importance of the level of exertion during exercise was maintained even after adjusting for energy expenditure. Finally, only physical activity measured in middle age as a college alumnus conferred protection against a heart attack and not participation in sport during youth either as a varsity athlete or in recreational non-varsity sports as a student for >5 hours week^{-1} (Figure 4.7). This last observation is notable as it addresses the issue of self-selection through the argument that former varsity athletes may have inherited a sturdy constitution but this was not protective as only recent – but not past – physical activity was beneficial for reducing risk (Paffenbarger et al. 1978).

On the opposite side of the Atlantic, a study of 17,944 middle-aged British civil servants, initially recruited between 1968 and 1970, replicated the finding from the Harvard Alumni study in showing that exercise intensity was an important factor in protection from CHD. Morris and colleagues adopted a five-minute-by-five-minute record of how

Figure 4.7 Age-adjusted rates of first heart attack in alumni reporting high (>8.37 MJ week^{-1}) and low (<8.37 MJ week^{-1}) levels of estimated gross energy expenditure in physical activity as adults, according to past participation in university sport.

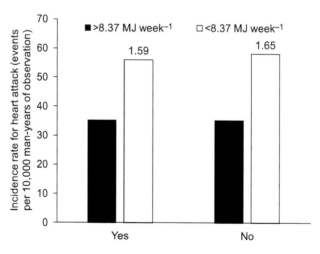

Source: Adapted from Paffenbarger et al. (1978).
Notes: Figures over bars show relative risk for the low activity group with the high activity group (>8.37 MJ week^{-1}) acting as the reference group.

these men spent the previous Friday and Saturday as the index of leisure-time physical activity at initial recruitment. The men were subsequently followed for 8.5 years and those reporting engaging in 30 minutes or more vigorous exercise (estimated as entailing peak rates of energy expenditure of 31.5 kJ min^{-1} (7.5 kcal min^{-1}) or more had an incidence of CHD less than half that of their sedentary counterparts who recorded no vigorous exercise (Morris et al. 1980). A later follow-up study in civil servants emphasised again the importance of vigorous activity with the most active men experiencing less than half the incidence of fatal and non-fatal heart attacks of the other men. Whilst vigorous activity included many sports it also equated to active transport in the form of walking at ≥6.4 km h^{-1} (4 mile h^{-1}) or cycling for approximately 40 km week^{-1} (25 miles week^{-1}) (Morris et al. 1990).

As explained in Chapter 2, examination of the influence of an exposure to a factor such as physical activity with a health-related outcome is often confounded in epidemiological studies by the presence of a third factor also associated with the health outcome. The studies of Harvard alumni and British civil servants attempted to address this issue by examining the interactions of both weekly energy expenditure in the alumni and exercise intensity in the civil servants with other risk factors for CHD. For those alumni whose physical activity energy expenditure >8.4 MJ week^{-1}, a reduced risk of heart attacks was maintained irrespective of factors such as smoking status, stature, body mass index (BMI), blood pressure, family history of the disease and participation in varsity sports (Paffenbarger et al. 1978). Similarly, in British civil servants, vigorous physical activity maintained its protective findings against CHD independently of confounding factors such as smoking, hypertension and high BMI (Morris et al. 1990) (Figure 4.8).

Building on the work of Morris and Paffenbarger

Since Morris and Paffenbarger's seminal studies, prospective epidemiological studies have consistently shown that regular physical activity is associated with a lower risk of CHD and CVD and this has been confirmed in a number of meta-analyses. One example is from Sattelmair and colleagues (2011) which included 645,087 individuals from 33 studies conducted between 1995 and 2009 assessing the relationship of physical activity with CHD. The overall risk reduction across all studies for individuals in the highest versus lowest category of physical activity was 25%. For leisure-time physical activity, individuals who completed 150 min week^{-1} of moderate-intensity physical activity, in line with the minimum recommended by public health guidelines, had a 14% reduction in CHD risk compared with those reporting no physical activity. Increasing this to 300 min week^{-1} lowered the risk by 20%. The data from this analysis are reassuringly similar to that reported in a meta-analysis of prospective CHD and CVD cohort studies in the Physical Activity Guidelines Advisory Committee Report 2008 (Physical Activity Guidelines Advisory Committee 2008) (Figure 4.9) and elsewhere (Arem et al. 2015; Nocon et al. 2008; Wahid et al. 2016) and collectively provide strong confirmation of the pioneering work of Morris and Paffenbarger.

Figure 4.8 Rates of CHD per 1,000 man-years of observation in English male civil servants grouped according to the frequency of vigorous aerobic exercise: (1) most frequent; (4) least frequent.

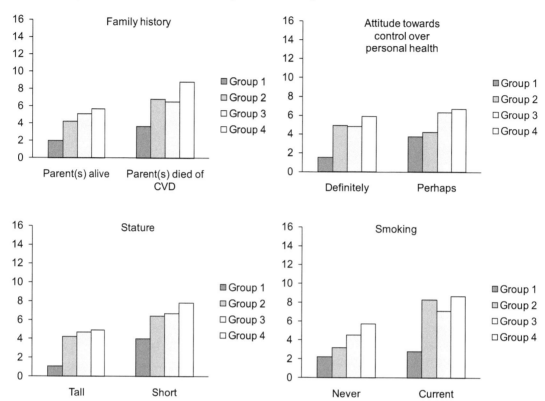

From Figure 4.9 it can be seen that the compelling evidence that physical activity affords protection against the risk of CHD in men extends to women as well. The Nurses' Health Study in the US is an example of one prospective study showing this. Data were collected on total physical activity, including walking, stair climbing and planned exercise, from 72,488 female nurses aged 40–65 years in 1986. Initial baseline information gathered in 1986 was updated every two years over eight years of follow-up. Comparable to observations in men, energy expended in physical activity was negatively associated with the number of coronary events in women, with those in the highest quintile of activity having less than half the risk of those in the lowest quintile even after adjusting for age, BMI, smoking status and parental history of the disease (Manson et al. 1999). Thus, for both sexes physically active individuals have a lower risk for CHD than their inactive counterparts.

The magnitude of risk reduction for CHD, however, appears to be greater in women than men. The aforementioned meta-analysis by Sattelmair and colleagues (2011) found that the relative risk reduction in the most active women was greater than that for the most active men by 0.10. Among studies assessing only leisure-time activity, those conducted in men showed a 22% reduction in risk from the most to least active

Figure 4.8 (continued)

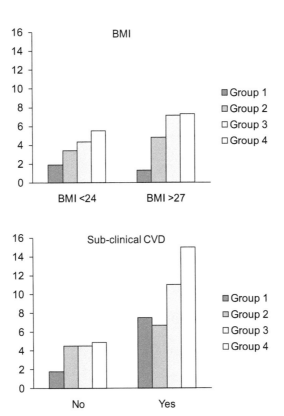

Source: Morris et al. (1990).
Notes: The association between vigorous aerobic exercise and low risk of CHD held across a variety of potentially confounding factors.

whereas for women it was 33%. This greater reduction in risk was also noted in the Physical Activity Guidelines Advisory Committee Report 2008 (see Figure 4.9) and by others (Shiroma and Lee 2010). Nevertheless, comparisons of risk reduction between the sexes have been difficult because different studies use varied questionnaires for assessment of physical activity and different categories of physical activity for analysis (e.g. energy expended, intensity of activities, duration or frequency). Moreover, this is also in part because activity levels of the least active women tend to be lower than those of the least active men. Thus, the category of physical activity used in analyses may represent different amounts and intensities of physical activity in women than men (Physical Activity Guidelines Advisory Committee 2008; Shiroma and Lee 2010). Another area not adequately addressed is whether the relationship between physical activity and CHD differs between pre- and post-menopausal women as studies have not distinguished the two groups.

As walking is the most common form of physical activity that adults perform and is acceptable and accessible to most individuals a number of large prospective studies

Figure 4.9 Median relative risk of CHD and CVD for men and women completing high intensity/amount or moderate intensity/amount of exercise in comparison with light intensity/amount of exercise.

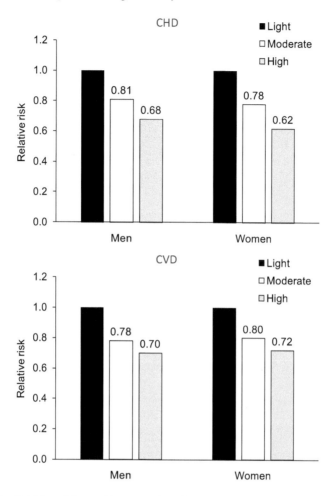

Source: Physical Activity Guidelines Advisory Committee (2008).
Notes: Data calculated from a meta-analysis of prospective cohort studies for CHD (men, n = 17 studies; women, n = 13 studies) and CVD (men, n = 10 studies; women, n = 12 studies). Relative risk includes risk ratio, odds ratio or hazard ratio.

have examined the importance of this activity independently of overall physical activity. In the US Nurses' Health Study, for example, both energy expended in walking and walking pace were negatively associated with coronary events and in terms of total energy expenditure, equivalent amounts of brisk walking and vigorous exercise appeared to confer the same magnitude of risk reduction and protective benefit (Manson et al. 1999). The Women's Health Study, also noted that time spent walking and walking pace were associated with lower CHD risk, although time was a more important variable in that study when analysed in a single model (Lee et al. 2001) (Figure 4.10). At least one meta-analysis of studies in women has confirmed the

Figure 4.10 Relative risk of CHD in US women involved in the Women's Health Study according to walking time (h week^{-1}) and walking speed (km h^{-1}).

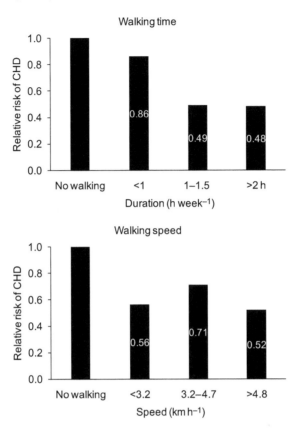

Source: Lee et al. (2001).
Notes: Data labels show relative risk with no walking group acting as the reference group. Relative risks are adjusted for age; randomised treatment assignment; smoking status; consumption of alcohol, saturated fat, fibre, and fruits and vegetables; menopausal status; use of postmenopausal hormones; and parental history of myocardial infarction at <60 years of age.

dose–response relationship of physical activity and walking with CHD events (Oguma and Shinoda-Tagawa 2004). A more recent study of data from the UK Biobank of 318,185 participants (54% women) aged 40–69 years with a mean of five years of follow-up looked at the association of walking pace and time with overall CVD. Compared with slow pace walkers, men and women who walked at an average or brisk pace had a reduced risk of CVD mortality and incidence. These associations were independent of other confounding factors including total physical activity. Furthermore, walking at a slow pace showed a higher hazard for CVD regardless of the time spent walking (Celis-Morales et al. 2019) (Figure 4.11). Collectively, these observations are supportive of the early findings from British civil servants and Harvard Alumni by Morris and Paffenbarger which emphasised the important of vigorous activity for the greatest protective benefit.

Figure 4.11 Hazard ratio for CVD mortality and incidence by walking pace and walking time tertiles in 244,093 men and women aged 40–69 years, recruited between 2007 and 2010 and followed to 2016, in the UK Biobank.

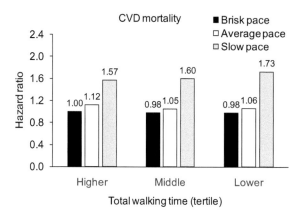

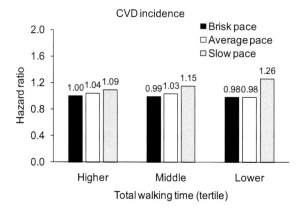

Source: Reprinted with permission from Wolters Kluwer Health, Inc: Celis-Morales, C.A. et al. (2019) 'Walking pace is associated with lower risk of all-cause and cause-specific mortality', *Medicine and Science in Sports and Exercise*, 51: 472–80. Available at: https://doi.org/10.1249/MSS.0000000000001795.

Notes: Data adjusted for month of recruitment, age, deprivation index, employment status, ethnicity, systolic blood pressure, medication for CVD, self-health rating, BMI categories, smoking, discretionary screen time, dietary intake (alcohol, red meat, processed meat, oily fish, processed meat and fruit and vegetables), hand-grip strength and moderate to vigorous physical activity. Slow pace walkers (<4.8 km h^{-1}; <3 mile h^{-1}), average pace (4.8–6.4 km h^{-1}; 3–4 mile h^{-1}) and brisk pace (>6.4 km h^{-1}; 4 mile h^{-1}). Higher risk of CVD mortality or incidence in all slow-pace walking groups, irrespective of walking time, in comparison with brisk pace and high walking time group.

One feature of many early studies examining the relationship of CHD with physical activity is that the populations studied were primarily of European descent or, where multi-ethnic populations were included, few had adequate sample sizes or number of events to be able to examine the ethnic associations between CHD and physical activity. Those that attempted such analyses were generally consistent in findings and outcomes with observations seen in individuals of European origin (Donahue et al. 1988; Hakim et al. 1999; Lam et al. 2004). More recently, two large multinational

Figure 4.12 Population-attributable risk (PAR) for myocardial infarction (MI) in different regions of the globe associated with <4 h week^{-1} of moderate or strenuous exercise.

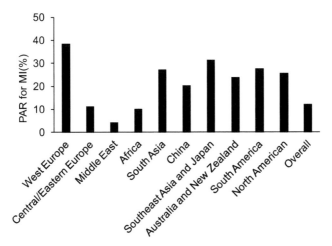

Source: Yusuf et al. (2004).
Notes: Overall data are adjusted for age, sex, smoking and other CVD risk factors.

studies demonstrated that physical activity affords protection across a range of ethnicities. The INTERHEART study examined the association of potentially modifiable coronary risk factors (please see below and Chapter 7) with myocardial infarction using data from case-control studies conducted in 52 countries. Physically active men and women, defined as those reporting doing >4 hours of moderate or vigorous intensity leisure-time physical activity each week, had a 14% lower risk of myocardial infarction than their inactive peers. The overall population-attributable risk from physical inactivity, calculated across all regions of the globe and adjusted for age, sex, smoking and other risk factors, was 12.2% (9.3% in men and 27.1% in women) (Yusuf et al. 2004) (Figure 4.12). Similarly, the Prospective Urban Rural Epidemiologic (PURE) study used the International Physical Activity Questionnaire (Chapter 2) to measure total physical activity time in 130,843 individuals from 17 countries spanning four continents. There was a graded reduction in major CVD events, CVD mortality and myocardial infarction over approximately seven years of follow-up in participants classified as low, moderate or high physical activity. Stratified by country income level, there was also a consistent reduction in risk with increasing total physical activity (Lear et al. 2017). Such data help confirm the dose-dependent benefits of physical activity on heart diseases across multi-ethnic cohorts in countries with varied income. Nevertheless, more studies providing direct cross-ethnic cohort comparisons of risk reduction from physical activity for CVD and CHD are needed, as studies in the US have found contrasting findings when comparing black and non-black men and women (Folsom et al. 1997; Manson et al. 2002).

Fewer studies have examined the relationship of physical activity with CHD incidence exclusively in older adults (>60 years). In the Honolulu Heart Program, which prospectively followed men of Japanese ancestry over 12 years, the most active men over 65 years had a 60% reduction in risk compared with the least active (Donahue et al. 1988). Moreover, those men aged 71–93 years who walked >2.4 km per day experienced half the CHD risk of those who walked less than this (Hakim et al. 1999). The ten-year Zutphen Elderly Study in the Netherlands found that men aged 64–84 years who walked or cycled at least three times weekly for 20 minutes each time experienced a 31% reduction in CHD mortality in comparison with their less active counterparts (Bijnen et al. 1998). Similarly, the Rancho Bernado study of community-dwelling individuals aged 50–90 years (82% of individuals were >60 years) from southern California showed that self-reported exercise at least three times per week reduced CHD incidence by 51% compared with a frequency of exercise less than this (Smith et al. 2007).

Most studies have assessed either only total or leisure-time physical activity but one meta-analysis including 13 prospective cohort studies has attempted to compare the protective effect of physical activity undertaken in different domains – occupational versus leisure time – on CHD. Both moderate and high levels of leisure time and occupational physical activity provided protective effects against CHD. For men, risk reductions with moderate-intensity leisure-time and occupational physical activity were comparable at 15% and 13%, respectively. Higher intensity leisure-time activity provided some further overall reduction in risk (21%) but not occupational activity (9%). For women, a similar pattern was seen, with no further reduction in risk between moderate (25%) and higher (20%) intensity occupational activity, whereas in the leisure-time domain the reduction in risk increased from 22% for moderate-intensity activity to 29% for higher-intensity activity (Li and Siegrist 2012). However, the data are overall supportive of the proposition that similar reductions in risk can be obtained through moderate-intensity activity in both men and women irrespective of which domain it is accrued in.

Finally, the studies described in this section have used either a single or multiple measures of self-report physical activity, which may have led to misclassification of the activity or recall bias. The prospective nature of the study designs means that this misclassification is most likely random and thus would tend to attenuate observed findings toward the null. Moreover, recall bias would probably be prevented as participants could not be influenced by the presence of the disease because they reported their physical activity before the onset of the disease (Shiroma and Lee 2010). Nevertheless, the emergence of more objective measures of physical activity in large-scale studies can overcome these potential criticisms and increase the accuracy of the data. A pioneering study, following 851 Swedish adults (56% women) aged ≥35 years for a mean duration of 14.2 years with 12,117 person-years of risk, examined the protective effect of physical activity measured using an accelerometer on CVD mortality. A total of 828 individuals (97%) had ≥4 valid days of accelerometer wear and 570 participants (66%) had one week of valid data. The average daily wear time was 14.5 hours. The hazard ratio, adjusted for confounding factors, showed that compared with individuals in the lowest tertile of moderate-to-vigorous physical activity each day, those in the middle and highest tertile had substantial reductions in CVD mortality (Dohrn et al. 2018) (Figure 4.13). These attenuations in risk are large compared with the approximate 30% reduction for high level of activity shown in Figure 4.9 at the start of this section and perhaps reflect improved assessment with more accurate measures of physical activity. Nevertheless, the number of overall cases of CVD (19 cases) in this objective report was low and the data need confirmation.

Figure 4.13 Hazard ratio for CVD mortality by tertile of accelerometer-determined moderate-to-vigorous physical activity for men and women in the Sweden Attitude Behavior and Change study.

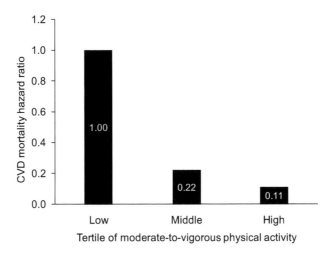

Source: Dohrn et al. (2018).
Notes: Data labels show CVD mortality hazard ratio with low tertile as the reference group. Mean moderate-to-vigorous physical activity in each tertile: low, 9.3 minutes day^{-1}; middle, 26.0 minutes day^{-1}; and high, 59.2 minutes day^{-1}. Data are adjusted for education, smoking and health conditions at baseline (hypertension, heart disease, cancer, diabetes).

SEDENTARY BEHAVIOUR AND CVD

The collective evidence from observational epidemiological studies in the previous section suggests that individuals who are regularly physically active are afforded some protection against CHD and CVD compared with their less active counterparts. In the studies highlighted individuals were classified as active or inactive based on measures, either self-reported or quantitative, of their physical activity level. Whilst this approach accounts for differences in physical activity among individuals it does not quantify the amount of time people spend in sedentary activities. Sedentary behaviour is not simply the time spent outside of physical activity as international definitions of physical activity define a minimal duration for each bout of activity as ten minutes and stipulate that activity should be moderate-to-vigorous intensity in nature. These definitions often do not account for time spent in light physical activities, such as slow walking or some household activities, which are distinct from sedentary behaviours such as sitting, lying down or screen time which do not substantially raise the metabolic rate. Although no consensus definition of sedentary behaviour is available, the two most prominent definitions are: (i) 'activities that involve energy expenditure at the level of 1.0–1.5 metabolic equivalents (METs)' (Pate et al. 2008); and (ii) 'any waking behaviour characterized by an energy expenditure ≤1.5 METs while in a sitting or reclining posture' (Sedentary Behaviour Research Network 2012). In both definitions, sedentary behaviour is considered ≤1.5 METs, which differs from light physical activity classified as 1.5–2.9 METs. The second definition also adds in an element of posture, however, which provides researchers the ability to test out hypotheses associated with this, such as whether standing is associated with better health outcomes than sitting.

Quantification of sedentary behaviours is considered important (Box 4.2) and a substantial body of research has emerged supporting the proposition that sedentary behaviours confer an independent risk for CVD. Whilst there are differences in reports about the prevalence of sedentary behaviours, with considerable variation by country and region (Bauman et al. 2011; Hallal et al. 2012), there may be underestimations in how much time populations spend sedentary as self-report questionnaires are poorly suited to measuring time spent in these behaviours each day. Moreover, there are reported declines in occupational and household physical activity in some countries (Church et al. 2011). One model of changes in physical activity-related energy expenditure and sedentary time suggested that time spent in sedentary activity increased from 26.4 to 37.7 h week^{-1} (42.7% increase) in the US and from 28.4 to 41.7 h week^{-1} (46.6% increase) in the UK between the early 1960s and the early 2000s (Ng and Popkin 2012).

The impact of these sedentary behaviours on CVD risk has been described in prospective studies and meta-analyses. One early prospective study analysed the impact of daily sitting time and leisure-time physical activity on CVD mortality in 17,103 Canadians aged 18–90 years who participated in the Canada Fitness Survey of 1981. Evaluation of daily sitting, measured by questionnaire, showed progressively increasing risk across the spectrum, with individuals who reported spending all their time seated approximately 1.5 times more likely to die from CVD than those who reported spending no time sitting. Importantly, the association held true for confounding factors including leisure-time physical activity (Katzmarzyk et al. 2009). Subsequent studies elsewhere have noted similar findings and two recent systematic reviews and meta-analyses have provided more confirmatory evidence. The first of these studies, encompassing 41 studies with 551,366 participants, found greater risk of CVD incidence and mortality associated with sedentary behaviours which remained significant after adjustment for physical activity (Biswas et al. 2015). The second examined the joint

---

BOX 4.2 REASONS TO QUANTIFY SEDENTARY BEHAVIOURS.

- Sedentary behaviours have become widespread as reductions in occupational physical activity have occurred.
- There is evidence from population-based studies in some countries that many people spend as much as half their waking day pursuing sedentary activities associated with prolonged sitting such as watching television and using computers (Matthews et al. 2008).
- Whilst physical activity confers protection against lifestyle diseases, such as CVD, sedentary behaviours such as sitting have deleterious health effects which are independent of physical activity.
- Sedentary behaviours and physical inactivity can be mutually exclusive. An individual can achieve international physical activity recommendations each day but spend the rest of their waking hours in sedentary activities. Conversely, other individuals may not meet physical activity recommendations but may spend substantial periods of each day in non-sedentary activities because of their workplace environment.

Figure 4.14 Hazard ratios for CVD mortality in relation to total physical activity and sitting time in 849,108 men and women pooled from nine studies.

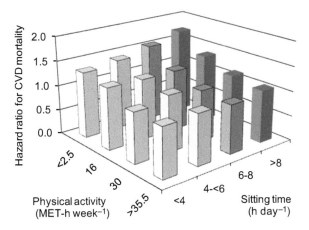

Source: Ekelund et al. (2016).
Notes: Data show hazard ratios in comparison with the reference group completing ≥35.5 MET-h week^{-1} of physical activity and sitting for <4 h day^{-1}. Data for physical activity are in quartiles. Note that sitting time did not increase risk of CVD mortality in individuals completing ≥35.5 MET-h week^{-1} of physical activity.

association of sedentary behaviour and physical activity with cardiovascular mortality. Compared with those who sat for less than four hours per day and were most active, cardiovascular mortality rates were 34% greater in the least active individuals who sat for <4 hours per day and 74% higher in the least active individuals who sat for >8 hours per day (Figure 4.14). A similar result was seen when television viewing time was used as a proxy measure of sedentary behaviour. One exception was that the associations of sedentary time with cardiovascular mortality were eliminated in individuals who reported the highest physical activity levels, i.e. >35.5 MET-h week^{-1}, which is equivalent to 60–75 minutes of moderate-intensity physical activity per day. Thus, very high levels of physical activity can offset some of the negative consequences of sedentary behaviour on CVD (Ekelund et al. 2016).

EPIDEMIOLOGY OF PHYSICAL FITNESS AND CHD

Some of the difficulties surrounding measures of physical activity were outlined in Chapter 2. Some investigators have sought to avoid these by measuring the characteristics exhibited by people who are physically active; that is, fitness, rather than the behaviour (physical activity/exercise) that leads to fitness. However, fitness is more than just a marker of physical activity habits. Several months of moderate-to-vigorous aerobic exercise can improve maximum oxygen uptake in previously sedentary adults by 15–25% whilst three weeks of bed rest leads to a 26% decrease in the same measure (Saltin et al. 1968; Skinner et al. 2000). Nevertheless, cardiorespiratory fitness is a result of interactions between environmental, constitutional and genetic factors with genes accounting for 40–50% of the between-person variation in the change in maximum oxygen uptake in response to endurance training (Bouchard et al. 1999; Bouchard et al. 2011; DeFina et al. 2015). Thus, as discussed later, it is possible for some individuals to have low activity levels but high fitness and vice versa.

A number of investigations have reported that low fitness appears to be a stronger risk factor for CHD than physical inactivity. An early report was from the Aerobic Center Longitudinal Study (the results of this study with respect to all-cause mortality are described in Chapter 3), where fitness was measured as time to exhaustion on a maximal treadmill test (a surrogate for maximal oxygen uptake) in more than 25,000 men. Steven Blair and colleagues found that the relative risk of low fitness (bottom quintile of study population versus all other men) was 1.70, a higher relative risk than often reported for physical inactivity. Based on comparisons within the same study population, the relative risk of low fitness was also higher than that observed for smoking (relative risk 1.57), systolic blood pressure ≥140 mm Hg (1.34), high cholesterol ≥6.2 mmol l^{-1} (1.65) or parental death from CHD (1.18). These estimates represent the independent risk associated with each factor as they are corrected for each other, as well as for body mass (Blair et al. 1996).

Other early studies supported the association of greater physical fitness with reduced risk of CHD (Ekelund et al. 1988; Lakka et al. 1994; Laukannen et al. 2001, 2004). One example was the Kuopio Ischemic Heart Disease Risk Factor Study in Eastern Finland, which made direct measurements of expired air during exercise to determine maximum oxygen uptake in 2,361 men aged 42–60 years. Fatal and non-fatal cardiac events were examined both in men with and without conventional cardiovascular risk factors, over a 13-year follow-up period. For both groups of men, each 1 MET (see Box 4.3) increase in maximum oxygen uptake translated to a 17–29% decrease in non-fatal and 28–51% decrease in fatal cardiac events, after adjustment for age (Laukannen et al. 2004). Other data on 854 men from the same study showed that a higher maximum oxygen uptake had a strong, inverse and graded association with increases in intima-media thickness of the carotid artery. This suggests that fitness is associated with a slower progression of clinical atherosclerosis as well as decreased risk of CHD/CVD events themselves (Lakka et al. 2001).

As with physical activity, many early studies on fitness focused on men. Although data now exist for women, there have been surprisingly few attempts to examine the sex-specific relationships between cardiorespiratory fitness and CHD. A meta-analysis of 24 eligible studies, including 84,323 men and women, noted that individuals in the lowest tertile of cardiorespiratory fitness had a relative risk for a CVD/CHD event of 1.40 and 1.47 compared with those in the high and intermediate tertiles of fitness (Kodama et al. 2009). However, no attempt was made to independently examine the results by sex. One investigation compared non-fatal CVD events in 20,728 men and 5,909 women who performed a maximal treadmill test in the Aerobic Center Longitudinal Study between 1971 and 2004 and found an inverse pattern of association between cardiorespiratory fitness with non-fatal CVD and CHD events in both men and women. However, in women the association did not remain significant after adjustment for confounding factors possibly because of the smaller number of events overall (Sui et al. 2007).

BOX 4.3 ENERGY EXPENDITURE DURING EXERCISE – RELATIONSHIPS WITH OXYGEN UPTAKE.

During sub-maximal exercise the majority of energy comes from the oxidation of fat and carbohydrate. The rate of oxygen uptake therefore reflects the rate of energy expenditure (metabolic rate). The exact energy expenditure per litre of oxygen depends on the proportion of fat and carbohydrate being oxidised, but if it is assumed that both contribute equally to energy metabolism, each litre of oxygen taken up is equivalent to an energy expenditure of 20.5 kJ (~5 kcal).
   Examples from the epidemiology:

- Morris's studies of male English civil servants defined exercise as vigorous if the rate of energy expenditure reached peaks of ≥ 31.4 kJ min^{-1} (7.5 kcal min^{-1}). This is equivalent to an oxygen uptake of $31.4/20.5 = 1.53$ l min^{-1}.
  Question – what does this mean in terms of exercise for these men?
  Answer – metabolic rate depends on body mass. For purposes of estimating and describing exercise intensity, metabolic rate has been defined as 3.5 ml of oxygen per kilogram of body mass per minute, that is, 3.5 ml kg^{-1} min^{-1} or 1 MET. If we assume that the civil servants typically weighed 78 kg, then an oxygen uptake of 1.53 l min^{-1} represents about 20 ml kg^{-1} min^{-1} or 5.7 METs. Activities such as easy cycling or doubles tennis typically demand this rate of oxygen uptake.
- In the Harvard Alumni Study, a threshold value for gross weekly energy expenditure in physical activity of 8.37 MJ (2,000 kcal) has often been used.
  Question – what does this equate to in terms that are readily understood?
  Answer – let us look at this from the point of view of, say, brisk walking. Walking briskly at 6.4 km h^{-1} (4 mile h^{-1}) demands about 4 METs, an oxygen uptake of (3.5 × 4) or 14 ml kg^{-1} min^{-1}. Assuming a body mass of 78 kg, this means 1.09 l min^{-1} and energy expenditure at a rate of (1.09 × 20.5) or 22.3 kJ min^{-1}. Thus, a total gross energy expenditure of 8.37 MJ per week is equivalent to: $8,370/22.3 = 375$ minutes (6 hours and 15 minutes) of brisk walking, about 40 km (25 miles).
- In the US Nurses' Health Study, walking is expressed in MET-h $week^{-1}$.
  Question – the median value for nurses in the top quintile for walking was 20 MET-h $week^{-1}$ (Manson et al. 1999). For how many hours did they walk?
  Answer – walking at a 'normal' speed of 4.8 km h^{-1} (3 mile h^{-1}) demands 3.5 METs. So, walking for one hour at this speed gives 3.5 MET-h and 20 MET-h $week^{-1}$ means walking for 5.7 hours during a week, covering 27.4 km (17 miles).

Thus, adjectives such as 'vigorous', 'heavy' or 'moderate' do not have precise meaning in the literature. For example, much of the work activity classified as 'heavy' in Paffenbarger's studies of dockworkers (Paffenbarger and Hale 1975) would have been well below the threshold for 'vigorous' exercise adopted in the studies of English civil servants (Morris et al. 1980, 1990).

Little information exists on how ethnicity effects the relationship between cardiorespiratory fitness and CHD. A study in Port of Spain in Trinidad in the West Indies followed 626 men of African, South Asian Indian and European origin, clinically free of CHD at study entry, over 7.6 years. When men were grouped into those with an age and fat-free mass adjusted maximum oxygen uptake level above and below the mean of 1.34 l min^{-1} (~5.3 METs), those below had a 2.36-fold increased risk of myocardial infarction. However, Indian ethnicity remained a predictor of myocardial infarction in men even after allowing for cardiorespiratory fitness (Miller et al. 2005). More evidence is needed to characterise the association of fitness with CHD in men and women of differing ethnicity.

Some data are available with respect to how ageing moderates the relationship between cardiorespiratory fitness and CVD/CHD mortality. Data from 11,049 men who underwent clinical examination before 1990 in the Aerobic Center Longitudinal Study and categorised into groups aged 40–49, 50–59 and 60–69 years showed that in all three groups lower levels of age- and sex-specific fitness were associated with higher lifetime risks for CVD death. However, the lowest and highest fitness levels showed considerable differences in the lifetime risks for CVD death at each age (Berry et al. 2011) (Figure 4.15). At the other end of the spectrum, the Coronary Artery Risk Development in Young Adults (CARDIA) study attempted to examine the prognostic value of cardiorespiratory fitness with clinical and subclinical CVD (coronary artery calcification) outcomes in 4,872 young adults in the US who underwent clinical treadmill testing. Each additional minute of baseline exercise test duration was associated with a 12% lower hazard risk for CVD but was not associated with coronary artery calcification (Shah et al. 2016).

Studies of fitness can make comparisons of CHD incidence among multiple ordinal fitness categories, thus providing new information on the level of fitness below which there seems to be an important increase in risk. A few investigations have attempted to identify such thresholds, which might be important for public health policy. For

Figure 4.15 Lifetime risk for CVD death to 90 years at age 45, 55 and 65 years stratified by fitness level in US men in the Cooper Center Longitudinal Study.

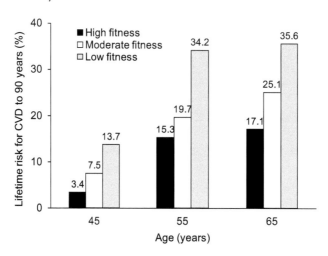

Source: Berry et al. (2011).
Notes: Data labels show percentage risk by fitness category within each age group (45 years: low fitness (mean), 8.4 METs; moderate, 10.8 METs, high, 13.9 METs; 55 years: low, 7.4 METs; moderate, 9.6 METs, high, 12.6 METs; 65 years: low, 5.9 METs; moderate, 8.3 METs, high, 11.2 METs).

middle-aged men, this is in the order of 8–9 METs (28–32 ml kg^{-1} min^{-1}). Based solely on the Aerobic Center Longitudinal Study, the comparable level for women is in the order of 6–7 METs (21–25 ml kg^{-1} min^{-1}). The aforementioned meta-analysis of 24 studies of cardiorespiratory fitness, suggested a minimum level of fitness associated with significantly lower CVD/CHD event rates in healthy men and women of 9 and 7 METs at 40 years, 8 and 6 METs at 50 years, and 7 and 5 METs at 60 years, respectively. From these data, it was suggested that men and women of ~50 years should be capable of continuous walking at 4 and 3 mile h^{-1}, respectively. Moreover, the same study found a 15% reduction in CVD/CHD risk brought about by each 1-MET increment in maximum aerobic capacity. This is comparable with reductions in waist circumference, systolic blood pressure, plasma triglyceride and fasting plasma glucose concentrations, respectively, of 7 cm, 5 mm Hg, 1 mmol l^{-1} and 1 mmol l^{-1} and an increase in high-density lipoprotein cholesterol of 0.2 mmol l^{-1} (Kodama et al. 2009). Other studies have found reassuringly similar reductions in risk (Celis-Morales et al. 2017; Khan et al. 2017). For example, treadmill test data from 54,720 individuals in the UK Biobank showed that each 1-MET decrease in fitness was associated with a 12% higher hazard ratio for CVD events after adjusting for confounding factors (Celis-Morales et al. 2017). A discussion of the potential of popular activities to elicit MET of values associated with improved public health is included in Chapter 14.

Finally, most recently, an attempt has been made to examine indicators of fitness other than cardiorespiratory measures with CHD/CVD risk. Grip strength in particular has emerged an appealing, simple, quick and inexpensive measure. The PURE study

Figure 4.16 Hazard ratios for CVD mortality and incidence for each 5 kg decrement of age- and sex-specific grip strength in 477,074 individuals (54% women) followed for a mean of 7.1 years in the UK Biobank.

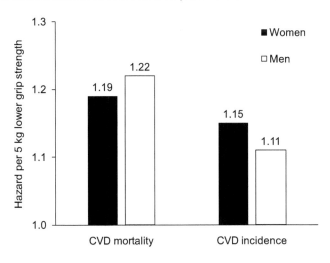

Source: Celis-Morales et al. (2018).
Notes: Data adjusted for age, deprivation index, ethnicity, month of recruitment, comorbidities (depression, diabetes, hypertension, long-standing illness, respiratory diseases, cancer and cardiovascular disease), height, body mass index categories, smoking, physical activity, sedentary behaviour and dietary intake (alcohol, fruit and vegetables, oily fish, red meat and processed meat) and excluding events in first two years after recruitment.

found that each 5 kg decrement in grip strength increased the risk of cardiovascular mortality by 17% and risk of a myocardial infarction by 7% in 139,691 participants from 17 countries followed up for a median duration of four years (Leong et al. 2015). Similarly, a large dataset of individuals from the UK Biobank showed that each 5 kg reduction in grip strength increased both CVD mortality and incidence after adjustment for confounding factors (Celis-Morales et al. 2018) (Figure 4.16). Other large prospective studies have reported similar associations between grip strength and CVD mortality (Celis-Morales et al. 2017; Yates et al. 2017). More recently, a retrospective ten-year analysis of a cohort of 1,107 career firefighters from the US showed that those able to complete >40 push-ups had a 96% reduction in incident CVD events compared with those able to complete <10 push-ups (Yang et al. 2019).

CHANGES IN PHYSICAL ACTIVITY AND FITNESS AND CHD

Many early studies on occupational and leisure-time physical activity and fitness referred to in this chapter used a single baseline measure of activity/fitness as an assessment of the exposure variable. This assumes, probably wrongly in many cases, that participants' levels of physical activity or fitness are rather stable over years and leads to misclassification. Studying activity or fitness on more than one occasion several years apart increases the precision with which exposure to inactivity or low fitness is measured. It also allows the hypothesis that changing exposure is associated with a change in risk to be tested.

Several cohort studies have been able to obtain repeated measurements of activity or fitness and findings from these studies were discussed in Chapter 3 in relation to all-cause mortality. Here we examine the findings for CVD/CHD. The first of these was the Harvard Alumni Study that reported deaths from CHD in men who returned questionnaires about their activity level in 1962 or 1966 and again in 1977. Previously inactive men who, over this period, increased their total physical activity $\geq$8.4 MJ week^{-1} had a 17% lower risk of death from CHD than those who remained sedentary (Paffenbarger et al. 1993). Even greater benefit was seen in the subgroup of men who took up moderately vigorous physical activity $\geq$4.5 METs with a 41% lower risk of death from CHD. This reduction in risk was similar to that seen among men who gave up cigarette smoking (44% lower risk than men who continued smoking) or who avoided becoming overweight for their height (41% lower risk than those whose BMI increased to >26 kg m^{-2}). Similar findings were reported among both healthy men and those already diagnosed with CVD in the British Regional Heart Study when changes in activity were assessed over 12–14 years (Wannamethee et al. 1998). A study in 7,553 postmenopausal older women (>65 years) followed up over a median of 5.7 years also found that increasing the level of physical activity was associated with a 35% reduction in overall CVD mortality but CHD mortality was not reported (Gregg et al. 2003) (Figure 4.17).

Improvements in fitness are also associated with lower risk of CVD. Findings from the Aerobic Center Longitudinal Study found that unfit men in the bottom quintile for performance on a maximal treadmill test on one assessment but who improved their fitness when assessed five years later had a 52% lower age-adjusted risk of CVD

Figure 4.17 Hazard ratio for CVD mortality associated with maintaining or changing activity in white US women (≥65 years) participating in the Study of Osteoporotic Fractures.

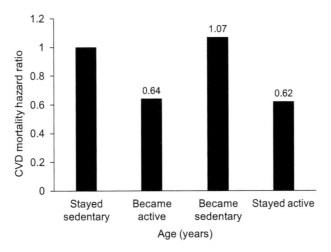

Source: Gregg et al. (2003).
Notes: Data labels show overall CVD mortality hazard ratio over 6.7 years of follow-up with women who stayed sedentary acting as reference group. Sedentary was defined as women in the lowest 40% of weekly energy expenditure (<595 kcal week^{-1}). The reduction in risk is only in individuals who became or stayed active during follow-up. Data controlled for age, smoking, BMI, stroke, diabetes, cancer, chronic obstructive pulmonary disease, incident hip fracture, self-rated health status and baseline physical activity.

mortality (CHD deaths were not reported separately) than men who remained unfit (Blair et al. 1995). The association between improved fitness and reduced risk of CVD mortality was not isolated to the least fit men but those designated as moderately fit at first assessment who improved their fitness when reassessed also had a 28% lower risk of CVD mortality. These findings were independent of confounding by other risk factors at baseline or by changes in risk factors during follow-up. Long-term follow-up over 11.4 years in men from the same study found a significant reduction in CVD mortality in men who were able to maintain (27%) or improve (42%) their cardio-respiratory fitness in comparison with those who lost fitness after the second fitness examination. Moreover, every 1-MET increase in fitness over time decreased CVD mortality by 19% (Lee et al. 2011). At least one other study in men has shown similar findings (Erikssen et al. 1998) but data confirming this relationship in women is needed. However, data from the CARDIA study, which included men and women, found that each one-minute reduction in fitness by year seven of follow-up was associated with a 20% increased hazard for CVD but change in fitness was not associated with coronary artery calcification (Shah et al. 2016).

Collectively, these findings suggest that the relationships between fitness or physical activity and cardiovascular mortality are not due solely to hereditary factors. They also partly address concerns that low fitness and inactivity may be a consequence in some individuals of undetected, pre-existing disease. These data, from cohort studies, do not prove a causal link with reduced CVD mortality, but they strengthen the argument that, if activity or fitness improves, risk is modified. Nevertheless, there are concerns that the change in fitness category noted in these studies may also be an artefact due to measurement error rather than any real association between improved fitness with CVD mortality. Measurement error of true values at initial baseline testing (for example from a treadmill test to exhaustion) can entirely account for movement in individuals on the boundary between categories (fit and unfit) and who have an intermediate mortality risk whereas those on the extremes at both measures probably represent the true values. This demonstrates the difficulty of inferring change from non-experimental data. This view also challenges the association between increased fitness and reduced CVD mortality and further suggests that the 50% heritability reported for fitness may be an underestimation since it includes the attenuating effects of measurement error. One way to overcome this criticism would be to provide two baseline measures of treadmill duration more accurately to assign an individual's fitness at the start of the follow-up period (Williams 2003).

DOSE–RESPONSE: WHAT LEVEL OF ACTIVITY OR FITNESS CONFERS PROTECTION AGAINST CHD?

This question is important for two reasons: first, if the relationship between physical activity or fitness and the risk of CHD is causal, then there should be a graded effect – more activity/higher fitness should be associated with greater benefit; and second, public health initiatives demand an understanding of what constitutes a sufficient level of activity or fitness to confer a worthwhile decrease in risk. Only studies where several gradations of physical activity or fitness are reported can help address dose–response issues. However, these are compelling in their consistency and in the steepness of the gradient across groups.

A notable example of a study demonstrating dose–response effects of physical activity is the Health Professionals Follow-Up Study which involved 44,452 US men followed up from 1986 to 1998 with physical activity assessed every two years between 1986 and 1996. Inverse dose–response relationships were found between CHD risk and the volume and intensity of physical activity, the duration and speed of walking and the duration of running and weight training (Tanasescu et al. 2002) (Figure 4.18). Rowing and racquet sports were also associated with a lower CHD risk. These findings were confirmed in the Nurses' Health Study which demonstrated inverse dose–response associations between both walking and vigorous exercise and the risk of CHD in 72,488 female nurses aged 40 to 65 years upon enrolment (Manson et al. 1999). In both of these studies the findings remained significant after controlling for a host of potentially confounding factors including age, BMI, alcohol intake, cigarette smoking, family history of CHD and nutrient intake.

Two papers from the Harvard Alumni Health Study provide further information regarding relationships between exercise duration and intensity and CHD risk. One examined the influence of the duration of exercise episodes, through the range <15 minutes in 15-minute increments to >60 minutes (Lee et al. 2000). Longer sessions of exercise did not have a different effect on the risk of CHD than shorter sessions, as long as the total energy expended was similar. The second paper examined the influence of the relative intensity of exercise (assessed using participants' ratings on the Borg scale of perceived exertion) and found a strong relationship with the risk of CHD that was independent of total energy expenditure (Lee, Sesso, Oguma and Paffenbarger 2003). This ties in well with evidence from laboratory studies that the physiological 'stress' of exercise depends on the proportion of an individual's maximal oxygen uptake it demands, rather than on its intensity measured in absolute terms.

A systematic review of 49 studies published between 1975 and 2007, all of which reported on at least three levels of physical activity, involving 726,474 participants with a total of 34,815 CVD events showed an overall reduction in CVD of 33% between active and non-active individuals and that energy expenditure equivalent to 4.2 MJ per week (1000 kcal; equivalent to 30 minutes' walking per day) produced substantial reductions in risk (Warburton et al. 2010). The previously mentioned meta-analysis of 33 prospective cohort studies was the first to examine the dose–response for physical activity and the risk of CHD (Sattelmair et al. 2011). As stated, individuals who met public health recommendations by performing 150 minutes of moderate-intensity physical activity each week demonstrated a 14% lower risk for CHD compared with those who did no leisure-time physical activity but this increased to a 20% risk reduction for individuals achieving 300 minutes per week. A more recent meta-analysis report on ischaemic heart

Figure 4.18 Age-adjusted relative risk of CHD in US men enrolled in the Health Professionals Follow-Up Study, according to overall physical activity (MET-h week^{-1}), physical activity intensity (METs), amount of running and weight lifting (both in hours per week), walking volume (MET-h week^{-1}) and walking intensity (miles h^{-1}).

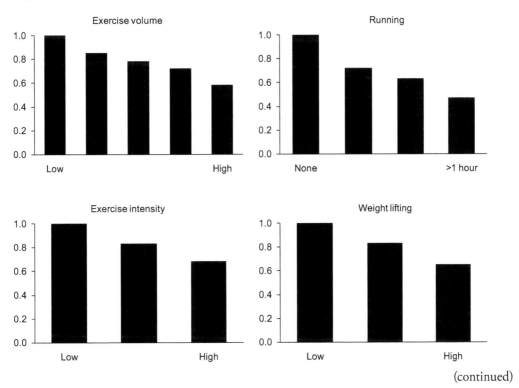

(continued)

Figure 4.18 (continued)

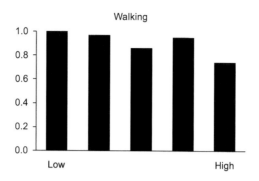

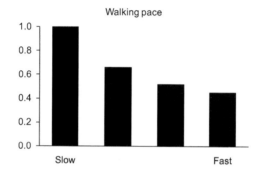

Source: Tanasescu et al. (2002).
Notes: Exercise volume quintile one: 0–6.32; quintile two: 6.33–14.49; quintile three: 14.50–25.08; quintile four: 25.09–41.98; quintile five: ≥41.99 MET-h week^{-1}. Exercise intensity tertile one: 1–3.9; tertile two: 4–5.9; tertile three: ≥6 METs. Running quartile one: none; quartile two: <0.5; quartile three: 0.5–1; quartile four: ≥1 h week^{-1}. Weight lifting tertile one: none; tertile two: <0.5; tertile three: ≥0.5 h week^{-1}. Walking volume quintile one: 0–1.19; quintile two: 1.20–3.49; quintile three: 3.50–6.99; quintile four: 7.00–14.74; quintile five: ≥14.75 MET-h week^{-1}. Walking pace quartile one: 2; quartile two: 2–3; quartile three: 3–4; quartile four: ≥4 miles h^{-1}. Displayed findings are age-adjusted relative risks, but findings remained significant in multivariate models.

disease including 43 prospective studies from several countries attempted to identify the upper limit of total physical activity that confers a protective benefit. Compared with a reference group doing <600 MET-minutes per week of activity (~4 hours of brisk walking), increasing volumes of total physical activity reduced the risk of ischaemic heart disease up to 8000 MET-min per week with no further worthwhile reduction thereafter (Kyu et al. 2016) (Figure 4.19). The equivalent changes in risk per MET increase or decrease in fitness have already been mentioned as have the dose–response thresholds for fitness (Celis-Morales et al. 2017; Khan et al. 2017; Kodama et al. 2009). Based on age, these are probably between 7 and 9 METs for men and between 5 and 7 METs for women (Kodama et al. 2009). Such data demonstrate that much of the benefit from physical activity and fitness on CHD can be obtained at levels that are achievable from a public health perspective (see Chapter 14).

Figure 4.19 Relative risk for ischaemic heart disease (IHD) based on the volume of total physical activity calculated from a pooled analysis of 43 studies.

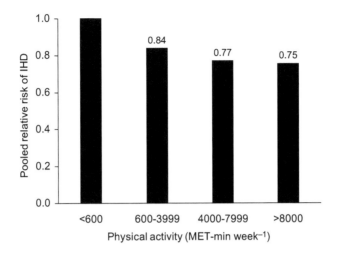

Source: Kyu et al. (2016).
Notes: Data labels show pooled relative risk from all studies with <600 MET-min week[-1] acting as the reference activity level.

Based on the available evidence, the conclusion may be drawn that, while moderate levels of physical activity or fitness confer a measurable decrease in the risk of CHD, more vigorous activity or higher levels of fitness confer a greater benefit. Often the greatest difference in risk is observed between those categorised as least active or fit and the next category up. The benefit levels off at the upper end of the continuum. However, as discussed later, the interactions between activity and fitness may moderate this association. Future studies need to provide detail on the associations between exercise and CHD risk for specific activities (e.g. running, swimming, cycling, racquet sports). Currently, sufficient data are available for confident recommendations only for walking. In relation to this Morris and colleagues observed a clear inverse gradient of risk according to reported walking speed in English civil servants, with a particularly low rate of disease in men claiming to be fast walkers ($\geq$4 mile h^{-1} or $\geq$6.4 km h^{-1}) (Morris et al. 1990). Similarly in the Women's Health Study in the US there were dose–response relationships with both walking duration and walking pace (Lee et al. 2001) and the Health Professionals Follow-Up Study (Tanasescu et al. 2002), the Nurses' Health Study (Manson et al. 1999), the Women's Health Initiative (Manson et al. 2002) and data from the UK Biobank (Celis-Morales et al. 2019) all reported inverse associations of walking pace and energy expenditure with CHD or CVD risk. The dose–response relationship between walking and overall CHD or CVD risk have been confirmed in meta-analyses (Hamer and Chida 2008; Oguma and Shinoda-Tagawa 2004). Thus, it can be assumed that a walking pace of $\geq$4 mile h^{-1} is required for optimal protection from CHD and, within certain limits, that the greater the volume of walking the greater the protection from CHD.

INTERACTION OF PHYSICAL ACTIVITY, FITNESS AND GENETICS WITH CVD RISK

The studies discussed thus far have demonstrated that physical activity, cardiovascular fitness and strength all exert independent effects on CHD and CVD risk. Increasing physical activity can improve both cardiovascular fitness and strength but, as noted previously, approximately half of the changes in fitness is genetic. It has been unclear whether the association of physical activity with CVD risk is therefore moderated or varies by these fitness measures. It is important to understand this interaction as many physical activity interventions target the least active segment of the population based on the data showing that the greatest decreases in CVD mortality occur in these individuals. This assumes, however, a constant association between physical activity and CVD irrespective of fitness. An examination of the interaction between physical activity and fitness can help better define the subgroup within the population who most benefit from any intervention. Published data from men and women aged 40–69 years in the UK Biobank have examined this interaction between activity and fitness. The study included physical activity and grip strength data on 495,786 participants and data on 67,702 participants for cardiorespiratory fitness, assessed using a six-minute incremental cycle ergometer ramp test. A higher hazard of CVD events with decreasing physical activity was only observed in the lowest tertile for grip strength (8% increase per one quintile change in physical activity) or cardiorespiratory fitness (10% increase per one quintile change in physical activity) (Celis-Morales et al. 2017). These data point toward fitness moderating the relationship of physical activity with CVD and future studies will contribute to these early findings.

A second area of recent examination has been the interaction of genetics with physical activity and fitness as the extent to which genetic risk for CVD can be compensated for by exercise has been uncertain. Again, data from the UK Biobank has helped address this by stratifying individuals with genome-wide genetic data into high, intermediate and low genetic risk categories based on genetic markers for CHD and atrial fibrillation (an abnormal heart rhythm resulting from disorganised electrical impulse in the atria of the heart and which increases the risk of stroke). Low, intermediate and high levels of physical activity (from accelerometer data), cardiorespiratory fitness and grip strength were examined in association to these genetic risk categories. After accounting for confounding factors, the individuals in the highest third for genetic risk had a hazard ratio of 1.73 for CHD events and 1.95 for atrial fibrillation compared with the lowest third. Moreover, for all three categories of grip strength and cardiorespiratory fitness, individuals at an intermediate or high level of strength or fitness had a reduced risk of CHD (Figure 4.20) and atrial fibrillation, with a similar trend being observed for physical activity across categories (Tikkanen et al. 2018).

ARE PHYSICAL INACTIVITY AND LOW FITNESS CAUSAL FACTORS FOR CHD?

The evidence discussed to this point strongly supports the proposition that physical inactivity and low fitness are causative factors for CHD. However, because of the

Figure 4.20 Hazard ratio for CHD events in individuals by tertile of genetic risk and grip strength (n = 468,095) and genetic risk and cardiorespiratory fitness (n = 66,438) aged 40–69 years, recruited between 2006 and 2010 and followed to 2016, in the UK Biobank.

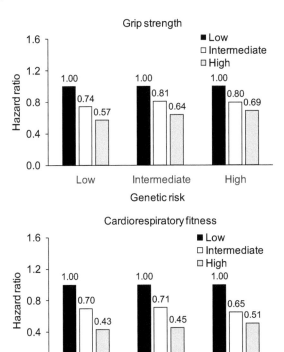

Source: Tikkanen et al. (2018).
Notes: Hazard data in comparison to lowest grip strength or cardiorespiratory fitness within each group. Data adjusted for age, sex, ethnicity, genotype array and ten principal components and stratified by region of the UK Biobank assessment centre.

enduring problem of self-selection and because people in whom disease is developing but undetected may be more likely to establish sedentary habits, epidemiological studies cannot by themselves determine causality. This limitation is nicely described in an editorial by Paul Thompson who states that:

all epidemiological examinations of occupational and recreational physical activity are plagued by the possibility that people who elect vigorous lifestyles are different physiologically, emotionally, or genetically from their less active peers. Selection according to such a 'hardiness factor' can only be addressed by a clinical trial.

(Thompson 2002, p. 755)

As pointed out in Chapter 2, a randomised, controlled trial with disease endpoints as the outcome measure is probably not feasible in healthy individuals partly because of the length of time that CHD takes to develop. Nevertheless, there are now some studies available which have examined how physical activity in combination with other healthy lifestyle factors effects the occurrence of CVD events in higher risk groups and these are discussed later in this chapter. For healthy individuals, complementary evidence that examines the ability of physical activity to affect the potential biological mechanisms for CHD is vital in supporting the relationship and is described in this chapter in brief but more thoroughly in Chapter 7. The features of epidemiological evidence that contribute towards establishing causality were explained in Chapter 2. The evidence discussed thus far in this chapter appears to fulfil these criteria (Box 4.4).

EPIDEMIOLOGY OF PHYSICAL ACTIVITY AND FITNESS WITH STROKE

There are good reasons why the hypothesis that physical activity reduces the risk of stroke is attractive. Clear evidence links physical inactivity to CHD, and thrombo-embolytic stroke (ischaemic stroke, the commonest type) and CHD share similar pathophysiology and risk factors (raised blood pressure, obesity, glucose intolerance, smoking).

Historically, the number of epidemiological studies examining the relationship between physical activity and stroke incidence is smaller than that for CHD. However, at least two meta-analyses support the protective effect of physical activity on stroke in both men and women. The first included 23 studies (18 cohort, 5 case-control) and found that highly active and moderately active individuals had a 27% and 20% lower stroke incidence or mortality, respectively (Lee, Folsom and Blair 2003). Reductions

---

BOX 4.4 FEATURES OF EVIDENCE FOR THE PROPOSITION THAT PHYSICAL ACTIVITY AND FITNESS CONFERS PROTECTION AGAINST CHD.

- Findings are remarkably consistent in diverse populations.
- Better studies are more likely than poorer studies to observe an inverse relationship.
- Good evidence is available in middle-aged men, women, older adults and racially diverse groups.
- The relationships between CHD risk and physical activity or fitness are inverse and graded. Whether intensity and/or frequency of sessions of physical activity have separate effects over and above that of the total energy expenditure is not yet clear, although these are issues of much research interest. It appears that 'vigorous' exercise confers optimal protection.
- The relative risk of inactivity or low fitness is at least two.
- Most studies have measured activity/fitness before the onset of CHD. This decreases the likelihood that participants were inactive/unfit because they had preclinical disease.
- The findings are not confounded by other major risk factors.
- Becoming more active or fit decreases risk compared with remaining inactive or of low fitness.

Figure 4.21 Relative risk of stroke incidence or mortality for high and moderately active individuals based on a pooled analysis of 18 cohort studies.

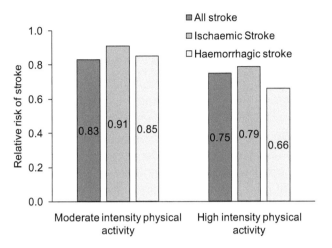

Source: Lee, Folsom and Blair (2003).
Notes: Data labels show pooled relative risk at each exercise intensity for all stroke, ischaemic stroke and haemorrhagic stroke compared with individuals in the pooled studies reporting a low intensity of physical activity as the reference group.

in risk remained significant for both activity groups when only cohort studies for both ischaemic and haemorrhagic stroke were analysed (Figure 4.21). The second analysis included 31 studies and found that moderate and intense leisure-time as well as occupational physical activity protected against total stroke and that higher levels of activity were protective in independent analyses of ischaemic and haemorrhagic stroke (Wendel-Vos et al. 2004). These analyses are supported by data published in the Physical Activity Guidelines Advisory Committee Report 2008 (Physical Activity Guidelines Advisory Committee 2008) where an examination of prospective and cohort studies published between 1995 and 2007 found a reduction in total stroke of 33% and 25% for moderate intensity/amount and higher intensity/amount activity, respectively. Similarly, a systematic review of 25 articles published between 1993 and 2007 for Canadian physical activity guidelines and including 479,336 participants with 12,361 reported cases of stroke showed an average risk reduction of 31% for active individuals (Warburton et al. 2010).

The relationship between physical activity and stroke risk appears similar in men and women. One Norwegian study found similar trends for total physical activity with stroke mortality in 32,872 men and 34,868 women and similar relative risk reductions for the highly active men and women (Vatten et al. 2006). Similarly, walking for more than one hour per day in Japanese men and women was associated with similar reductions in risk for ischaemic stroke after adjustment for multiple risk factors of 29% and 27%, respectively (Noda et al. 2005). Stroke rates tend to be higher in black men and women than other ethnicities, but few data make any ethnic comparison of stroke risk in relation to physical activity. Data from the first National Health and Nutrition Examination Survey I (NHANES I) noted that low levels of non-recreational activity were associated with an increased risk of stroke in white women aged 65–74 years with similar associations in men and black people (Gillum et al. 1996). Comparably, engaging in any physical activity (light to moderate or heavy) was protective in whites, blacks and Hispanics in the Northern Manhattan Stroke Study with reductions in risk of 56%, 67% and 73%, respectively, compared with their inactive counterparts (Sacco et al. 1998). More recently, however, data from the Atherosclerosis Risk in Communities Study in the US found a clearer protective association of physical activity with total stroke and several stroke subtypes in black than white Americans (Autenreith et al. 2013). More studies need to clarify the associations of physical activity, ethnicity and stroke.

As with CHD, some attempt has been made to quantify the nature of the dose–response relationship of physical activity with stroke. One meta-analysis of 26 studies of ischaemic stroke from several countries reported that, compared with individuals completing <600 MET-min week^{-1}, increasing total physical activity reduced the risk of ischaemic stroke by 16%, 19% and 26% at total volumes of physical activity of 600–3999, 4000–7999, and ≥8000 MET-min week^{-1} (Kyu et al. 2016). The dose–response effect with walking has been isolated in some instances. In the US Nurses' Health Study reports on total physical activity level and walking activity were gathered and averaged over eight years prior to the assessment of total stroke incidence and adjusted for age and for other potentially confounding factors (Figure 4.22). The relationship for total physical activity was inverse, graded and statistically significant and although adjustment for potentially confounding factors – including alcohol, which is an important risk factor for stroke but not CHD – somewhat attenuated the risk, this remained significant. For walking, the multivariate analysis was adjusted for participation in vigorous exercise, so these findings can be regarded as describing the association of the risk of stroke with walking *per se* (Hu et al. 2000). In another example, older men aged 60–79 years who walked 4–7 hours and 8–14 hours each week had 11% and 37% reductions in risk, respectively, compared with those who reported walking 0–3 hours each week independent of walking pace as well as established and novel risk factors (Jefferis et al. 2014). Fewer studies, however, have allowed estimation of the separate effects of exercise intensity or frequency. One – a case control study in Manhattan – found a significant effect of both intensity (light to moderate versus heavy) and duration (<2 h week^{-1} versus >2–<5 h week^{-1} versus ≥5 h week^{-1}) of exercise (Sacco et al. 1998).

Several studies of fitness and stroke incidence are available. The Aerobic Center Longitudinal Study analysed stroke mortality incidence among 16,878 men during a ten-year follow-up (Lee and Blair 2002). Compared with the least-fit 20% of men, the relative risk of stroke mortality was 0.37 in those with moderate fitness (next 40%) and 0.32 in those designated as high fitness (top 40%) suggesting that, as for CHD, little extra protection is conferred at high levels of fitness. However, only 32 cases of stroke were recorded overall, many fewer than for CHD, illustrating the difficulty of examining different types of stroke separately (it is possible that activity/fitness is not related in the same way to both thromboembolytic (ischaemic) and haemorrhagic stroke). Data from a larger population tested for the Aerobic Center Longitudinal Study with >1 million person-years of follow-up has since been published (Hooker et al. 2008). After

Figure 4.22 Relative risk of stroke in 72,488 US women aged 40–65 years followed from 1986 to 1992 in the Nurses' Health Study according to quintiles of total physical activity measured in MET-h week^{-1} and walking activity measured in MET-h week^{-1}.

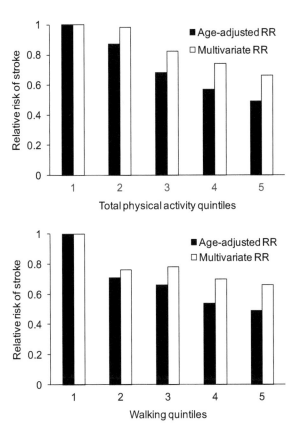

Source: Hu et al. (2000).
Notes: Multivariate risks adjusted for age, smoking, BMI, menopausal status, parental history of myocardial infarction, alcohol consumption, aspirin use and history of hypertension, diabetes or hypercholesterolaemia. For walking activity, the multivariate model was adjusted for vigorous exercise in addition to the other factors listed above.

adjustment for confounding risk factors, men in the highest quartile of fitness had a 50%, 38% and 40% reduced risk of fatal, non-fatal and total stroke, respectively, compared with the least fit men (Figure 4.23). For women, there was a 43% and 44% reduction in total and non-fatal stroke, but the relationship did not hold true for fatal stroke. A cardiorespiratory fitness threshold of 7 to 8 METs was associated with substantially reduced incidence of total stroke in both men and women compared with <5 METs but with little survival gain beyond 8 METs.

The findings of the Aerobic Center Longitudinal Study were confirmed by the Kuopio Ischemic Heart Disease Risk Factor Study in Eastern Finland. This study involved 2,011 men and an average of 11 years of follow-up. Maximum oxygen uptake was determined directly using a cycle ergometer test. The relative risk of stroke (all types) was 3.2 in men

Figure 4.23 Relative risk of stroke in 46,505 men and 15,282 women aged 18–100 years, followed from 1982 to 2004, in the Cooper Center Longitudinal Study in the US according to quartiles of cardiorespiratory fitness measured in METs.

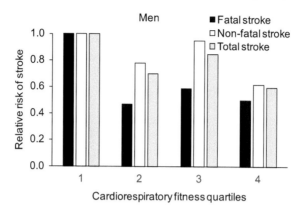

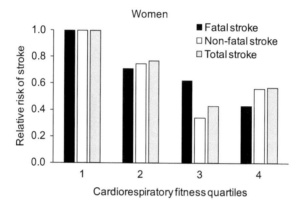

Source: Hooker et al. (2008).
Notes: Data for fatal, non-fatal and total stroke significant in men (P < 0.05); only data for non-fatal and total stroke significant in women (P < 0.05). Data adjusted for age, examination year, smoking, alcohol intake, family history of CVD and abnormal exercise electrocardiogram responses, BMI, and personal history of hypertension, diabetes or hypercholesterolaemia. Mean fitness men quartile one: 8.6 METs; quartile two: 10.8 METs; quartile three: 12.4 METs; quartile four: 15.0 METs. Mean fitness women quartile one: 6.8 METs; quartile two: 8.5 METs; quartile three: 10.1 METs; quartile four: 12.6 METs.

in the lowest quartile for fitness ($\dot{V}O_2$max <25 ml kg^{-1} min^{-1}, 7.2 METs) compared with those in the highest quartile ($\dot{V}O_2$max >35.3 ml kg^{-1} min^{-1}, 10.1 METs). These findings remained significant after adjustment for a variety of potentially confounding factors and the risk of low fitness was comparable to that of established risk factors for stroke, including hypertension, obesity, alcohol consumption, smoking and elevated low-density lipoprotein (Kurl et al. 2003). Finally, the PURE study across 17 countries noted that each 5 kg reduction in grip strength was associated with a 9% increase in risk for stroke (Leong et al. 2015). Thus, collectively there is good evidence to demonstrate that low levels of physical activity and physical fitness increase the risk of stroke.

EPIDEMIOLOGY FOR THE PREVENTION OF OTHER CARDIOVASCULAR DISEASES

The studies described in this chapter have examined the epidemiology of physical activity and fitness with the two most predominant CVDs – CHD and stroke. These account for by far the greatest number of CVD-related deaths worldwide but other forms of CVD have substantial impacts on the population and are important. Recent epidemiological studies are attempting to address the lack of information on these other CVDs and examine the associations of physical activity and fitness with their occurrence. One example is heart failure, a condition where the heart is unable to pump blood around the body at a rate sufficient to meet the metabolic demands because of an impaired left ventricular function (see Box 4.1). This impact of this disease is becoming more important as ageing populations are characteristic of many developed countries and secondly because of improved survival after CHD events in patients.

Several studies have examined the effect of physical activity on heart failure in disease-free cohorts. One example is the Copenhagen City Heart Study, a prospective cohort study in 8,422 men and 9,931 women aged 20–80 years, where self-assessed leisure-time physical activity was related to subsequent hospitalisation or death from heart failure (Saevereid et al. 2014). Both light and moderate physical activity produced 40–50% reductions in the risk for hospitalisation or death by heart failure, although these reductions were somewhat attenuated by confounding factors. Importantly, from a public health standpoint, in a sub-analysis of 9,937 participants for whom there was data on walking speed and duration, walking speed in particular was associated with reductions in risk for death or hospitalisation (Figure 4.24). The Atherosclerosis Risk in Communities Study (ARICS) examined how changes in physical activity affect heart failure (Florido et al. 2018). This study evaluated physical activity via questionnaire in 11,351 participants aged 45–64 years at five intervals between initial recruitment in 1987–89 until 2011–13. During a median 19 years of follow-up, those individuals who consistently met recommended activity levels had a cumulative 31% reduction in heart failure. The individuals whose physical activity levels increased from poor to the recommended amount over time showed a 22% reduction in risk. Increasing physical activity by 512 MET-minutes each week – equivalent to approximately four 30-minute brisk walks – resulted in an 11% decrease in the risk of incident heart failure. Findings from these cohort studies have been confirmed in a meta-analysis of 12 prospective studies with 20,203 heart failure events among 370,460 participants (53.5% women; median follow-up 13 years). The highest levels of physical activity reduced the risk of heart failure by 30% compared with the lowest level. Participants who met the minimal level of recommended physical activity each week (500 MET-min week^{-1}) had a 10% reduction in risk compared with those who reported no leisure-time physical activity. The reduction in risk increased to 19% and 35% in individuals who did twice (1,000 MET-min week^{-1}) and four (2,000 MET-min week^{-1}) times the recommended physical activity level (Pandey et al. 2015).

Physical fitness is also associated with decreased risk of heart failure. Data from the Aerobic Center Longitudinal Study collected over 20 years in 44,674 men free from CVD at the outset found that cardiorespiratory fitness, determined using duration of treadmill time to exhaustion, was strongly and inversely related with heart failure

Figure 4.24 Hospital admission or death from heart failure in relation to speed of walking in 9,937 men and women enrolled in the Copenhagen City Heart Study between 1976 and 2003.

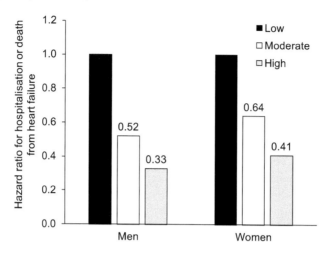

Source: Saevereid et al. (2014).
Notes: Data show hazard ratios in comparison with the lowest walking speed in each sex. Data adjusted for the following confounders and mediators: age, smoking, alcohol consumption, years of education, household income, family history of CVD, atrial fibrillation, impaired lung function, diabetes, systolic blood pressure, resting heart rate, total cholesterol, triglycerides and BMI.

mortality, with those in the lowest category of fitness almost four times as likely to experience a death from heart failure. This held true regardless of the number of heart failure risk factors present (Farrell et al. 2013). Further data from the same study in 20,642 men and women showed not only improved survival from fatal events but that each 1-MET increase in cardiorespiratory fitness achieved in midlife was associated with an approximate 20% reduction in risk for heart failure hospitalisation after the age of 65 years (Berry et al. 2013). Given the associated costs of heart failure, such data are important considerations for governments searching for a 'best buy' in public health (see Chapter 14).

RISK FACTORS FOR CVD

Epidemiological evidence collected over many decades has helped identify several major risk factors for CVD. These risk factors are separated into two major types: (i) modifiable risk factors that can be changed via lifestyle intervention and (ii) non-modifiable risk factors. The importance of these risk factors lies not only in the prevention and management of the disease but is useful because intervention studies can be conducted to examine the effects of physical activity on these factors. As highlighted, it is very difficult to perform randomised controlled trials for the prevention of CVD due to ethical and practical constraints. If it can be demonstrated that exercise has positive outcomes on these risk factors, this provides support for the associations between inactivity/low

Table 4.1 Major risk factors for cardiovascular disease.	
MODIFIABLE RISK FACTORS	NON-MODIFIABLE RISK FACTORS
Dyslipidaemia: elevated total cholesterol or low-density lipoprotein cholesterol concentrations, depressed high-density lipoprotein cholesterol concentrations, elevated triglyceride concentrations	Family history: risk is increased in first-degree relatives (parents, siblings and offspring) of people with premature atherosclerotic disease (men <55 years and women <65 years)
Hypertension	Age: higher risk in older individuals
Cigarette smoking	Gender: higher risk in males than females
Obesity (particularly central/abdominal obesity)	Ethnic background: higher risk in South Asians,
Hyperglycaemia or diabetes	although this may be due to the higher prevalence of diabetes in this group

Note: For further information on CVD risk factors please see Chapter 7.

fitness with CVD and helps affirm the link that the evidence collected in epidemiological studies is causal. Moreover, if exercise is able to ameliorate these risk factors it would suggest that CVD incidence can be reduced because studies have demonstrated that favourable changes in these risk factors reduce the risk of CVD.

Table 4.1 lists the major risk factors for CVD, many of which were identified from early cohort studies conducted in the 30–40 years after the Second World War. The list is not comprehensive, and newer or emerging risk factors have been identified in the past two decades including those associated with abnormal body fat distribution (central/visceral fat distribution; liver fat; adipose tissue biomarkers), lipids (apolipoprotein B, non-high-density lipoprotein cholesterol and small low-density lipoproteins), markers of insulin resistance, markers of abnormal vascular function and regulation (endothelial function; microalbuminuria), pro-inflammatory markers (C-reactive protein; adiponectin), indicators of a pro-thrombotic state (clotting factors) and hormonal factors (pituitary-adrenal axis). Note also that physical inactivity and low physical fitness are not listed in Table 4.1. It could be argued that they should be since the evidence discussed previously indicates that low levels of physical activity and physical fitness are independently related to CVD risk. In view of this there is an argument for including activity and/or fitness assessments routinely in clinical practice. Chapter 7 will provide a comprehensive examination of the evidence that physical activity favourably influences many of the major modifiable risk factors for CVD.

COMBINED HEALTHY LIFESTYLE BEHAVIOURS

Thus far the evidence for the role of physical activity alone in reducing the risk of CVD has been described. Some studies have investigated the association between combined healthy lifestyle behaviours and the risk of CVD. One example is the Health Ageing: A Longitudinal Study in Europe (HALE) project. The main outcome of interest in this study was all-cause mortality, but the study also identified relative risks of 0.27 and 0.33 for CHD and CVD, respectively, in participants who adhered to four healthy lifestyle behaviours compared with participants who reported either none or only one of these behaviours. The healthy lifestyle behaviours examined in this study were Mediterranean diet, physical activity, non-smoking and moderate alcohol consumption (Knoops et al. 2004).

Another study investigating the association between CHD and lifestyle is the Nurses' Health Study. One finding was that nurses who reported five low-risk factors (healthy diet, non-smoking, regular exercise, BMI <25 kg m^{-2} and moderate alcohol consumption ≥ 5 g day^{-1}) had an 83% lower risk of CHD (relative risk 0.17) over 14 years of follow-up compared with all other women. The population-attributable risk for nurses in this group suggested that 82% of coronary events among nurses in the study could have been prevented if all women had been in the low-risk group (Stampfer et al. 2000) (Figure 4.25). Thus, although the focus of this book is on physical activity, it is

Figure 4.25 Relative risk of CHD and the population-attributable risk (PAR) according to lifestyle factors in 84,129 women participating in the Nurses' Health Study.

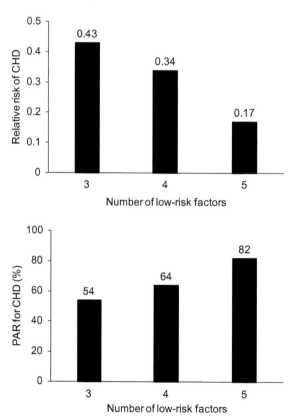

Source: Stampfer et al. (2000).
Notes: Lifestyle factors included were: three low-risk factors, healthy diet, non-smoking and exercise (≥ 30 min day^{-1}); four low-risk factors, healthy diet, non-smoking, exercise (≥ 30 min day^{-1}) and a BMI <25 kg m^{-2}; five low-risk factors, healthy diet, non-smoking, exercise (≥ 30 min day^{-1}), BMI <25 kg m^{-2} and moderate alcohol consumption (≥ 5 g day^{-1}).

important to emphasise that a combination of healthy lifestyle behaviours is necessary for optimal protection from CVD/CHD.

HEALTHY LIFESTYLE AND CVD PREVENTION IN HIGH-RISK GROUPS

As discussed earlier and in Chapter 2, data obtained from prospective epidemiological studies alone make it difficult to attribute a protective effect of physical activity on CVD as causal because of potential underlying genetic or constitutional factors separating individuals who choose to exercise from their sedentary peers. Only randomised controlled trials, which remove the influence of genetics at the outset of an investigation, can address this criticism. However, the slow rate of progression to primary events for CVD along with the large number of individuals needed makes conducting, funding and performing such trials in healthy populations unviable.

Individuals with type 2 diabetes mellitus (see Chapter 5) have an increased risk of cardiovascular events compared with those in the general population and cardiovascular risk factors are often found to cluster together (see Chapter 7) in people with this disease. They therefore form a population where the potential to address the effect of a lifestyle intervention on CVD events or outcomes is viable. Nevertheless, CVD events are slow to occur, given that a 20% ten-year risk of a CVD event is classified as high. This means that the number of randomised trials is rare. One smaller trial in Denmark randomised 160 patients with type 2 diabetes to either a conventional standard treatment for cardiovascular risk factors from general practitioners or intensive treatment, which included lifestyle behaviour modification. Lifestyle modification centred on reductions in total and saturated fat, three to five times per week of light-to-moderate physical activity for 30 minutes each time and smoking cessation, in addition to vitamin supplementation and pharmacological therapy. During eight years of follow-up, the intensive treatment group experienced a 53% reduction in cardiovascular events compared with the conventional-treatment group (Gaede et al. 2003).

A larger intervention trial on CVD in individuals with type 2 diabetes mellitus took place in the US more recently. The Look AHEAD (Action for Health in Diabetes) Trial was a multi-centre randomised, controlled trial reporting on deaths from cardiovascular events, non-fatal heart attacks, non-fatal stroke and hospitalisation for angina pectoris in 5,145 obese patients with type 2 diabetes mellitus. Patients in the intervention group underwent intensive lifestyle treatment, which included maintaining a weight loss of 7% of initial body mass via reduced energy intake of 1200–1800 kcal per day (less than 30% of calories from fat and more than 15% from protein) and at least 175 minutes of moderate intensity physical activity each week. Patients in the control arm of the trial received education on diet and exercise and social support three times per year for the first four years of the study and subsequently once annually. Perhaps surprisingly, the study was terminated early after 9.6 years of follow-up with approximately 20% of patients in both intervention and control groups meeting a primary event endpoint (Look AHEAD Research Group 2013). One positive outcome emerged in a secondary analysis of data. Those patients, irrespective of the treatment group they were in, who had achieved the greatest increases in physical fitness in the first year of the study (≥ 2 METs) had a 23% reduction in a composite risk calculated from fatal

Figure 4.26 Hazard ratios for 4,406 participants in the Look AHEAD (Action for Health in Diabetes) Trial showing the association of fitness change in the first year with risk of occurrence of non-fatal myocardial infarction, stroke, hospitalised angina and CVD death.

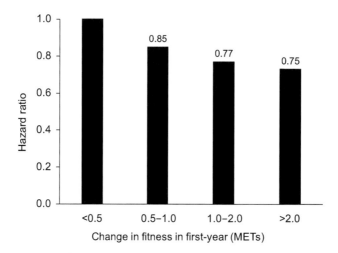

Source: Look AHEAD Research Group (2016).
Notes: Data labels show hazard ratios with reference group being those individuals whose fitness changed <0.5 METs. Reduction in risk is significant only for individuals whose fitness improved >2 METs. Data were adjusted for sex, age, baseline weight, baseline fitness, CVD history, insulin use, diabetes duration, smoking status, low-density lipoprotein, systolic blood pressure and diastolic blood pressure.

and non-fatal CVD occurrences and CVD-related hospital treatments. There were also reductions in risk for secondary outcomes of non-fatal myocardial infarction, stroke, hospitalised angina, CVD death and total mortality (Look AHEAD Research Group 2016) (Figure 4.26). Thus, the study may not have achieved great enough changes in fitness – and weight loss for which there were similar secondary analyses – to affect CVD incidence.

In contrast, long-term findings from a randomised, controlled trial initially conducted in 1986 in Da Qing in northern China were more positive. The study was initially designed to investigate the effect of lifestyle interventions on prevention of type 2 diabetes mellitus in 577 individuals at high risk for the disease through impaired glucose tolerance (see Chapter 5). Individuals enrolled at 33 clinics and were assigned to a diet, exercise, diet plus exercise or control group at baseline. The exercise prescription for the study was to increase physical activity by 20–40 minutes per day of moderate intensity activity such as brisk walking or 10–20 minutes per day of more vigorous activity such as jogging. The intervention lasted six years, and long-term follow-up of the patients after two decades, in 2009, was conducted to assess cardiovascular mortality. Cumulative incidence of cardiovascular deaths over the 23 years of follow-up was 11.9% in the intervention groups collectively versus 19.6% in the control group (Li et al. 2014) (Figure 4.27). Several points may explain the contrasting results between the differing outcomes observed in the Look AHEAD and Da Qing study. Underlying patient differences may be one explanation as individuals in the Look AHEAD trial

Figure 4.27 Cumulative incidence of cardiovascular disease mortality over 23 years of follow-up in 576 individuals from Da Qing in China with impaired glucose tolerance, enrolled to a control (black line, n = 138) or lifestyle intervention (blue line, n = 438) group in 1986 and followed for 23 years.

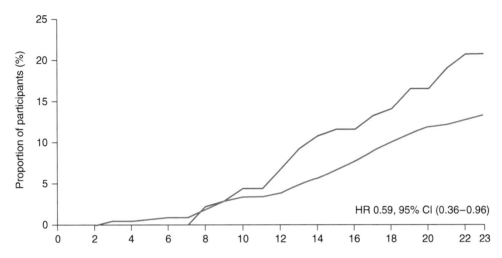

Source: Reprinted from *The Lancet Diabetes and Endocrinology*, 2: 474–80, Li, G. et al., 'Cardiovascular mortality, all-cause mortality, and diabetes incidence after lifestyle intervention for people with impaired glucose tolerance in the Da Qing Diabetes Prevention Study: a 23-year follow-up study', page 477, copyright © 2014, with permission from Elsevier.
Note: The difference between the control and intervention becomes obvious after >10 years of follow-up.

already had type 2 diabetes mellitus at the outset whereas initial recruitment into the Da Qing study was for individuals only at high risk of the disease and a delayed onset of the disease was associated with significantly lower cardiovascular mortality. Intensive medical management of cardiovascular risk factors, such as increased use of statins to manage low-density-lipoprotein cholesterol levels in the control group, in the Look AHEAD trial may explain why the intervention did not provide additional benefit. Finally, the longer follow-up period may be essential as the difference in cumulative cardiovascular mortality between the intervention and control groups only started to become apparent in the Da Qing study after 12 years of follow-up, and only became significantly different after 23 years of follow-up – aptly demonstrating why so few randomised controlled trials of physical activity and CVD are available.

PHYSICAL ACTIVITY AND SECONDARY PREVENTION OF CVD

This chapter has reviewed the evidence that physical activity provides a protective effect against CVD in individuals free of the disease. However, physical activity and fitness are also important for preventing recurrence and improving the survival of individuals who have already experienced a myocardial infarction or stroke. Indeed, exercise has been used in clinical settings as a treatment for patients with CVD since the 1950s.

Observational studies have quantified the amount of activity or level of fitness providing protection against secondary CVD events. The British Regional Heart Study found that the amount of weekly recreational activity, number of minutes spent walking each day, and intensity of gardening all reduced the risk of mortality in men diagnosed with CHD (Wannamethee et al. 2000) (Figure 4.28). In the US, the Women's Health Initiative-Observational Study studied changes in physical activity and sitting time in postmenopausal women who had experienced a first myocardial infarction in relation to subsequent mortality. Compared with those women who maintained only low physical activity after the first event (<7.5 MET-h week^{-1}), women who increased or maintained higher physical activity (≥7.5 MET-h week^{-1}) during follow-up reduced the risk of mortality by 46% and 48%, respectively. Moreover, for women who had low physical activity prior to the first event, every 1 MET-h week^{-1} increase translated to an 8% decreased risk of all-cause mortality, 16% decreased risk of CHD mortality and 9% decreased risk of CVD mortality. The same increase for women with higher levels of activity pre-myocardial infarction translated to an 8% decreased risk of CHD mortality. Reductions in risk for walking were similar to that for physical activity when analysed independently but stronger. For sitting, women who had pre-event sitting times of <8 hours per day had a 9% higher risk of all-cause mortality for every 1 hour per day of increased sitting time post-event (Gorczyca et al. 2017).

In terms of fitness levels, the National Exercise and Heart Disease Project (NEHDP) found that every 1-MET increase in work capacity was associated with an 8–14% reduction in the risk of all-cause mortality in male myocardial infarction patients over 19 years of follow-up (Dorn et al. 1999). A more recent report on the relationship between fitness and survival in patients with a first myocardial infarction support these data.

Figure 4.28 Relative risk of CVD mortality associated with the amount of weekly recreational activity, number of minutes spent walking each day, and intensity of gardening in 772 men diagnosed with CHD in the British Regional Heart Study.

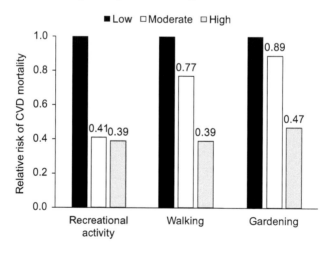

Source: Wannamethee et al. (2000).
Notes: Data labels show relative risk in comparison with the low volume/intensity activity. Recreational activity: low, <4 h weekend^{-1}; moderate, 4 h weekend^{-1}; high, >4 h weekend^{-1}. Walking: low, 0 min day^{-1}; moderate, 1–40 min day^{-1}; high, >40 min day^{-1}. Gardening: low, none; moderate, light; high, moderate/heavy. Reductions in risk significant for moderate and high recreational activities, high levels of walking and high intensity of gardening. Data adjusted for age, smoking, social class, obesity, self-rated health, history of myocardial infarction, stroke and diabetes.

Individuals whose fitness levels were high pre-event (men ≥ 22 ml kg^{-1} min^{-1}; women 19 ml kg^{-1} min^{-1}) had the lowest risk of death. However, individuals whose fitness improved from a middle to high level showed no difference in risk from those who started at a high level and maintained their fitness post-event (Barons et al. 2015).

Individuals who have experienced a first cardiovascular event have a high rate of mortality and are more likely to have a second event. Thus, randomised controlled trials to examine the effects of physical activity on CVD mortality and occurrence of secondary events in these individuals can be performed and helps to provide a clearer causal link than that seen from observational studies examining primary prevention in healthy populations. Evidence for the effectiveness of exercise in cardiac rehabilitation is provided by a meta-analysis of 48 randomised controlled trials involving 8,940 patients with CHD. The findings of this analysis revealed a 20% reduction in all-cause mortality risk and a 26% reduction in cardiac mortality in patients assigned to exercise rehabilitation compared with usual care (Taylor et al. 2004). A more recent systematic review published by the Cochrane Library of 63 trials randomising 14,486 male and female CHD patients to exercise-based cardiac rehabilitation or usual care confirms these findings (Anderson et al. 2016). Exercise reduced cardiovascular mortality by 26% and risk of hospital admissions by 18%. However, there were no reductions in the risk for myocardial infarction, coronary artery bypass graft (a procedure to bypass a blocked coronary artery using a healthy artery or vein), or percutaneous transluminal coronary angioplasty (a procedure to open up a blocked artery using a catheter). These findings are supported by other data (Lawler et al. 2011; O'Connor et al. 1989).

The effect of physical activity on secondary prevention and survival after stroke is less well documented. A recent meta-analysis reported the effect of lifestyle interventions, with or without exercise programmes on cardiovascular events in patients who had a stroke or transient ischaemic attack. Twenty-two randomised controlled trials with 2,574 patients were examined, including five studies with 1,800 patients which used a cardiovascular exercise intervention exclusively and five studies with 222 patients using a combined lifestyle intervention. Collectively, there were no significant reductions for cardiovascular events or mortality although there was a mean reduction in systolic blood pressure, a major risk factor for stroke, of -3.6 mm Hg. Subgroup analyses found no difference in these findings among therapies including exercise (Deijle et al. 2017). This finding supports a meta-analysis from the Cochrane Library stating that the effect of exercise training on stroke mortality is presently unclear (Saunders et al. 2016).

For chronic heart failure an early meta-analysis from nine randomised controlled trial datasets including 801 patients concluded that mortality and admission to hospital are significantly reduced after exercise training in chronic heart failure patients (Piepoli et al. 2004). These data are supported by a large randomised multi-centre controlled trial of 2,331 medically stable patients in the US which found that, after adjustment for baseline prognostic characteristics, there were modest reductions in all-cause mortality and all-cause hospitalisation with regular moderate-intensity exercise at 60–70% of heart rate reserve (O'Connor et al. 2009).

Exercise can be more effective than some surgical techniques for treating CVD. One example is a study involving 101 male patients with stable coronary artery disease who were randomly assigned to 12 months of exercise training (20 minutes of cycling each day) or to percutaneous (through the skin) coronary stenting (which involves inserting a plastic or metal mesh into an artery to reopen it or keep it open). Maximum oxygen uptake increased by 16% in the exercise training group (from 22.7 ml kg^{-1} min^{-1} at baseline to 26.2 ml kg^{-1} min^{-1} at 12 months) while remaining unchanged in those who underwent surgery (22.3 ml kg^{-1} min^{-1} at baseline versus 22.8 ml kg^{-1} min^{-1} at 12 months). Exercise training was associated with a higher event-free survival than surgery (88% versus 70% respectively) and was cheaper. The estimated costs of delivering the exercise programme were US$3,708 per patient per year compared with US$6,086 for percutaneous coronary intervention. Notable here are the reduced costs due to rehospitalisation and repeat surgery in the exercise group compared with the group who underwent surgery (Hambrecht et al. 2004). Similarly, a recent analysis examined the effectiveness of exercise versus drug interventions on mortality outcomes for CHD, stroke and heart failure. No statistically relevant differences were evident in the effectiveness of drug versus exercise for secondary prevention of CHD, and for secondary prevention of stroke physical activity was more effective than drug treatments. For heart failure only diuretics were a more effective treatment in preventing deaths than exercise (Naci and Ioannidis 2015).

The mechanisms via which exercise improves outcomes for patients with CVD are uncertain, but are thought to involve improvements in myocardial perfusion. These may result from improved endothelial function – the ability of the endothelium to interact with vascular smooth muscle and influence blood flow – as well as the growth of coronary collaterals within the heart (Gielen et al. 2001). It is also possible that exercise training may lead to reversal (regression) of coronary atherosclerosis. There is limited evidence to support this suggestion, but intervention trials involving multiple lifestyle factors (diet, exercise, stress management and smoking cessation) have shown that regression of coronary atherosclerosis is possible (Ornish et al. 1998).

PHYSICAL ACTIVITY AS THERAPY FOR CVD

Physical activity and fitness are also therapies for those afflicted with CVD. Areas where physical activity has proven effective are stroke rehabilitation, claudication, heart failure and hypertension (for hypertension see Chapter 7). A meta-analysis from the Cochrane Library points toward cardiorespiratory training or mixed training (including resistance exercise) interventions being effective for improving maximum walking speed, preferred gait speed and walking capacity in stroke survivors, with mixed training also improving balance (Saunders et al. 2016). Other meta-analyses have supported these findings with improvements in mobility documented in long-term stroke survivors after aerobic exercise interventions lasting between two and six months (Kendall and Gothe 2016) and improved balance outcomes (van Duijnhoven et al. 2016). For balance, specific balance and/or weight-shifting and gait training were identified as producing successful improvements suggesting that targeted exercise therapies are required for this outcome.

There has been growing interest in the effects of physical activity on post-stroke cognitive function. Several cellular and molecular mechanisms may explain the influence of physical activity here. These include factors related to the survival and growth of

Figure 4.29 Distance to onset of claudication pain, distance to maximal claudication pain, and six-minute walk distance in patients with peripheral arterial disease and intermittent claudication before and after six months of exercise rehabilitation (*n* = 28) or control (*n* = 24) treatment.

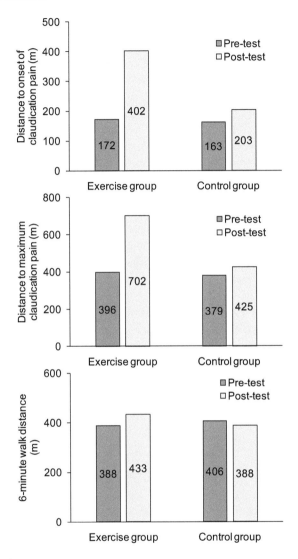

Source: Gardner et al. (2001).

neurons (brain-derived neurotropic factor), the formation of synapses (synaptogenesis), the formation of new dendrites to create synapses (dendritic branching), reducing the lesion volume in affected areas of the brain, and protecting tissue from inflammation and oxidative damage. A meta-analysis of 14 randomised controlled trials with 736 participants showed that combined aerobic and strength training programmes generated the largest cognitive gains and that this occurred even in the chronic post-stroke phase. The biggest effect was on attention and processing speeds rather than executive function (a set of processes which includes the ability to switch between concepts and prevent impulsive actions) or working memory (being able to keep information in mind) (Oberlin et al. 2017).

Claudication is the primary symptom of peripheral vascular disease and is defined as walking-induced pain in one or both legs (primarily affecting the calves) that does not go away with continued walking and is only relieved by rest (Stewart et al. 2002). Training studies have shown that exercise may ameliorate the severity of claudication and increase maximal walking time (Gardner and Poehlman 1995; Gardner et al. 2001) (Figure 4.29) and there are suggestions that exercise training may outweigh peripheral angioplasty in improving exercise tolerance (Whyman and Ruckley 1998) although more evidence is needed. A variety of mechanisms may account for the improvements with exercise including improved endothelial function, vascular angiogenesis (growth of new capillaries), enhanced muscle metabolic capacity and improved walking economy.

Exercise can also reduce the debilitating symptoms (breathlessness and fatigue) of chronic heart failure. Mean increase in peak oxygen uptake in 15 randomised controlled trials of exercise training that included 426 heart failure patients was 20.5% and despite varying exercise prescription the range of increase in peak oxygen uptake was between 12% and 31% (Piña et al. 2003). These data are supported by a large randomised multi-centre trial in the US showing improvement in six-minute walk capacity, cardiopulmonary exercise time, peak oxygen consumption (O'Connor et al. 2009), along with self-reported health status in exercise trained versus usual care patients with chronic heart failure (Flynn et al. 2009). Exercise training can also affect several other outcomes in individuals with heart failure including maximal cardiac output, mitochondrial size and density, skeletal muscle oxidative enzymes and improved quality of life in both men and women (Thompson et al. 2003).

SUMMARY

- CVDs are a major cause of mortality and morbidity in developed countries and their prevalence is increasing in developing countries.
- Atherosclerosis is the major cause of CVD. It has a long clinical history and may be well progressed before symptoms occur.
- Evidence that inactivity and low fitness are strong risk factors for CHD is compelling. Both confer an increase in risk similar to that associated with smoking, hypertension and high blood cholesterol.
- Sedentary activities have become widespread and are an independent risk for CVD beyond that of physical inactivity.
- Good evidence has emerged showing that being physically active or fit reduces the risk of having a stroke. There is some dose–response effect with higher levels of activity/fitness conferring a greater protective effect.
- Recent epidemiological studies have demonstrated that physical activity/fitness can afford protection against heart failure.

- Randomised controlled trials show that combined healthy lifestyle interventions can reduce the occurrence of CVD in healthy individuals and in some high-risk groups.
- There is strong evidence supporting the effectiveness of physical activity for secondary prevention of CVD and as a central component of cardiac rehabilitation programmes. Exercise training may be particularly effective in this regard because it enhances myocardial perfusion and hence oxygen delivery to the heart.
- Exercise is beneficial for rehabilitating stroke patients and reducing the symptoms of claudication and heart failure.

STUDY TASKS

1 Provide arguments centred on the debate of whether atherosclerosis is a disease of 'nature' or 'nurture'.

2 Using the data in Table 4.2, calculate the relative risk of death from CHD associated with different levels of fitness. Express this first with the low fitness group as the reference category and then with the high fitness group as the reference category. As well as working out the figures, put each relative risk into words as if you were explaining the findings to someone else. In addition, explain: (a) why it is necessary to use person-years as the units for the death rate; (b) why the death rates were adjusted for age; and (c) why the person-years of follow-up are not simply ten times the numbers of subjects in the fitness group.

Table 4.2 Deaths from CHD over an average follow-up period of ten years.

	NUMBER OF SUBJECTS	PERSON-YEARS OF FOLLOW-UP	NUMBER OF DEATHS	DEATH RATE PER 10,000 PERSON-YEARS*
Low fitness	5,130	46,098	112	20.70
High fitness	5,075	45,650	44	8.25

Note: *Adjusted for age

3 In the example given in Box 4.3 the women in the top quintile for walking in the US Nurses' Health Study completed an average of 20 MET-h of walking each week. It is estimated that this meant about 5.7 h of walking at a 'normal' pace (assumed to be 4.8 km h^{-1} or 3 mile h^{-1}). Estimate the gross weekly energy expenditure of these nurses in walking, assuming an average body mass of 60 kg.

4 In what ways could the design of epidemiological studies be improved to provide stronger evidence that physical inactivity and low fitness are causal factors for CHD in healthy individuals? Discuss the problems that would have to be faced in seeking this information.

5 What is the difference between physical inactivity and sedentary behaviour? Why is it important to examine sedentary behaviours separately from physical activity?

6 Provide reasons for the contrasting findings for CVD from the Look AHEAD Trial with the long-term outcomes from the Da Qing Study.

7 Describe the advantages of exercise training compared with percutaneous coronary stenting for the treatment of stable coronary artery disease as indicated in the study by Hambrecht and colleagues (2004).

8 In what way is the evidence supporting the role of exercise in treating CHD stronger than the evidence indicating that regular physical activity prevents CHD?

FURTHER READING

Gibbs, B.B., Hergenroeder, A.L., Katzmarzyk, P.T., Lee, I.-M. and Jakicic, J.M. (2015) Definition, measurement, and health risks associated with sedentary behavior. *Medicine and Science in Sports and Exercise* 47: 1295–300.

Gill, J.M., Celis-Morales, C.A. and Ghouri, N. (2014) Physical activity, ethnicity and cardiometabolic health: does one size fit all? *Atherosclerosis* 232: 319–33.

Hamer, M. and Chida, Y. (2008) Walking and primary prevention: a meta-analysis of prospective cohort studies. *British Journal of Sports Medicine* 42: 238–43.

Harber, M.P., Kaminsky, L.A., Arena, R., Blair, S.N., Franklin, B.A., Myers, J. and Ross, R. (2017) Impact of cardiorespiratory fitness on all-cause and disease-specific mortality: advances since 2009. *Progress in Cardiovascular Diseases* 60: 11–20.

Pate, R.R., O'Neill, J.R. and Lobelo, F. (2008) The evolving definition of "sedentary". *Exercise and Sport Sciences Reviews* 36: 173–8.

Ross, R., Blair, S.N., Arena, R., Church, T.S., Després, J.P., Franklin, B.A. et al.; American Heart Association Physical Activity Committee of the Council on Lifestyle and Cardiometabolic Health; Council on Clinical Cardiology; Council on Epidemiology and Prevention; Council on Cardiovascular and Stroke Nursing; Council on Functional Genomics and Translational Biology; Stroke Council. (2016) Importance of assessing cardiorespiratory fitness in clinical practice: a case for fitness as a clinical vital sign: a scientific statement from the American Heart Association. *Circulation* 134: e653–99.

Shiroma, E.J. and Lee, I.-M. (2010) Physical activity and cardiovascular health: lessons learned from epidemiological studies across age, gender, and race/ethnicity. *Circulation* 122: 743–52.

Stewart, K.J., Hiatt, W.R., Regensteiner, J.G. and Hirsch, A.T. (2002) Exercise training for claudication. *New England Journal of Medicine* 347: 1941–51.

Swift, D.L., Lavie, C.J., Johannsen, N.M., Arena, R., Earnest, C.P., O'Keefe, J.H. et al. (2013) Physical activity, cardiorespiratory fitness, and exercise training in primary and secondary coronary prevention. *Circulation Journal* 77: 281–92.

REFERENCES

Anderson, L., Thompson, D.R., Oldridge, N., Zwisler, A.D., Rees, K., Martin, N. and Taylor, R.S. (2016) Exercise-based cardiac rehabilitation for coronary heart disease. *Cochrane Database of Systematic Reviews* 1: CD001800. doi: 10.1002/14651858.CD001800.pub3.

Arem, H., Moore, S.C., Patel, A., Hartge, P., Berrington de Gonzalez, A., Visvanathan, K. et al. (2015) Leisure time physical activity and mortality: a detailed pooled analysis of the dose–response relationship. *Journal of the American Medical Association Internal Medicine* 175: 959–67.

Autenrieth, C.S., Evenson, K.R., Yatsuya, H., Shahar, E., Baggett, C. and Rosamond, W.D. (2013) Association between physical activity and risk of stroke subtypes: the atherosclerosis risk in communities study. *Neuroepidemiology* 40: 109–16.

Barons, M.J., Turner, S., Parsons, N., Griffiths, F., Bethell, H., Weich, S. and Thorogood, M. (2015) Fitness predicts long-term survival after a cardiovascular event: a prospective cohort study. *British Medical Journal Open* 5(10): e007772. doi: 10.1136/bmjopen-2015–007772.

Bauman, A., Ainsworth, B.E., Sallis, J.F., Hagströmer, M., Craig, C.L., Bull, F.C. et al.; IPS Group. (2011) The descriptive epidemiology of sitting: a 20-country comparison using the International Physical Activity Questionnaire (IPAQ). *American Journal of Preventive Medicine* 41: 228–35.

Berry, J.D., Pandey, A., Gao, A., Leonard, D., Farzaneh-Far, R., Ayers, C. et al. (2013) Physical fitness and risk for heart failure and coronary artery disease. *Circulation: Heart Failure* 6: 627–34.

Berry, J.D., Willis, B., Gupta, S., Barlow, C.E., Lakoski, S.G., Khera, A. et al. (2011) Lifetime risks for cardiovascular disease mortality by cardiorespiratory fitness levels measured at ages 45, 55, and 65 years in men. The Cooper Center Longitudinal Study. *Journal of the American College of Cardiology* 57: 1604–10.

Bijnen, F.C., Caspersen, C.J., Feskens, E.J., Saris, W.H., Mosterd, W.L. and Kromhout, D. (1998) Physical activity and 10-year mortality from cardiovascular diseases and all causes: the Zutphen Elderly Study. *Archives of Internal Medicine* 158: 1499–505.

Biswas, A., Oh, P.I., Faulkner, G.E., Bajaj, R.R., Silver, M.A., Mitchell, M.S. and Alter, D.A. (2015) Sedentary time and its association with risk for disease incidence, mortality, and hospitalization in adults: a systematic review and meta-analysis. *Annals of Internal Medicine* 162: 123–32.

Blair, S.N., Kampert, J.B., Kohl, H.W. III, Barlow, C.E., Macera, C.A., Paffenbarger, R.S. Jr. and Gibbons, L.W. (1996) Influences of cardiorespiratory fitness and other precursors on cardiovascular disease and all-cause mortality in men and women. *Journal of the American Medical Association* 276: 205–10.

Blair, S.N., Kohl, H.W. III, Barlow, C.E., Paffenbarger, R.S. Jr, Gibbons, L.W. and Macera, C.A. (1995) Changes in physical fitness and all-cause mortality: a prospective study of healthy and unhealthy men. *Journal of the American Medical Association* 273: 1093–8.

Boden, W.E., O'Rourke, R.A., Teo, K.K., Hartigan, P.M., Maron, D.J., Kostuk, W.J. et al.; COURAGE Trial Research Group. (2007) Optimal medical therapy with or without PCI for stable coronary disease. *New England Journal of Medicine* 356: 1503–16.

Bouchard, C., An, P., Rice, T., Skinner, J.S., Wilmore, J.H., Gagnon, J. et al. (1999) Familial aggregation of VO(2max) response to exercise training: results from the HERITAGE Family Study. *Journal of Applied Physiology* 87: 1003–8.

Bouchard, C., Sarzynski, M.A., Rice, T.K., Kraus, W.E., Church, T.S., Sung, Y.J. et al. (2011) Genomic predictors of the maximal O_2 uptake response to standardized exercise training programs. *Journal of Applied Physiology* 110: 1160–70.

Celis-Morales, C.A., Gray, S., Petermann, F., Iliodromiti, S., Welsh, P., Lyall, D.M., et al. (2019) Walking pace is associated with lower risk of all-cause and cause-specific mortality. *Medicine and Science in Sports and Exercise* 51: 472–80.

Celis-Morales, C.A., Lyall, D.M., Anderson, J., Iliodromiti, S., Fan, Y., Ntuk, U.E. et al. (2017) The association between physical activity and risk of mortality is modulated by grip strength and cardiorespiratory fitness: evidence from 498 135 UK-Biobank participants. *European Heart Journal* 38: 116–22.

Celis-Morales, C.A., Welsh, P., Lyall, D.M., Steell, L., Petermann, F., Anderson, J. et al. (2018) Associations of grip strength with cardiovascular, respiratory, and cancer outcomes and all-cause mortality: prospective cohort study of half a million UK Biobank participants. *British Medical Journal* 361: k1651. doi: 10.1136/bmj.k1651.

Church, T.S., Thomas, D.M., Tudor-Locke, C., Katzmarzyk, P.T., Earnest, C.P., Rodarte, R.Q. et al. (2011) Trends over 5 decades in U.S. occupation-related physical activity and their associations with obesity. *PLoS One* 6: e19657. doi: 10.1371/journal.pone.0019657.

DeFina, L.F., Haskell, W.L., Willis, B.L., Barlow, C.E., Finley, C.E., Levine, B.D. and Cooper, K.H. (2015) Physical activity versus cardiorespiratory fitness: two (partly) distinct components of cardiovascular health? *Progress in Cardiovascular Diseases* 57: 324–9.

Deijle, I.A., Van Schaik, S.M., Van Wegen, E.E., Weinstein, H.C., Kwakkel, G. and Van den Berg-Vos, R.M. (2017) Lifestyle interventions to prevent cardiovascular events after stroke and transient ischemic attack: systematic review and meta-analysis. *Stroke* 48: 174–9.

Donahue, R.P., Abbott, R.D., Reed, D.M. and Yano, K. (1988) Physical activity and coronary heart disease in middle-aged and elderly men: the Honolulu Heart Program. *American Journal of Public Health* 78: 683–5.

Dohrn, I.M., Sjöström, M., Kwak, L., Oja, P. and Hagströmer, M. (2018) Accelerometer-measured sedentary time and physical activity: a 15 year follow-up of mortality in a Swedish population-based cohort. *Journal of Science and Medicine in Sport* 21: 702–7.

Dorn, J., Naughton, J., Imamura, D. and Trevisan, M. (1999) Results of a multicenter randomized clinical trial of exercise and long-term survival in myocardial infarction patients: the National Exercise and Heart Disease Project (NEHDP). *Circulation* 100: 1764–9.

Ekelund, L.G., Haskell, W.L., Johnson, J.L., Whaley, F.S., Criqui, M.H. and Sheps, D.S. (1988) Physical fitness as a predictor of cardiovascular mortality in asymptomatic North American men: the Lipid Research Clinics Mortality Follow-up Study. *New England Journal of Medicine* 319: 1379–84.

Ekelund, U., Steene-Johannessen, J., Brown, W.J., Fagerland, M.W., Owen, N., Powell, K.E. et al.; Lancet Physical Activity Series 2 Executive Committee; Lancet Sedentary Behaviour Working Group. (2016) Does physical activity attenuate, or even eliminate, the detrimental association of sitting time with mortality? A harmonised meta-analysis of data from more than 1 million men and women. *The Lancet* 388: 1302–10.

Enos, W.F. Jr, Beyer, J.C. and Holmes, R.H. (1955) Pathogenesis of coronary disease in American soldiers killed in Korea. *Journal of the American Medical Association* 158: 912–14.

Enos, W.F., Holmes, R.H. and Beyer, J. (1953) Coronary disease among United States soldiers killed in action in Korea; preliminary report. *Journal of the American Medical Association* 152: 1090–3.

Erikssen, G., Liestøl, K., Bjørnholt, J., Thaulow, E., Sandvik, L. and Erikssen, J. (1998) Changes in physical fitness and changes in mortality. *The Lancet* 352: 759–62.

Farrell, S.W., Finley, C.E., Radford, N.B. and Haskell, W.L. (2013) Cardiorespiratory fitness, body mass index, and heart failure mortality in men: Cooper Center Longitudinal Study. *Circulation: Heart Failure* 6: 898–905.

Florido, R., Kwak, L., Lazo, M., Nambi, V., Ahmed, H.M., Hegde, S.M. et al. (2018) Six-year changes in physical activity and the risk of incident heart failure: ARIC Study. *Circulation* 137: 2142–51.

Flynn, K.E., Piña, I.L., Whellan, D.J., Lin, L., Blumenthal, J.A., Ellis, S.J. et al.; HF-ACTION Investigators. (2009) Effects of exercise training on health status in patients with chronic heart failure: HF-ACTION randomized controlled trial. *Journal of the American Medical Association* 301: 1451–9.

Folsom, A.R., Arnett, D.K., Hutchinson, R.G., Liao, F., Clegg, L.X. and Cooper, L.S. (1997) Physical activity and incidence of coronary heart disease in middle-aged women and men. *Medicine and Science in Sports and Exercise* 29: 901–9.

Gaede, P., Vedel, P., Larsen, N., Jensen, G.V., Parving, H.H. and Pedersen, O. (2003) Multifactorial intervention and cardiovascular disease in patients with type 2 diabetes. *New England Journal of Medicine* 348: 383–93.

Gardner, A.W., Katzel, L.I., Sorkin, J.D., Bradham, D.D., Hochberg, M.C., Flinn, W.R. and Goldberg, A.P. (2001) Exercise rehabilitation improves functional outcomes and peripheral circulation in patients with intermittent claudication: a randomized controlled trial. *Journal of the American Geriatrics Society* 49: 755–62.

Gardner, A.W. and Poehlman, E.T. (1995) Exercise rehabilitation programs for the treatment of claudication pain: a meta-analysis. *Journal of the American Medical Association* 274: 975–80.

Gielen, S., Schuler, G. and Hambrecht, R. (2001) Exercise training in coronary artery disease and coronary vasomotion. *Circulation* 103: E1–6.

Gillum, R.F., Mussolino, M.E. and Ingram, D.D. (1996) Physical activity and stroke incidence in women and men: the NHANES I Epidemiologic Follow-up Study. *American Journal of Epidemiology* 143: 860–9.

Gorczyca, A.M., Eaton, C.B., LaMonte, M.J., Manson, J.E., Johnston, J.D., Bidulescu, A. et al. (2017) Change in physical activity and sitting time after myocardial infarction and mortality among postmenopausal women in the Women's Health Initiative-Observational Study. *Journal of the American Heart Association* 6: e005354. doi: 10.1161/JAHA.116.005354.

Gregg, E.W., Cauley, J.A., Stone, K., Thompson, T.J., Bauer, D.C., Cummings, S.R. and Ensrud, K.E.; Study of Osteoporotic Fractures Research Group. (2003) Relationship of changes in physical activity and mortality among older women. *Journal of the American Medical Association* 289: 2379–86.

Hakim, A.A., Curb, J.D., Petrovitch, H., Rodriguez, B.L., Yano, K., Ross, G.W. et al. (1999) Effects of walking on coronary heart disease in elderly men: the Honolulu Heart Program. *Circulation* 100: 9–13.

Hallal, P.C., Andersen, L.B., Bull, F.C., Guthold, R., Haskell, W. and Ekelund, U.; Lancet Physical Activity Series Working Group. (2012) Global physical activity levels: surveillance progress, pitfalls, and prospects. *The Lancet* 380: 247–57.

Hambrecht, R., Walther, C., Möbius-Winkler, S., Gielen, S., Linke, A., Conradi, K. et al. (2004) Percutaneous coronary angioplasty compared with exercise training in patients with stable coronary artery disease: a randomized trial. *Circulation* 109: 1371–8.

Hamer, M. and Chida, Y. (2008) Walking and primary prevention: a meta-analysis of prospective cohort studies. *British Journal of Sports Medicine* 42: 238–43.

Hansson, G.K. (2005) Inflammation, atherosclerosis, and coronary artery disease. *New England Journal of Medicine* 352: 1685–95.

Heady, J.A., Morris, J.N., Kagan, A. and Raffle, P.A. (1961) Coronary heart disease in London busmen. A progress report with particular reference to physique. *British Journal of Preventive and Social Medicine* 15: 143–53.

Hochman, J.S., Lamas, G.A., Buller, C.E., Dzavik, V., Reynolds, H.R., Abramsky, S.J. et al.; Occluded Artery Trial Investigators. (2006) Coronary intervention for persistent occlusion after myocardial infarction. *New England Journal of Medicine* 355: 2395–407.

Hooker, S.P., Sui, X., Colabianchi, N., Vena, J., Laditka, J., LaMonte, M.J. and Blair, S.N. (2008) Cardiorespiratory fitness as a predictor of fatal and nonfatal stroke in asymptomatic women and men. *Stroke* 39: 2950–7.

Hu, F.B., Stampfer, M.J., Colditz, G.A., Ascherio, A., Rexrode, K.M., Willett, W.C. and Manson, J.E. (2000) Physical activity and risk of stroke in women. *Journal of the American Medical Association* 283: 2961–7.

Jefferis, B.J., Whincup, P.H., Papacosta, O. and Wannamethee, S.G. (2014) Protective effect of time spent walking on risk of stroke in older men. *Stroke* 45: 194–9.

Kaplan, H., Thompson, R.C., Trumble, B.C., Wann, L.S., Allam, A.H., Beheim, B. et al. (2017) Coronary atherosclerosis in indigenous South American Tsimane: a cross-sectional cohort study. *The Lancet* 389: 1730–9.

Katzmarzyk, P.T., Church, T.S., Craig, C.L. and Bouchard, C. (2009) Sitting time and mortality from all causes, cardiovascular disease, and cancer. *Medicine and Science in Sports and Exercise* 41: 998–1005.

Kendall, B.J. and Gothe, N.P. (2016) Effect of aerobic exercise interventions on mobility among stroke patients: a systematic review. *American Journal of Physical Medicine and Rehabilitation* 95: 214–24.

Khan, H., Jaffar, N., Rauramaa, R., Kurl, S., Savonen, K. and Laukkanen, J.A. (2017) Cardiorespiratory fitness and nonfatal cardiovascular events: a population-based follow-up study. *American Heart Journal* 184: 55–61.

Knoops, K.T., de Groot, L.C., Kromhout, D., Perrin, A.E., Moreiras-Varela, O., Menotti, A. and van Staveren, W.A. (2004) Mediterranean diet, lifestyle factors, and 10-year mortality in elderly European men and women: the HALE project. *Journal of the American Medical Association* 292: 1433–9.

Kodama, S., Saito, K., Tanaka, S., Maki, M., Yachi, Y., Asumi, M. et al. (2009) Cardiorespiratory fitness as a quantitative predictor of all-cause mortality and cardiovascular events in healthy men and women: a meta-analysis. *Journal of the American Medical Association* 301: 2024–35.

Kurl, S., Laukkanen, J.A., Rauramaa, R., Lakka, T.A., Sivenius, J. and Salonen, J.T. (2003) Cardiorespiratory fitness and the risk for stroke in men. *Archives of Internal Medicine* 163: 1682–8.

Kyu, H.H., Bachman, V.F., Alexander, L.T., Mumford, J.E., Afshin, A., Estep, K. et al. (2016) Physical activity and risk of breast cancer, colon cancer, diabetes, ischemic heart disease, and ischemic stroke events: systematic review and dose–response meta-analysis for the Global Burden of Disease Study 2013. *British Medical Journal* 354: i3857. doi: 10.1136/bmj.i3857.

Lakka, T.A., Laukkanen, J.A., Rauramaa, R., Salonen, R., Lakka, H.M., Kaplan, G.A. and Salonen, J.T. (2001) Cardiorespiratory fitness and the progression of carotid atherosclerosis in middle-aged men. *Annals of Internal Medicine* 134: 12–20.

Lakka, T.A., Venäläinen, J.M., Rauramaa, R., Salonen, R., Tuomilehto, J. and Salonen, J.T. (1994) Relation of leisure-time physical activity and cardiorespiratory fitness to the risk of acute myocardial infarction. *New England Journal of Medicine* 330: 1549–54.

Lam, T.H., Ho, S.Y., Hedley, A.J., Mak, K.H. and Leung, G.M. (2004) Leisure time physical activity and mortality in Hong Kong: case-control study of all adult deaths in 1998. *Annals of Epidemiology* 14: 391–8.

Laukkanen, J.A., Kurl, S., Salonen, R., Rauramaa, R. and Salonen, J.T. (2004) The predictive value of cardiorespiratory fitness for cardiovascular events in men with various risk profiles: a prospective population-based cohort study. *European Heart Journal* 25: 1428–37.

Laukkanen, J.A., Lakka, T.A., Rauramaa, R., Kuhanen, R., Venäläinen, J.M., Salonen, R. and Salonen, J.T. (2001) Cardiovascular fitness as a predictor of mortality in men. *Archives of Internal Medicine* 161: 825–31.

Lawler, P.R., Filion, K.B. and Eisenberg, M.J. (2011) Efficacy of exercise-based cardiac rehabilitation post-myocardial infarction: a systematic review and meta-analysis of randomized controlled trials. *American Heart Journal* 162: 571–584.e2.

Lear, S.A., Hu, W., Rangarajan, S., Gasevic, D., Leong, D., Iqbal, R. et al. (2017) The effect of physical activity on mortality and cardiovascular disease in 130 000 people from 17 high-income, middle-income, and low-income countries: the PURE study. *The Lancet* 390: 2643–54.

Lee, C.D. and Blair, S.N. (2002) Cardiorespiratory fitness and stroke mortality in men. *Medicine and Science in Sports and Exercise* 34: 592–5.

Lee, C.D., Folsom, A.R. and Blair, S.N. (2003) Physical activity and stroke risk: a meta-analysis. *Stroke* 34: 2475–81.

Lee, D.C., Sui, X., Artero, E.G., Lee, I.-M., Church, T.S., McAuley, P.A. et al. (2011) Long-term effects of changes in cardiorespiratory fitness and body mass index on all-cause and cardiovascular disease mortality in men: the Aerobics Center Longitudinal Study. *Circulation* 124: 2483–90.

Lee, I.-M., Rexrode. K.M., Cook, N.R., Manson, J.E. and Buring, J.E. (2001) Physical activity and coronary heart disease in women: is "no pain, no gain" passé? *Journal of the American Medical Association* 285: 1447–54.

Lee, I.-M., Sesso, H.D., Oguma, Y. and Paffenbarger, R.S. Jr. (2003) Relative intensity of physical activity and risk of coronary heart disease. *Circulation* 107: 1110–16.

Lee, I.-M., Sesso, H.D. and Paffenbarger, R.S. Jr. (2000) Physical activity and coronary heart disease risk in men: does the duration of exercise episodes predict risk? *Circulation* 102: 981–6.

Leong, D.P., Teo, K.K., Rangarajan, S., Lopez-Jaramillo, P., Avezum, A. Jr., Orlandini, A. et al.; Prospective Urban Rural Epidemiology (PURE) Study investigators. (2015) Prognostic value of grip strength: findings from the Prospective Urban Rural Epidemiology (PURE) study. *The Lancet* 386: 266–73.

Li, J. and Siegrist, J. (2012) Physical activity and risk of cardiovascular disease – a meta-analysis of prospective cohort studies. *International Journal of Environmental Research and Public Health* 9: 391–407.

Li, G., Zhang, P., Wang, J., An, Y., Gong, Q., Gregg, E.W. et al. (2014) Cardiovascular mortality, all-cause mortality, and diabetes incidence after lifestyle intervention for people with impaired glucose tolerance in the Da Qing Diabetes Prevention Study: a 23-year follow-up study. *Lancet Diabetes and Endocrinology* 2: 474–80.

Libby, P. (2013) Mechanisms of acute coronary syndromes and their implications for therapy. *New England Journal of Medicine* 368: 2004–13.

Look AHEAD Research Group; Gregg, E.W., Jakicic, J.M., Blackburn, G., Bloomquist, P., Bray, G.A., Clark, J.M. et al. (2016) Association of the magnitude of weight loss and changes in physical fitness with long-term cardiovascular disease outcomes in overweight or obese people with type 2 diabetes: a post-hoc analysis of the Look AHEAD randomised clinical trial. *The Lancet Diabetes and Endocrinology* 4: 913–21.

Look AHEAD Research Group; Wing, R.R., Bolin, P., Brancati, F.L., Bray, G.A., Clark, J.M., Coday, M. et al. (2013) Cardiovascular effects of intensive lifestyle intervention in type 2 diabetes. *New England Journal of Medicine* 369: 145–54.

Manson, J.E., Greenland, P., LaCroix, A.Z., Stefanick, M.L., Mouton, C.P., Oberman, A. et al. (2002) Walking compared with vigorous exercise for the prevention of cardiovascular events in women. *New England Journal of Medicine* 347: 716–25.

Manson, J.E., Hu, F.B., Rich-Edwards, J.W., Colditz, G.A., Stampfer, M.J., Willett, W.C. et al. (1999) A prospective study of walking as compared with vigorous exercise in the prevention of coronary heart disease in women. *New England Journal of Medicine* 341: 650–8.

Matthews, C.E., Chen, K.Y., Freedson, P.S., Buchowski, M.S., Beech, B.M., Pate, R.R. and Troiano, R.P. (2008) Amount of time spent in sedentary behaviors in the United States, 2003–2004. *American Journal of Epidemiology* 167: 875–81.

McNamara, J.J., Molot, M.A., Stremple, J.F. and Cutting, R.T. (1971) Coronary artery disease in combat casualties in Vietnam. *Journal of the American Medical Association* 216: 1185–7.

Miller, G.J., Cooper, J.A. and Beckles, G.L. (2005) Cardiorespiratory fitness, all-cause mortality, and risk of cardiovascular disease in Trinidadian men – the St James survey. *International Journal of Epidemiology* 34: 1387–94.

Morris, J.N., Clayton, D.G., Everitt, M.G., Semmence, A.M. and Burgess, E.H. (1990) Exercise in leisure time: coronary attack and death rates. *British Heart Journal* 63: 325–34.

Morris, J.N., Everitt, M.G., Pollard, R., Chave, S.P. and Semmence, A.M. (1980) Vigorous exercise in leisure-time: protection against coronary heart disease. *The Lancet* 2: 1207–10.

Morris, J.N., Heady, J.A., Raffle, P.A., Roberts, C.G. and Parks, J.W. (1953) Coronary heart-disease and physical activity of work. *The Lancet* 265: 1111–20.

Naci, H. and Ioannidis, J.P. (2015) Comparative effectiveness of exercise and drug interventions on mortality outcomes: metaepidemiological study. *British Journal of Sports Medicine* 49: 1414–22.

Napoli, C., D'Armiento, F.P., Mancini, F.P., Postiglione, A., Witztum, J.L., Palumbo, G. and Palinski, W. (1997) Fatty streak formation occurs in human fetal aortas and is greatly enhanced by maternal hypercholesterolemia: intimal accumulation of low density lipoprotein and its oxidation precede monocyte recruitment into early atherosclerotic lesions. *Journal of Clinical Investigation* 100: 2680–90.

Narula, J., Nakano, M., Virmani, R., Kolodgie, F.D., Petersen, R., Newcomb, R. et al. (2013) Histopathologic characteristics of atherosclerotic coronary disease and implications of the findings for the invasive and noninvasive detection of vulnerable plaques. *Journal of the American College of Cardiology* 61: 1041–51.

Ng, S.W. and Popkin, B.M. (2012) Time use and physical activity: a shift away from movement across the globe. *Obesity Reviews* 13: 659–80.

Nichols, M., Townsend, N., Luengo-Fernandez, R., Leal, J., Gray, A., Scarborough, P. and Rayner, M. (2012) *European Cardiovascular Disease Statistics 2012*. Brussels: European Heart Network; Sophia Antipolis: European Society of Cardiology.

Nocon, M., Hiemann, T., Müller-Riemenschneider, F., Thalau, F., Roll, S. and Willich, S.N. (2008) Association of physical activity with all-cause and cardiovascular mortality: a systematic review and meta-analysis. *European Journal of Cardiovascular Prevention and Rehabilitation* 15: 239–46.

Noda, H., Iso, H., Toyoshima, H., Date, C., Yamamoto, A., Kikuchi, S. et al.; JACC Study Group. (2005) Walking and sports participation and mortality from coronary heart disease and stroke. *Journal of the American College of Cardiology* 46: 1761–7.

Oberlin, L.E., Waiwood, A.M., Cumming, T.B., Marsland, A.L., Bernhardt, J. and Erickson, K.I. (2017) Effects of physical activity on poststroke cognitive function: a meta-analysis of randomized controlled trials. *Stroke* 48: 3093–100.

O'Connor, G.T., Buring, J.E., Yusuf, S., Goldhaber, S.Z., Olmstead, E.M., Paffenbarger, R.S. Jr. and Hennekens, C.H. (1989) An overview of randomized trials of rehabilitation with exercise after myocardial infarction. *Circulation* 80: 234–44.

O'Connor, C.M., Whellan, D.J., Lee, K.L., Keteyian, S.J., Cooper, L.S., Ellis, S.J. et al.; HF-ACTION Investigators. (2009) Efficacy and safety of exercise training in patients with chronic heart failure: HF-ACTION randomized controlled trial. *Journal of the American Medical Association* 301: 1439–50.

Oguma, Y. and Shinoda-Tagawa, T. (2004) Physical activity decreases cardiovascular disease risk in women: review and meta-analysis. *American Journal of Preventive Medicine* 26: 407–18.

Ornish, D., Scherwitz, L.W., Billings, J.H., Brown, S.E., Gould, K.L., Merritt, T.A. et al. (1998) Intensive lifestyle changes for reversal of coronary heart disease. *Journal of the American Medical Association* 280: 2001–7.

Paffenbarger, R.S. and Hale, W.E. (1975) Work activity and coronary heart mortality. *New England Journal of Medicine* 292: 545–50.

Paffenbarger, R.S. Jr, Hyde, R.T., Wing, A.L., Lee, I.-M., Jung, D.L. and Kampert, J.B. (1993) The association of changes in physical-activity level and other lifestyle characteristics with mortality among men. *New England Journal of Medicine* 328: 538–45.

Paffenbarger, R.S. Jr, Wing, A.L. and Hyde, R.T. (1978) Physical activity as an index of heart attack risk in college alumni. *American Journal of Epidemiology* 108: 161–75.

Pandey, A., Garg, S., Khunger, M., Darden, D., Ayers, C., Kumbhani, D.J. et al. (2015) Dose–response relationship between physical activity and risk of heart failure: a meta-analysis. *Circulation* 132: 1786–94.

Pate, R.R., O'Neill, J.R. and Lobelo, F. (2008) The evolving definition of "sedentary". *Exercise and Sport Sciences Reviews* 36: 173–8.

Physical Activity Guidelines Advisory Committee (2008) *Physical Activity Guidelines Advisory Committee Report, 2008*. Washington, DC: US Department of Health and Human Services.

Piepoli, M.F., Davos, C., Francis, D.P. and Coats, A.J.; ExTraMATCH Collaborative. (2004) Exercise training meta-analysis of trials in patients with chronic heart failure (ExTraMATCH). *British Medical Journal* 328: 189. doi: 10.1136/bmj.37938.645220.EE.

Piña, I.L., Apstein, C.S., Balady, G.J., Belardinelli, R., Chaitman, B.R., Duscha, B.D. et al.; American Heart Association Committee on exercise, rehabilitation, and prevention. (2003) Exercise and heart failure: a statement from the American Heart Association Committee on exercise, rehabilitation, and prevention. *Circulation* 107: 1210–25.

Ross, R. (1993) The pathogenesis of atherosclerosis: a perspective for the 1990s. *Nature* 362: 801–9.

Ross, R. (1999) Atherosclerosis – an inflammatory disease. *New England Journal of Medicine* 340: 115–26.

Roth, G.A., Johnson, C., Abajobir, A., Abd-Allah, F., Abera, S.F., Abyu, G. et al. (2017) Global, regional, and national burden of cardiovascular diseases for 10 Causes, 1990 to 2015. *Journal of the American College of Cardiology* 70: 1–25.

Rothberg, M.B. (2013) Coronary artery disease as clogged pipes: a misconceptual model. *Circulation: Cardiovascular Quality and Outcomes* 6: 129–32.

Sacco, R.L., Gan, R., Boden-Albala, B., Lin, I.F., Kargman, D.E., Hauser, W.A. et al. (1998) Leisure-time physical activity and ischemic stroke risk: the Northern Manhattan Stroke Study. *Stroke* 29: 380–7.

Saevereid, H.A., Schnohr, P. and Prescott, E. (2014) Speed and duration of walking and other leisure time physical activity and the risk of heart failure: a prospective cohort study from the Copenhagen City Heart Study. *PLoS One* 9: e89909. doi: 10.1371/journal.pone.0089909.

Saltin, B., Blomqvist, G., Mitchell, J.H., Johnson, R.L., Wildenthal, K. and Chapman, C.B. (1968) Response to exercise after bed rest and after training. *Circulation* 38: VII1–78.

Sattelmair, J., Pertman, J., Ding, E.L., Kohl, H.W., Haskell, W. and Lee, I.-M. (2011) Dose response between physical activity and risk of coronary heart disease: a meta-analysis. *Circulation* 124: 789–95.

Saunders, D.H., Sanderson, M., Hayes, S., Kilrane, M., Greig, C.A., Brazzelli, M. and Mead, G.E. (2016) Physical fitness training for stroke patients. *Cochrane Database of Systematic Reviews* 3: CD003316. doi: 10.1002/14651858.CD003316.pub6.

Sedentary Behaviour Research Network. (2012) Letter to the editor: standardized use of the terms "sedentary" and "sedentary behaviours". *Applied Physiology Nutrition and Metabolism* 37: 540–2.

Shah, R.V., Murthy, V.L., Colangelo, L.A., Reis, J., Venkatesh, B.A., Sharma, R. et al. (2016) Association of fitness in young adulthood with survival and cardiovascular risk: the Coronary Artery Risk Development in Young Adults (CARDIA) Study. *Journal of the American Medical Association Internal Medicine* 176: 87–95.

Shiroma, E.J. and Lee, I.-M. (2010) Physical activity and cardiovascular health: lessons learned from epidemiological studies across age, gender, and race/ethnicity. *Circulation* 122: 743–52.

Skinner, J.S., Wilmore, K.M., Krasnoff, J.B., Jaskólski, A., Jaskólska, A., Gagnon, J. et al. (2000) Adaptation to a standardized training program and changes in fitness in a large, heterogeneous population: the HERITAGE Family Study. *Medicine and Science in Sports and Exercise* 32: 157–61.

Smith, T.C., Wingard, D.L., Smith, B., Kritz-Silverstein, D. and Barrett-Connor, E. (2007) Walking decreased risk of cardiovascular disease mortality in older adults with diabetes. *Journal of Clinical Epidemiology* 60: 309–17.

Stampfer, M.J., Hu, F.B., Manson, J.E., Rimm, E.B. and Willett, W.C. (2000) Primary prevention of coronary heart disease in women through diet and lifestyle. *New England Journal of Medicine* 343: 16–22.

Stewart, K.J., Hiatt, W.R., Regensteiner, J.G. and Hirsch, A.T. (2002) Exercise training for claudication. *New England Journal of Medicine* 347: 1941–51.

Strong, J.P., Malcom, G.T., McMahan, C.A., Tracy, R.E., Newman, W.P. III, Herderick, E.E. and Cornhill, J.F. (1999) Prevalence and extent of atherosclerosis in adolescents and young adults: implications for prevention from the Pathobiological Determinants of Atherosclerosis in Youth Study. *Journal of the American Medical Association* 281: 727–35.

Sui, X., LaMonte, M.J. and Blair, S.N. (2007) Cardiorespiratory fitness as a predictor of nonfatal cardiovascular events in asymptomatic women and men. *American Journal of Epidemiology* 165: 1413–23.

Tanasescu, M., Leitzmann, M.F., Rimm, E.B., Willett, W.C., Stampfer, M.J. and Hu, F.B. (2002) Exercise type and intensity in relation to coronary heart disease in men. *Journal of the American Medical Association* 288: 1994–2000.

Taylor, R.S., Brown, A., Ebrahim, S., Jolliffe, J., Noorani, H., Rees, K. et al. (2004) Exercise-based rehabilitation for patients with coronary heart disease: systematic review and meta-analysis of randomized controlled trials. *American Journal of Medicine* 116: 682–92.

Thompson, P.D. (2002) Additional steps for cardiovascular health. *New England Journal of Medicine* 347: 755–6.

Thompson, P.D., Buchner, D., Piña, I.L., Balady, G.J., Williams, M.A., Marcus, B.H. et al.; American Heart Association Council on Clinical Cardiology Subcommittee on Exercise, Rehabilitation, and Prevention; American Heart Association Council on Nutrition, Physical Activity, and Metabolism Subcommittee on Physical Activity. (2003) Exercise and physical activity in the prevention and treatment of atherosclerotic cardiovascular disease: a statement from the Council on Clinical Cardiology (Subcommittee on Exercise, Rehabilitation, and Prevention) and the Council on Nutrition, Physical Activity, and Metabolism (Subcommittee on Physical Activity). *Circulation* 107: 3109–16.

Thompson, R.C., Allam, A.H., Lombardi, G.P., Wann, L.S., Sutherland, M.L., Sutherland, J.D. et al. (2013) Atherosclerosis across 4000 years of human history: the Horus study of four ancient populations. *The Lancet* 381: 1211–22.

Tikkanen, E., Gustafsson, S. and Ingelsson, E. (2018) Associations of fitness, physical activity, strength, and genetic risk with cardiovascular disease: longitudinal analyses in the UK Biobank Study. *Circulation* 137: 2583–91.

van Duijnhoven, H.J., Heeren, A., Peters, M.A., Veerbeek, J.M., Kwakkel, G., Geurts, A.C. and Weerdesteyn, V. (2016) Effects of exercise therapy on balance capacity in chronic stroke: systematic review and meta-analysis. *Stroke* 47: 2603–10.

Vatten, L.J., Nilsen, T.I., Romundstad, P.R., Drøyvold, W.B. and Holmen, J. (2006) Adiposity and physical activity as predictors of cardiovascular mortality. *European Journal of Cardiovascular Prevention and Rehabilitation* 13: 909–15.

Wahid, A., Manek, N., Nichols, M., Kelly, P., Foster, C., Webster, P. et al. (2016) Quantifying the association between physical activity and cardiovascular disease and diabetes: a systematic review and meta-analysis. *Journal of the American Heart Association* 5: e002495. doi: 10.1161/JAHA.115.002495.

Wannamethee, S.G., Shaper, A.G. and Walker, M. (1998) Changes in physical activity, mortality, and incidence of coronary heart disease in older men. *The Lancet* 351: 1603–8.

Wannamethee, S.G., Shaper, A.G. and Walker, M. (2000) Physical activity and mortality in older men with diagnosed coronary heart disease. *Circulation* 102: 1358–63.

Warburton, D.E., Charlesworth, S., Ivey, A., Nettlefold, L. and Bredin, S.S. (2010) A systematic review of the evidence for Canada's Physical Activity Guidelines for Adults. *International Journal of Behavioral Nutrition and Physical Activity* 7: 39. doi: 10.1186/1479–5868-7–39.

Wendel-Vos, G.C., Schuit, A.J., Feskens, E.J., Boshuizen, H.C., Verschuren, W.M., Saris, W.H. and Kromhout, D. (2004) Physical activity and stroke. A meta-analysis of observational data. *International Journal of Epidemiology* 33: 787–98.

Whyman, M.R. and Ruckley, C.V. (1998) Should claudicants receive angioplasty or just exercise training? *Cardiovascular Surgery* 6: 226–31.

Williams, P.T. (2003) The illusion of improved physical fitness and reduced mortality. *Medicine and Science in Sports and Exercise* 35: 736–40.

World Health Organization (2011) *Global Atlas on Cardiovascular Disease Prevention and Control*, Mendis, S., Puska, P., Norrving, B. editors. Geneva: WHO.

Yang, J., Christophi, C.A., Farioli, A., Baur, D.M., Moffatt, S., Zollinger, T.W. and Kales, S.N. (2019) Association between push-up exercise capacity and future cardiovascular events among active adult men. *Journal of the American Medical Association Network Open* 2: e188341. doi: 10.1001/jamanetworkopen.2018.8341.

Yates, T., Zaccardi, F., Dhalwani, N.N., Davies, M.J., Bakrania, K., Celis-Morales, C.A. et al. (2017) Association of walking pace and handgrip strength with all-cause, cardiovascular, and cancer mortality: a UK Biobank observational study. *European Heart Journal* 38: 3232–40.

Yusuf, S., Hawken, S., Ounpuu, S., Dans, T., Avezum, A., Lanas, F. et al.; INTERHEART Study Investigators. (2004) Effect of potentially modifiable risk factors associated with myocardial infarction in 52 countries (the INTERHEART study): case-control study. *The Lancet* 364: 937–52.

5 Type 2 diabetes

Jason M.R. Gill

INTRODUCTION

Diabetes mellitus, often referred to as diabetes, refers to several metabolic conditions characterised by chronic hyperglycaemia (raised blood glucose concentrations). It occurs because the body cannot produce any, or produces insufficient amounts, of the hormone insulin or because the body's tissues become resistant to effects of the insulin it produces. Diabetes is a major public health concern, with an estimated 463 million people aged 20–79 years worldwide – 9.3% of the world's population in this age range – living with the condition (International Diabetes Federation 2019). It is a major cause of morbidity – increasing risk of complications including cardiovascular disease, eye disease and blindness, cancer, chronic kidney disease, neurological disorders and peripheral vascular disease in the lower limbs, pregnancy complications and adverse oral health – and increases risk of mortality (International Diabetes Federation 2019). A meta-analysis of 97 prospective studies which included 820,900 participants (123,205 deaths) and 12.3 million person-years of observation, reported that people with diabetes had a hazard ratio for mortality of 1.80 (95% confidence interval 1.71–1.90) compared to people without diabetes (Seshasai et al. 2011). To put this into perspective, these data indicate that a 50-year-old with diabetes has about a six-year lower life expectancy than a counterpart without diabetes (Seshasai et al. 2011). In 2019, it was estimated that approximately 4.2 million deaths in people aged 20–79 years (11.3% of global deaths in this age range) were caused by diabetes and its complications and worldwide diabetes-related health expenditure was estimated to be ~US$760 billion. Worldwide prevalence of diabetes tripled from 2000 to 2019, and is projected to increase further to ~700 million people worldwide by 2045 (International Diabetes Federation 2019). This secular trend is due to two key factors, first, population growth and an ageing population (risk of diabetes increases with age); and second, increasing prevalence of lifestyle-related risk factors, principally levels of obesity and physical inactivity.

WHAT IS DIABETES?

Diabetes is defined by hyperglycaemia (high blood sugar) and has traditionally been diagnosed based on a fasting plasma glucose measurement or from an oral glucose tolerance test, in which a 75 g oral glucose load is consumed and plasma glucose concentrations are monitored for two hours. More recently, diabetes has also been diagnosed based on glycated haemoglobin (HbA1c) concentrations. This is possible because glucose in the bloodstream bonds irreversibly with haemoglobin in proportion to average plasma glucose concentrations. As the life of red blood cells is approximately three months, the HbA1c concentration represents a weighted average of plasma glucose concentrations over this period (weighted more to glucose concentrations preceding days and weeks). This has the advantage of not requiring a person to be fasted for measurement, or to undertake a time-consuming oral glucose tolerance test. Between normal glucose concentrations (normoglycaemia) and diabetes, there are intermediate conditions (impaired fasting glucose, impaired glucose tolerance, impaired glucose regulation) which are often termed 'pre-diabetes'. Diagnostic criteria for diabetes and pre-diabetes (American Diabetes Association 2016; World Health Organization 2006, 2011) are shown in Box 5.1.

There are two major types of diabetes: type 1 and type 2. However there are several other forms of the disease which do not fall into one of these two broad classifications including gestational diabetes (hyperglycaemia in pregnancy in women without a previous history of diabetes), maturity onset diabetes of the young or MODY (caused by single gene mutations affecting insulin production, sometimes called monogenic diabetes) and latent autoimmune diabetes in adults or LADA (a form of diabetes that occurs in adulthood which has characteristics of both type 1 and type 2 diabetes, and is sometimes referred to as 'type 1.5 diabetes'). Discussing these further is beyond the scope of this chapter; for more information about diabetes subtypes, Tuomi and colleagues provide an excellent summary (Tuomi et al. 2014).

BOX 5.1 DIAGNOSIS OF DIABETES MELLITUS.

Diabetes mellitus is defined by hyperglycaemia. It may be diagnosed from a fasting plasma glucose measurement, from an oral glucose tolerance test involving consumption of a 75 g glucose load after which plasma glucose concentrations are monitored for two hours, or from the measurement of glycated haemoglobin (HbA1c) concentrations. Intermediate stages between normoglycaemia (normal glucose) and diabetes have also been defined by groups such as the World Health Organization (WHO) and American Diabetes Association (ADA).

		Fasting plasma glucose concentration	Plasma glucose concentration two hours after glucose load	HbA1c concentration
Normoglycaemia		< 6.0 mmol.l^{-1}(< 110 mgdl^{-1}) WHO	< 7.8 mmol.l^{-1}	<42 mmol.mol^{-1} ($<6.0\%$) WHO
		< 5.6 mmol.l^{-1} (< 100 mg.dl^{-1}) ADA	< 140 mg.dl^{-1}	<39 mmol.mol^{-1} ($<5.6\%$) ADA
Impaired glucose regulation/pre-diabetes	Impaired fasting glucose	6.0–6.9 mmol.l^{-1} (110–125 mg.dl^{-1}) WHO 5.6–6.9 mmol.l^{-1} (100–125 mg.dl^{-1}) ADA		
	Impaired glucose tolerance		≥ 7.8 to <11.1 mmol.l^{-1} ≥ 140 to <200 mg.dl^{-1}	
				42–47 mmol.mol^{-1} (6.0–6.4%) WHO 39–47 mmol.mol^{-1} (5.6–6.4%) ADA
Diabetes mellitus		≥ 7.0 mmol.l^{-1} ≥ 126 mg.dl^{-1}	≥ 11.1 mmol.l^{-1} ≥ 200 mg.dl^{-1}	≥ 48 mmol.mol^{-1} ($\geq 6.5\%$)

Source: American Diabetes Association (2016), World Health Organization (2006) and World Health Organization (2011).

Notes:

1 The WHO and ADA use different thresholds to define normoglycaemia and pre-diabetes.

2 In the absence of symptoms, diagnosis of diabetes must be confirmed by a repeat test on a separate day.

Type 1 diabetes (referred to as insulin-dependent diabetes mellitus (IDDM) in older literature) is caused by an autoimmune destruction of the pancreatic beta cells (in the islets of Langerhans). As a result, the pancreas is unable to produce insulin and this hormone must be injected regularly to control blood glucose concentrations (insulin cannot be given orally because gastrointestinal enzymes would digest it). Type 1 diabetes usually occurs before adulthood, and for this reason is sometimes referred to as juvenile-onset diabetes. In contrast with type 2 diabetes, risk of developing type 1 diabetes is not affected by lifestyle factors such as physical activity or obesity. Type 1 diabetes is associated with increased risk of both macrovascular disease (diseases of large blood vessels, principally CHD and stroke) and of microvascular complications (damage to small blood vessels, commonly occurring in eyes (retinopathy), kidneys (nephropathy) and nerves of the hands, feet, arms and legs (peripheral neuropathy)). The influence of physical activity on risk of these outcomes in people with type 1 diabetes has been relatively understudied, but the available evidence from prospective cohort studies suggests that being physically active is associated with lower risk of all-cause and CVD mortality (Moy et al. 1993; Tielemans et al. 2013; Tikkanen-Dolenc et al. 2017), as is the case for people without diabetes. More limited evidence suggests that physical activity may be associated with lower risk of retinopathy (Tikkanen-Dolenc et al. 2020) and nephropathy (Wadén et al. 2015). In addition, intervention studies have shown that exercise training programmes improve risk factors for CVD in people with type 1 diabetes (Wu et al. 2019). Physical activity can also play an important role in the management of glycaemia in type 1 diabetes, and reduce daily insulin requirements, but it is important to recognise that different types of physical activity have different effects on glucose control, with continuous aerobic activities generally decreasing glycaemia and high-intensity anaerobic activities increasing glycaemia (Riddell et al. 2017). Thus, both type and duration of activity needs to be taken into account when considering insulin requirements and food intake around exercise. For more information on this topic, the consensus statement on *Exercise Management in Type 1 Diabetes* by Riddell and colleagues is an excellent resource (Riddell et al. 2017).

Type 2 diabetes (referred to as non-insulin-dependent diabetes mellitus (NIDDM) in older literature) is characterised by poor responsiveness (insensitivity) of cells in the body (primarily in skeletal muscle, liver and adipose tissue) to the effects of insulin, known as insulin resistance. This means that greater levels of insulin secretion by the pancreatic beta cells, leading to higher circulating insulin concentrations, are needed to maintain blood glucose concentrations in the normal range. This combination of insulin resistance with high insulin secretion can often be maintained for several years, but when the beta cells become unable to maintain the high level of insulin secretion needed to compensate for this insulin resistance, blood glucose levels rise leading to type 2 diabetes (Rydén et al. 2013) (Figure 5.1). It is important to recognise that risk of macrovascular complications is elevated by insulin resistance *per se* so can be evident in normoglycaemic insulin resistant individuals and in individuals with pre-diabetes several years prior to the onset of type 2 diabetes. In contrast, risk of microvascular complications only increases substantially with the onset of diabetes.

Type 2 diabetes is the most common form of diabetes, accounting for about 90% of all diabetes cases worldwide (International Diabetes Federation 2019). The International Diabetes Federation estimates that in 2019 the prevalence of diabetes amongst adults aged 20–79 years was 10.4% (95.2 million people) in high-income countries, 9.5% (353.3 million people) in middle-income countries and 4.0% (14.5 million) in low-income countries (International Diabetes Federation 2019). The countries with the highest numbers of diabetes cases and the highest prevalence of diabetes amongst adults in 2019 are shown in Table 5.1. It is estimated that a further 374 million adults aged 20–79 worldwide have impaired glucose tolerance, with 104.1 million (11.4% of population) in high-income countries, 239.6 million (6.5%) in middle-income countries and 30.2 million (8.3%) in low-income countries having the condition (International Diabetes Federation 2019). Thus, it is estimated that 16.8% of the world's population have either diabetes or impaired glucose tolerance.

JASON M.R. GILL

Figure 5.1 Time-course of changes in glycaemia, insulin resistance and secretion, and microvascular and macrovascular disease risk.

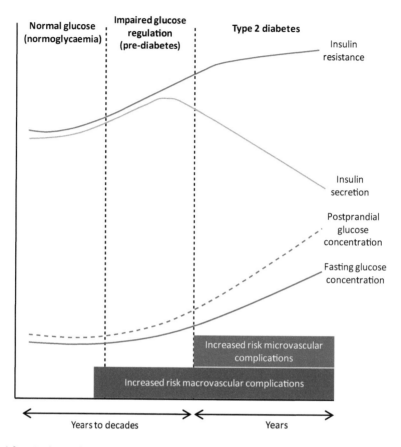

Source: Adapted from Rydén et al. (2013).

WHAT ARE THE CONSEQUENCES OF INSULIN RESISTANCE?

Although there are defects in insulin secretion in type 2 diabetes, the feature which distinguishes it from type 1 diabetes, as mentioned above, is insulin resistance. One indication of insulin resistance is fasting hyperinsulinaemia (high fasting insulin concentration) in the presence of either normal or elevated blood glucose concentrations. Insulin resistance also leads to a larger postprandial rise in insulin concentrations, and both fasting insulin concentrations and postprandial insulin responses (often in response to a standardised 75 g oral glucose load) can be used to assess insulin resistance. For example, Figure 5.2 shows glucose and insulin responses to a mixed test meal containing 70 g carbohydrate and 80 g fat in lean insulin sensitive and centrally obese insulin resistant, but non-diabetic, middle-aged men (Gill et al. 2004). This clearly shows higher insulin concentrations, and moderately raised glucose concentrations, in the insulin resistant group. The gold-standard method for assessing insulin resistance is the euglycaemic hyperinsulinaemic clamp, which involves intravenous (via a vein)

	DIABETES CASES IN ADULTS (20–79 YEARS)		DIABETES PREVALENCE IN ADULTS (20–79 YEARS)	
RANK	COUNTRY	NUMBER OF DIABETES CASES (MILLIONS)	COUNTRY	AGE-ADJUSTED DIABETES PREVALENCE (%)
1	China	116.4	Marshall Islands	30.5
2	India	77.0	Kiribati	22.5
3	United States	31.0	Sudan	22.1
4	Pakistan	19.4	Tuvalu	22.1
5	Brazil	16.8	Mauritius	22.0
6	Mexico	12.8	New Caledonia	22.8
7	Indonesia	10.7	Pakistan	19.9
8	Germany	9.5	French Polynesia	19.5
9	Egypt	8.9	Solomon Islands	19.0
10	Bangladesh	8.4	Guam	18.7

Table 5.1 Countries with the highest numbers of diabetes cases and highest age-adjusted rates of diabetes prevalence in 2019.

Source: International Diabetes Federation (2019).

Figure 5.2 Glucose and insulin concentrations in the fasted state and in response to consumption of a meal containing 70 g of carbohydrate and 80 g of fat in lean insulin sensitive and centrally obese insulin resistant middle-aged men.

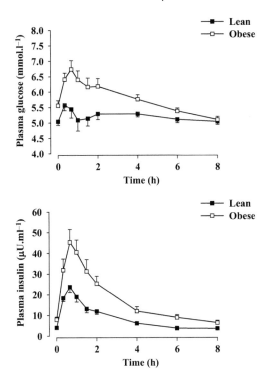

Source: Reprinted from the *Journal of the American College of Cardiology*, 44: 2375–82, Gill, J.M.R. et al., 'Effects of prior moderate exercise on postprandial metabolism and vascular function in lean and centrally obese men', page 2378, copyright © 2004, with permission from Elsevier.

infusion of insulin at a predefined rate with glucose simultaneously infused at the rate needed to maintain euglycaemia (normal blood glucose concentration). In this test, a higher required glucose infusion rate indicates greater insulin sensitivity (i.e. less insulin resistance). This concept is described in more detail in Chapter 7.

Insulin resistance influences regulation of blood glucose concentrations in two ways. Firstly, resistance of peripheral tissues (principally skeletal muscle) to the effects of insulin means that less glucose is cleared from the blood for a given concentration of insulin. Secondly, insulin resistance in the liver means that insulin is less effective at suppressing hepatic glucose production when this is metabolically appropriate (for example after a meal). Thus, insulin resistance can both prevent downregulation of glucose production by the liver and impair glucose clearance from the circulation into muscle.

In addition to its role in glucose metabolism, insulin also exerts multiple influences on lipid metabolism, which collectively promote the uptake and storage of fatty acids in adipose tissue, inhibit their mobilisation from adipose tissue and decrease secretion of very low-density lipoproteins (VLDL) from the liver. This is illustrated in Figure 5.3. Thus, when insulin resistance develops, insulin's normal effects are impaired. This results in increased hepatic VLDL secretion, and decreased clearance of VLDL and (in the postprandial state) chylomicrons from the circulation, which results in higher plasma triglyceride concentrations. A consequence of this is increased neutral lipid exchange between triglyceride-rich chylomicrons and VLDL with cholesterol-rich high-density lipoproteins (HDL) and low-density lipoproteins (LDL). This depletes HDL of cholesterol and leads to small, dense LDL particles, a combination termed the 'atherogenic lipoprotein phenotype' which is associated with increased CVD risk (see Chapter 7 for a more detailed description of lipid and lipoprotein metabolism). In addition, insulin resistance in adipocytes make them insensitive to the antilipolytic (resisting the breakdown of fat) effects of insulin. Thus, triglycerides within adipocytes are catabolised, leading to the release of non-esterified fatty acids (NEFAs) and glycerol into the circulation. Elevated NEFA release, resulting in increased plasma NEFA concentrations, is desirable in some circumstances (e.g. during exercise or prolonged fasting). However, in insulin resistance NEFA concentrations are often elevated at inappropriate times (e.g. after a meal). These elevated NEFAs compromise the tissues' ability to clear glucose, thereby exacerbating insulin resistance. Figure 5.4 shows the markedly higher triglyceride and NEFA concentrations in both the fasted and postprandial states in insulin resistant compared with insulin sensitive middle-aged men (Gill et al. 2004).

In addition to effects on glucose and lipid metabolism, insulin resistance can lead to disturbances in many other body systems. This clustering of metabolic dysfunction around insulin resistance is sometimes described as the 'metabolic syndrome', which was conceptualised by Gerald Reaven in his 1988 Banting Lecture (named after Sir Frederick Banting, who co-discovered insulin) where he described a 'Syndrome X' clustered around insulin resistance including glucose intolerance, hyperinsulinaemia, increased VLDL triglyceride, decreased HDL cholesterol and hypertension (Reaven 1988). Over subsequent years, understanding of the breadth of body systems affected by insulin resistance and the metabolic syndrome has increased and it has become clear that obesity (particularly abdominal obesity) is a key driver of these adverse metabolic effects. Thus, beyond effects on glucose, lipids and blood pressure, insulin resistance is

Figure 5.3 Influence of insulin on lipid metabolism to promote lipid synthesis and storage.

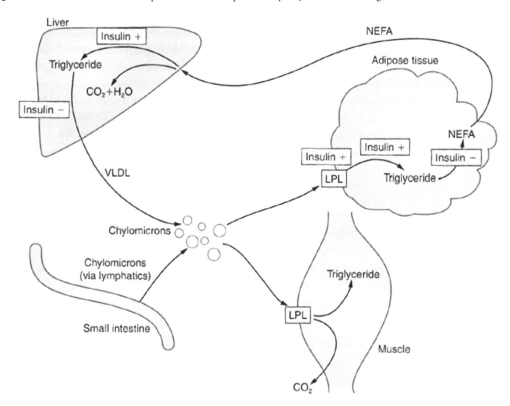

Source: Republished with permission of John Wiley and Sons, from *Metabolic regulation: a human perspective*, Frayn K.N., 2nd edition, copyright © 2003; permission conveyed through Copyright Clearance Center, Inc.

mechanistically linked to a range of metabolic abnormalities including endothelial dysfunction, increased inflammation, increased thrombotic risk, androgen disturbances, renal dysfunction, non-alcoholic fatty liver disease and appetite dysregulation (Laaksonen et al. 2004; Rask-Madsen and Kahn 2012).

Various attempts have been made to provide diagnostic criteria for the metabolic syndrome to help clinicians assess patients and improve their management. The current internationally agreed criteria for clinical diagnosis of the metabolic syndrome is the presence of three out of the following five criteria: 1) elevated waist circumference (with population- and country-specific definitions); 2) elevated triglycerides (≥ 1.7 mmol l^{-1}); 3) reduced HDL cholesterol (<1.3 mmol l^{-1} for men, <1.0 mmol l^{-1} for women); 4) elevated blood pressure (systolic ≥ 130 and/or diastolic ≥ 85 mm Hg); 5) elevated fasting glucose (>5.5 mmol l^{-1}) (Alberti et al. 2009). Based on these criteria, it has been estimated that ~35–40% of US adults have the metabolic syndrome (Alberti et al. 2009). The use of the metabolic syndrome as a diagnostic tool has received criticism in some quarters as it has been argued that the syndrome does not predict cardiovascular events or progression any better than the sum of its components (Eckel et al. 2010) and that, although having the metabolic syndrome is associated with an approximately five-fold

Figure 5.4 Triglyceride and NEFA concentrations in the fasted state and in response to consumption of a meal containing 70 g of carbohydrate and 80 g of fat in lean insulin sensitive and centrally obese insulin resistant middle-aged men.

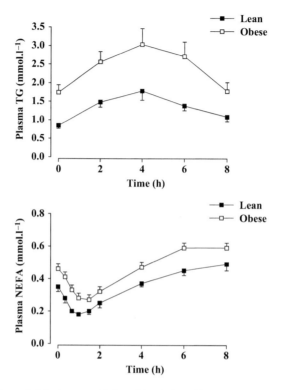

Source: Reprinted from the *Journal of the American College of Cardiology*, 44: 2375–82, Gill, J.M.R. et al., 'Effects of prior moderate exercise on postprandial metabolism and vascular function in lean and centrally obese men', page 2378, copyright © 2004, with permission from Elsevier.

increased risk of developing type 2 diabetes, it is unclear whether it improves diabetes prediction beyond measuring fasting glucose alone (Ford et al. 2008). However, these arguments do not detract from the key concept that there is a cluster of metabolic abnormalities centred on insulin resistance which increase the risk of cardio-metabolic disease and thus interventions which improve insulin sensitivity – such as physical activity or weight loss – can elicit a wide range of interlinked metabolic benefits.

NON-MODIFIABLE RISK FACTORS FOR TYPE 2 DIABETES

Risk factors for type 2 diabetes can be classed as modifiable and non-modifiable. The strongest non-modifiable risk factor is age: in 2019 global prevalence of diabetes was ~4% amongst adults aged 30–34 years, ~14% at age 50–54 years, and ~20% at age 70–74 years (International Diabetes Federation 2019). Risk of type 2 diabetes also differs according sex, with prevalence being higher in men than women, and men also developing the disease at lower levels of body mass index (Logue et al. 2011). Ethnicity is a further key risk factor: in the UK and USA, adults who are of Afro-Caribbean or

African American ethnicity have about twice the risk, and adults who are of South Asian origin have two to three times the risk of developing diabetes, compared with adults of white European ethnic origin (Cheng et al. 2019; Sproston and Mindell 2006). Family history of type 2 diabetes also has a strong influence on diabetes risk. In the EPIC-Interact study of 13,869 individuals who had available data on diabetes family history, having any first-degree relative (parent or sibling) with diabetes led to a 2.7-fold increase in type 2 diabetes risk and having two parents with diabetes resulted in a 5.1-fold increase in risk (InterAct Consortium 2013). Risks associated with sex, ethnicity and family history may interact with modifiable lifestyle-related risk factors. For example, the increase in type 2 diabetes risk associated with increasing body mass index appears to be higher in South Asian, Chinese and Black adults compared with adults of White European origin (Ntuk et al. 2014).

OBESITY AS A RISK FACTOR FOR TYPE 2 DIABETES

Obesity appears to be the most important modifiable risk factor for type 2 diabetes. A meta-analysis of 18 prospective studies including a total of 590,251 participants, of which 16,107 developed diabetes over follow-up period of 2–27 years, found that, compared with individuals of normal weight, individuals who were overweight (defined as BMI 25–29.99 kg m^{-2} in most of the included studies) had a relative risk of diabetes of 2.99 (95% confidence interval: 2.42 to 3.71), and those who were obese (defined an BMI ≥30 kg m^{-2} in most studies) had a relative risk of 7.19 (95% confidence interval: 5.74 to 9.00) (Abdullah et al. 2010). Weight gain in adulthood, particularly early adulthood, is also a strong risk factor for type 2 diabetes, as evidenced by meta-analysis of 15 eligible studies, by Kodama and colleagues, which examined the association between weight gain in early adulthood (aged 18–24 years) and later adulthood (from age 25 onwards) on risk of incident type 2 diabetes. Weight gain corresponding to a 5 kg m^{-2} increase in BMI in early adulthood was associated with three-fold increase (relative risk 3.07, 95% confidence interval 2.49 to 3.79) in risk of type 2 diabetes, with similar weight gain after age 25 being associated with a doubling of type 2 diabetes risk (relative risk 2.12, 95% confidence interval 1.74 to 2.58) (Kodama et al. 2014).

While BMI has the advantage of being easy to measure, it is sometimes criticised as being a relatively crude measure of adiposity (as it does not distinguish between fat and lean mass, and gives no indication of fat distribution). Thus, it is important to consider whether other anthropometric measures, particularly ones which specifically provide indices of abdominal obesity (such as waist circumference, waist-to-hip or waist-to-height ratio) provide a better index of type 2 diabetes risk. A meta-analysis of 15 studies, including 120,012 participants, of which 6,472 developed diabetes over mean follow-up period of six years, compared the strength of association of different anthropometric obesity indicators on risk of type 2 diabetes, finding that the difference of one standard deviation increment in BMI was associated with an increment in the relative risk of diabetes of 1.55 (95% confidence interval 1.43 to 1.69), whereas one standard deviation increments in waist circumference, waist-to-hip ratio and waist-to-height ratio were associated with relative risks of 1.63 (95% confidence interval 1.49 to 1.79), 1.52 (95% confidence interval 1.40 to 1.66), and 1.62 (95% confidence interval 1.48 to 1.78), respectively (Kodama et al. 2012). One difficulty in interpreting the relative importance of these measures is that these adiposity variables are highly correlated. For example, the correlation coefficient for the relationship between BMI and waist circumference in this meta-analysis was 0.96. Thus, most people with large BMIs also have large waists and vice versa. One way to try to disentangle this is to stratify the study population according to both BMI and waist circumference. This was done in an analysis of data from the Health Professionals Follow-Up Study of 27,270 male health professionals who were followed up for 13 years (Wang et al. 2005). This indicated that both overall BMI and waist circumference (or waist-to-hip ratio) independently predicted type 2 diabetes risk (Figure 5.5).

It is likely that the relationship between adiposity and type 2 diabetes risk is causal. One line of evidence comes from genetic studies. For example, individuals who possess the high-risk variants of the FTO (fat mass and obesity-associated protein) gene, which leads to ~3 kg higher body weight on average, have increased risk of type 2 diabetes which has been shown to be mediated by the effect of the gene on BMI (Frayling et al. 2007). In addition, recent data from randomised clinical trials (i.e. gold-standard evidence) indicates that substantial weight loss can lead to diabetes remission, i.e. plasma glucose HbA1c concentrations being sustained long term in the non-diabetic range, in at least some patients with type 2 diabetes. In the Diabetes Remission Clinical Trial (DiRECT), 298 patients with type 2 diabetes were randomised to 'usual care' or an intensive structured weight-management programme involving 12 weeks of an approximately 800 kcal day^{-1} total diet replacement intervention, followed by gradual food reintroduction over two months and then ongoing weight management support

Figure 5.5 Relative risk of type 2 diabetes by BMI and waist circumference in 27,270 men in the Health Professionals Follow-Up Study.

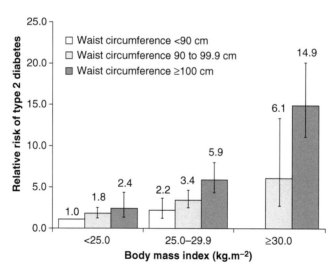

Source: Wang, Y. et al., 'Comparison of abdominal adiposity and overall obesity in predicting risk of type 2 diabetes among men', *American Journal of Clinical Nutrition*, 2005, 81: 555–63, reproduced by permission of Oxford University Press.
Notes: Error bars represent 95% confidence intervals. There were too few men with BMI ≥30 kg.m^{-2} and waist circumference <90 cm to estimate the relative risk in this category. The findings were adjusted for age, physical activity, smoking, alcohol and cereal fibre intake.

(Lean et al. 2019). Average weight loss was 10 kg at 12 months and 7.6 kg at 24 months, with more than 45% of patients achieving diabetes remission at 12 months, which persisted until 24 months in more than 35% of patients. Higher levels of weight loss increased the chances of attaining diabetes remission, with 64% of patients maintaining at least 10 kg weight loss at 24 months achieving sustained diabetes remission (Lean et al. 2019).

While obesity is a strong risk factor for type 2 diabetes, not everyone with obesity develops the disease, whereas some normal weight individuals do. The 'adipose tissue overflow' hypothesis provides a potential explanation. This postulates that subcutaneous (under the skin) adipose tissue is the primary storage depot for fat, and once this becomes 'full', fat accumulating from positive energy balance spills over into visceral (around internal organs) and ectopic fat within the liver, pancreas and skeletal muscle (Sniderman et al. 2007). Subcutaneous adipose is a relatively 'safe' depot for fat storage, but individuals' capacity to store fat in this depot varies. Thus, individuals with high subcutaneous fat storage capacity can attain very high BMIs without accumulating substantial visceral and ectopic fat, and remain metabolically healthy (Stefan et al. 2008), whereas at the other extreme individuals with the condition lipodystrophy, who have an impaired ability to store subcutaneous fat, accumulate substantial visceral and ectopic fat with even modest weight gain, and develop severe insulin resistance and type 2 diabetes while remaining outwardly very lean (Huang-Doran et al. 2010). Most people lie somewhere on this continuum, and it has been hypothesised that one reason for ethnic and sex differences in the association between adiposity and type 2 diabetes risks relates to differences in the extent to which weight gain leads to ectopic fat accumulation (Sattar and Gill 2014). This concept is illustrated in Figures 5.6 and 5.7.

Figure 5.6 The adipose tissue overflow hypothesis. Magnetic resonance imaging (MRI) scans of the abdomen at different stages of abdominal obesity.

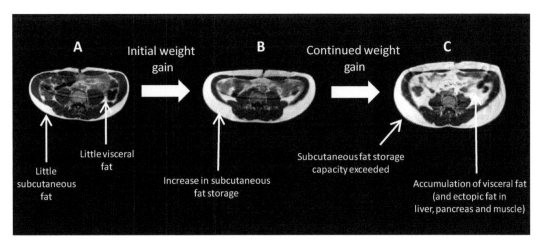

Source: MRI images from Thomas, E.L. et al., 'Excess body fat in obese and normal-weight subjects', *Nutrition Research Reviews*, 2012, 25: 150–61; reproduced with permission.
Notes: In (A) there is little subcutaneous or visceral fat. With initial weight gain (B), fat mostly accumulates subcutaneously. As weight gain continues (C), subcutaneous fat storage capacity is exceeded, and fat starts to 'overflow' and accumulate in visceral and ectopic depots.

Figure 5.7 Healthy and unhealthy fat accumulation. Magnetic resonance imaging (MRI) scans of the abdomen showing different pathways for fat accumulation with weight gain.

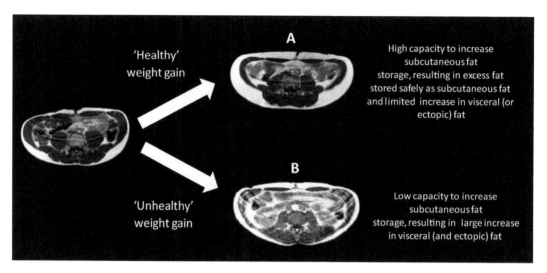

Source: MRI images from Thomas, E.L. et al., 'Excess body fat in obese and normal-weight subjects', *Nutrition Research Reviews*, 2012, 25: 150–61; reproduced with permission.

Notes: Individuals with a large capacity for subcutaneous fat storage (A) can have 'healthy' weight gain with limited accumulation of visceral and ectopic fat. In contrast, individuals with low subcutaneous fat storage capacity (B) accumulate visceral and ectopic fat even with limited weight gain.

PHYSICAL ACTIVITY AND SEDENTARY BEHAVIOUR AS RISK FACTORS

There is a substantial body of evidence which indicates that physical inactivity is an important risk factor for type 2 diabetes, with robust evidence beginning to emerge in the 1990s in the form of prospective cohort studies. One of the first involved 5,990 male alumni of the University of Pennsylvania, followed from 1962 to 1976. This study reported an inverse association between weekly self-reported energy expenditure in walking, stair climbing and sports activity and the risk of developing type 2 diabetes and concluded that each 500 kcal week^{-1} increment in energy expenditure was associated with a 6% lower age-adjusted risk of developing diabetes (Helmrich et al. 1991). This observation has since been confirmed in a large number of prospective cohort studies which have been summarised in multiple meta-analyses (Aune et al. 2015; Jeon et al. 2007; Smith et al. 2016). The most recent of these analyses by Smith and colleagues included 28 eligible cohort studies with a total of 1,261,991 participants and 84,134 incident cases of type 2 diabetes over follow-up periods ranging from 3 to 23 years (Smith et al. 2016). This analysis revealed a non-linear relationship between level of self-reported leisure-time physical activity and risk of type 2 diabetes with the largest benefit occurring with increments of physical activity at the lower end of the volume range (Figure 5.8). Compared with inactive individuals, those achieving 11.25 MET-h week^{-1} of physical activity (equivalent to 150 min week^{-1} of MVPA) had a 26% lower risk (95% confidence interval 20% to 31%), of developing type 2 diabetes, whereas

Figure 5.8 Dose–response relationship between self-reported leisure-time physical activity and incidence of type 2 diabetes from a meta-analysis of 28 prospective cohort studies.

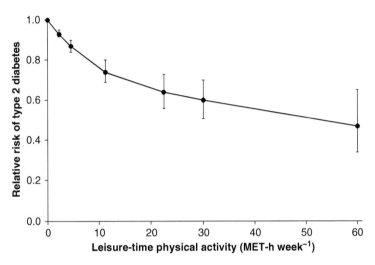

Source: Reprinted and adapted from 'Physical activity and incident type 2 diabetes mellitus: a systematic review and dose-response meta-analysis of prospective cohort studies', Smith, A.D. et al., *Diabetologia*, 2016, 59: 2527–45. Article distributed under the terms of the Creative Commons Attribution 4.0 International Licence (https://creativecommons.org/licenses/by/4.0/).
Notes: Error bars represent 95% confidence intervals. The analysis included the maximally adjusted model from each study.

those achieving twice this amount of physical activity had a 36% lower risk (95% confidence interval 27% to 46%) (Smith et al. 2016). A key factor to consider when examining the relationship between physical activity and risk of type 2 diabetes is the extent to which the benefit of physical activity might be mediated by lower adiposity in physically active individuals. Some studies have attempted to address this by adjusting for BMI in their analysis. The meta-analysis by Jeon and colleagues, which examined the association between moderate intensity physical activity and risk of type 2 diabetes in 10 prospective cohort studies including 310,221 participants and 9,367 with incident type 2 diabetes, compared risk in those reporting the highest versus lowest levels of moderate-intensity physical activity in analyses with and without adjustment for BMI (Jeon et al. 2007) (Figure 5.9). BMI-adjustment attenuated the risk reduction associated with undertaking a high level of moderate-intensity physical activity from 31% (95% confidence interval 17% to 42%) to 17% (95% confidence interval 10% to 24%), but the association remained statistically significant. These data indicate that the association between physical activity and risk of diabetes is partially independent of, and partially mediated by, the effects of physical activity on BMI.

Level of physical activity is associated with risk of type 2 diabetes at all levels of BMI. For example, Hu and colleagues reported that, in a study of 4,369 Finnish adults, with 120 incident cases of type 2 diabetes over a mean 9.4 year follow-up, higher levels of self-reported physical activity were associated with lower type 2 diabetes risk in subgroups with BMI <30, and ≥30 kg.m^{-2} (Hu et al. 2004) (Figure 5.10). However, it is important to note that while a high level of physical activity can attenuate the excess risk

Figure 5.9 Forest plot from meta-analysis of ten prospective cohort studies showing relative risk for incident type 2 diabetes comparing highest versus lowest reported level of total moderate intensity physical activity for individual cohort studies and all studies combined. Panel a shows analyses without adjustment for BMI and panel b shows analyses with this adjustment.

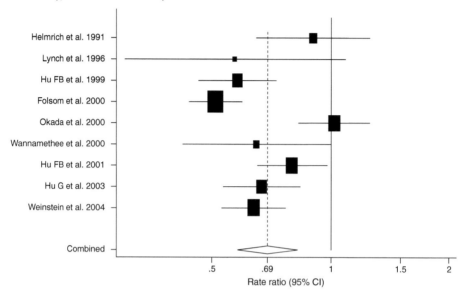

a RR of type 2 diabetes without adjustment for BMI

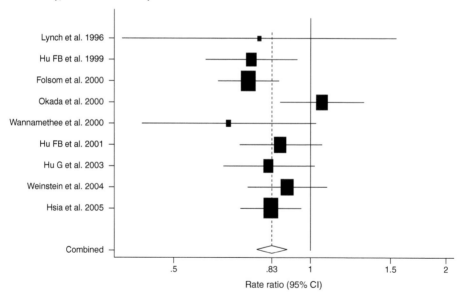

b RR of type 2 diabetes with adjustment for BMI

Notes: Horizontal bars represent 95% confidence intervals for individual studies; width of diamond represents 95% confidence interval for combined analysis. The size of the squares corresponds to the study weighting in the meta-analysis.

Figure 5.10 Relative risk of type 2 diabetes according to level of physical activity and BMI in 4,369 Finnish adults.

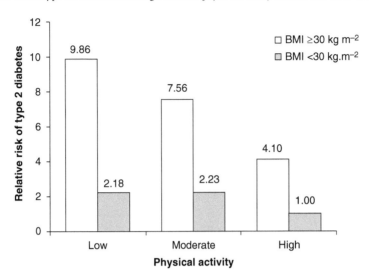

Notes: Analyses were adjusted for age, sex, study year, systolic blood pressure, smoking status, education and BMI.

of type 2 diabetes in overweight and obese individuals, diabetes risk remains high in active individuals with a high BMI. Thus, in individuals who are overweight or obese a combination of weight loss and increased physical activity should generally be encouraged to minimise type 2 diabetes risk.

Fewer studies have investigated the association between participation in muscle strengthening resistance exercise and risk of type 2 diabetes. Grøntved and colleagues undertook a prospective cohort study of 32,002 US men from the Health Professionals Follow-up Study, who were followed up for 18 years, during which time there were 2,278 new cases of type 2 diabetes. At baseline, the men were asked to report participation in weight training and other forms of physical activity. In analyses adjusted for a comprehensive range of covariates including age, smoking, diet, TV viewing, participation in weight training and aerobic exercise were associated with lower risk of type 2 diabetes in a dose-dependent manner (p-value for trend <0.001) (Grøntved et al. 2012) (Figure 5.11). Further adjustment for BMI attenuated the association slightly but the trend remained statistically significant. Similar findings were reported in a study of 99,316 middle-aged and older women from the Nurses' Health Study and Nurses' Health Study II who were followed up for eight years, during which time 3,491 cases of type 2 diabetes were documented. Here, women who reported undertaking 1–29, 30–59, 60–150 and >150 minutes per week of muscle strengthening and conditioning activities had relative risks of type 2 diabetes of 0.83 (0.75–0.92), 0.93 (0.83–1.04), 0.75 (0.67–0.85) and 0.60 (0.50–0.72), respectively, compared with women engaging in none of these activities, in analyses adjusted for multiple covariates including participation in aerobic activities (p-value for trend <0.001) (Grøntved et al. 2014).

Figure 5.11 Relative risk of type 2 diabetes according to level of weight training and aerobic exercise undertaken in 32,002 US men from the Health Professionals Follow-up Study.

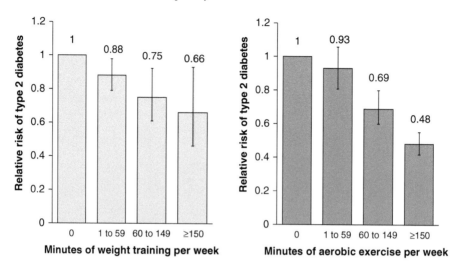

Source: Grøntved et al. (2012).
Notes: Error bars represent 95% confidence intervals. Analyses were adjusted for age, smoking, alcohol consumption, coffee intake, race (white vs non-white), family history of diabetes, dietary factors and TV viewing. Analyses for weight training were additionally adjusted for participation in aerobic exercise, and analyses for aerobic exercise were additionally adjusted for participation in weight training.

Thus, the available evidence indicates that muscle-strengthening activity and aerobic physical activity appear to be independently associated with type 2 diabetes risk.

There is an accumulating body of prospective cohort studies which have examined the association between sedentary behaviour and risk of type 2 diabetes. A recent meta-analysis, by Patterson and colleagues, which included four studies using self-reported total sitting (total n = 271,724; 10,246 diabetes cases) and seven studies using television viewing (total n = 182,568; 7,306 diabetes cases) as the sedentary behaviour exposure has summarised these data (Patterson et al. 2018). In analyses adjusted for a range of covariates, including physical activity, risk of type 2 diabetes increased by 1% for every hour per day increase in total sitting (relative risk 1.01 (1.00–1.01)), and by 9% for every hour per day increase in television viewing (1.09 (1.07–1.12)). The stronger association with type 2 diabetes risk observed for television viewing, compared with total sitting, is similar to that observed for all-cause mortality described in Chapter 3, and may reflect that there is a clustering of several other adverse risk factors around television viewing (such as unhealthy diet and lower socio-economic status) which may not be fully adjusted for in statistical analyses (Stamatakis et al. 2019). Thus, in terms of potential strategies to reduce type 2 diabetes risk, focusing on reducing television viewing may be a stronger target than overall time spent sitting. However, given the observational nature of these data, intervention trials are needed to confirm this suggestion.

Although the findings from prospective cohort studies are consistent in reporting an inverse association between physical inactivity and diabetes risk, these studies have limitations. Assessments of physical activity were based on self-report and therefore liable to inaccuracy (see Chapter 2 for more details), and in several studies diabetes was determined by self-report of a diagnosis, which may lead to inaccuracies due to undiagnosed cases. The majority of studies have also come from Europe and North America mainly including participants of white European origin, with relatively few from Asia (none from South Asia), and none from Africa. Thus, there are limited data examining the dose–response relationship between physical activity and diabetes risk amongst the non-white populations who are at highest risk of type 2 diabetes. Preliminary findings from cross-sectional studies comparing the association between physical activity and metabolic risk factors between South Asian and white European adults suggests that South Asians may require higher levels of physical activity than white Europeans to achieve favourable metabolic profiles for insulin sensitivity and glycaemia (Celis-Morales et al. 2013; Iliodromiti et al. 2016), but substantial further work is needed to understand ethnic differences in the association between physical activity and type 2 diabetes risk more fully. Finally, as explained in Chapter 2, observational studies cannot prove cause and effect. This requires intervention studies, which are discussed later in this chapter.

CARDIORESPIRATORY FITNESS AND MUSCULAR STRENGTH AS RISK FACTORS

Several studies have examined the association between cardiorespiratory fitness and risk of type 2 diabetes. One of the earliest reports was from the Aerobics Center Longitudinal Study which involved 8,633 men, who were free from diabetes at baseline, and had fitness measured via a maximal treadmill exercise test. Over a six-year follow-up, during which time 149 participants developed type 2 diabetes, men with low fitness (the least fit 20% of the cohort), had a 1.9-fold higher risk of developing impaired fasting glucose, and a 3.7-fold higher risk of developing type 2 diabetes compared with highly fit men (the most fit 40% of the cohort). This association between low fitness and higher risk of type 2 diabetes was present in both younger (<45 year) and older (≥45 year), in men with and without a parental history of diabetes, in men with both high (≥27 kg m^{-2}) and low (<27 kg m^{-2}) BMI, and in those with both normal and impaired fasting glucose at baseline (Wei et al. 1999). Recently, a meta-analysis has summarised the evidence on the association between cardiorespiratory fitness and risk of type 2 diabetes (Qiu et al. 2019). Based on an analysis of eight studies, including 54,074 participants, each 1-MET increase in cardiorespiratory fitness was associated with 10% lower risk of developing type 2 diabetes (hazard ratio 0.90 (0.86–0.94)). A further analysis of six studies, including 37,169 participants, examined the joint association of cardiorespiratory fitness and BMI with risk of type 2 diabetes. This showed that, compared with a fit (top two-thirds or top three-quarters of the population for fitness depending on the study) and normal weight reference group, those who were unfit and normal weight; fit and overweight or obese; and unfit and overweight or obese had hazard ratios for type 2 diabetes of 1.26 (1.06–1.50), 2.05 (1.55–2.70) and 2.98 (1.97–4.50), respectively. Thus, fitness and BMI are independently associated with type 2 diabetes and, while being fit is associated with a substantially lower diabetes risk in the overweight and obese, there is still substantial excess diabetes risk amongst those who are fit but overweight or obese.

Further evidence linking cardiorespiratory fitness to the risk of diabetes comes from studies using an experimental model comprising rats artificially selected for the trait of high or low fitness, which was described in Chapter 3. Here, rats were selectively bred for high or low fitness over several generations, by repeatedly interbreeding 'high capacity' and 'low capacity' runners. By generation 11, the low-capacity runners had 58% lower maximum oxygen uptake ($\dot{V}O_2$max) than the high-capacity runners, and exhibited several features of metabolic dysfunction associated with insulin resistance including 131% higher fasting insulin and 20% higher fasting glucose concentrations, as well as elevated circulating concentrations of triglyceride and NEFA (Wisløff et al. 2005). This suggests that the biological mechanisms underpinning low cardiorespiratory fitness and poor metabolic function are likely to be causally linked. In humans, $\dot{V}O_2$max is a strong predictor of whole-body insulin sensitivity (Bruce et al. 2003), and it is interesting to note that relatives of patients with type 2 diabetes, who are more insulin resistant and at increased risk of developing diabetes than their counterparts with no diabetes family history, have ~10–15% lower $\dot{V}O_2$max values than age- and BMI-matched controls (Nyholm et al. 2004; Thamer et al. 2003). Furthermore South Asian adults, who are more insulin resistant and at increased diabetes risk compared with adults of white European adults, have been shown in several studies to have lower $\dot{V}O_2$max values (Ghouri et al. 2013; Hall et al. 2010). Mechanistically, the link between cardiorespiratory fitness and insulin resistance and diabetes risk is likely to be mediated via effects on skeletal muscle mitochondrial function, which has been strongly implicated in the pathogenesis of insulin resistance and type 2 diabetes (Schrauwen and Hesselink 2004). For example, one study found that patients with type 2 diabetes had smaller mitochondria than a lean non-diabetic control group, and that mitochondrial size correlated strongly with insulin sensitivity assessed by euglycaemic hyperinsulinemic clamp (Kelley et al. 2002). The mechanisms involved have not been fully elucidated but one hypothesis is that lower mitochondrial oxidative capacity leads to an impaired ability of skeletal muscle to oxidise fat (Horowitz 2007; Petersen et al. 2004). This, in turn, leads to an accumulation of intramuscular lipid intermediates which impairs insulin signalling, resulting in insulin resistance.

A growing body of evidence indicates that, like cardiorespiratory fitness, muscular strength is also associated with risk of type 2 diabetes. These findings were summarised in a recent meta-analysis by Tarp and colleagues of 11 studies, which included 1,713,468 participants and 39,233 incident cases of type 2 diabetes (Tarp et al. 2019). In analyses controlled for adiposity, each standard deviation increase in muscular strength (assessed using grip strength in most studies) was associated with a 13% (95% confidence interval 6% to 19%) lower relative risk of type 2 diabetes.

LIFESTYLE INTERVENTION TRIALS FOR DIABETES PREVENTION

There is a substantial body of evidence which indicates that interventions to increase physical activity can improve insulin sensitivity and glucose control, which is likely to be the key mechanism by which activity affects risk of type 2 diabetes. For aerobic-type physical activity interventions this is likely to be mediated by a combination of chronic effects of training on cardiorespiratory fitness and oxidative capacity in skeletal muscle, and acute effects of single exercise sessions on insulin sensitivity and insulin-independent glucose uptake (Gill and Malkova 2006). Effects of physical activity on adiposity, particularly on visceral fat and ectopic fat in the liver, are also likely to contribute (Sabag et al. 2017; Sargeant et al. 2018). These adiposity changes can occur even in the absence of weight loss (Lee et al. 2005). Fewer studies have examined the effects of resistance exercise training on insulin sensitivity and glucose control: the available evidence suggests a likely benefit, but the overall quality of this evidence is quite low (Ashton et al. 2020), and further study is needed. The effects of physical activity interventions on pancreatic beta-cell function have not been widely studied, but limited recent evidence suggests that exercise training may be able to reduce ectopic fat in the pancreas and improve beta-cell function in pre-diabetic individuals as well as people with type 2 diabetes (Heiskanen et al. 2018). The mechanisms by which physical activity affects insulin sensitivity and glucose tolerance are discussed in more detail in Chapter 7. The focus of the remainder of this section is on interventions which had the primary outcome of reducing the risk of developing type 2 diabetes in individuals known to be at high risk.

In the late 1990s and early 2000s, a series of gold-standard randomised controlled trials demonstrated that lifestyle intervention including increased physical activity, together with dietary changes to induce weight loss and improve diet quality were effective at preventing type 2 diabetes in populations with impaired glucose regulation. A summary of some the key lifestyle intervention focused diabetes prevention trials is shown in Table 5.2 (Diabetes Prevention Program Research Group 2015; Gong et al. 2019; Knowler et al. 2002; Lindström et al. 2013; Pan et al. 1997; Ramachandran et al. 2006; Tuomilehto et al. 2001). Over the initial follow-up periods of 2.8 to 6 years, lifestyle intervention in these trials reduced incidence of type 2 diabetes by 28–63% compared with control groups (Knowler et al. 2002; Pan et al. 1997; Ramachandran

Table 5.2 Selected major lifestyle diabetes prevention trials which incorporated a physical activity component.

TRIAL	PARTICIPANTS	FOLLOW-UP DURATION	LIFESTYLE INTERVENTION	MAIN FINDINGS
Da Qing Diabetes Prevention Study Pan et al. (1997) Gong et al. (2019)	577 Chinese adults with impaired glucose tolerance randomly assigned according to clinic attended to Control, Exercise, Diet or Diet plus Exercise groups.	Six-year follow-up in original trial; continued follow-up until 30 years	*Exercise intervention:* Increase leisure-time exercise by at least 1 unit per day, where 1 unit ≡ 30 mins of mild exercise (e.g. slow walking) or 20 mins of moderate exercise (e.g. brisk walking) or 10 mins of strenuous exercise (e.g. slow running or climbing stairs) or 5 mins of very strenuous exercise (e.g. jumping rope, basketball).	**Six-year follow-up:** Mean cumulative incidence of diabetes over follow-up was 65.9% for Control clinics, 44.2% for Exercise clinics, 47.1% for Diet clinics and 44.6% for Diet plus Exercise clinics. Thus, Exercise, Diet and Diet plus Exercise reduced diabetes incidence by 46%, 31% and 42% respectively, relative to control.

(Continued)

TRIAL	PARTICIPANTS	FOLLOW-UP DURATION	LIFESTYLE INTERVENTION	MAIN FINDINGS
			Diet intervention: Participants with BMI < 25 kg.m^{-2} prescribed diet containing 25–30 kcal per kg body weight, with 55–65% energy from carbohydrate, 10–15% protein, and 25–30% fat, and encouraged to consume more vegetables, control alcohol intake and reduce sugar intake. Those with BMI ≥ 25 kg m^{-2} also encouraged to lose wight until they achieved BMI 23 kg m^{-2}.	**30-year follow-up:** Exercise, Diet or Diet plus Exercise interventions groups were combined as 'Intervention' and compared to the control group in analysis. Compared to control, the intervention reduced incidence of diabetes by 39% (hazard ratio 0.61, 95% confidence interval 0.45–0.83); incidence of cardiovascular disease events by 26% (hazard ratio 0.74 (0.59–0.92)); incidence of microvascular disease by 35% (hazard ratio 0.65 (0.45–0.95)); cardiovascular disease deaths by 33% (hazard ratio 0.67 (0.48–0.94)); and all-cause mortality by 26% (hazard ratio 0.74 (0.61–0.89)).
Finnish Diabetes Prevention Study Tuomilehto et al. (2001) Lindström et al. (2013)	522 Finnish adults with impaired glucose tolerance randomly assigned to Control or Intervention groups.	Mean follow-up 3.2 years in original trial; continued follow-up until 13 years.	**Intervention goals:** • Reduce body mass by ≥ 5%. • Increase moderate exercise by ≥ 30 mins per day. • Reduce total fat intake to ≤ 30%. • Reduce saturated fat intake to ≤ 10%. • Increase fibre intake to ≥ 15 g per 1000 kcal.	**3.2-year follow-up:** Incidence of diabetes was 78 cases per 1000 person-years in the Control group and 32 cases per 1000 person-years in the Intervention group. Cumulative incidence of diabetes was 58% lower in the Intervention group than the Control group. In the Intervention group, among participants who lost less than 5% of body mass, those who increased exercise by more than four hours per week, had an odds ratio for diabetes of 0.3 (95% confidence interval 0.1–0.7) compared to those who did not achieve this exercise target after adjusting for baseline BMI. **13-year follow-up:** Risk of diabetes was 38.6% lower in the Intervention group compared to the Control group over 13 years of follow-up (hazard ratio 0.614 (0.478–0.789).

| US Diabetes Prevention Program Knowler et al. (2002) Diabetes Prevention Program Outcomes Study Diabetes Prevention Program Research Group (2015) | 3,234 US adults with impaired glucose tolerance randomly assigned to Placebo, Metformin*, or Lifestyle groups. * Metformin is a diabetes drug which improves insulin sensitivity and reduces glucose production by the liver. | Mean follow-up 2.8 years in original Diabetes Prevention Program trial; continued follow-up until 15 years in Diabetes Prevention Program Outcomes Study | *Lifestyle intervention goals:* • Reduce body mass by ≥ 7%. • Increase moderate intensity physical activity by ≥ 150 mins per week. | **2.8-year follow-up:** Incidence of diabetes was 11.0, 7.8 and 4.8 cases per 100 person-years for Placebo, Metformin and Lifestyle intervention groups. Incidence of diabetes in the Lifestyle group was 58% lower than the Placebo group and 39% lower than the Metformin group. Effects of Lifestyle intervention were similar in men and women, across ethnic groups and throughout the BMI and age range. **15-year follow-up:** Compared to the Placebo group, diabetes incidence was reduced by 27% (hazard ratio 0.73 (0.65–0.83)) in the Lifestyle intervention group and by 18% (hazard ratio 0.82 (0.72–0.93)) in the Metformin group over 15 years of follow-up. |
| **Indian Diabetes Prevention Programme** Ramachandran et al. (2006) | 531 Asian Indian adults with impaired glucose randomised to Control, Lifestyle, Metformin and Lifestyle plus Metformin intervention groups | Three years | *Lifestyle intervention:* Increase walking by ≥ 30 mins per day if sedentary or engaged in light physical activity at baseline. Maintain activity if walking or cycling > 30 mins per day or involved in physical labour at baseline. Dietary advice given on to reduce total calories, refined sugars and fats, avoid sugar and increase fibre-rich foods. | Cumulative incidences of diabetes at year 3 were 55.0%, 39.3%, 40.5% and 39.5% in the Control, Lifestyle, Metformin and Lifestyle plus Metformin intervention groups. Compared to the Control group, incidence of diabetes was 28.5% lower in the Lifestyle group, 28.2% lower in the Lifestyle plus Metformin group and 26.4% lower in the Metformin group. |

et al. 2006; Tuomilehto et al. 2001) and, in studies where follow-up continued over an extended period after completion of the initial trial, the sustained benefit in terms of reduced incidence of type 2 diabetes has been observed to persist for up to 30 years (Diabetes Prevention Program Research Group 2015; Gong et al. 2019; Lindström et al. 2013). An important observation is that in studies where the effect of lifestyle and diabetes drug Metformin on diabetes prevention was compared, lifestyle intervention was either more effective than (in the US Diabetes Prevention Program), or similarly effective to (in the Indian Diabetes Prevention Programme) Metformin in preventing incident diabetes cases. Long-term follow-up in the Da Qing study also revealed that lifestyle intervention led to reductions in the incidence of overall microvascular complications (Gong et al. 2019), and lower incidence of retinopathy was similarly observed with long-term follow-up in the Finnish Diabetes Prevention study (Aro et al. 2019). In contrast, a significant effect of lifestyle intervention on aggregate microvascular complications was only evident in women in the Diabetes Prevention Program Outcomes Study (Diabetes Prevention Program Research Group 2015). In the Da Qing study, which was the earliest of these trials to start and therefore has had the longest follow-up, lifestyle intervention reduced the hazard ratio for all-cause mortality by 26%, for cardiovascular disease incidence by 35% and for cardiovascular disease mortality by 33%, over the 30-year follow-up period (Gong et al. 2019) (Figure 5.12). Thus, the Da Qing study is the first gold-standard randomised controlled trial to demonstrate that lifestyle intervention can be effective in reducing mortality risk. It is noteworthy that a significant effect of the intervention on cardiovascular disease and all-cause-mortality risk only became apparent after 23 years of follow-up (Li et al. 2014), showing the need for extremely long trials robustly to demonstrate benefit on cardiovascular outcomes, which contrasts with the relatively shorter follow-up period needed to demonstrate the effectiveness of lifestyle interventions on diabetes incidence, at least in populations with impaired glucose tolerance.

It is difficult to disentangle the separate effects of increased physical activity *per se* versus weight loss in mediating the diabetes prevention effects of these lifestyle interventions. Greater risk reductions at the end of the initial follow-up were observed in the US Diabetes Prevention Program and Finnish Diabetes Prevention Study (Knowler et al. 2002; Tuomilehto et al. 2001), which induced substantial weight loss, compared with the Da Qing study and Indian Diabetes Prevention Programme (Pan et al. 1997; Ramachandran et al. 2006), in which weight loss was more modest. Nevertheless, lifestyle intervention in the Indian Diabetes Prevention Programme led to a 28.5% reduction in diabetes incidence without weight loss or change in waist circumference (Ramachandran et al. 2006), and in the exercise intervention arm of the Da Qing study, a 46% reduction in diabetes risk was achieved in the absence of weight loss (Pan et al. 1997). Furthermore, a secondary analysis of the Finnish Diabetes Prevention Study found that participants who increased their physical activity by the largest amounts had the largest reductions in diabetes risk (Laaksonen et al. 2005). However, in contrast, a secondary analysis of the US Diabetes Prevention Study found that the reduction in risk of diabetes in the lifestyle intervention arm was largely attributable to weight loss (Hamman et al. 2006). However, while the argument concerning the relative importance of increased physical activity versus weight loss may be of academic interest, in practical terms, it is clear that a combination of increased physical activity and weight loss yields the best outcomes, and thus optimal lifestyle intervention programmes to reduce risk of type 2 diabetes should include both components.

The effectiveness of lifestyle intervention in the prevention of type 2 diabetes amongst individuals with impaired glucose regulation has led to implementation of these programmes as standard care within some health-care systems. For example, in the UK, the English National Diabetes Prevention Programme was launched in 2016. By December 2018 over 324,699 people had been referred to the programme, and

Figure 5.12 Kaplan–Meier plots of cumulative incidence of diabetes (a), cardiovascular disease events (b), composite microvascular disease (c), cardiovascular disease deaths (d), and all-cause mortality (e) during 30 years of follow-up in the Da Qing Diabetes Prevention Outcome Study.

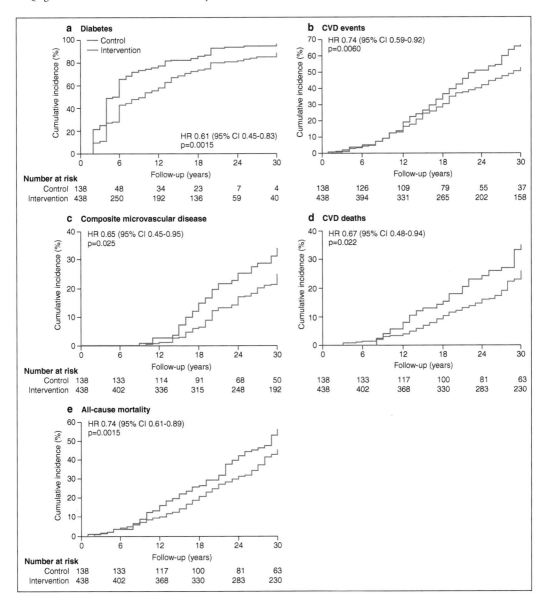

Source: Reprinted from *The Lancet Diabetes and Endocrinology*, 7: 452–61, Gong, Q. et al., 'Morbidity and mortality after lifestyle intervention for people with impaired glucose tolerance: 30-year results of the Da Qing Diabetes Prevention Outcome Study', page 456, copyright © 2019, with permission from Elsevier.
Notes: Cardiovascular disease (CVD) events were defined as non-fatal or fatal myocardial infarction or sudden death, hospital admission for heart failure, or non-fatal or fatal stroke. Composite microvascular disease was defined as the aggregate outcome retinopathy, nephropathy and neuropathy. CVD deaths were defined as death due to myocardial infarction, sudden death, heart failure or stroke. HR = hazard ratio (intervention vs control).

amongst the 32,665 who had sufficient time to complete the nine-month behaviour change intervention programme focused on increased physical activity, weight loss and improved diet quality, a mean weight loss of 2.3 kg and a reduction in HbA1c of 1.3 mmol.mol^{-1} was observed in an intention-to-treat analysis (Valabhji et al. 2020). The extent of weight loss and HbA1c reduction was strongly associated with attendance at the intervention sessions, with participants who attended all sessions having a mean weight loss of 5.1 kg and reduction in HbA1c of 3.3 mmol.mol^{-1}. This clearly illustrates the need to ensure that participants actively engage with a lifestyle intervention programme to ensure successful outcomes and facilitating this is a real challenge to implementation of lifestyle interventions in 'real-world' settings.

LIFESTYLE INTERVENTION IN THE MANAGEMENT OF TYPE 2 DIABETES

There is an increasing body of epidemiological evidence demonstrating that amongst people with type 2 diabetes, high levels of physical activity (Kodama et al. 2013), cardiorespiratory fitness (Chacko et al. 2008; Church et al. 2004, 2005) and muscular strength (as assessed by grip strength) (Celis-Morales et al. 2017) are associated with lower risk of all-cause mortality, and incidence of, and mortality from cardiovascular disease. In addition, a large body of evidence from intervention studies also demonstrates that both aerobic and resistance exercise training are effective at improving glucose control, reducing HbA1c concentrations, and improving markers of metabolic health amongst people with type 2 diabetes (Gordon et al. 2009; Snowling and Hopkins 2006; Umpierre et al. 2011), with a combination of aerobic and resistance training inducing larger glycaemic benefits than either aerobic or resistance exercise alone (Church et al. 2010; Sigal et al. 2007). These studies and the mechanisms underpinning these effects are discussed further in Chapter 7. As a consequence, physical activity is a cornerstone of the management of type 2 diabetes, with the American Diabetes Association recommending that people with type 2 diabetes undertake daily exercise, and ideally perform both aerobic and resistance exercise training for optimal glycaemic and health outcomes (Colberg et al. 2016). A number of different exercise approaches have been shown to be efficacious at improving insulin sensitivity, glucose control and other markers of metabolic health in people with type 2 diabetes, including continuous moderate intensity physical activity interventions (Snowling and Hopkins 2006), high-intensity interval training (Jelleyman et al. 2015; Ross et al. 2016), and 'exercise snacking' approaches involving repeated small amounts of aerobic or resistance exercise spread throughout the day (Dempsey et al. 2016; Francois et al. 2014). A key challenge with all of these approaches is long-term sustainability of these interventions – compliance with supervised exercise over several weeks in a laboratory or gym setting, and long-term sustained adherence are likely to differ substantially – and long-term maintenance of physical activity behaviour change is one of the key challenges facing the field going forwards. There is now increasing research interest in how to develop and deliver interventions that are sustainable and therefore show long-term effectiveness in improving health outcomes (Bullard et al. 2019; Gray et al. 2016; Sansano-Nadal et al. 2019). Individual preference is likely to play a role here and thus, irrespective of the relative benefits of different types of physical activity interventions when they are completed as prescribed, it is unlikely that a single 'one-size-fits-all' approach will be optimal.

While there is considerable evidence that physical activity interventions improve glycaemia and other aspects of cardio-metabolic health in patients with type 2 diabetes, it has been unclear whether this translates to reduction in risk of cardiovascular events. The Look AHEAD (Action for Health in Diabetes) study aimed to answer this question. In the largest ever randomised controlled trial of a lifestyle intervention, costing over US$250 million (Ryan 2005), 5,145 overweight or obese patients with type 2 diabetes in the US were randomised to 'Intensive Lifestyle Intervention' (n = 2,570) and 'Diabetes Support and Education' (n = 2,575) intervention arms (Look AHEAD Research Group 2013). Participants in the Diabetes Support and Education arm – the 'control' arm of the study – received three group educational sessions per year focused on diet, physical activity and social support for the first 4.0 to 6.5 years of the study. It is of note that the intensity of intervention offered to these participants was similar to that seen in the 'intervention' arm of several other lifestyle intervention studies. Participants in the Intensive Lifestyle Intervention arm received a diet and physical activity intervention with the aim of undertaking at least 175 minutes of moderate intensity physical activity per week, and target of at least 7% of body weight loss in the first year and weight loss maintenance thereafter. To support them in achieving these goals, participants attended individual or group sessions conducted by nutritionists, exercise specialists and behaviour therapists every week during the first six months, and three times per month for the next six months. For the next three years they continued to receive individual sessions at least once per month and also received a support phone call or email at least monthly. The primary outcome in the trial was a composite of death from cardiovascular disease, non-fatal myocardial infarction, non-fatal stroke and hospitalisation for angina over an intended 13.5-year follow-up period. However, the trial stopped early after an interim analysis conducted after 9.6 years found that it was unlikely for a significant difference in groups to become evident by the planned study end-date (Look AHEAD Research Group 2013). At this point, the hazard ratio for the primary outcome in the intervention compared to control group was 0.95 (95% confidence interval 0.83 to 1.09). There are a number of potential reasons for the negative outcome in this trial. These include a lower than expected rate of cardiovascular events reducing power to detect any differences between groups; the relatively intensive intervention provided to the control group (who lost 3.5% body weight on average over the 9.6 years of the trial) which would act to attenuate any potential differences between groups; diminishing compliance to the intervention over time in the intervention group; and the greater use of diabetes, blood pressure and lipid-lowering drugs over the course of the trial in the control group (Look AHEAD Research Group 2013). Furthermore, given that a significant effect on cardiovascular disease mortality only became apparent after 23 years of follow-up in the Da Qing study (Li et al. 2014), it is possible that the Look AHEAD study was simply too short to detect a clear effect of lifestyle intervention on cardiovascular disease outcomes. There were, however, several benefits seen in the intervention compared with the control group. Despite not increasing life expectancy, the intervention was effective at compressing the period of morbidity at the end of the lifespan, with a reduced incidence of physical disability in the intervention group compared with control (incidence rate ratio 0.88

(95% confidence interval 0.81 to 0.96), translating to 0.9 more disability-free life years for a 60-year-old (Gregg et al. 2018). Prevalence of diabetes remission was also higher in the intervention study arm (11.5% of participants (95% confidence interval 10.1% to 12.8%) in year 1; and 7.3% of participants (6.2%–9.4%) in year 4) than the control arm (2.0% of participants (1.4%–2.6%) in year 1; 2.0% of participants (1.5%–2.7%) in year 4) (Gregg et al. 2012). Furthermore, in a post-hoc analysis of the data, participants who lost most than 10 kg body weight had a 21% lower risk of an adverse cardiovascular outcome (primary outcome as defined above) (hazard ratio 0.78 (95% confidence interval 0.60–1.03)), and greater increases in fitness were significantly associated with a lower incidence of adverse cardiovascular events (Look AHEAD Research Group 2016). Thus, it appears that the Look AHEAD intervention was efficacious in reducing cardiovascular events in participants who managed to comply with the intervention well, particularly in those who managed to maintain substantial weight loss. However, despite the intensive support offered to participants in the intervention arm, many were unable to sustain the intervention long-term. This highlights the key challenge of facilitating long-term adherence and sustainability of lifestyle interventions, which is an area where much further research is needed.

SUMMARY

- Type 2 diabetes is a disease characterised by insulin resistance and defective insulin secretion leading to chronic hyperglycaemia.
- Type 2 diabetes increases risk of mortality and of several comorbidities including microvascular (retinopathy, nephropathy, neuropathy) and macrovascular (CHD and stroke) disease.
- Progression to type 2 diabetes is generally preceded by years or decades of insulin resistance. Insulin resistance can lead to a cluster of adverse changes to glucose metabolism, lipid metabolism, vascular function and inflammation which are associated with increased macrovascular disease risk.
- Obesity is the most important modifiable risk factor for type 2 diabetes, and substantial weight loss in people with type 2 diabetes can put disease into remission.
- Prospective observational studies demonstrate an association between low levels of physical activity, low cardiovascular fitness and low muscular strength and increased risk of type 2 diabetes.
- Randomised controlled trials of lifestyle interventions incorporating physical activity and dietary change demonstrate that they are effective at preventing type 2 diabetes. Longer-term follow-up in these trials indicates that this benefit persists for up to 30 years, and may also extend to reductions in risk of microvascular complications and mortality.
- Physical activity in patients with type 2 diabetes improves glycaemic and other health outcomes, with a combination of aerobic and resistance exercise inducing larger benefits to HbA1c reduction than either type of exercise alone.
- The Look AHEAD study found that an intensive lifestyle intervention did not reduce risk of cardiovascular events in patients with type 2 diabetes. This may have

been because the period of follow-up was too short for benefits to become apparent. However, participants who lost the most weight and had the largest gains in fitness did have lower risk of adverse cardiovascular disease outcomes highlighting the key challenge of developing new approaches to facilitate long-term adherence to lifestyle interventions.

STUDY TASKS

1 Explain how insulin resistance can increase risk of cardiovascular disease even when normoglycaemia is maintained.
2 Describe the evidence suggesting that the association between obesity and type 2 diabetes is causal. Explain why the relationship between adiposity and metabolic dysfunction is not the same for everyone.
3 Summarise the epidemiological evidence indicating an association between physical activity and risk of type 2 diabetes. Based on this evidence, what amounts of physical activity would you recommend to minimise type 2 diabetes risk? What are the limitations of this evidence? How might these limitations affect your recommendations?
4 With reference to the epidemiological evidence, explain the extent to which the association between physical activity/cardiorespiratory fitness and risk of type 2 diabetes is independent of effects on adiposity and the extent to which being active and fit can offset the increased diabetes risk associated with obesity. If an inactive and obese friend or colleague approached you asking how they could reduce their diabetes risk, what would your recommendation be, and why?
5 Describe the major lifestyle-based diabetes prevention trials and summarise their key findings. Explain why randomised controlled trials such as these represent gold-standard evidence.
6 The American Diabetes Association recommend that people with type 2 diabetes undertake daily exercise, ideally performing both aerobic and resistance exercise. Explain the evidence behind this recommendation.
7 Describe the Look AHEAD study and its major findings. Critically reflect on the implications of these findings and the further challenges which remain for lifestyle interventions in people with type 2 diabetes.

FURTHER READING

Ashton, R.E., Tew, G.A., Aning, J.J., Gilbert, S.E., Lewis, L. and Saxton, J.M. (2020) Effects of short-term, medium-term and long-term resistance exercise training on cardiometabolic health outcomes in adults: systematic review with meta-analysis. *British Journal of Sports Medicine* 54: 341–8.

Colberg, S.R., Sigal, R.J., Yardley, J.E., Riddell, M.C., Dunstan, D.W., Dempsey, P.C. et al. (2016) Physical activity/exercise and diabetes: a position statement of the American Diabetes Association. *Diabetes Care* 39: 2065–79.

Diabetes Prevention Program Research Group. (2015) Long-term effects of lifestyle intervention or metformin on diabetes development and microvascular complications over 15-year follow-up: the Diabetes Prevention Program Outcomes Study. *The Lancet Diabetes and Endocrinology* 3: 866–75.

Gong, Q., Zhang, P., Wang, J., Ma, J., An, Y., Chen, Y. et al. and Da Qing Diabetes Prevention Study Group. (2019) Morbidity and mortality after lifestyle intervention for people with impaired glucose tolerance: 30-year results of the Da Qing Diabetes Prevention Outcome Study. *The Lancet Diabetes and Endocrinology* 7: 452–61.

Lindström, J., Peltonen, M., Eriksson, J.G., Ilanne-Parikka, P., Aunola, S., Keinänen-Kiukaanniemi, S. et al. (2013) Improved lifestyle and decreased diabetes risk over 13 years: long-term follow-up of the randomised Finnish Diabetes Prevention Study (DPS). *Diabetologia* 56: 284–93.

Look AHEAD Research Group; Wing, R.R., Bolin, P., Brancati, F.L., Bray, G.A., Clark, J.M., Coday, M. et al. (2013) Cardiovascular effects of intensive lifestyle intervention in type 2 diabetes. *New England Journal of Medicine* 369: 145–54.

Qiu, S., Cai, X., Yang, B., Du, Z., Cai, M., Sun, Z. et al. (2019) Association between cardiorespiratory fitness and risk of type 2 diabetes: a meta-analysis. *Obesity* 27: 315–24.

Rydén, L., Grant, P.J., Anker, S.D., Berne, C., Cosentino, F., Danchin, N. et al., Document Reviewers. (2013) ESC Guidelines on diabetes, pre-diabetes, and cardiovascular diseases developed in collaboration with the EASD: the Task Force on diabetes, pre-diabetes, and cardiovascular diseases of the European Society of Cardiology (ESC) and developed in collaboration with the European Association for the Study of Diabetes (EASD). *European Heart Journal* 34: 3035–87.

Sattar, N. and Gill, J.M.R. (2014) Type 2 diabetes as a disease of ectopic fat? *BMC Medicine* 12: 123. doi: 10.1186/s12916-014-0123-4.

Smith, A.D., Crippa, A., Woodcock, J. and Brage, S. (2016) Physical activity and incident type 2 diabetes mellitus: a systematic review and dose-response meta-analysis of prospective cohort studies. *Diabetologia* 59: 2527–45.

Umpierre, D., Ribeiro, P.A., Kramer, C.K., Leitão, C.B., Zucatti, A.T., Azevedo et al. (2011) Physical activity advice only or structured exercise training and association with HbA1c levels in type 2 diabetes: a systematic review and meta-analysis. *Journal of the American Medical Association* 305: 1790–9.

Valabhji, J., Barron, E., Bradley, D., Bakhai, C., Fagg, J., O'Neill, S. et al. (2020) Early outcomes from the English National Health Service Diabetes Prevention Programme. *Diabetes Care* 43: 152–60.

REFERENCES

Abdullah, A., Peeters, A., de Courten, M. and Stoelwinder, J. (2010) The magnitude of association between overweight and obesity and the risk of diabetes: a meta-analysis of prospective cohort studies. *Diabetes Research and Clinical Practice* 89: 309–19.

Alberti, K.G., Eckel, R.H., Grundy, S.M., Zimmet, P.Z., Cleeman, J.I., Donato et al. (2009) Harmonizing the metabolic syndrome: a joint interim statement of the International Diabetes Federation Task Force on Epidemiology and Prevention; National Heart, Lung, and Blood Institute; American Heart Association; World Heart Federation; International Atherosclerosis Society; and International Association for the Study of Obesity. *Circulation* 120: 1640–5.

American Diabetes Association. (2016) 2. Classification and diagnosis of diabetes. *Diabetes Care* 39(Suppl. 1): S13–22.

Aro, A., Kauppinen, A., Kivinen, N., Selander, T., Kinnunen, K., Tuomilehto, J. et al. (2019) Life-style intervention improves retinopathy status: the Finnish Diabetes Prevention Study. *Nutrients* 11: 1691. doi: 10.3390/nu11071691.

Ashton, R.E., Tew, G.A., Aning, J.J., Gilbert, S.E., Lewis, L. and Saxton, J.M. (2020) Effects of short-term, medium-term and long-term resistance exercise training on cardiometabolic health outcomes in adults: systematic review with meta-analysis. *British Journal of Sports Medicine* 54: 341–8.

Aune, D., Norat, T., Leitzmann, M., Tonstad, S. and Vatten, L.J. (2015) Physical activity and the risk of type 2 diabetes: a systematic review and dose-response meta-analysis. *European Journal of Epidemiology* 30: 529–42.

Bruce, C.R., Anderson, M.J., Carey, A.L., Newman, D.G., Bonen, A., Kriketos, A.D. et al. (2003) Muscle oxidative capacity is a better predictor of insulin sensitivity than lipid status. *Journal of Clinical Endocrinology and Metabolism* 88: 5444–51.

Bullard, T., Ji, M., An, R., Trinh, L., Mackenzie, M. and Mullen, S.P. (2019) A systematic review and meta-analysis of adherence to physical activity interventions among three chronic conditions: cancer, cardiovascular disease, and diabetes. *BMC Public Health* 19: 636. doi: 10.1186/s12889-019-6877-z.

Celis-Morales, C.A., Ghouri, N., Bailey, M.E., Sattar, N. and Gill, J.M. (2013) Should physical activity recommendations be ethnicity-specific? Evidence from a cross-sectional study of South Asian and European men. *PLoS One* 8: e82568. doi: 10.1371/journal.pone.0082568.

Celis-Morales, C.A., Petermann, F., Hui, L., Lyall, D.M., Iliodromiti, S., Mclaren, J. et al. (2017) Associations between diabetes and both cardiovascular disease and all-cause mortality are modified by grip strength: evidence from UK Biobank, a prospective population-based cohort study. *Diabetes Care* 40: 1710–18.

Chacko, K.M., Bauer, T.A., Dale, R.A., Dixon, J.A., Schrier, R.W. and Estacio, R.O. (2008) Heart rate recovery predicts mortality and cardiovascular events in patients with type 2 diabetes. *Medicine and Science in Sports and Exercise* 40: 288–95.

Cheng, Y.J., Kanaya, A.M., Araneta, M.R.G., Saydah, S.H., Kahn, H.S., Gregg, E.W. et al. (2019) Prevalence of diabetes by race and ethnicity in the United States, 2011–2016. *Journal of the American Medical Association* 322: 2389–98.

Church, T.S., Blair, S.N., Cocreham, S., Johannsen, N., Johnson, W., Kramer, K. et al. (2010) Effects of aerobic and resistance training on hemoglobin A1c levels in patients with type 2 diabetes: a randomized controlled trial. *Journal of the American Medical Association* 304: 2253–62.

Church, T.S., Cheng, Y.J., Earnest, C.P., Barlow, C.E., Gibbons, L.W., Priest, E.L. and Blair, S.N. (2004) Exercise capacity and body composition as predictors of mortality among men with diabetes. *Diabetes Care* 27: 83–8.

Church, T.S., Lamonte, M.J., Barlow, C.E. and Blair, S.N. (2005) Cardiorespiratory fitness and body mass index as predictors of cardiovascular disease mortality among men with diabetes. *Archives of Internal Medicine* 165: 2114–20.

Colberg, S.R., Sigal, R.J., Yardley, J.E., Riddell, M.C., Dunstan, D.W., Dempsey, P.C. et al. (2016) Physical activity/exercise and diabetes: a position statement of the American Diabetes Association. *Diabetes Care* 39: 2065–79.

Dempsey, P.C., Larsen, R.N., Sethi, P., Sacre, J.W., Straznicky, N.E., Cohen et al. (2016) Benefits for type 2 diabetes of interrupting prolonged sitting with brief bouts of light walking or simple resistance activities. *Diabetes Care* 39: 964–72.

Diabetes Prevention Program Research Group. (2015) Long-term effects of lifestyle intervention or metformin on diabetes development and microvascular complications over 15-year follow-up: the Diabetes Prevention Program Outcomes Study. *The Lancet Diabetes and Endocrinology* 3: 866–75.

Eckel, R.H., Alberti, K.G., Grundy, S.M. and Zimmet, P.Z. (2010) The metabolic syndrome. *The Lancet* 375: 181–3.

Ford, E.S., Li, C. and Sattar, N. (2008) Metabolic syndrome and incident diabetes: current state of the evidence. *Diabetes Care* 31: 1898–904.

Francois, M.E., Baldi, J.C., Manning, P.J., Lucas, S.J., Hawley, J.A., Williams, M.J. and Cotter, J.D. (2014) 'Exercise snacks' before meals: a novel strategy to improve glycaemic control in individuals with insulin resistance. *Diabetologia* 57: 1437–45.

Frayling, T.M., Timpson, N.J., Weedon, M.N., Zeggini, E., Freathy, R.M., Lindgren, C.M. et al. (2007) A common variant in the FTO gene is associated with body mass index and predisposes to childhood and adult obesity. *Science* 316: 889–94.

Frayn, K.N. (2003) *Metabolic regulation: a human perspective.* 2nd edn, Oxford: Blackwell Science Ltd.

Ghouri, N., Purves, D., McConnachie, A., Wilson, J., Gill, J.M. and Sattar, N. (2013) Lower cardiorespiratory fitness contributes to increased insulin resistance and fasting glycaemia in middle-aged South Asian compared with European men living in the UK. *Diabetologia* 56: 2238–49.

Gill, J.M.R., Al-Mamari, A., Ferrell, W.R., Cleland, S.J., Packard, C.J., Sattar, N. et al. (2004) Effects of prior moderate exercise on postprandial metabolism and vascular function in lean and centrally obese men. *Journal of the American College of Cardiology* 44: 2375–82.

Gill, J.M.R. and Malkova, D. (2006) Physical activity, fitness and cardiovascular disease risk in adults: interactions with insulin resistance and obesity. *Clinical Science* 110: 409–25.

Gong, Q., Zhang, P., Wang, J., Ma, J., An, Y., Chen, Y. et al. and Da Qing Diabetes Prevention Study Group. (2019) Morbidity and mortality after lifestyle intervention for people with impaired glucose tolerance: 30-year results of the Da Qing Diabetes Prevention Outcome Study. *The Lancet Diabetes and Endocrinology* 7: 452–61.

Gordon, B.A., Benson, A.C., Bird, S.R. and Fraser, S.F. (2009) Resistance training improves metabolic health in type 2 diabetes: a systematic review. *Diabetes Research and Clinical Practice* 83: 157–75.

Gray, S.R., Ferguson, C., Birch, K., Forrest, L.J. and Gill, J.M. (2016) High-intensity interval training: key data needed to bridge the gap from laboratory to public health policy. *British Journal of Sports Medicine* 50: 1231–2.

Gregg, E.W., Chen, H., Wagenknecht, L.E., Clark, J.M., Delahanty, L.M., Bantle, J. et al. (2012) Association of an intensive lifestyle intervention with remission of type 2 diabetes. *Journal of the American Medical Association* 308: 2489–96.

Gregg, E.W., Lin, J., Bardenheier, B., Chen, H., Rejeski, W.J., Zhuo, X. et al. and the Look AHEAD Study Group. (2018) Impact of intensive lifestyle intervention on disability-free life expectancy: The Look AHEAD Study. *Diabetes Care* 41: 1040–8.

Grøntved, A., Pan, A., Mekary, R.A., Stampfer, M., Willett, W.C., Manson, J.E. and Hu, F.B. (2014) Muscle-strengthening and conditioning activities and risk of type 2 diabetes: a prospective study in two cohorts of US women. *PLoS Medicine* 11: e1001587. doi: 10.1371/journal.pmed.1001587.

Grøntved, A., Rimm, E.B., Willett, W.C., Andersen, L.B. and Hu, F.B. (2012) A prospective study of weight training and risk of type 2 diabetes mellitus in men. *Archives of Internal Medicine* 172: 1306–12.

Hall, L.M., Moran, C.N., Milne, G.R., Wilson, J., MacFarlane, N.G., Forouhi, N.G. et al. (2010) Fat oxidation, fitness and skeletal muscle expression of oxidative/lipid metabolism genes in South Asians: implications for insulin resistance? *PLoS One* 5: e14197. doi: 10.1371/journal.pone.0014197.

Hamman, R.F., Wing, R.R., Edelstein, S.L., Lachin, J.M., Bray, G.A., Delahanty, L. et al. (2006) Effect of weight loss with lifestyle intervention on risk of diabetes. *Diabetes Care* 29: 2102–7.

Heiskanen, M.A., Motiani, K.K., Mari, A., Saunavaara, V., Eskelinen, J.J., Virtanen, K.A. et al. (2018) Exercise training decreases pancreatic fat content and improves beta cell function regardless of baseline glucose tolerance: a randomised controlled trial. *Diabetologia* 61: 1817–28.

Helmrich, S.P., Ragland, D.R., Leung, R.W. and Paffenbarger, R.S. (1991) Physical activity and reduced occurrence of non-insulin-dependent diabetes mellitus. *New England Journal of Medicine* 325: 147–52.

Horowitz, J.F. (2007) Exercise-induced alterations in muscle lipid metabolism improve insulin sensitivity. *Exercise and Sport Sciences Reviews* 35: 192–6.

Hu, G., Lindström, J., Valle, T.T., Eriksson, J.G., Jousilahti, P., Silventoinen, K. et al. (2004) Physical activity, body mass index, and risk of type 2 diabetes in patients with normal or impaired glucose regulation. *Archives of Internal Medicine* 164: 892–6.

Huang-Doran, I., Sleigh, A., Rochford, J.J., O'Rahilly, S. and Savage, D.B. (2010) Lipodystrophy: metabolic insights from a rare disorder. *Journal of Endocrinology* 207: 245–55.

Iliodromiti, S., Ghouri, N., Celis-Morales, C.A., Sattar, N., Lumsden, M.A. and Gill, J.M. (2016) Should physical activity recommendations for South Asian adults be ethnicity-specific? Evidence from a cross-sectional study of South Asian and White European men and women. *PLoS One* 11: e0160024. doi: 10.1371/journal.pone.0160024.

InterAct Consortium; Scott, R.A., Langenberg, C., Sharp, S.J., Franks, P.W., Rolandsson, O., Drogan, D. et al. (2013) The link between family history and risk of type 2 diabetes is not explained by anthropometric, lifestyle or genetic risk factors: the EPIC-InterAct study. *Diabetologia* 56: 60–9.

International Diabetes Federation. (2019). *IDF Diabetes Altas*. 9th edn, Brussels: International Diabates Federation.

Jelleyman, C., Yates, T., O'Donovan, G., Gray, L.J., King, J.A., Khunti, K. and Davies, M.J. (2015) The effects of high-intensity interval training on glucose regulation and insulin resistance: a meta-analysis. *Obesity Reviews* 16: 942–61.

Jeon, C.Y., Lokken, R.P., Hu, F.B. and van Dam, R.M. (2007) Physical activity of moderate intensity and risk of type 2 diabetes: a systematic review. *Diabetes Care* 30: 744–52. doi: 10.2337/dc06-1842

Kelley, D.E., He, J., Menshikova, E.V. and Ritov, V.B. (2002) Dysfunction of mitochondria in human skeletal muscle in type 2 diabetes. *Diabetes* 51: 2944–50.

Knowler, W.C., Barrett-Connor, E., Fowler, S.E., Hamman, R.F., Lachin, J.M., Walker, E.A. and Nathan, D.M. (2002) Reduction in the incidence of type 2 diabetes with lifestyle intervention or metformin. *New England Journal of Medicine* 346: 393–403.

Kodama, S., Horikawa, C., Fujihara, K., Heianza, Y., Hirasawa, R., Yachi, Y. et al. (2012) Comparisons of the strength of associations with future type 2 diabetes risk among anthropometric obesity indicators, including waist-to-height ratio: a meta-analysis. *American Journal of Epidemiology* 176: 959–69.

Kodama, S., Horikawa, C., Fujihara, K., Yoshizawa, S., Yachi, Y., Tanaka, S. et al. (2014) Quantitative relationship between body weight gain in adulthood and incident type 2 diabetes: a meta-analysis. *Obesity Reviews* 15: 202–14.

Kodama, S., Tanaka, S., Heianza, Y., Fujihara, K., Horikawa, C., Shimano, H. et al. (2013) Association between physical activity and risk of all-cause mortality and cardiovascular disease in patients with diabetes: a meta-analysis. *Diabetes Care* 36: 471–9.

Laaksonen, D.E., Lindström, J., Lakka, T.A., Eriksson, J.G., Niskanen, L., Wikström, K., et al. (2005) Physical activity in the prevention of type 2 diabetes: the Finnish diabetes prevention study. *Diabetes* 54: 158–65.

Laaksonen, D.E., Niskanen, L., Lakka, H.M., Lakka, T.A. and Uusitupa, M. (2004) Epidemiology and treatment of the metabolic syndrome. *Annals of Medicine* 36: 332–46.

Lean, M.E.J., Leslie, W.S., Barnes, A.C., Brosnahan, N., Thom, G., McCombie, L. et al. (2019) Durability of a primary care-led weight-management intervention for remission of type 2 diabetes: 2-year results of the DiRECT open-label, cluster-randomised trial. *The Lancet Diabetes and Endocrinology* 7: 344–55.

Lee, S., Kuk, J.L., Davidson, L.E., Hudson, R., Kilpatrick, K., Graham, T.E. and Ross, R. (2005) Exercise without weight loss is an effective strategy for obesity reduction in obese individuals with and without type 2 diabetes. *Journal of Applied Physiology* 99: 1220–5.

Li, G., Zhang, P., Wang, J., An, Y., Gong, Q., Gregg, E.W. et al. (2014) Cardiovascular mortality, all-cause mortality, and diabetes incidence after lifestyle intervention for people with impaired glucose tolerance in the Da Qing Diabetes Prevention Study: a 23-year follow-up study. *The Lancet Diabetes and Endocrinology* 2: 474–80.

Lindström, J., Peltonen, M., Eriksson, J.G., Ilanne-Parikka, P., Aunola, S., Keinänen-Kiukaanniemi, S. et al. (2013) Improved lifestyle and decreased diabetes risk over 13 years: long-term follow-up of the randomised Finnish Diabetes Prevention Study (DPS). *Diabetologia* 56: 284–93.

Logue, J., Walker, J.J., Colhoun, H., Leese, G.P., Lindsay, R.S., Mcknight, J.A. et al. (2011) Do men develop type 2 diabetes at lower body mass indices than women? *Diabetologia* 54: 3003–6.

Look AHEAD Research Group; Gregg, E.W., Jakicic, J.M., Blackburn, G., Bloomquist, P., Bray, G.A., Clark, J.M., et al. (2016) Association of the magnitude of weight loss and changes in physical fitness with long-term cardiovascular disease outcomes in overweight or obese people with type 2 diabetes: a post-hoc analysis of the Look AHEAD randomised clinical trial. *The Lancet Diabetes Endocrinol*ogy 4: 913–21.

Look AHEAD Research Group; Wing, R.R., Bolin, P., Brancati, F.L., Bray, G.A., Clark, J.M., Coday, M. et al. (2013) Cardiovascular effects of intensive lifestyle intervention in type 2 diabetes. *New England Journal of Medicine* 369: 145–54.

Moy, C.S., Songer, T.J., Laporte, R.E., Dorman, J.S., Kriska, A.M., Orchard, T.J. et al. (1993) Insulin-dependent diabetes mellitus, physical activity, and death. *American Journal of Epidemiology* 137: 74–81.

Ntuk, U.E., Gill, J.M., Mackay, D.F., Sattar, N. and Pell, J.P. (2014) Ethnic-specific obesity cutoffs for diabetes risk: cross-sectional study of 490,288 UK biobank participants. *Diabetes Care* 37: 2500–7.

Nyholm, B., Nielsen, M.F., Kristensen, K., Nielsen, S., Østergård, T., Pedersen, S.B. et al. (2004) Evidence of increased visceral obesity and reduced physical fitness in healthy insulin-resistant first-degree relatives of type 2 diabetic patients. *European Journal of Endocrinology* 150: 207–14.

Pan, X.R., Li, G.W., Hu, Y.H., Wang, J.X., Yang, W.Y., An, Z.X. et al. (1997) Effects of diet and exercise in preventing NIDDM in people with impaired glucose tolerance: the Da Qing IGT and Diabetes Study. *Diabetes Care* 20: 537–44.

Patterson, R., McNamara, E., Tainio, M., de Sá, T.H., Smith, A.D., Sharp, S.J. et al. (2018) Sedentary behaviour and risk of all-cause, cardiovascular and cancer mortality, and incident type 2 diabetes: a systematic review and dose response meta-analysis. *European Journal of Epidemiology* 33: 811–29.

Petersen, K.F., Dufour, S., Befroy, D., Garcia, R. and Shulman, G.I. (2004) Impaired mitochondrial activity in the insulin-resistant offspring of patients with type 2 diabetes. *New England Journal of Medicine* 350: 664–71.

Qiu, S., Cai, X., Yang, B., Du, Z., Cai, M., Sun, Z. et al. (2019) Association between cardiorespiratory fitness and risk of type 2 diabetes: a meta-analysis. *Obesity* 27: 315–24.

Ramachandran, A., Snehalatha, C., Mary, S., Mukesh, B., Bhaskar, A.D. and Vijay, V. (2006) The Indian Diabetes Prevention Programme shows that lifestyle modification and metformin prevent type 2 diabetes in Asian Indian subjects with impaired glucose tolerance (IDPP-1). *Diabetologia* 49: 289–97.

Rask-Madsen, C. and Kahn, C.R. (2012) Tissue-specific insulin signaling, metabolic syndrome, and cardiovascular disease. *Arteriosclerosis, Thrombosis and Vascular Biology* 32: 2052–9.

Reaven, G.M. (1988) Role of insulin resistance in human disease. *Diabetes* 37: 1595–607.

Riddell, M.C., Gallen, I.W., Smart, C.E., Taplin, C.E., Adolfsson, P., Lumb, A.N. et al. (2017) Exercise management in type 1 diabetes: a consensus statement. *The Lancet Diabetes Endocrinology* 5: 377–90.

Ross, L.M., Porter, R.R. and Durstine, J.L. (2016) High-intensity interval training (HIIT) for patients with chronic diseases. *Journal of Sport and Health Science* 5: 139–44.

Ryan, D. (2005) Risks and benefits of weight loss: challenges to obesity research. *European Heart Journal* 7(Suppl. L): L27–31.

Rydén, L., Grant, P.J., Anker, S.D., Berne, C., Cosentino, F., Danchin, N. et al., ESC Committee for Practice Guidelines (CPG); De Backer, G., Sirnes, P.A., Ezquerra, E.A., Avogaro, A., Badimon, L., Baranova, E. et al., Document Reviewers. (2013) ESC Guidelines on diabetes, pre-diabetes, and cardiovascular diseases developed in collaboration with the EASD: the Task Force on diabetes, pre-diabetes, and cardiovascular diseases of the European Society of Cardiology (ESC) and developed in collaboration with the European Association for the Study of Diabetes (EASD). *European Heart Journal* 34: 3035–87.

Sabag, A., Way, K.L., Keating, S.E., Sultana, R.N., O'Connor, H.T., Baker, M.K. et al. (2017) Exercise and ectopic fat in type 2 diabetes: a systematic review and meta-analysis. *Diabetes Metabolism* 43: 195–210.

Sansano-Nadal, O., Giné-Garriga, M., Brach, J.S., Wert, D.M., Jerez-Roig, J., Guerra-Balic, M. et al. (2019) Exercise-based interventions to enhance long-term sustainability of physical activity in older adults: a systematic review and meta-analysis of randomized clinical trials. *International Journal of Environmental Research and Public Health* 16: 2527. doi: 10.3390/ijerph16142527.

Sargeant, J.A., Gray, L.J., Bodicoat, D.H., Willis, S.A., Stensel, D.J., Nimmo, M.A. et al. (2018) The effect of exercise training on intrahepatic triglyceride and hepatic insulin sensitivity: a systematic review and meta-analysis. *Obesity Reviews* 19: 1446–59.

Sattar, N. and Gill, J.M. (2014) Type 2 diabetes as a disease of ectopic fat? *BMC Medicine* 12: 123. doi: 10.1186/s12916-014-0123-4.

Schrauwen, P. and Hesselink, M.K. (2004) Oxidative capacity, lipotoxicity, and mitochondrial damage in type 2 diabetes. *Diabetes* 53: 1412–17.

Seshasai, S.R., Kaptoge, S., Thompson, A., Di Angelantonio, E., Gao, P., Sarwar, N. et al. (2011) Diabetes mellitus, fasting glucose, and risk of cause-specific death. *New England Journal of Medicine* 364: 829–41.

Sigal, R.J., Kenny, G.P., Boulé, N.G., Wells, G.A., Prud'homme, D., Fortier, M. et al. (2007) Effects of aerobic training, resistance training, or both on glycemic control in type 2 diabetes: a randomized trial. *Annals of Internal Medicine* 147: 357–69.

Smith, A.D., Crippa, A., Woodcock, J. and Brage, S. (2016) Physical activity and incident type 2 diabetes mellitus: a systematic review and dose-response meta-analysis of prospective cohort studies. *Diabetologia* 59: 2527–45.

Sniderman, A.D., Bhopal, R., Prabhakaran, D., Sarrafzadegan, N. and Tchernof, A. (2007) Why might South Asians be so susceptible to central obesity and its atherogenic consequences? The adipose tissue overflow hypothesis. *International Journal of Epidemiology* 36: 220–5.

Snowling, N.J. and Hopkins, W.G. (2006) Effects of different modes of exercise training on glucose control and risk factors for complications in type 2 diabetic patients: a meta-analysis. *Diabetes Care* 29: 2518–27.

Sproston, K. and Mindell, J. (eds). (2006) *Health Survey for England 2004: the health of minority ethnic groups*. London: National Centre for Social Research.

Stamatakis, E., Ekelund, U., Ding, D., Hamer, M., Bauman, A.E. and Lee, I.-M. (2019) Is the time right for quantitative public health guidelines on sitting? A narrative review of sedentary behaviour research paradigms and findings. *British Journal of Sports Medicine* 53: 377–82.

Stefan, N., Kantartzis, K., Machann, J., Schick, F., Thamer, C., Rittig, K. et al. (2008) Identification and characterization of metabolically benign obesity in humans. *Archives of Internal Medicine* 168: 1609–16.

Tarp, J., Støle, A.P., Blond, K. and Grøntved, A. (2019) Cardiorespiratory fitness, muscular strength and risk of type 2 diabetes: a systematic review and meta-analysis. *Diabetologia* 62: 1129–42.

Thamer, C., Stumvoll, M., Niess, A., Tschritter, O., Haap, M., Becker, R. et al. (2003) Reduced skeletal muscle oxygen uptake and reduced beta-cell function: two early abnormalities in normal glucose-tolerant offspring of patients with type 2 diabetes. *Diabetes Care* 26: 2126–32.

Thomas, E.L., Frost, G., Taylor-Robinson, S.D. and Bell, J.D. (2012) Excess body fat in obese and normal-weight subjects. *Nutrition Research Reviews* 25: 150–61.

Tielemans, S.M., Soedamah-Muthu, S.S., De Neve, M., Toeller, M., Chaturvedi, N., Fuller, J.H. and Stamatakis, E. (2013) Association of physical activity with all-cause mortality and incident and prevalent cardiovascular disease among patients with type 1 diabetes: the EURODIAB Prospective Complications Study. *Diabetologia* 56: 82–91.

Tikkanen-Dolenc, H., Wadén, J., Forsblom, C., Harjutsalo, V., Thorn, L.M., Saraheimo, M. et al. and FinnDiane Study Group. (2017) Physical activity reduces risk of premature mortality in patients with type 1 diabetes with and without kidney disease. *Diabetes Care* 40: 1727–32.

Tikkanen-Dolenc, H., Wadén, J., Forsblom, C., Harjutsalo, V., Thorn, L.M., Saraheimo, M. et al. and FinnDiane Study Group. (2020) Frequent physical activity is associated with reduced risk of severe diabetic retinopathy in type 1 diabetes. *Acta Diabetologica* 57: 527–34.

Tuomi, T., Santoro, N., Caprio, S., Cai, M., Weng, J. and Groop, L. (2014). The many faces of diabetes: a disease with increasing heterogeneity. *The Lancet* 383: 1084–94.

Tuomilehto, J., Lindström, J., Eriksson, J.G., Valle, T.T., Hämäläinen, H., Ilanne-Parikka, P. et al. (2001) Prevention of type 2 diabetes mellitus by changes in lifestyle among subjects with impaired glucose tolerance. *New England Journal of Medicine* 344: 1343–50.

Umpierre, D., Ribeiro, P.A., Kramer, C.K., Leitão, C.B., Zucatti, A.T., Azevedo, M.J. et al. (2011) Physical activity advice only or structured exercise training and association with HbA1c levels in type 2 diabetes: a systematic review and meta-analysis. *Journal of the American Medical Association* 305: 1790–9.

Valabhji, J., Barron, E., Bradley, D., Bakhai, C., Fagg, J., O'Neill, S. et al. (2020) Early outcomes from the English National Health Service Diabetes Prevention Programme. *Diabetes Care* 43: 152–60.

Wadén, J., Tikkanen, H.K., Forsblom, C., Harjutsalo, V., Thorn, L.M., Saraheimo, M. et al. and FinnDiane Study Group. (2015). Leisure-time physical activity and development and progression of diabetic nephropathy in type 1 diabetes: the FinnDiane Study. *Diabetologia* 58: 929–36.

Wang, Y., Rimm, E.B., Stampfer, M.J., Willett, W.C. and Hu, F.B. (2005) Comparison of abdominal adiposity and overall obesity in predicting risk of type 2 diabetes among men. *American Journal of Clinical Nutrition* 81: 555–63.

Wei, M., Gibbons, L.W., Mitchell, T.L., Kampert, J.B., Lee, C.D. and Blair, S.N. (1999) The association between cardiorespiratory fitness and impaired fasting glucose and type 2 diabetes mellitus in men. *Annals of Internal Medicine* 130: 89–96.

Wisløff, U., Najjar, S.M., Ellingsen, O., Haram, P.M., Swoap, S., Al Share, Q. et al. (2005) Cardiovascular risk factors emerge after artificial selection for low aerobic capacity. *Science* 307: 418–20.

World Health Organization. (2006) Definition and diagnosis of diabetes mellitus and intermediate hyperglycaemia [online], available at: https://www.who.int/diabetes/publications/diagnosis_diabetes2006/en/ (accessed 25 October 2020).

World Health Organization. (2011) Use of glycated haemoglobin (HbA1c) in the diagnosis of diabetes mellitus [online], available at: https://www.who.int/diabetes/publications/diagnosis_diabetes2011/en/ (accessed 25 October 2020).

Wu, N., Bredin, S.S.D., Guan, Y., Dickinson, K., Kim, D.D., Chua, Z. et al. (2019) Cardiovascular health benefits of exercise training in persons living with type 1 diabetes: a systematic review and meta-analysis. *Journal of Clinical Medicine* 8: 253. doi: 10.3390/jcm8020253.

6 Obesity

James A. King

▌ INTRODUCTION

Obesity is a highly emotive and contentious topic that receives significant attention in newspaper headlines and the wider popular press on almost a daily basis. In recent years, increasing resources have been directed to help understand both the fundamental principles governing body weight regulation and practical strategies to help individuals manage their body weight. Unfortunately, despite this investment and significant advancement in knowledge it has brought, levels of obesity remain high across the globe and continue to increase in many nations (Non-Communicable Disease Risk Factor Collaboration 2016). This relative lack in progress is rooted in the complex aetiology of obesity which is influenced by genetic, metabolic, psychological, environmental and sociocultural variables that are inextricably intertwined.

Most fundamentally, obesity develops when individuals sustain a positive energy balance for a prolonged period; i.e. when daily energy intake consistently exceeds energy expenditure. With the recognition that exercise increases energy expenditure, it would seem quite logical to expect that the instruction to 'move more' would be an effective therapy for weight management. Unfortunately, this interpretation is a little oversimplified as it does not consider: 1) whether an individual is able to regularly perform enough exercise to meaningfully influence energy balance; 2) whether the act of performing exercise elicits compensatory behavioural or metabolic responses that may constrain the energy deficit produced. This issue is complicated further by the growing recognition that a significant degree of individual variability exists in relation to these factors which is a key consideration when working with individuals. Fortunately, over the last three decades, collaborative research efforts between experts within the biomedical and behavioural sciences have improved our understanding of these issues; and this knowledge has helped to refine lifestyle recommendations for the management of obesity and related chronic diseases.

In this chapter we examine a variety of topics relating to obesity, including the definition of obesity, how obesity develops and its prevalence and health risks. After this, the two major issues explored within this chapter are:

1   evidence that sedentary behaviour and physical inactivity contributes to the development of obesity;
2   the role of exercise as a therapeutic intervention for those with obesity.

The final section of this chapter examines contemporary physical activity recommendations for weight control. This chapter will not address the topic of childhood obesity which is covered in Chapter 11. By the end of this chapter the reader should appreciate that obesity is a complex condition which remains a global problem despite the high levels of attention it receives from scientists, governments and policy makers.

DEFINITION

The World Health Organization (WHO) defines overweight and obesity as an abnormal or excessive fat accumulation that presents a risk to health (World Health Organization, 2016). The most frequently used method for assessing obesity is the body mass index (BMI). This is calculated by dividing weight in kilograms by height (in metres) squared. Table 6.1 shows the BMI cut-points used to classify individuals as underweight, normal weight, overweight and obese. These boundaries were originally defined by the WHO to reflect the J- or U-shaped relationship which has been identified between BMI and mortality (World Health Organization, 1998). Given the inability to distinguish between fat and fat-free mass, it is often stated that the BMI provides a simple way to assess obesity levels at a population scale but has limitations on a personal basis. This issue is only problematic, however, for a small segment of the population who may be heavily muscular. Moreover, evidence suggests that the BMI is as good as any other measurement of adiposity in classifying disease risk (Taylor et al. 2010) whilst some evidence also indicates that the combination of BMI and waist circumference improve disease risk prediction (Emerging Risk Factor Collaboration 2011). For an in-depth discussion of techniques used to assess body composition the interested reader is referred to Gatterer and colleagues (2017).

Table 6.1 Classification of overweight and obesity by BMI, waist circumference and associated disease risks

	BMI (KG M^{-2})	OBESITY CLASS	DISEASE RISK* RELATIVE TO NORMAL WEIGHT AND WAIST CIRCUMFERENCE	
			MEN 102 CM (40 IN) OR LESS / WOMEN 88 CM (35 IN OR LESS)	MEN > 102 CM (40 IN) / WOMEN > 88 CM (35 IN)
Underweight	< 18.5		–	–
Normal+	18.5–24.9		–	–
Overweight	25.0–29.9		Increased	High
Obesity	30.0–34.9	I	High	Very high
	35.0–39.9	II	Very high	Very high
Extreme obesity	40 +	III	EXTREMELY HIGH	EXTREMELY HIGH

* Disease risk for type 2 diabetes, hypertension and CVD; increased waist circumference also can be a marker for enhanced risk, even in persons of normal weight.

Source: National Heart, Lung, and Blood Institute; National Institutes of Health; U.S. Department of Health and Human Services.

One issue to consider when using the BMI is that traditional BMI classifications may not be appropriate for all individuals. Asian populations represent one example of this whereby BMI thresholds of ≥ 23 kg m^{-2} and ≥ 25 kg m^{-2} are now recommended as criteria of overweight and obesity, respectively (Misra 2015). These population specific thresholds have been defined given the earlier presentation of cardio-metabolic risk factors in South Asian populations (Gray et al. 2011; Tillin et al. 2015).

PREVALENCE

One of the reasons why the field of obesity attracts so much attention is because its prevalence is high in many areas of the world. The inception of what has frequently been described as an 'obesity epidemic' by many is thought to have begun in the latter half of the twentieth century – with a relatively rapid increase in prevalence occurring across many continents in subsequent decades (Imes and Burke 2014). It is relevant to note that some of the most recent data available has indicated that levels of obesity may be starting to plateau in some high-income nations whilst levels have risen dramatically in many low-income nations.

When looking back over the last 40 years, the most comprehensive data available suggests that population levels of obesity have increased markedly across large sections of the world during this time (Non-Communicable Disease Risk Factor Collaboration 2016. In the Non-Communicable Disease Risk Factor Collaboration's recent global analysis, which pooled data from 186 nations (covering 99% of the world's population), it was estimated that the age-standardised mean BMI increased between 1975 and 2014 from 21.7 to 24.2 kg m^{-2} and 22.1 to 24.4 kg m^{-2} in men and women, respectively. This corresponds to a 1.5 kg per decade increase in average body weight. In actual terms, the number of individuals with obesity (BMI $\geq$ 30 kg m^{-2}) worldwide increased from 34 million men and 71 million women in 1975, to 266 million and 375 million in 2014. Notably, in 2014, 21.8% and 33.6% of obese men and women were classified as being severely obese (defined as BMI $\geq$ 35 kg m^{-2} in this analysis[1]) which is thought to confer an especially high disease burden. In these global data, it is important to recognise the marked geographical variation in both the current obesity prevalence and trends over time. For example, in men, the mean population BMI in 2014 ranged from 21.4 kg m^{-2} in Central Africa to 29.2 in South Asia and Micronesia. In women, the lowest mean BMI was seen in South Asia (21.8 kg m^{-2}) and the highest in Polynesia and Micronesia (32.2 kg m^{-2}). For men, the steepest increase in mean BMI in the observation period occurred in high-income English-speaking nations, whilst for women, the most marked increase has been witnessed in Central Latin America. Table 6.2 details the top ten nations which currently have the highest levels of obesity and

Table 6.2 Countries with the largest population percentage of obesity and morbid obesity globally in 2014.

OBESITY

Rank	Men		Women	
1	Nauru	59.9	American Samoa	65.3
2	American Samoa	58.8	Nauru	64.8
3	Cook Islands	54.0	Cook Islands	60.9
4	Palau	53.1	Palau	60.5
5	Marshall Islands	49.8	Marshall Islands	59.0
6	French Polynesia	48.9	Tuvalu	57.9
7	Tuvalu	48.5	French Polynesia	56.9
8	Niue	46.2	Niue	56.8
9	Kiribati	42.9	Samoa	56.6
10	Tonga	42.7	Tonga	56.1

SEVERE OBESITY

Rank	Men		Women	
1	Nauru	14.1	Nauru	19.9
2	American Samoa	13.9	American Samoa	18.7
3	Cook Islands	10.8	Cook Islands	16.6
4	Palau	9.5	Samoa	14.5
5	French Polynesia	9.1	Palau	14.3
6	Marshall Islands	8.7	French Polynesia	14.1
7	Tuvalu	8.6	Marshall Islands	13.8
8	Tokelau	8.1	Tuvalu	13.7
9	Micronesia (FS)	8.0	Micronesia	13.3
10	Niue	7.6	Niue	13.3

Source: Non-Communicable Disease Risk Factor Collaboration (n.d.).
Notes: Obesity defined as BMI $\geq$ 30 kg m^{-2} and morbid obesity as BMI $\geq$ 40 kg m^{-2}. For reference, the percentage of men and women in the UK with obesity is 27.9 and 29.7%; whilst the prevalence of morbid obesity is 2.1 and 4.7%.

morbid obesity worldwide. It is notable that this list is dominated by Pacific Island nations where it has been suggested that modernisation and urbanisation have facilitated population overconsumption (Hawley and McGarvey 2015).

In recent years, some commentators have described obesity as a 'pandemic' (Meldrum et al. 2017), which refers to a disease that affects a wide proportion of individuals over a large geographical area. Although it is possible that trends in total levels of obesity may be flattening out in some high-income nations, it is important to recognise that obesity prevalence remains high and the proportion of those who are severely obese (BMI $\geq$ 40 kg m^{-2}) may actually be increasing (Kral et al. 2012). The next section examines how various levels of overweight and obesity are likely to impact on the health of individuals.

HEALTH RISKS

One of the main reasons why the issue of obesity receives so much attention is because of the adverse health consequences arising from excess adiposity. This is of concern to individuals and governments as the health consequences of obesity have many direct (health care) and indirect (productivity, social, economic) costs.

Although most people would probably think that being overweight or obese is detrimental to health, and may affect life expectancy, this issue has been debated intensely within recent years. In 2013, Flegal and colleagues famously published a systematic review of evidence reporting hazard ratios (HR) between BMI classifications and all-cause mortality in adults. These analyses included data from 97 prospective cohort studies that collectively provided information on more than 2.88 million individuals. The authors somewhat controversially concluded that possessing a BMI in the overweight range (25–29.9 kg m^{-2}) was associated with a lower risk of mortality as compared with a BMI in the 'healthy' range (18.5–24.9 kg m^{-2}). Furthermore, class one obesity (BMI 30–34.9 kg m^{-2}) was reported to confer no additional mortality risk than a healthy BMI. Instead, an augmented mortality risk only became visible with a BMI $\geq$ 35 kg m^{-2}. Since the publication of this research, others have challenged the validity of the findings based on methodological grounds. Most prominently, 'reverse causation' is one crucial issue that may have been overlooked (Willet et al. 2013). In observational research, reverse causality is a term which refers to a direction of cause and effect that is contrary to a common presumption. In the present context, it is likely that the inclusion of sick, elderly and current or past smokers (which are each associated with lower body weight) may have inflated the mortality risk in the healthy body weight range; therefore, masking the adverse impact of overweight and obesity.

More recent studies have accounted for the issue of reverse causality by excluding data collected during the first five years of follow-up as well as that from smokers and individuals with morbidity (Global BMI Mortality Collaboration 2016). In what is currently the largest analysis to date, including data from 189 prospective studies across the world (3.95 million individuals), the Global BMI Mortality Collaboration (2016) identified a heightened risk of mortality in both the lower and upper range of overweight (Figure 6.1). Furthermore, mortality risk increased progressively throughout classes of obesity. These findings therefore suggest that the health risks associated

Figure 6.1 The association between BMI and all-cause mortality.

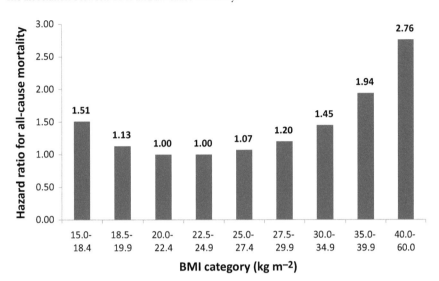

Source: Global BMI Mortality Collaboration (2016).
Notes: This figure includes data from a pooled analysis of 189 cohorts; 3,951,455 participants (never smokers, without chronic disease at baseline); 385,879 deaths. The reference group is BMI 22.5–24.9 kg m^{-2}. All analyses were adjusted for age and sex and excluded the first five years of follow-up.

with excess adiposity begin in the overweight range and progress in step-wise fashion as BMI increases.

The findings from another high-profile study lend further support to the notion that the health risks associated with an elevated BMI begin in the overweight range (Kivimäki et al. 2017). Specifically, Kivimäki and colleagues (2017) examined the link between BMI and risk of developing cardio-metabolic multi-morbidity which was defined as diagnoses of more than one of the following: coronary heart disease, stroke and type 2 diabetes. This outcome is particularly important given that the risk of premature death is greater when multiple cardio-metabolic conditions are present simultaneously (Emerging Risk Factor Collaboration 2015). In this analysis of 16 cohort studies (120,813 adults, mean follow-up of 10.7 years), compared to a healthy BMI, the odds ratio of developing cardio-metabolic multi-morbidity was 2.0 for an overweight BMI (25–29.9 kg m^{-2}), 4.5 for class one obesity (BMI 30–34.9 kg m^{-2}) and 14.5 for a BMI $\geq$ 35 kg m^{-2}. The balance of evidence appears to suggest that the mortality risk associated with an elevated BMI begins in the overweight range and progresses across the BMI spectrum. This knowledge has important implications for health care where reducing excess adiposity is likely to provide therapeutic benefit for anyone with a BMI in the overweight or obese range.

The evidence discussed in this section prompts the question about how an elevated BMI, or excess adiposity, provokes premature mortality. In this regard, the Global Burden of Disease Collaboration (2017) identified 20 health conditions where robust evidence suggests an association with BMI (Table 6.3). Within these analyses the

Table 6.3 20 health conditions where convincing evidence suggests an association with high BMI.

CANCERS

Oesophageal
Colon and rectal
Liver
Gallbladder and biliary tract
Pancreatic
Breast cancer (post-menopause)
Breast cancer (pre-menopause)
Uterine
Ovarian
Kidney
Thyroid
Leukaemia

CARDIOVASCULAR AND CARDIOMETABOLIC DISEASES

Ischaemic heart disease
Ischaemic stroke
Haemorrhage stroke
Hypertensive heart disease
Diabetes mellitus
Chronic kidney disease

MUSCULOSKELETAL CONDITIONS

Osteoarthritis
Low back pain

Source: Global Burden of Disease Collaborators (2017).
Note: For all conditions, a dose–response relationship is apparent with a high BMI and the link is biologically plausible.

strongest association was found for type 2 diabetes which is a long-term condition whose pathophysiology is intricately linked to obesity (see Chapter 5 for discussion of the aetiology of this disease).

The specific mechanisms through which excess adiposity leads to adverse health outcomes have been reviewed recently in an excellent review in the *New England Journal of Medicine* (Heymsfield and Wadden 2017). The metabolic and anatomical pathways linking excess adiposity and cardio-metabolic disease can be seen in Figure 6.2. The development of a chronic inflammatory state and dyslipidaemia are key players within the adverse metabolic profile seen in individuals with obesity (Gregor and Hotamisligil 2011; Schulman 2014). These derangements promote insulin resistance which is a primary defect within the pathophysiology of cardiovascular disease and type 2 diabetes (see Chapters 4 and 5, respectively).

Figure 6.2 Pathways through which excess adiposity leads to major risk factors and chronic health conditions.

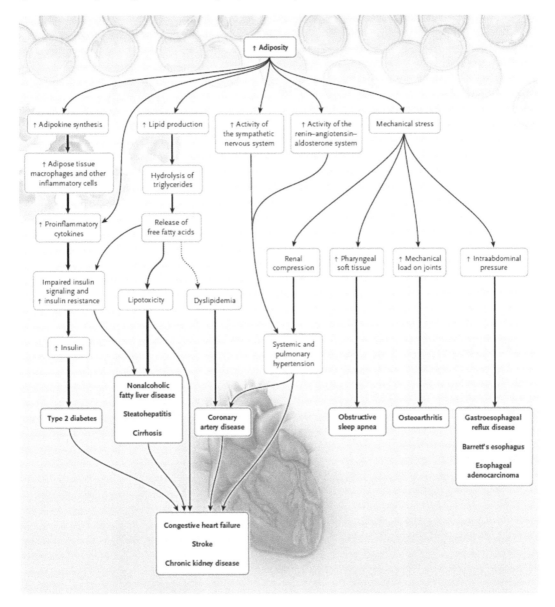

When talking about adipose tissue and its link to health, it is important to recognise that the influence of adiposity is dependent on both the quantity of fat present and the storage location. Specifically, when an individual has a healthy amount of body fat, the majority is typically stored in subcutaneous regions, e.g. around the hips, thighs and upper arms. Fat in these peripheral areas is essential for good health as it facilitates 'safe triglyceride storage' and metabolic homeostasis. Indeed, animal studies have shown that the absence of this essential fat is associated with the same metabolic problems seen in obesity (Gavrilova et al. 2000). In contrast, during the progression to overweight and obesity, an increasing amount of adipose tissue is stored in central regions which is associated with poor cardio-metabolic health. This is because fat stored in ectopic regions interferes with the normal metabolic function of affected tissues; principally via insulin resistance and chronic low-grade inflammation (Fabbrini et al. 2009; Schulman 2014). The most important areas where ectopic fat is commonly located include the abdominal cavity (visceral fat), liver, heart and pancreas.

The variable nature of adipose tissue distribution can be visualised with reference to Figure 6.3 which contains images of four magnetic resonance imaging (MRI) scans of men who differ with regards to their BMI and the proportion of intra-abdominal versus subcutaneous adipose tissue. It is important to note that individuals with these phenotypes have very different metabolic health profiles and future morbidity and

Figure 6.3 MRI images of men classified according to their adipose tissue distribution: (a) lean control (BMI 25.5 kg m^{-2}, IAAT = 1.0 L; (b) TOFI BMI 25.8 kg m^{-2}, IAAT = 4.6 L; (c) obese control BMI 36.9 kg m^{-2}, IAAT = 5.6 L; (d) MHO BMI 36.4 kg m^{-2}, IAAT = 0.9 L.

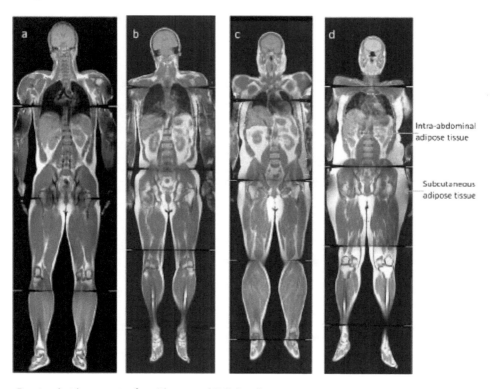

Source: Reprinted with permission from Thomas and Bell (2014).
Notes: IAAT = intra-abdominal adipose tissue; MHO = metabolically healthy obesity; TOFI = thin on the outside, fat on the inside.

mortality risk. Indeed, at any given BMI, individuals with a greater proportion of central fat possess the poorest health outcomes. Within Figure 6.3, image 'b' shows the body fat distribution profile for an individual with a relatively healthy BMI (albeit just in the overweight range) but a large proportion of fat stored centrally. Such profiles have been described as 'thin-on-the-outside-fat-on-the-inside'. Despite their relatively healthy BMI, this individual is more likely to experience poorer metabolic health outcomes than their counterpart in image 'a' who has a similar BMI but little central fat. The same principle also applies to the individuals depicted in images 'c' and 'd.' Notably, the profile shown in image 'd' is often described as 'metabolically healthy obesity' given the preponderance of peripheral fat. Evidence has shown that this body fat profile is protective against common metabolic health problems in obesity (see Stefan et al. 2018 for an excellent review of this topic). The phenomenon of metabolically healthy obesity is a widely debated issue and may have implications for health-care resource prioritisation. It is important to note, however, that only 10–34% of obese individuals are classed as metabolically healthy (Muñoz-Garach et al. 2016). Moreover, longitudinal data suggests that in such individuals the appearance of obesity-related health problems may be delayed, rather than prevented entirely (Hamer et al. 2015).

The importance of adipose tissue distribution also helps explain differing obesity-related metabolic health risks between the sexes and ethnicities. Specifically, men typically possess more adiposity in the upper body whereas women store a greater proportion of fat in the lower body. These are often referred to android and gynoid obesity, respectively (Vague 1956). Similarly, as described at the beginning of this chapter, the adverse health effects of obesity are more severe in individuals with South Asian heritage than in white Europeans. A reduced capacity to store adipose tissue subcutaneously, resulting in lipid 'spillover', is thought to contribute to this effect in South Asians (Sniderman et al. 2007).

AETIOLOGY

The concept of energy balance is fundamental to any discussion about the causes of obesity. In particular, it is crucial to appreciate that human physiology complies with the first law of thermodynamics, which states that energy can be transformed from one form to another but cannot be created or destroyed (Hall et al. 2012). In essence, human energy balance is determined by the matching between chemical energy entering the body via food and drink versus thermal and kinetic energy expended through metabolism and movement. This concept is often abbreviated in the following equation:

Energy intake (food and drink) = energy expenditure (resting metabolic rate, diet-induced thermogenesis, physical activity) ± energy stored (fat, protein and carbohydrate) (Box 6.1 details common methods used to assess energy intake and energy expenditure).

On this basis, body weight will remain stable when energy intake and energy expenditure are equal. Conversely, body weight will deviate if there is a mismatch between these components over a prolonged period. The time element is important in this scenario because on a day-to-day basis there are likely to be large variations between energy intake and energy expenditure (Champagne et al. 2013). Over many weeks,

---

BOX 6.1 COMMON TECHNIQUES USED TO ASSESS ENERGY INTAKE AND COMPONENTS OF ENERGY EXPENDITURE.

ENERGY INTAKE

	Weighed food record	Individuals weigh and record all food and energy containing beverages consumed over a period of three to seven days. The burden imposed on participants (to record) and researchers (to analyse) often limits the use of this method to studies with small sample sizes.
	Food frequency questionnaire	Habitual consumption of foods and drinks are assessed by an individual self-reporting their usual consumption. This technique is often used in studies with large samples.
	24-hour recall	Used to obtain a snapshot of an individual's habitual food intake. Often used in studies with large samples.

ENERGY EXPENDITURE

Resting metabolic rate	Breath-by-breath gas analysis, ventilated hood, whole-room calorimeter	When rested, in a supine position, and in the post-absorptive state, collections of expired air are made over 30 minutes to measure oxygen uptake and carbon dioxide production (indirect calorimetry). The first 10 mins of measurements are often discarded to eliminate any habituation artefact.
Diet-induced thermogenesis	Breath-by-breath gas analysis, ventilated hood, whole-room calorimeter	The increase in energy expenditure following food consumption is ascertained from postprandial measurements of expired air. Indirect calorimetry is used to measure energy expenditure before and after (several hours) the consumption of a standardised meal. The elevation in metabolism is quantified by contrasting measurements made either before and after a meal or, on separate days, with and without meal consumption.
Physical activity energy expenditure	Self-report	Metabolic equivalents can be applied to self-reported activity data to provide an estimation of physical activity energy expenditure. Knowledge about the type of activity, its duration and frequency are needed to permit these calculations (see https://sites.google.com/site/compendiumofphysicalactivities/home).
	Breath-by-breath expired air analysis	In controlled laboratory settings, expired air can be sampled from stationary or portable metabolic carts which directly measure energy expenditure via indirect calorimetry.
	Accelerometery	Free-living energy expenditure can be measured objectively using movement sensors that are worn by individuals for several days. Proprietary algorithms are used to derive energy expenditure estimates from acceleration data.

however, this variability evens out in individuals who are not experiencing chronic positive or negative energy balance. Another consideration important to appreciate is that energy balance can be established with variable levels of energy intake, energy expenditure and adiposity. This concept can be seen clearly with reference to Figure 6.4, which shows the contribution of factors to daily energy intake and energy expenditure

Figure 6.4 Influence of activity status and BMI on factors contributing to daily energy intake and energy expenditure in a female example.

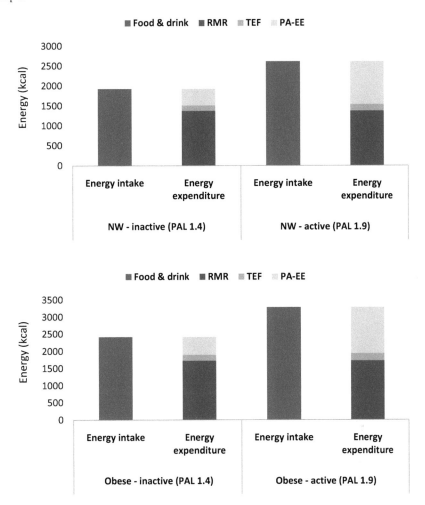

Notes: Top panel – values calculated for 35-year-old women with a BMI of 22.5 kg m^{-2}. Bottom panel – values calculated for 35-year-old women with a BMI of 34.6 kg m^{-2}. NW = normal weight; TEF = thermic effect of feeding; PA-EE = physical activity energy expenditure; RMR = resting metabolic rate; PAL = physical activity level.

in 35-year-old women whose physical activity and BMI have been manipulated. The important point to note in these examples is that energy intake and energy expenditure are balanced despite the higher energy intake requirement provoked by an active lifestyle and a larger body tissue mass.

Alongside energy balance, another important relationship to appreciate is that between macronutrient balance and body composition. Herein, body composition will remain constant when the rate of macronutrient intake is equal to the rate of macronutrient expenditure (carbohydrate, fat, protein, alcohol). Conversely, changes in body composition will occur if macronutrient balance is not achieved, even if energy balance is maintained. As explained later in this chapter, the capacity for exercise to increase fat oxidation can therefore induce negative fat balance and lead to reduced body fat, even if total body weight remains constant.

Figure 6.4 shows the relative contribution of discrete factors to daily energy intake and energy expenditure. A discussion about the multitude of factors which influence appetite and energy intake is beyond the scope of this chapter; instead, the interested reader is referred to Blundell and colleagues (2015). One notable development in this area, however, is the recognition that a strong association exists between an individual's resting metabolic rate (RMR) and their daily energy intake (Hopkins et al. 2016). An individual's RMR is the rate at which the body expends energy when at complete rest and represents the sum of each tissue's basic energetic requirements. Given that fat-free mass, or lean mass, is the primary determinant of RMR, these data suggest that lean mass drives daily energy needs. At present, however, the mechanisms linking lean mass and eating behaviour are poorly understood.

As well as influencing energy intake, RMR is also a key determinant of daily energy expenditure. In fact, in non-athletes, RMR typically accounts for 60–80% of total energy expenditure each day. As alluded to above, RMR is related to body size but is also influenced by our age and sex. Within this, it is important to appreciate that the contribution of each bodily tissue to RMR is not equal. Indeed, despite representing ~2% of total body mass, the high metabolic activity of the liver and brain means that each contribute ~20% to RMR (Wang et al. 2011). This contrasts with skeletal muscle which typically comprises one-third of body mass and ~20% of RMR. On this basis it should be recognised that RMR can be altered by changes in the quantity or metabolic activity of bodily tissue. The potential for physical activity to influence RMR is discussed later in this chapter; however, at this point it is important to comment on the role of RMR in the aetiology of obesity.

It is sometimes assumed that obesity results from a low RMR. Given that RMR contributes significantly to total daily energy expenditure, this question has received much attention. Cross-sectional studies have repeatedly shown that RMR is higher in obese individuals owing to their greater lean mass (James et al. 1978; Ravussin et al. 1982; Schutz et al. 1984). Consequently, low RMR is not responsible for sustaining obesity once it has developed. The trickier question to answer is whether a low RMR is responsible for the initial development of obesity. Longitudinal studies are needed to answer this question whereby RMR is measured over several years so that comparisons can be made between those who do and do not gain weight. Unfortunately, although several of these studies have been completed, the findings have been mixed, with some studies confirming a predictive role of RMR in weight gain (Buscemi et al. 2005; Ravussin et al. 1988; Roberts et al. 1988) and others refuting the suggestion (Katzmarzyk et al. 2000; Seidell et al. 1992). Differences in the populations examined and methodological details likely explain these discrepant outcomes, and further research is needed to provide more clarity.

The two other components of daily energy expenditure are diet-induced thermogenesis and physical activity energy expenditure. Diet-induced thermogenesis represents the energy expended in the act of digesting and processing food and energy containing drinks. Humans have no voluntary control over this parameter which is principally determined by the amount of energy consumed at each meal and its nutrient composition

(Westerterp 2004). Diet-induced thermogenesis contributes only 10–15% of daily energy expenditure, and under normal circumstances, differences between people are not thought to contribute to the development of obesity.

Movement, or physical activity, is the most variable component of daily energy expenditure which can vary from zero (e.g. bed rest) to several thousand kilocalories (e.g. endurance cycling or artic trekking). This component of daily energy expenditure encompasses all forms of muscle contraction, including standing, ambulation and low-, moderate- and high-intensity physical activity (Levine 2003). For many years, academics have debated intensely whether obesity is a problem that relates most predominantly to a lack of movement (sedentary behaviour and physical inactivity) or an excessive energy intake (Blair et al. 2013; Luke and Cooper 2013; Prentice and Jebb 1995). This debate has famously been referred to as 'gluttony' verses 'sloth' and the interested reader is referred to an excellent review article on this topic (Millward 2013).

Proponents supporting the view that recent trends in obesity are predominantly due to diet often cite data suggesting that population levels of physical activity have not changed, or may have even increased, during the years when obesity levels have been rising (Luke and Cooper 2013; Swinburn et al. 2009). Population-level data have also been used to argue that increased food consumption explains changes in BMI. For example, across the 1970s and 2000s, Swinburn and colleagues (2009) contrasted US food supply and population body weight data and concluded that an increase in estimated energy intake during these years was more than enough to explain documented weight changes in adults and children. Furthermore, Luke and Cooper (2013) support their view about the dominant influence of diet by citing cross-sectional studies which show that total daily energy expenditure is no different between traditional 'hunter-gatherer' and rural populations (who have active lifestyles) as compared with those in high-income nations (Luke et al. 2009; Pontzer et al. 2012). These latter findings are noteworthy given that the highly accurate doubly labelled water technique was used to measure free-living energy expenditure in these studies (see Box 2.4).

In contrast, Stephen Blair has argued that a lack of movement has been central to population-wide obesity in recent decades. In fact, he has directly criticised several assumptions inherent within the aforementioned data relating to diet (Blair 2015). Specifically, based on analyses conducted by his group, he has argued that conclusions based on population dietary intake data are invalid due to widespread inaccuracy in energy intake reporting (Archer, Hand and Blair 2013). Furthermore, he has suggested that changes in occupational activity, rather than leisure time, are more relevant to the present discussion. Indeed, using US population data over 50 years, Church and colleagues reported that declining occupational energy expenditure accurately predicted changes in body weight over the same period (Church et al. 2011). Similar decrements in energy expenditure within the household, and for transportation, have supported this contention (Archer, Lavie, McDonald et al. 2013).

The perspectives outlined above provide a dichotomous viewpoint about the fundamental causes of obesity; however, most things in life are rarely clear-cut and it is most likely that the global obesity pandemic has developed due to a combination of increasing energy consumption and reduced energy expenditure (Hall 2018). The specific role of sedentary behaviour and physical inactivity as risk factors for obesity are examined later in this chapter. At this point, however, it is important to highlight factors which have influenced energy intake in recent decades.

Before discussing this issue, it is relevant to note that humans have the capacity to influence 100% of their daily energy intake through their eating behaviour. Conversely, our capacity to modulate energy expenditure is much smaller given that movement typically contributes just 20–25% of daily energy output. Thus, through our eating behaviour, we have the ability significantly to modulate energy balance each day. However, behaviour is often shaped by factors within our environment and this is problematic when our environment appears to facilitate overconsumption (Swinburn et al. 2011).

In this regard, some of the most important factors that have been highlighted include the widespread availability of foods dense in energy, fat, sugar and salt that have been designed to taste good and have been marketed aggressively to the public (Harris et al. 2009; Johnson and Wardle 2014). Furthermore, unrestricted access to these foods may have adversely influenced normative eating behaviours, e.g. larger portion sizes and snacking in between meals (Hall 2018; Livingstone and Pourshahidi 2014). Within contemporary 'Western diets', fat may be especially problematic because its energy density is more than twice that of protein and carbohydrate (9 vs 4 kcal g^{-1}). Furthermore, fat is less satiating and provokes a smaller influence on postprandial energy expenditure than the other macronutrients. Increased consumption of carbohydrate, particularly refined carbohydrates and added sugars, have also been flagged as contributors to rising levels of obesity. Simple sugars foster passive overconsumption but may also contribute by altering the endocrine regulation of adipose tissue. This has been termed the 'carbohydrate-insulin model of obesity' and the interested reader is referred to Hall (2017) for a comprehensive discussion about this model. A complete discussion about the interaction between the food environment and obesity is beyond the scope of this chapter but those who are interested may like to read a series of excellent articles in this area that were commissioned by the American Society for Nutrition and the Obesity Society (for all citations see Mattes and Foster 2014).

One of the greatest problems with obesity is that once it has developed it is incredibly difficult for individuals to lose a clinically relevant amount of weight; and even more so, to maintain the weight loss in the long term (Mann et al. 2007; Ochner et al. 2015). This statement is supported by the findings from several intervention studies (Anderson et al. 2001; Wadden 1993) and one recent population-based cohort study in the UK (Fildes et al. 2015). Using the electronic health records of 278,982 adults over a period of nine years, the latter investigation showed that the annual probability of attaining a normal weight was incredibly low (1 in 210 men; 1 in 124 women) for individuals with obesity (BMI 30–34.9 kg m^{-2}) and even less likely for individuals with morbid obesity (1 in 1,290 men; 1 in 1,677 women). The explanation for this phenomenon is rooted in the fundamental importance of energy balance and nutrient supply for humans; and the complex regulatory systems that have evolved to ensure their viability (Greenway 2015). Consequently, any deliberate attempt to induce a negative energy balance is met by several compensatory responses that seek to attenuate the energy deficit and maintain body weight. This concept is referred to as adaptive thermogenesis and it affects both the energy intake (appetite, food cravings; Figure 6.5) (Rosenbaum et al. 2008; Sumithran et al. 2011) and energy expenditure (RMR,

Figure 6.5 Meal-related appetite responses measured before and after 13.5 kg of weight loss; and subsequently following 12 months of weight maintenance.

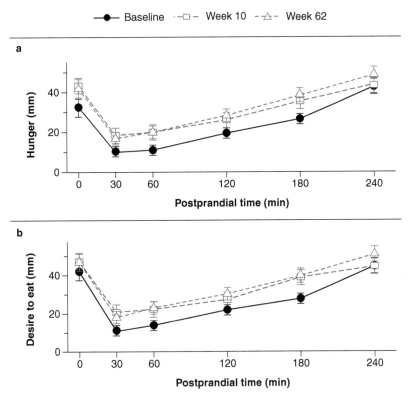

Source: From the *New England Journal of Medicine*, Sumithran, P. et al., 'Long-term persistence of hormonal adaptations to weight loss', 365: 1597–604. Copyright © 2011 Massachusetts Medical Society. Reprinted with permission from Massachusetts Medical Society.

diet-induced thermogenesis, spontaneous physical activity, mechanical movement efficiency) (Leibel et al. 1995; Nelson et al. 1992; Rosenbaum et al. 2003; Weyer et al. 2000) side of the energy balance equation. Some excellent reviews have been written about this topic (Dullo et al. 2012; MacLean et al. 2015).

GENETIC CONTRIBUTION

In the previous section the important contribution of lifestyle to obesity was highlighted; however, it is becoming clearer that a prominent genetic component influences the risk of developing an obese phenotype (Albuquerque et al. 2015). Hereditary factors may therefore have an important role in determining an individual's level of susceptibility or resistance to 'obesogenic environments'.

A genetic contribution to body weight control was originally defined in twin and family studies. Two of the most famous investigations in this area are the twin and adoption studies led by the late Albert Stunkard (Stunkard, Fich and Hrubec 1986; Stunkard, Sorensen, Hanis et al. 1986). In one investigation, high concordance rates among monozygotic (identical) twins for height, weight and BMI were identified, both at 20 years old (intra-pair r = 0.91, 0.85 and 0.81, respectively) and after 25 years of follow-up (r = 0.88, 0.74 and 0.67 respectively) (Stunkard, Fich and Hrubec 1986). In a second study, the investigators compared the BMI of adult adoptees (n = 540) in a Danish cohort with that of their biological and adoptive parents (Stunkard, Sorensen, Hanis et al. 1986) (Figure 6.6). Importantly, 90% of adoptees had been placed in their adoptive homes within the first year of life, which limited the opportunity for early socialisation with biological parents. In this study, a clear relationship was seen between the BMI of the biological parents and adoptees, but not between adoptive parents and their adopted children. These data suggest that hereditary factors exerted a greater impact on the adiposity of the adopted children than social or environmental influences.

Further support for a genetic contribution to adiposity has been provided by rare cases of extreme obesity that develop early on in childhood and are typically linked to endocrine disorders (Farooqi and O'Rahilly 2006; Ramachandrappa and Farooqi 2011). These examples are referred to as monogenic forms of obesity given that these phenotypes are related to a defect in a single gene. The most well-characterised monogenic cases are those relating to the leptin-melanocortin signalling pathway in the hypothalamus which causes extreme hyperphagia (overeating) and severe obesity (Dubern and Clement 2012).

Rare single gene defects cannot, however, explain the high prevalence of obesity in society. Instead, the genetic contribution to adiposity is likely to be related to the

Figure 6.6 The association between the BMI of adopted children and that of their biological parents (left panel) and their adoptive parents (right panel).

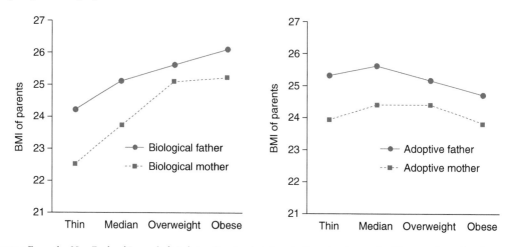

Source: From the *New England Journal of Medicine*, Stunkard, A.J. et al., 'An adoption study of human obesity', 314: 193–8. Copyright © 1986 Massachusetts Medical Society. Reprinted with permission from Massachusetts Medical Society.
Notes: The BMI of the adopted children is strongly associated with that of their biological parents, but shows no association with that of their adoptive parents, indicating a strong genetic effect.

simultaneous presence of many subtle gene variations (polygenic obesity) that cluster in some people. Recent advances in biotechnology have provided scientists with more powerful tools to identify the location of common gene variants that are associated with obesity-related traits. In a recent analysis, 97 BMI-associated loci were identified which account for 2.7% of variation in BMI (Locke et al. 2015). This information has been used to develop equations that can predict obesity risk based on an individual's genotype (Wang et al. 2017, 2018). To date, the three most robustly associated single gene variants for BMI within populations of European ancestry are those found within the *FTO* (fat-mass and obesity associated) gene and in proximity to the *TMEM18* (transmembrane protein 18) and *MC4R* (melanocortin-4 receptor) genes (Waalen 2014). Of all obesity susceptibility gene loci identified, variations in *FTO* have the largest effect on obesity-related traits (weight, BMI, body fat). Moreover, *FTO* variants are common in populations of European ancestry with 43% and 20% of Europeans possessing either one or two obesity susceptibility alleles, respectively (Abecasis et al. 2012). Notably, the possession of each allele is additively associated with a 0.39 kg m^{-2} increase in BMI or 1.2-fold increased risk of obesity (Speliotes et al. 2010). Recent data suggests that this effect of *FTO* is related to alterations in the homeostatic and hedonic (conferring pleasure) control of eating (Karra et al. 2013) (Figure 6.7).

As alluded to above, the combination of all identified obesity risk alleles explains <3% of the heredity contribution to BMI. Thus, a significant gap exists between ex-plained genetic variance and known variance identified in twin and family studies. A lot therefore remains to be learnt about the contribution of hereditary to obesity. The study of epigenetics (lifestyle-related alterations in gene expression) is one important and potentially fruitful area of investigation that is likely to provide greater clarity in this area within the next decade (Cordero et al. 2015). One fact that has become clear is

Figure 6.7 Ratings of perceived hunger (left) and plasma concentrations of acylated ghrelin (hunger-stimulating hormone) before and after the consumption of a test meal in individuals with an AA (grey) and TT (blue) FTO genotype. Attenuated postprandial responses in AA's indicate weaker satiety responsiveness.

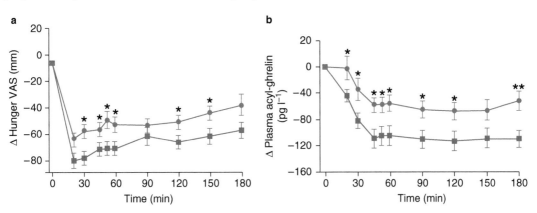

Source: Republished with permission of the American Society for Clinical Investigation, from 'A link between FTO, ghrelin, and impaired brain food-cue responsivity', Karra, E. et al., 123, copyright © 2013; permission conveyed through Copyright Clearance Center, Inc.

that an individual's environment can potently influence their hereditary risk of obesity. This issue has recently been demonstrated in two large observational studies which examined changes in participants' BMI over 20 years of follow-up (Wang et al. 2017, 2018). In these studies, the maintenance of a physically active lifestyle, or the consumption of a high-quality diet, were found to attenuate weight gain in those with a genetic predisposition (based on genetic risk scores). Collectively, these findings show that the maintenance of a healthy lifestyle can help mitigate against the risk of obesity in those who are genetically susceptible.

PHYSICAL INACTIVITY AS A RISK FACTOR

The role of physical inactivity in the pathogenesis of obesity has been debated widely for many years because of the important contribution of movement to daily energy expenditure. More recently, changing patterns of work and leisure have generated great curiosity about this issue which has been amplified by a contemporary focus on sedentary behaviour (sitting time) as an independent risk factor for chronic metabolic disease (Biswas et al. 2015; Henson et al. 2016). Usefully, this interest in habitual, or non-structured physical activity, has catalysed the development of objective monitoring devices (accelerometers and inclinometers) that permit improved assessment of daily sedentary time and physical activity. These new tools help overcome the issue of self-reporting physical activity and enable us to define the relationship between movement, weight gain and obesity more precisely. In this section we will examine evidence from a variety of observational sources relating to sedentary behaviour, physical activity and the risk of obesity.

An increasing number of studies have sought to examine the relationship between sedentary time and measures of obesity (e.g. BMI, waist circumference, body fat). In a cross-sectional analysis, a positive association was found between sitting time (assessed by questionnaire) and BMI in a population of 15,000 men and women across Europe (Martinez-Gonzalez et al. 1999). Individuals who spent more than 35 hours per week of their leisure time sitting down had a 61% higher risk of obesity (BMI > 30 kg m^{-2}) than with those who sat for less than 15 hours. This finding has been replicated in more recent studies that have utilised accelerometers to measure sedentary time. For instance, a positive association was identified between sedentary time and several obesity markers (body weight, fat mass, body fat percentage) in a group of 231 UK adults with parental history of type 2 diabetes (Golubic et al. 2015). These relationships were independent of moderate-to-vigorous physical activity (MVPA) and it was identified that every additional 1.5 hour per day of sedentary time was associated with a 1.5 kg higher body weight. Further support for a role of sedentary time as a risk factor for obesity has been provided by studies which have shown that breaks in sitting time (assessed by accelerometer) were negatively associated with waist circumference (Healy et al. 2011) (Figure 6.8) and BMI (Healy et al. 2015), independent of MVPA. In contrast to these findings, other studies have found no relationship between sedentary time and obesity-related traits, either when assessed by questionnaire (Pulsford et al. 2013) or more objectively (Van Dyck et al. 2015). These mixed findings show that at present the relationship between sedentary behaviour and obesity risk is not entirely clear. One

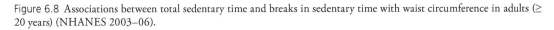

Figure 6.8 Associations between total sedentary time and breaks in sedentary time with waist circumference in adults (≥ 20 years) (NHANES 2003–06).

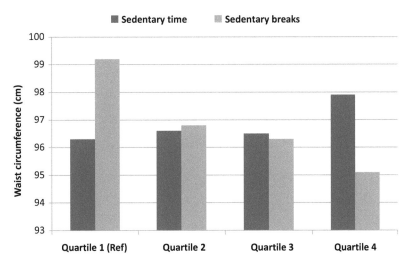

Source: Healy et al. (2011).
Notes: Quartile cut-points corrected for wear time are 7.24, 8.51, 9.57 h day^{-1} for total sedentary time; 470, 559, 645 for breaks in sedentary time (moving from < 100 counts per minute to ≥ 100 counts per min). $P = 0.049$ and < 0.001 for trends across quartiles for total sedentary time and breaks in sedentary time.

issue which makes the interpretation even more difficult is that of 'bi-directionality' – where the possibility exists that it is weight gain and obesity driving increasing sedentary time, rather than vice versa (Golubic et al. 2015).

In contrast to sedentary behaviour, the relationship between physical activity and obesity risk is more consistent, demonstrating that lower levels of physical activity are associated with an elevated risk of obesity. This outcome has been reported in cross-sectional studies that have assessed physical activity using questionnaires (Besson et al. 2009; Lahti-Koski et al. 2002; Martinez-Gonzalez et al. 1999) and accelerometers (Van Dyck et al. 2015). In the latter study, habitual physical activity data were collected in a sample of 5,712 adults across ten countries and the results showed that BMI and obesity risk decreased linearly as MVPA increased from zero minutes per day to 150 minutes per day. After this point, greater amounts of MVPA had no further benefit. These findings provide convincing evidence that physical activity is associated with lower BMI and obesity prevalence; however, as these data are cross-sectional they provide no information on the direction of association between variables and cannot be used to infer causality. Further insight into the relationship between physical activity and obesity risk has been sought through longitudinal studies with multiple assessment points over time.

Hankinson and colleagues (2010) examined the influence of changes in physical activity on BMI and waist circumference over a period of 20 years (1985/86 to 2005/06) in a sample of American adults (n = 3,554) who were aged between 18 and 30 years at baseline. In this study, participants' physical activity scores were divided into tertiles at inception and the researchers examined movement between categories during follow-up. Over time, the results showed that men and women who consistently remained in the most active tertiles had smaller gains in BMI and waist circumference than those in the lowest activity tertile (Figure 6.9). These findings are consistent with those from another investigation which pooled data from three prospective cohort studies to yield 1,570,808 person-years of follow-up (Mozaffarian et al. 2011). In this study, the authors assessed weight change and lifestyle behaviours at four-year intervals and divided individuals into quintiles based on participants' change in physical activity over time. Compared with the worst quintile who decreased their activity levels by

Figure 6.9 Average annual changes in BMI and waist circumference for young adults (18 to 30 years at baseline) by long-term activity tertiles.

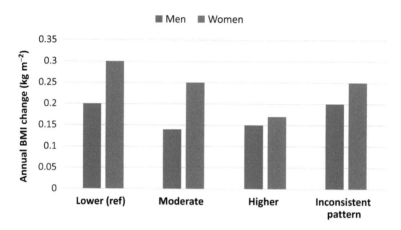

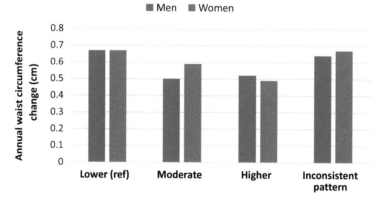

Source: Hankinson et al. (2010).

Notes: Individuals designated to lower, moderate or higher physical activity categories were required to hold that sex-specific tertile classification for two-thirds of assessments during 20 years of follow-up. The lower activity tertile is the reference group in this analysis.

For reference: lower activity, less than 340 exercise units (men) and 192 (women); moderate activity, 340 to 607 exercise units (men) and 192 to 397 (women); higher activity, at least 608 exercise units (men) and 398 exercise units (women); inconsistent patterns, all other activity patterns. Note that 300 exercise units equates to meeting generic health-oriented physical activity guidelines (150 minutes of MVPA).

16.3 MET-h week^{-1}, the quintile who increased activity levels the most (23.2 MET-h week^{-1}) maintained their body weight 0.8 kg lower across each interval. In another study, Hamer and colleagues (2013) examined the influence of meeting the UK physical activity guidelines (150 mins of MVPA or 75 mins vigorous physical activity) on BMI and waist circumference during an 11-year period of follow-up in the Whitehall II study (4,880 participants). Dose–response relationships were identified between the consistency in meeting the guidelines and changes in BMI and waist circumference. More recently, these findings have been reinforced by a study that measured physical activity at two time points (one and seven years) after baseline assessments using accelerometers (Golubic et al. 2015). In this study, MVPA was negatively associated with body weight and adiposity. In effect, undertaking an extra 16 minutes of MVPA per day was associated with a 0.5 and 1.4 kg lower body weight after a one- and seven-year follow-up, respectively. The authors of this research suggest that the strengthening of these associations over the seven years of observation may be related to physically active individuals being more health conscious and adopting overall healthier lifestyles.

Within the aforementioned study, an important observation to recognise is that the association between MVPA and obesity-related traits were three times stronger when MVPA was the outcome rather than the exposure variable. In a tangible sense, this means that body weight and/or adiposity may be influencing MVPA to a greater extent than MVPA influences body weight and/or adiposity. This finding is consistent with the recognition that the performance of physical activity becomes increasingly difficult as body weight is gained due to musculoskeletal and respiratory problems. These data highlight the bi-directionality in the relationship between physical activity and obesity; and underscore the inability of observational studies to determine causal influence.

Another consideration with observational research studies, such as those described above, is that they do not account for the interaction between different domains of physical activity. Specifically, in real life, changing the amount of time dedicated to one activity behaviour will directly impact on time allocation for another. For example, if an individual reduces their sedentary time by one hour per day, this inevitably means that they will have increased their daily light physical activity (LPA) or MVPA. Moreover, the therapeutic effect of activity reallocation will depend entirely on which activity behaviours are replaced and instilled. In recent years, academics have attempted to account for this by statistically modelling the effect of behaviour reallocation using a technique called iso-temporal substitution modelling (Mekary et al. 2009). This method simulates the expected outcome of long-term behaviour change using cross-sectional data. In relation to physical activity, this method has been used in a handful of studies to assess the anticipated effect of exchanging time spent in sedentary behaviour for light physical activity and MVPA (Bumen et al. 2014; Falconer et al. 2015; Hamer et al. 2014; Healy et al. 2015). The consensus from this body of work appears to show that favourable changes in adiposity-related traits occur when sedentary time is replaced by MVPA but not necessarily by standing or LPA. As an example, using data from the Whitehall II epidemiological cohort (445 healthy men and women), Hamer and colleagues (2014) modelled the effect of reallocating 10 minute blocks of sedentary time to either LPA or MVPA. The findings showed that BMI decreased by 0.39 kg m^{-2} for every 10 mins of sedentary time that was exchanged for MVPA. Conversely, replacing sedentary time with LPA had no impact on BMI. This evidence highlights the potential benefit to be gained from replacing sedentary behaviours with active pursuits; however, when considering this evidence, it is important to remember that energy balance is dynamic, and the effects of behavioural substitution may be oversimplified in these statistical models.

EXERCISE AS THERAPY

Many studies have examined the effectiveness of exercise, either alone or in combination with diet, as a therapy for overweight and obesity. In this area of investigation it is important to appreciate from the outset that obesity is a heterogeneous condition, and consequently the effectiveness of exercise is likely to differ depending on the severity of obesity along with the presence or absence of comorbidities and medications. Crucially, these factors will affect an individual's capacity to engage in exercise and therefore the prescription that is accomplishable.

Earlier in this chapter the concepts of energy and macronutrient balance were introduced. In summary, for body weight and body composition to remain stable, the intake of energy and individual macronutrients must match their utilisation. Any mismatch between these variables will induce changes to body weight and/or composition. This knowledge provides a platform to discuss the therapeutic effects of exercise for weight management. To provide a thorough understanding of this issue, this section will separately discuss the effects of single and repeated (training) bouts of exercise on energy balance and body weight.

Acute effect of exercise

All forms of bodily movement are fuelled by the breakdown of adenosine triphosphate (ATP) which provides an immediate source of energy to fuel skeletal muscle contraction. The ability to sustain exercise is dependent on the capacity to continually replenish ATP through a combination of aerobic and anaerobic metabolic pathways. The oxidation of carbohydrate and fat are central to this process which means that single bouts of exercise have the capacity to modulate both energy and substrate balance.

The amount of energy expended during an acute bout of exercise is a product of the rate of energy expenditure and the duration of exercise. The exercise modality and intensity are the primary determinants of the rate at which energy is expended (an individual's movement efficiency has a lesser influence). Within this, forms of exercise that recruit a large muscle mass (e.g. rowing) and/or are weight bearing (e.g. running), will elicit a greater amount of energy expenditure than those that use a small muscle mass (e.g. arm ergometry) and/or are weight supported (e.g. cycling). With reference to the present discussion, this means that heavier individuals will expend more energy than lighter individuals when performing the same weight-bearing activity. This concept is demonstrated in Figure 6.10, which shows how body weight and exercise intensity combine to influence energy expenditure during walking. With regards to running, it is relevant to note that a linear relationship exists between running speed and oxygen uptake. Therefore, the energy expended to cover a certain distance is approximately

Figure 6.10 Impact of walking speed and body mass on the rate of energy expenditure.

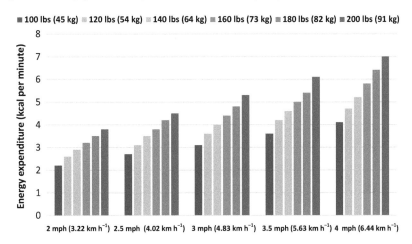

Source: Passmore and Durnin (1955).

the same regardless of the speed at which it is completed. In effect, running faster will simply mean that the distance is completed more quickly. As a rule of thumb, the energy expenditure of running can be estimated as: one kilocalorie per kilogram (of body weight) per kilometre (distance covered). Thus, a 75 kg individual would expend approximately 750 kcal running 10 kilometres. To cover the same distance, an individual weighing 100 kg would expend an additional 250 kcal.

In addition to influencing the rate of energy expenditure, exercise intensity also modulates the pathways used to replenish ATP and therefore the mix of substrate oxidised. During exercise, the oxidation of protein contributes only a small amount to energy production. A blend of carbohydrate and fat therefore provide the predominant substrate for ATP regeneration. Because fat can only be oxidised through aerobic metabolism, whereas carbohydrate can be oxidised aerobically or anaerobically, the relative contribution of fat and carbohydrate to energy provision vary depending on the intensity of exercise (Figure 6.11).

After the transition from rest to low-intensity exercise, an increase in adipose tissue blood flow and adipocyte lipolysis (stimulated by the sympathetic nervous system and adrenaline) augment circulating levels of non-esterified fatty acids (NEFA) which facilitate an increase in fat oxidation within skeletal muscle. As intensity progresses, the percentage of fat oxidised increases to a maximum which occurs at around 64% of maximum oxygen uptake (Achten et al. 2002). This point is sometimes referred to as the 'fat max' (Jeukendrup and Achten 2001). After this point, as intensity increases further, a reduced availability of oxygen and redistribution of blood to skeletal muscle reduce the contribution of fat to energy metabolism. Instead, the contribution of carbohydrate increases.

The duration of exercise, training status of the individual and diet will all influence substrate metabolism during exercise. Specifically, during steady-state exercise,

Figure 6.11 Percentage contribution of substrates to total energy expenditure during cycling at low, moderate and high intensity.

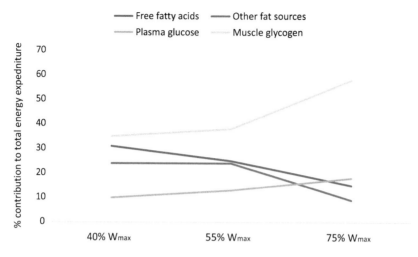

Source: Van Loon et al. (2001).
Notes: Data derived from eight male cyclists. W_{max}, maximal workload.

the relative contribution of fat to energy metabolism will increase as the limited stores of carbohydrate in the liver (60–120 g) and skeletal muscle (200–500 g) are depleted (Flatt 1995). Trained individuals will also be able to rely more on the plentiful supplies of fat during exercise, and therefore spare the more limited supplies of carbohydrate. Metabolic adaptations within skeletal muscle are central to this shift, including increases in mitochondria, capillaries and oxidative enzymes. Finally, an individual's recent dietary intake and their habitual diet consumption will influence the substrate oxidised during exercise. Most importantly, glucose and insulin supress adipose tissue lipolysis and skeletal muscle fat oxidation. The consumption of food or energy containing drinks, before or during exercise, therefore suppresses fat oxidation. More chronically, research has shown that a habitual diet that is high in fat can augment fat oxidation; however, studies of the impact of this adaption on exercise performance have produced mixed results (see Achten and Jeukendrup 2004 for a thorough review of this issue).

The impact of exercise on substrate metabolism has relevance to macronutrient balance and body composition. At first glance, the aforementioned knowledge suggests that exercise at a low to moderate intensity is the optimum prescription for the purpose of fat loss and body weight control. However, in this context it is important to consider the relative vs absolute contribution of substrate to energy metabolism. Specially, although the relative contribution of fat (percentage) predominates at low exercise intensities, the absolute amount of fat oxidised (grams) will be small when low-intensity exercise is performed. Thus, increasing the intensity of exercise, and the overall rate of energy expenditure, will increase the amount of fat oxidised. On top of this, we also need to consider what happens over the period after exercise. In particular, after a bout of hard exercise that predominantly relies on carbohydrate as substrate, if this is not replenished and stores remain depleted, the energy deficit will subsequently be met through an increase in fat metabolism. Consequently, for the purpose of weight loss, a focus on the overall energy expended during exercise may be more relevant than the contribution of individual macronutrients.

In addition to the energy expended during exercise, researchers have also investigated whether a single bout of exercise affects resting metabolic rate, and therefore energy expenditure, in the hours afterwards. This issue is often referred to as excess post-exercise oxygen consumption (EPOC) (Gaesser and Brooks 1984) and is thought to reflect a heightened rate of metabolism elicited during the post-exercise recovery process. The impact of exercise on EPOC has been studied over several decades and a mixture of findings have been reported (see Børsheim and Bahr 2003 for overview). In some instances, considerable increases in EPOC have been identified within several hours after exercise. For example, LaForgia and colleagues (1997) reported an EPOC of 15 L (~75 kcal) within several hours after 20 minutes of interval training. Additionally, others have found metabolic rate to be elevated on the morning after exercise (~5%, Melby et al. 1993). In contrast, others have reported no effect, or very minor responses (Kelly et al. 2013). Discrepancies in findings are likely related to methodological differences between studies, including the methods used to assess metabolic rate/oxygen consumption and standardisation of confounding factors (e.g. room temperature, time of day, food intake). On balance, however, although exercise of higher intensity and longer duration is more likely to influence EPOC, consensus suggests that typical bouts of exercise that most people are able to complete are unlikely to raise post-exercise energy expenditure substantially.

As mentioned previously, energy intake is wholly determined by an individual's eating behaviour. Consequently, humans possess the capacity to drastically perturb daily energy balance by varying the consumption of food and energy containing drinks. Recognition of this fact has promoted researchers to investigate whether exercise influences appetite and energy intake. The importance of this question is emphasised when considering that even a subtle change in appetite and food intake has the potential to exert a far greater effect on energy balance than is elicited by a single bout of exercise.

Initial research within this area sought to investigate the strength of the relationship between exercise-related energy expenditure, appetite control and energy intake in the short-term. That is, researchers wanted to know whether performing exercise automatically led to increases in appetite and energy intake in order to replace the energy expended during physical exertion. Such a tight coupling has been shown to occur when an energy deficit is induced via food restriction (Hubert et al. 1998; King et al. 2011). In stark contrast, a large body of research has shown that single bouts of exercise do not increase appetite or energy intake (Stensel 2010). This lack of response has been replicated in many different populations, with different modalities of exercise, and holds true even when the energy expenditure induced by exercise is large (King et al. 2010). In fact, research has actually demonstrated that moderate- to high-intensity exercise suppresses appetite. However, this response is typically brief and does not influence subsequent eating behaviour (Schubert et al. 2013). Taken collectively, individual bouts of exercise are able to induce a relative energy deficit which may contribute to weight management (Deighton and Stensel 2014). In relation to this issue, it is important to be aware that the assessment of eating behaviour in controlled laboratory settings may not provide the most ecologically valid data. Furthermore, a generic limitation of many studies in this field is that assessments have commonly been limited to the day of exercise. Such trials are not able to identify subtle changes in eating behaviour that may occur over a longer period of time, which may contribute to the re-establishment of energy balance.

Chronic effect of exercise (training) on body weight and composition

One of the most important conclusions to have emerged from the evidence base in relation to exercise and weight management is the recognition that performing an amount of exercise consistent with standard physical activity and health guidelines (Haskell et al. 2007; Department of Health 2011) will produce moderate weight loss at best (< 3 kg) (Donnelly et al. 2009; Swift et al. 2014). As an example, Richardson et al. (2008) performed a meta-analysis of nine pedometer-based walking interventions in overweight and obese adults (mean duration 16 weeks) and found a pooled weight loss of 1.27 kg. This notion is also supported by the findings from several chronic exercise intervention studies which collectively showed that weight loss was ≤ 2.2 kg in all instances (Church et al. 2007, 2010; Kraus et al. 2002; Sigal et al. 2007). Importantly, these findings are recognised as being robust given that: each study included large samples of individuals with overweight and obesity; had supervised exercise training sessions with strong adherence; and made comparisons with control groups (Swift et al. 2014).

Additional studies have sought to determine whether greater amounts of exercise are able to facilitate clinically relevant (typically defined as ≥ 5%) weight loss in individuals with overweight and obesity. Donnelly et al. (2013) sought to address this issue using a large sample (n = 141) of overweight and obese men and women. In this study, researchers randomised participants to a ten-month intervention of control or supervised aerobic exercise training requiring an energy expenditure of 400 or 600 kcal per training session (five days per week). Participants experienced a weight loss of 3.9 kg (4.3%) and 5.2 kg (5.7%) in the 400 kcal and 600 kcal groups, respectively. This response was consistent between men and women and was composed almost entirely of body fat loss (Figure 6.12). Other studies have shown that substantial amounts of weight can be lost through exercise training without dietary modification if the exercise regimen is of sufficient volume and participants are adherent to the exercise prescription. As an example, Ross et al. (2000) observed a 7.5 kg (8%) weight loss in a sample of men with obesity who undertook exercise every day (700 kcal energy expenditure) for 12 weeks. A response of similar magnitude was also found in a sample of women in an identical study protocol (Ross et al. 2004). These findings support the efficacy of exercise in weight management; however, it must be appreciated that these studies were rigorously controlled and included motivated participants and research staff. Most notably, many people may not be able to perform such high volumes of exercise on a daily basis and one must therefore be cautious about extrapolating these findings to real-world settings.

Another important finding to emerge from the research evidence is that weight loss responses seem to be most related to the exercise volume and energy expenditure rather

Figure 6.12 Changes in body weight and fat mass in male and female participants in the Midwest Exercise 2 study.

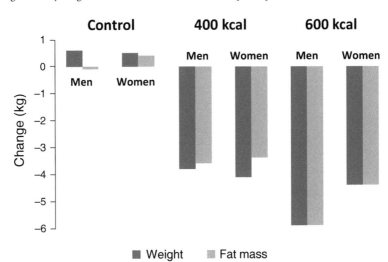

Source: Donnelly et al. (2013).
Note: 400 and 600 kcal refers to the amount of energy expended during each exercise training session (five days per week, ten months) in each study group

than to the exercise intensity or modality (Donnelly et al. 2009; Ross et al. 2000, 2015). This explains why weight loss is typically negligible with resistance training interventions as the energy expenditure elicited by intermittent bouts of this type of activity is low (Fenkci et al. 2006; Schmitz et al. 2007). The final section of this chapter examines the specific volume and energy expenditure required to elicit weight loss through exercise training and will therefore not be discussed any further at this point. An important issue to recognise, however, is that as greater amounts of exercise are undertaken it becomes more likely that compensatory behavioural (e.g. dietary choices, spontaneous activity, exercise adherence) and metabolic responses (RMR, exercise efficiency) will occur that will attenuate the energy deficit and weight loss induced by exercise (King et al. 2007). Furthermore, the extent to which these responses occur may vary considerably between individuals. For example, in one study involving 35 men and women with overweight or obesity, 12 weeks of supervised aerobic exercise training reduced body mass by 3.7 kg; however, responses ranged from −14.7 to +1.7 kg (King et al. 2008). Further scrutiny of these data showed that those who lost less body weight than expected experienced increased appetite and energy intake after the intervention, whilst RMR tended to decline. These findings highlight the need to be aware of dietary changes during physical activity interventions and to recognise that not all individuals will respond in the same way.

From a compensatory perspective, the influence of physical activity on movement outside of formal activity sessions is another issue that has received attention in recent years. The advent of technologies capable of measuring sitting time, physical activity and energy expenditure in free-living environments have facilitated this research which has been reviewed recently (Melanson 2017). To date, based on short-term studies lasting up to 16 days, there is little evidence that structured physical activity reduces free-living activity. Conversely, data from longer studies which have used doubly labelled water to measure total daily energy expenditure have suggested that physical activity compensation may occur, especially in populations of older adults. It should be recognised, however, that this conclusion assumes that the fact that total energy expenditure does not increase in line with greater amounts of physical activity is due solely to declining movement outside of formal activity sessions. This assumption may not be correct. Indeed, it has recently been hypothesised that total daily energy expenditure may be a regulated variable and that, during periods of high physical activity, energy may be reallocated away from other energetically expensive processes, e.g. growth, repair and reproductive function (Pontzer 2015). This developing hypothesis has key implications for the role of physical activity in weight management as it suggests that simply doing more may not automatically increase total energy expenditure.

It is generally accepted that to maximise weight loss, reductions in energy intake are needed. The optimal dietary approach for weight loss is beyond the scope of this chapter, but it is of interest to note that a meta-analysis by Johnston and colleagues (2014), including 59 studies with 7,286 participants, found that low-fat and low-carbohydrate diets were equally effective for weight loss at 12 months. A key question is whether the addition of exercise on top of dietary restriction elicits further benefits. The available guidance for those seeking to lose weight commonly identifies exercise as an accompaniment to a reduced energy diet (Raynor and Champagne 2016; National Institute for Health and Care Excellence 2014) and this prompts the question whether exercise training can facilitate weight loss alongside dietary induced energy deficits.

Schwingshackl and colleagues (2014) tackled this question directly through a network meta-analysis of studies which had directly compared interventions of diet versus diet plus exercise training lasting longer than 12 months. This comprehensive analysis identified a benefit of adding exercise to a dietary regimen; however, the effect was small (1.38 kg). Furthermore, a detailed review of the evidence on behalf of the American College of Sports Medicine (ACSM) has concluded that the addition of exercise to an energy restricted diet will enhance weight loss only if the degree of energy restriction is modest, but not severe (Donnelly et al. 2009). This evidence should be considered by practitioners when tailoring weight loss interventions to individuals.

The primary outcome discussed in this section has been body weight; however, this focus ignores the distinct influence of exercise on body fat and fat-free mass. The separate effects of exercise on these individual tissues are important given that it is excess adiposity that is ultimately responsible for the higher cardio-metabolic risk experienced by individuals with obesity. Furthermore, low fat-free mass is increasingly recognised as a risk factor for impaired metabolic health and poor functional capacity, especially in older adults.

The ability of exercise training to modify body fat stems from its capacity to influence both energy and fat balance. With particular regard to fat balance, research has shown that in the absence of an energy deficit and weight loss, exercise training interventions can reduce adiposity (Lee et al. 2005; Ross et al. 2000, 2004). As one example, Lee and colleagues (2005) used MRI to compare changes in total and regional body fat between three groups, i.e. lean men, obese men and obese men with type 2 diabetes, after 13 weeks of supervised exercise training (60 mins per session, five times per week at 60% of $\dot{V}O_2$ peak). Reductions in total and abdominal body fat were observed in each group (Figure 6.13). Notably, the relative change in abdominal fat was much greater than the relative change in total adiposity. This probably reflects the proportionally smaller central fat depot, and/or the greater sensitivity of visceral fat to beta-adrenergic stimulatory effects during exercise (Arner et al. 1990). The greater capacity of the trained skeletal muscle to enhance fat oxidation during exercise, and also possibly at rest, underpins these changes in fat balance (Thompson et al. 2012).

Figure 6.13 Absolute (top panel) and relative (bottom panel) changes in total and abdominal body fat following 13 weeks of supervised exercise training in lean men and in obese men with or without type 2 diabetes.

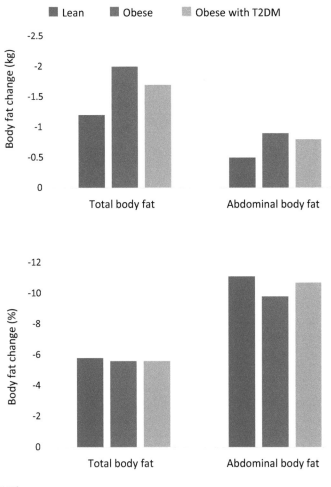

Source: Lee et al. (2005).

As alluded to already within this section, exercise training typically induces a negative energy balance which results in a certain degree of weight loss. In both men and women, research has shown that when substantial weight loss (6.5–8%) is induced exclusively by exercise, the loss of body fat is greater than when an equivalent energy deficit is induced by dietary energy restriction alone (Ross et al. 2000, 2004). It is important to appreciate, however, that this difference in fat loss is small, and may only be detectable when using the most sensitive body composition measurement techniques (whole body MRI was used in these studies). Additionally, in more typical scenarios where exercise is added to dietary energy restriction, fat loss is very similar when the total energy deficit is the same (Larson-Mayer et al. 2010; Villareal et al. 2017). In these situations, it is likely that the greater contribution of diet to the energy deficit overrides the influence of exercise.

One consistent finding within the research literature is that including exercise within weight loss regimens helps to attenuate the loss of fat-free mass which occurs during sustained periods of negative energy balance (Villareal et al. 2011; Weiss et al. 2017). This effect is particularly relevant to individuals with obesity who also possess low muscle mass, a condition which has been termed 'sarcopenic obesity'. This condition is more common in older adults and is linked to insulin resistance and chronic low-grade inflammation (Cleasby et al. 2016). In response to a 12-month weight loss intervention (9–10% body weight loss) in older adults with obesity, it was shown that the reduction of fat-free mass was halved (–1.7 vs 3.5 kg) when an exercise programme consisting of aerobic and resistance training was added to dietary energy restriction. Recent research by the same group has shown that this effect is principally mediated by the resistance exercise component of the intervention (Villareal et al. 2017). These findings are supported by others which show that exercise training can also protect against the loss of bone mineral density during weight loss interventions (Villareal et al. 2006) and show that a combination of exercise and diet is needed to optimise changes in body composition during weight-reduction interventions.

Despite the evidence presented in this section, a common problem in weight management is that few people can maintain their weight loss after successful interventions. As previously mentioned, this problem occurs because the body robustly defends against negative energy balance and weight loss. This issue has prompted the suggestion that individuals who have lost significant amounts of weight should be treated as having 'obesity in remission' (Ochner et al. 2015).

Observational evidence has shown that greater amounts of exercise are associated with better weight-loss maintenance (Catenacci et al. 2008, 2011; Thomas et al. 2014) and these data are supported by the results from experimental trials (Swift et al. 2014). For instance, Jeffery and colleagues (2003) investigated whether the prescription of higher levels of physical activity than normally recommended in weight loss studies (i.e. energy expenditure > 1000 kcal week^{-1}) would improve long-term weight loss. In this study, 202 men and women were randomised to one of two behavioural therapy interventions which included weekly energy expenditure targets of 1000 or 2500 kcal week^{-1}. At six months, both interventions reduced body weight substantially (8–9%); however, greater weight loss was sustained over the course of an additional 12 months in those with the greater exercise energy expenditure (6.7 vs 4.1 kg). These findings suggest that high volumes of exercise can facilitate weight-loss maintenance.

Unfortunately, in this study it is impossible to tease apart the effect of exercise and other lifestyle changes that formed part of the behavioural therapy programme, particularly dietary changes. Furthermore, this study did not directly address the question of weight maintenance because participants were not randomised to exercise groups after weight loss occurred. The initial weight loss induced by the interventions will have influenced weight changes over the course of the whole study.

The importance of exercise volume for weight loss maintenance has been highlighted in another study which randomised 191 women with overweight or obesity to one of four, 24-month-long exercise interventions, based on intensity (moderate vs vigorous) and duration (moderate, 1000 kcal week^{-1} vs high, 2000 kcal week^{-1}) (Jakicic et al. 2008). In this study, the interventions were equally effective at reducing weight at 6 months (–9.3% across all arms); however, 50% of lost weight was regained by 24 months. The most interesting findings from this trial came from a retrospective analysis of the data which examined how adherence to exercise influenced long-term weight change. The results showed that those completing more minutes of exercise each week, or expending greater amounts of energy, were more likely to maintain a higher proportion of weight loss. In fact, those undertaking more than 300 mins per week, or expending more than 2000 kcal week^{-1}, were able to maintain more than 10% of their weight loss at 24 months. In contrast, those performing <150 mins per week, or expending less than 1000 kcal week^{-1}, maintained less than 4% of their weight loss at 24 months. Again, these findings are limited by the failure to randomise participants after weight loss. The retrospective nature is also problematic as it is possible that those who performed more exercise were more motivated to also make dietary changes.

These limitations will be overcome in the ongoing MET POWeR study (clinical trial identifier NCT01664715) which has randomised overweight and obese men and women to one of four trial arms (control, 150, 225 and 300 minutes of exercise per week) lasting 12 months after diet-induced weight loss (≥5%) (Szabo et al. 2013). The findings from this study will be published shortly and will provide greater clarity about the amount of exercise necessary to prevent weight regain after successful weight loss.

PHYSICAL ACTIVITY RECOMMENDATIONS

From reading this chapter it should be clear that a substantial body of scientific evidence has been amassed in relation to the interaction between physical activity, energy balance and weight control. This information has been used by experts to develop evidence-based recommendations concerning the utilisation of exercise in weight management. Most specifically, practical guidelines have been produced outlining the type and amount of exercise needed to: (1) prevent weight gain; (2) induce weight loss; (3) prevent weight regain after successful weight loss. It is important to appreciate that these recommendations are based on careful consideration of the best scientific evidence available at the time of development and may evolve as new evidence emerges. Furthermore, by nature, generic guidelines assume a 'one-size-fits-all' approach when, in reality, large variation within individuals' weight-related responses to physical activity will exist (King et al. 2007). It is therefore essential to consider the individual when developing weight-management strategies.

The most widely recognised recommendations regarding physical activity and weight management are those endorsed by the ACSM (Donnelly et al. 2009). These guidelines suggest that 150 to 250 minutes of moderate-intensity physical activity per week is necessary to prevent weight gain. This amount of physical activity is equivalent to an energy expenditure of some 1200 to 2000 kcal week^{-1} or the completion of 20 miles' walking/running. Notably, however, it is suggested that this amount of physical activity is sufficient to induce only a modest amount of weight loss (2–3kg). Instead, >225 to 420 minutes of physical activity per week are recognised as necessary to induce a clinically relevant level of weight loss of 5 to 7.5 kg. Importantly, the ACSM state that current physical activity recommendations for general health (150 mins week^{-1}) are likely to produce minimal weight loss whereas a higher amount of physical activity (200–300 mins week^{-1}) may be necessary to prevent weigh regain after successful weight loss. It is important to note that despite conferring positive effects on lean mass, the ACSM state with confidence that resistance training is not an effective means of facilitating weight loss.

The ACSM recommendations have been supported in an updated review of the literature (Swift et al. 2014). Within this review the importance of exercise volume or total energy expenditure is emphasised, as opposed to concern over exercise intensity. The authors also reinforce the ACSM's view that meeting physical activity guidelines for general health and wellbeing are unlikely to have an important impact on body weight control.

SUMMARY

- Over the last 70 years, a pandemic of obesity has arisen which poses significant health and economic challenges for individuals and governments.
- Obesity results from positive energy balance, where energy consumed in food and drink surpasses that expended through basal metabolism, diet-induced thermogenesis and movement, over a sustained period.
- Obesity risk is a product of genetic and environmental influences which interact.
- The role of sedentary behaviour (sitting time) as a risk factor for obesity is not clear at present, with the possibility that weight gain may drive greater sedentary time.
- Convincing evidence shows that physical activity is inversely related to obesity and obesity-related traits.
- As a therapy, the ability of exercise to influence obesity is related to the accumulated effects of each individual bout on energy and substrate balance.
- Exercise training can provoke clinically relevant weight loss if a sufficiently large amount of energy is expended, and energy compensation does not occur.

STUDY TASKS

1 Explain the fundamental principles of human energy balance.
2 Discuss whether nature (genes) or nurture (environment) has the greater impact on obesity risk.
3 Outline the mechanisms through which excess adiposity leads to chronic disease.

4 Define 'metabolically healthy obesity' and discuss the potential implications for the provision of health-care resources.

5 Critically discuss the merits and pitfalls of exercise as an obesity-management therapy.

NOTE

1 The standard definition of morbid or severe obesity is 40 kg m^{-2}.

FURTHER READING

Albuquerque, D., Stice E, Rodríguez-López, R., Manco, L. and Nóbrega, C. (2015) Current review of genetics of human obesity: from molecular mechanisms to an evolutionary perspective. *Molecular Genetics and Genomics* 290: 1191–221.

Bluher, M. (2019) Obesity: global epidemiology and pathogenesis. *Nature Reviews Endocrinology* 15: 288–98.

Blundell, J.E., Gibbons, C., Caudwell, P., Finlayson, G. and Hopkins M. (2015) Appetite control and energy balance: impact of exercise. *Obesity Reviews*: 16(Suppl. 1): 67–76.

Chin, S.-H., Kahathuduwa, C.N. and Binks, M. (2016) Physical activity and obesity: what we know and what we need to know. *Obesity Reviews* 17: 1226–44.

Donnelly, J.E., Blair, S.N., Jakicic, J.M., Manore, M.M., Rankin, J.W. and Smith, B.K., American College of Sports Medicine (2009) American College of Sports Medicine position stand: appropriate physical activity intervention strategies for weight loss and prevention of weight regain. *Medicine and Science in Sports and Exercise* 41: 459–71.

Dullo, A.G., Jacquet, J., Montani, J.P. and Schutz, Y. (2012) Adaptive thermogenesis in human body weight regulation: more of a concept than a measurable entity? *Obesity Reviews* 13: 105–21.

Hall, K.D. and Guo, J. (2017) Obesity energetics: body weight regulation and the effects of diet composition. *Gastroenterology* 152: 1718–27.

Heymsfield, S.B. and Wadden, T.A. (2017) Mechanisms, pathophysiology, and management of obesity. *New England Journal of Medicine* 376: 254–66.

National Institute for Health and Care Excellence. (2014) Obesity: identification, assessment and management [online], available at: https://www.nice.org.uk/guidance/cg189.

Ross, R., Freeman, J.A. and Janssen, I. (2000) Exercise alone is an effective strategy for reducing obesity and related co-morbidities. *Exercise and Sport Science Reviews* 28: 165–70.

Stefan, N., Häring, H.U. and Schulze, M.B. (2018) Metabolically healthy obesity: the low-hanging fruit in obesity treatment? *The Lancet Diabetes and Endocrinology* 6: 249–58.

Swift, D.L., Johannsen, N.M., Lavie, C.J., Earnest, C.P. and Church, T.S. (2014) The role of exercise and physical activity in weight loss and maintenance. *Progress in Cardiovascular Diseases* 56: 441–7.

REFERENCES

Abecasis, G.R., Auton, A., Brooks, L.D., DePristo, M.A., Durbin, R.M., Handsaker, R.E. et al. (2012) An integrated map of genetic variation from 1,092 human genomes. *Nature* 491: 56–65.

Achten, J., Gleeson, M. and Jeukendrup, A.E. (2002) Determination of the exercise intensity that elicits maximal fat oxidation. *Medicine and Science in Sports and Exercise* 34: 92–7.

Achten, J. and Jeukendrup, A.E. (2004) Optimizing fat oxidation through exercise and diet. *Nutrition* 20: 716–27.

Albuquerque, D., Stice E, Rodríguez-López, R., Manco, L. and Nóbrega, C. (2015) Current review of genetics of human obesity: from molecular mechanisms to an evolutionary perspective. *Molecular Genetics and Genomics* 290: 1191–221.

Anderson, J.W., Konz, E.C., Frederich, R.C. and Wood, C.L. (2001) Long-term weight-loss maintenance: a meta-analysis of US studies. *American Journal of Clinical Nutrition* 74: 579–84.

Archer, E., Hand, G.A. and Blair, S.N. (2013) Validity of US nutritional surveillance: National Health and Nutrition Examination Survey caloric energy intake data, 1971–2010. *PLoS One* 8: e76632. doi: 10.1371/journal.pone.0076632.

Archer, E., Lavie, C.J., McDonald, S.M., Thomas, D.M., Hébert, J.R., Taverno Ross, S.E. et al. (2013) Maternal inactivity: 45-year trends in mothers' use of time. *Mayo Clinical Proceedings* 88: 1368–77.

Arner, P., Kriegholm, E., Engfeldt, P. and Bolinder, J. (1990) Adrenergic regulation of lipolysis in situ at rest and during exercise. *Journal of Clinical Investigation* 85: 893–8.

Besson, H., Ekelund, Luan, J., May, A.M., Sharp, S., Travier, N. et al. (2009) A cross-sectional analysis of physical activity and obesity in European participants of the EPIC-PANACEA study. *International Journal of Obesity* 33: 497–506.

Biswas, A., Oh, P.I., Faulkner, G.E., Bajaj, R.R., Silver, M.A., Mitchell, M.S. and Alter, D.A. (2015) Sedentary time and its association with risk for disease incidence, mortality, and hospitalization in adults: a systematic review and meta-analysis. *Annals of Internal Medicine* 162: 123–32.

Blair, S.N. (2015) Physical inactivity and obesity is not a myth: Dr Steven Blair comments on Dr Aseem Malhotra's editorial. *British Journal of Sports Medicine* 49: 968–9.

Blair, S.N., Archer, E. and Hand, G.A. (2013) Luke and Cooper are wrong: physical activity has a crucial role in weight management and determinants of obesity. *International Journal of Epidemiology* 42: 1836–8.

Blundell, J.E., Gibbons, C., Caudwell, P., Finlayson, G. and Hopkins M. (2015) Appetite control and energy balance: impact of exercise. *Obesity Reviews*: 16(Suppl. 1): 67–76.

Børsheim, E. and Bahr, R. (2003) Effect of exercise intensity, duration and mode on post-exercise oxygen consumption. *Sports Medicine* 33: 1037–60.

Bumen, M.P., Winkler, E.A., Kurka, J.M., Hekler, E.B., Baldwin, C.M., Owen, N. et al. (2014) Reallocating time to sleep, sedentary behaviours, or active behaviours: associations with cardiovascular disease risk biomarkers, NHANES 2005–2006. *American Journal of Epidemiology* 179: 323–34.

Buscemi, S., Verga, S., Caimi, G. and Cerasola, G. (2005) Low relative metabolic rate and body weight gain in adult Caucasian Italians. *International Journal of Obesity* 29: 287–91.

Catenacci, V.A., Grunwald, G.K., Ingebrigtsen, J.P., Jakicic, J.M., McDermott, M.D., Phelan, S., et al. (2011) Physical activity patterns using accelerometry in the National Weight Control Registry. *Obesity* 19: 1163–70.

Catenacci, V.A., Ogden, L.G., Stuht, J., Phelan, S., Wing, R.R., Hill, J.O. and Wyatt, H.R. (2008) Physical activity patterns in the National Weight Control Registry. *Obesity* 16: 153–61.

Champagne, C.M., Han, H., Bajpeyi, S., Rood, J., Johnson, W.D., Lammi-Keefe, C.J. et al. (2013) Day-to-day variation in food intake and energy expenditure in healthy women: the dietician II study. *Journal of the Academy of Nutrition and Dietetics* 113: 1532–8.

Church, T.S., Earnest, C.P., Skinner, J.S. and Blair, S.N. (2007) Effects of different doses of physical activity on cardiorespiratory fitness among sedentary, overweight or obese postmenopausal women with elevated blood pressure: a randomised controlled trial. *Journal of the American Medical Association* 297: 2081–91.

Church, T.S., Earnest, C.P., Thompson, A.M., Priest, E.L., Rodarte, R.Q., Saunders, T. et al. (2010) Exercise without weight loss does not reduce C-reactive protein: the INFLAME study. *Medicine and Science in Sports and Exercise* 42: 708–16.

Church, T.S., Thomas, D.M., Tudor-Locke, C., Katzmarzyk, P.T., Earnest, C.P., Rodarte, R.Q. et al. (2011) Trends over 5 decades in U.S. occupation-related physical activity and their associations with obesity. *PLoS One* 6: e19657. doi: 10.1371/journal.pone.0019657.

Cleasby, M.E., Jamieson, P.M. and Atherton, P.J. (2016) Insulin resistance and sarcopenia: mechanistic links between common co-morbidities. *Journal of Endocrinology* 229: 67–81.

Cordero, P., Li, J. and Oben, J.A. (2015) Epigenetics of obesity: beyond the genome sequence. *Current Opinion in Clinical Nutrition and Metabolic Care* 18: 361–6.

Deighton, K. and Stensel, D.J. (2014) Creating an acute energy deficit without stimulating compensatory increases in appetite: is there an optimal exercise protocol? *Proceedings of the Nutrition Society* 73: 352–8.

Department of Health (2011) Physical activity guidelines for adults (19–64 years) [online], available at: https://www.gov.uk/government/publications/uk-physical-activity-guidelines (accessed 21 July 2017).

Donnelly, J.E., Blair, S.N., Jakicic, J.M., Manore, M.M., Rankin, J.W. and Smith, B.K., American College of Sports Medicine (2009) American College of Sports Medicine position stand: appropriate physical activity intervention strategies for weight loss and prevention of weight regain. *Medicine and Science in Sports and Exercise* 41: 459–71.

Donnelly, J.E., Honas, J.J., Smith, B.K., Mayo, M.S., Gibson, C.A., Sullivan, D.K. et al. (2013) Aerobic exercise alone results in clinically significant weight loss for men and women: Midwest exercise trial. *Obesity* 21: 219–28.

Dubern, B. and Clement, K. (2012) Leptin and leptin receptor-related monogenic obesity. *Biochimie* 94: 2111–15.

Dullo, A.G., Jacquet, J., Montani, J.P. and Schutz, Y. (2012) Adaptive thermogenesis in human body weight regulation: more of a concept than a measurable entity? *Obesity Reviews* 13: 105–21.

Emerging Risk Factor Collaboration (2011) Separate and combined associations of body-mass index and abdominal adiposity with cardiovascular disease: collaborative analysis of 58 prospective studies. *The Lancet* 377: 1085–95.

Emerging Risk Factor Collaboration (2015) Association of cardiometabolic multimorbidity with mortality. *Journal of the American Medical Association* 314: 52–60.

Fabbrini, E., Magkos F., Mohammed, B.S., Pietka T., Abumrad, N.A., Patterson, B.W. et al. (2009) Intrahepatic fat, not visceral fat, is linked with metabolic complications of obesity. *Proceedings of the National Academy of Sciences USA* 106: 15430–5.

Falconer, C.L., Page, A.S., Andrews, R.C. and Cooper, A.R. (2015) The potential impact of displacing sedentary time in adults with type 2 diabetes. *Medicine and Science in Sports and Exercise* 47: 2070–5.

Farooqi, S. and O'Rahilly, S. (2006) Genetics of human obesity. *Endocrine Reviews* 27: 710–18. doi: 10.1210/er.2006-0040.

Fenkci, S., Sarsan, A., Rota, S. and Ardic, F. (2006) Effects of resistance or aerobic exercises on metabolic parameters in obese women who are not on a diet. *Advances in Therapy* 23: 404–13.

Fildes, A., Charlton, J., Ridisill, C., Littlejohns, P., Prevost, A.T. and Guilliford, M.C. (2015) Probability of an obese person attaining normal body weight: cohort study using electronic health records. *American Journal of Public Health* 105: e54–9.

Flatt, J.P. (1995) Use and storage of carbohydrate and fat. *American Journal of Clinical Nutrition* 61: 952–9.

Flegal, K.M., Kit, B.K., Orpana, H. and Graubard, B.I. (2013) Association of all-cause mortality with overweight and obesity using standard body mass index categories: a systematic review and meta-analysis. *Journal of the American Medical Association* 309: 71–82.

Gaesser, G.A. and Brooks, G.A. (1984) Metabolic bases of excess post-exercise oxygen consumption: a review. *Medicine and Science in Sports and Exercise* 16: 29–43.

Gatterer, H., Shenk, K. and Burtscher, M. (2017) Assessment of human body composition: methods and limitations, in H.C. Lukaski (ed.) *Body composition: health and performance in exercise and sport*, Boca Raton, FL: CRC Press, pp. 13–26.

Gavrilova, O., Marcus-Samuels, B., Graham, D., Kim, J.K., Shulman, G.I., Castle, A.L. et al. (2000) Surgical implantation of adipose tissue reverses diabetes in lipoatrophic mice. *Journal of Clinical Investigation* 105: 271–8.

Global BMI Mortality Collaboration. (2016) Body-mass index and all-cause mortality: individual participant-data meta-analysis of 239 prospective studies in four continents. *The Lancet* 388: 776–86.

Global Burden of Disease Collaboration. (2017) Health effects of overweight and obesity in 195 countries over 25 years. *New England Journal of Medicine* 377: 13–27.

Golubic, R., Wijndaele, K., Sharp, S.J., Simmons, R.K., Griffin, S.J., Wareham, N.J. et al., on behalf of the ProActive study group. (2015) Physical activity, sedentary time and gain in overall and central body fat: 7-year follow-up of the ProActive cohort. *International Journal of Obesity* 39: 142–8.

Gray, L.J., Yates, T., Davies, M.J., Brady E., Webb, D.R., Sattar, N. and Khunti, K. (2011) Defining obesity cut-points for migrant South Asians. *PLoS One* 6: e26464. doi: 10.1371/journal.pone.0026464.

Greenway, F.L. (2015) Physiological adaptations to weight loss and factors favouring weight regain. *International Journal of Obesity* 39: 1188–96.

Gregor, M.F. and Hotamisligil, G.S. (2011) Inflammatory mechanisms in obesity. *Annual Review of Immunology* 29: 415–45.

Hall, K.D. (2017) A review of the carbohydrate-insulin model of obesity. *European Journal of Clinical Nutrition* 71: 323–6.

Hall, K.D. (2018) Did the food environment cause the obesity epidemic? *Obesity* 26: 11–13.

Hall, K.D., Heymsfield, S.B., Kemnitz, J.W., Klein, S., Schoeller, D.A. and Speakman, J.R. (2012) Energy balance and its components: implications for body weight regulation. *American Journal of Clinical Nutrition* 95: 989–94.

Hamer, M., Bell, J.A., Sabia, S., Batty, G.D. and Kivimäki, M. (2015) Stability of metabolically healthy obesity over 8 years: the English Longitudinal Study of Ageing. *European Journal of Endocrinology* 173: 703–8.

Hamer, M., Brunner, E.J., Bell, J., Batty, G.D., Shipley, M., Akbaraly, T. et al. (2013) Physical activity patterns over 10 years in relation to body mass index and waist circumference: the Whitehall II cohort study. *Obesity* 21: E755–61.

Hamer, M., Stamatakis, E. and Steptoe, A. (2014) Effects of substituting sedentary time with physical activity on metabolic risk. *Medicine and Science in Sports and Exercise* 46: 1946–50.

Hankinson, A.L., Daviglus, M.L., Bouchard, C., Carnethon, M., Lewis, C.E., Schreiner, P.J., et al. (2010) Maintaining a high physical activity level over 20 years and weight gain. *Journal of the American Medical Association* 304: 2603–10.

Harris, J.L., Pomeranz, J.L., Lobstein, T. and Brownell, K.D. (2009) A crisis in the marketplace: how food marketing contributes to childhood obesity and what can be done. *Annual Review of Public Health* 30: 211–25.

Haskell, W.L., Lee, I.-M., Pate, R.R., Powell, K.E., Blair, S.N., Franklin, B.A. et al. (2007) Physical activity and public health: updated recommendations for adults from the American College of Sports Medicine and the American Heart Association. *Medicine and Science in Sports and Exercise* 39: 1423–34.

Hawley, N.L. and McGarvey, S.T. (2015) Obesity and diabetes in Pacific Islanders: the current burden and the need for urgent action. *Current Diabetes Reports* 15: 29. doi: 10.1007/s11892-015-0594-5.

Healy, G.N., Matthews, C.E., Dunstan, D.W., Winkler, E.A. and Owen, N. (2011) Sedentary time and cardio-metabolic biomarkers in US adults: NHANES 2003–06. *European Heart Journal* 32: 590–7.

Healy, G.N., Winkler, E.A., Brakenridge, C.L., Reeves, M.M. and Eakin, E.G. (2015) Accelerometer-derived sedentary and physical activity time in overweight/obese adults with type 2 diabetes: cross-sectional associations with cardiometabolic biomarkers. *PLoS One* 10: e0119140. doi: 10.1371/journal.pone.0119140.

Henson, J., Dunstan, D.W., Davies, M.J. and Yates, T. (2016) Sedentary behaviour as a new behavioural target in the prevention and treatment of type 2 diabetes. *Diabetes/Metabolism Research Reviews* 32: 213–20.

Heymsfield, S.B. and Wadden, T.A. (2017) Mechanisms, pathophysiology, and management of obesity. *New England Journal of Medicine* 376: 254–66.

Hopkins, M., Finlayson, G., Duarte, C., Whybrow, S., Ritz, P., Horgan, G.W. et al. (2016) Modelling the associations between fat-free mass, resting metabolic rate and energy intake in the context of total energy balance. *International Journal of Obesity* 40: 312–18.

Hubert, P., King, N.A. and Blundell, J.E. (1998) Uncoupling the effects of energy expenditure and energy intake: appetite response to short-term energy deficit induced by meal omission and physical activity. *Appetite* 31: 9–19.

Imes, C.C. and Burke, L.E. (2014) The obesity epidemic: the United States as a cautionary tale for the rest of the world. *Current Epidemiology Reports* 1: 82–8.

Jakicic, J.M., Marcus, B.H., Lang, W. and Janney, C. (2008) Effect of exercise on 24-month weight loss maintenance in overweight women. *Archives of Internal Medicine* 168: 1550–9.

James, W.P.T., Bailes, J., Davies, H.L. and Dauncy, M.J. (1978) Elevated metabolic rates in obesity. *The Lancet* 311: 1122–5.

Jeffery, R.W., Wing, R.R., Sherwood, N.E. and Tate, D.F. (2003) Physical activity and weight loss: does prescribing higher physical activity goals improve outcome? *American Journal of Clinical Nutrition* 78: 684–9.

Jeukendrup, A. and Achten, J. (2001) Fatmax: a new concept to optimize fat oxidation during exercise? *European Journal of Sport Science* 5: 1–5.

Johnson, F. and Wardle, J. (2014) Variety, palatability, and obesity. *Advances in Nutrition* 5: 851–9.

Johnston, B.C., Kanters, S., Bandayrel, K., Wu, P., Naji, F., Siemieniuk, R.A. et al. (2014) Comparison of weight loss among named diet programs in overweight and obese adults: a meta-analysis. *Journal of the American Medical Association* 312: 923–33.

Karra, E., O'Daly, O.G., Choudhury, A.I., Yousseif, A., Millership, S., Neary, M.T. et al. (2013) A link between FTO, ghrelin, and impaired brain food-cue responsivity. *Journal of Clinical Investigation* 123: 3539–51.

Katzmarzyk, P.T., Pérusse, L., Tremblay, A. and Bouchard, C. (2000) No association between resting metabolic rate or respiratory exchange ratio and subsequent changes in body mass and fatness: 5½ year follow-up of the Québec family study. *European Journal of Clinical Nutrition* 54: 610–14.

Kelly, B., King, J.A., Goerlach, J. and Nimmo, M.A. (2013) The impact of high-intensity intermittent exercise on resting metabolic rate in healthy males. *European Journal of Applied Physiology* 113: 3039–47.

King, J.A., Miyashita, M., Wasse, L.K. and Stensel, D.J. (2010) Influence of prolonged treadmill running on appetite, energy intake and circulating concentrations of acylated ghrelin. *Appetite* 54: 492–8.

King, J.A., Wasse, L.K., Ewens, J., Crystallis, K., Emmanuel, J., Batterham, R.L. and Stensel, D.J. (2011) Differential acylated ghrelin, peptide YY3-36, appetite and food intake responses to equivalent energy deficits created by exercise and food restriction. *Journal of Clinical Endocrinology and Metabolism* 96: 1114–21.

King, N.A., Caudwell, P., Hopkins, M., Byrne, N.M., Colley, R., Hills, A.P. et al. (2007) Metabolic and behavioural compensatory responses to exercise interventions: barriers to weight loss. *Obesity* 15: 1373–83.

King, N.A., Hopkins, M., Caudwell, P., Stubbs, R.J. and Blundell, J.E. (2008) Individual variability following 12 weeks of supervised exercise: identification and characterization of compensation for exercise-induced weight loss. *International Journal of Obesity* 32: 177–84.

Kivimäki, M., Kuosma, E., Ferrie, J.E., Luukkonen, R., Nyberg, S.T., Alfredsson, L. et al. (2017) Overweight, obesity, and risk of cardiometabolic multimorbidity: pooled analysis of individual-level data for 120,813 adults from 16 cohort studies from the USA and Europe. *The Lancet Public Health* 2: e277–85.

Kral, J.G., Kava, R.A., Catalano, P.M. and Moore, B.J. (2012) Severe obesity: the neglected epidemic. *Obesity Facts* 5: 254–69.

Kraus, W.E., Houmard, J.A., Duscha, B.D., Knetzger, K.J., Wharton, M.B., McCartney, J.S. et al. (2002) Effects of the amount and intensity of exercise on plasma lipoproteins. *New England Journal of Medicine* 347: 1483–92.

Laforgia, J., Withers, R.T., Shipp, N.J. and Gore, C.J. (1997) Comparison of energy expenditure elevations after submaximal and supramaximal running. *Journal of Applied Physiology* 82: 661–6.

Lahti-Koski, M., Pietinen, P., Heliövaara, M. and Vartiainen, E. (2002) Associations of body mass index and obesity with physical activity, food choices, alcohol intake, and smoking in the 1982–1997 FINRISK studies. *American Journal of Clinical Nutrition* 75: 809–17.

Larson-Meyer, D.E., Redman, L., Heilbronn, L.K., Martin, C.K. and Ravussin, E. (2010) Caloric restriction with or without exercise: the fitness verses fatness debate. *Medicine and Science in Sports and Exercise* 42: 152–9.

Lee, S., Kuk, J.L., Davidson, L.E., Hudson, R., Kilpatrick, K., Graham, T.E. and Ross, R. (2005) Exercise without weight loss is an effective strategy for obesity reduction in obese individuals with and without type 2 diabetes. *Journal of Applied Physiology* 99: 1220–5.

Leibel, R.L., Rosenbaum, M. and Hirsch, J. (1995) Change in energy expenditure resulting from altered body weight. *New England Journal of Medicine* 332: 621–8.

Levine, J.A. (2003) Non-exercise activity thermogenesis. *Proceedings of the Nutrition Society* 62: 667–79.

Livingstone, M.B. and Pourshahidi, L.K. (2014) Portion size and obesity. *Advances in Nutrition* 5: 829–34.

Locke, A.E., Kahali, B., Berndt, S.I. et al. (2015) Genetic studies of body mass index yield new insights for obesity biology. *Nature* 518: 197–206.

Luke A. and Cooper, R.S. (2013) Physical activity does not influence obesity risk: time to clarify the public health message. *International Journal of Epidemiology* 42: 1831–6.

Luke, A., Dugas, L.R., Ebersole, K., Durazo-Arvizu, R.A., Cao, G., Schoeller, D.A. et al. (2009) Energy expenditure does not predict weight change in either Nigerian or African American women. *American Journal of Clinical Nutrition* 89: 169–76.

MacLean, P.S., Higgins, J.A., Giles, V.D., Sherk, V.D. and Jackman, M.R. (2015) The role of adipose tissue in weight regain after weight loss. *Obesity Reviews* 16: 45–54.

Mann, T., Tomivama, A.J., Westling, E., Lew, A.M., Samuels, B. and Chatman, J. (2007) Medicare's search for effective obesity treatments: diets are not the answer. *The American Psychologist* 62: 220–33.

Martinez-Gonzalez, M.A., Martinez, J.A., Hu, F.B., Gibney, M.J. and Kearney, J. (1999) Physical inactivity, sedentary lifestyle and obesity in the European Union. *International Journal of Obesity and Related Metabolic Disorders* 23: 1192–201.

Mattes, R. and Foster, G.D. (2014) Research issues: the food environment. *Advances in Nutrition* 100: 1663–5.

Mekary, R.A., Willet, W.C., Hu, F.B. and Ding, E.L. (2009) Isotemporal substitution paradigm for physical activity and weight change. *American Journal of Epidemiology* 170: 519–27.

Melanson, E.L. (2017) The effect of exercise on non-exercise physical activity and sedentary behaviour in adults. *Obesity Reviews* 18: 40–9.

Melby, C., Scholl, C., Edwards, G., Bullough, R. (1993) Effect of acute resistance exercise on post-exercise energy expenditure and resting metabolic rate. *Journal of Applied Physiology* 75: 1847–53.

Meldrum, D.R., Morris, M.A. and Gambone, J.C. (2017) Obesity pandemic: causes, consequences, and solutions – but do we have the will? *Fertility and Sterility* 107: 833–9.

Millward, J. (2013) Energy balance and obesity: a UK perspective on the gluttony v. sloth debate. *Nutrition Research Reviews* 26: 89–109.

Misra, A. (2015) Ethnic-specific criteria for classification of body mass index: a perspective for Asian Indians and American Diabetes Association Position Statement. *Diabetes Technology and Therapeutics* 17: 667–71.

Mozaffarian, D., Hao, T., Rimm, E.B., Willet, W.C. and Hu, F.B. (2011) Changes in diet and lifestyle and long-term weight gain in women and men. *New England Journal of Medicine* 364: 2392–404.

Muñoz-Garach, A., Cornejo-Pareja, I. and Tinahones, F.J. (2016) Does metabolically healthy obesity exist? *Nutrients* 8: 320. doi: 10.3390/nu8060320.

National Heart, Lung and Blood Institute; National Institutes of Health; U.S. Department of Health and Human Services. (n.d.) Classification of overweight and obesity by BMI, waist circumference, and associated disease risks [online], available at: https://www.nhlbi.nih.gov/health/educational/lose_wt/BMI/bmi_dis.htm (accessed 18 July 2017).

National Institute for Health and Care Excellence. (2014) Weight management: lifestyle services for overweight or obese adults [online], available at: https://www.nice.org.uk/guidance/ph53/resources (accessed 16 July 2017).

Nelson, K.M., Weinsier, R.L., James, L.D., Darnell, B., Hunter, G. and Long, C.L. (1992) Effect of weight reduction on resting energy expenditure, substrate utilization, and the thermic effect of food in moderately obese women. *American Journal of Clinical Nutrition* 55: 924–32.

Non-Communicable Disease Risk Factor Collaboration. (n.d.) Obesity statistics [online], available at: http://www.ncdrisc.org/index.html (accessed 14 March 2019).

Non-Communicable Disease Risk Factor Collaboration. (2016) Trends in adult body-mass index in 200 countries from 1975 to 2014: a pooled analysis of 1698 population-based measurement studies with 19.2 million participants. *The Lancet* 387: 1377–96.

Ochner, C.N., Tsai, A.G., Kushner, R.F. and Wadden, T.A. (2015) Taking obesity seriously: when recommendations for lifestyle change confront biological adaptations. *The Lancet* 3: 232–4.

Passmore, P. and Durnin, J.V.G.A. (1955) Human energy expenditure. *Physiological Reviews* 35: 801–40.

Pontzer, H., Raichlen D.A., Wood, B.M., Mabulla, A.Z.P., Racette, S.B. and Marlowe, F.W. (2012) Hunter-gatherer energetics and human obesity. *PLoS One* 7: e40503. doi: 10.1371/journal. pone.0040503.

Pontzer, H. (2015) Constrained total energy expenditure and the evolutionary biology of energy balance. *Exercise and Sport Science Reviews* 43: 110–16.

Prentice, A.M. and Jebb, S.A. (1995) Obesity in Britain: gluttony or sloth? *British Medical Journal* 311: 437–9.

Pulsford, R.M., Stamatakis, E., Britton, A.R., Brunner, E.J. and Hillsdon, M.M. (2013) Sitting behaviour and obesity: evidence from the Whitehall II study. *American Journal of Preventive Medicine* 44: 132–8.

Ramachandrappa, S. and Farooqi, I.S. (2011) Genetic approaches to understanding human obesity. *Journal of Clinical Investigation* 121: 2080–6.

Ravussin, E., Burnand, B., Schutz, Y. and Jequier, E. (1982) Twenty-four-hour energy expenditure and resting metabolic rate in obese, moderately obese, and control subjects. *American Journal of Clinical Nutrition* 35: 566–73.

Ravussin, E., Lillioja, S., Knowler, W.C., Christin, L., Freymond, D., Abbott, W.G. et al. (1988) Reduced rate of energy expenditure as a risk factor for body-weight gain. *New England Journal of Medicine* 318: 467–72.

Raynor, H.A. and Champagne, C.M. (2016) Position of the academy of nutrition and dietetics: interventions for the Treatment of overweight and obesity in adults. *Journal of the Academy of Nutrition and Dietetics* 116: 129–47.

Richardson, C.R., Newton, T.L., Abraham, J.J., Sen, A., Jimbo, M. and Swartz, A.M. (2008) A meta-analysis of pedometer-based walking interventions and weight loss. *Annals of Family Medicine* 6: 69–77.

Roberts, S.B., Savage, J., Coward, W.A., Chew, B. and Lucas, A. (1988) Energy expenditure and intake in infants born to lean and obese mothers. *New England Journal of Medicine* 318: 461–6.

Rosenbaum, M., Sy, M., Pavlovich, K., Leibel, R.L. and Hirsh, J. (2008) Leptin reverses weight loss induced changes in regional neural activity responses to visual food stimuli. *Journal of Clinical Investigation* 118: 2583–91.

Rosenbaum, M., Vandenborne, K., Goldsmith, R., Simoneu, J., Heymsfield, S., Joanisse, D.R. et al. (2003) Effects of experimental weight perturbation on skeletal muscle work efficiency in human subjects. *American Journal of Physiology – Regulatory, Integrative and Comparative* 285: 183–92.

Ross, R., Dagnone, D., Jones, P.J., Smith, H., Paddags, A., Hudson, R. and Janssen, I. (2000) Reduction in obesity and related comorbid conditions after diet-induced weight loss or exercise-induced weight loss in men: a randomized, controlled trial. *Annals of Internal Medicine* 133: 92–103.

Ross, R., Hudson, R., Stotz, P.J. and Lam, M. (2015) Effects of exercise amount and intensity on abdominal obesity and glucose tolerance in obese adults: a randomized trial. *Annals of Internal Medicine* 162: 325–34.

Ross, R., Janssen, I., Dawson, J., Kungl, A.M., Kuk, J.L., Wong, S.L. et al. (2004) Exercise-induced reduction in obesity and insulin resistance in women: a randomized controlled trial. *Obesity Research* 12: 789–98.

Schmitz, K.H., Hannan, P.J., Stovitz, S.D., Bryan, C.J., Warren, M. and Jensen, M.D. (2007) Strength training and adiposity in premenopausal women: Strong, Healthy, and Empowered study. *American Journal of Clinical Nutrition* 86: 566–72.

Schubert, M.M., Desbrow, B., Sabapathy, S. and Leveritt, M. (2013) Acute exercise and subsequent energy intake. *Appetite* 63: 92–104.

Schulman, G.I. (2014) Ectopic fat in insulin resistance, dyslipidemia, and cardiometabolic disease. *New England Journal of Medicine* 37: 1131–41.

Schutz, Y., Bessard, T. and Jequier, E. (1984) Diet-induced thermogenesis measured over a whole day in obese and nonobese women. *American Journal of Clinical Nutrition* 40: 542–52.

Schwingshackl, L., Dias, S. and Hoffmann, G. (2014) Impact of long-term lifestyle programmes on weight loss and cardiovascular risk factors in overweight/obese participants: a systematic review and network meta-analysis. *Systematic Reviews* 3: 130. doi: 10.1186/2046-4053-3-130.

Seidell, J.C., Muller, D.C., Sorkin, J.D. and Andres R. (1992) Fasting respiratory exchange ratio and resting metabolic rate as predictors of weight gain: the Baltimore Longitudinal Study on Aging. *International Journal of Obesity and Related Metabolic Disorders* 16: 667–74.

Sigal, R.J., Kenny, G.P., Boulé, N.G., Wells, G.A., Prud'homme, D., Fortier, M. et al. (2007) Effects of aerobic training, resistance training, or both on glycemic control in type 2 diabetes: a randomized trial. *Annals of Internal Medicine* 147: 357–69.

Sniderman, A.D., Bhopal, R., Prabhakaran, D., Sarrafzadegan, N. and Tchernof, A. (2007) Why might South Asians be so susceptible to central obesity and its atherogenic consequences? The adipose tissue overflow hypothesis. *International Journal of Epidemiology* 36: 220–5.

Speliotes, E.K., Willer, C.J., Berndt, S.I. et al. (2010) Association analyses of 249,796 individuals reveal 18 new loci associated with BMI. *Nature Genetics* 42: 937–48.

Stefan, N., Häring, H.U. and Schulze, M.B. (2018) Metabolically healthy obesity: the low-hanging fruit in obesity treatment? *The Lancet Diabetes and Endocrinology* 6: 249–58.

Stensel, D.J. (2010) Exercise, appetite and appetite-regulating hormones: implications for food intake and weight control. *Annals of Nutrition and Metabolism* 57: 36–42.

Stunkard, A.J., Fich, T.T. and Hrubec, Z. (1986) A twin study of human obesity. *Journal of the American Medical Association* 256: 51–4.

Stunkard, A.J., Sorensen, T.I.A., Hanis, C., Teasdale, T.W., Chakraborty, R., Schull, W.J. and Schulsinger, F. (1986) An adoption study of human obesity. *New England Journal of Medicine* 314: 193–8.

Sumithran, P., Prendergast, L.A., Delbridge, E., Purcell, K., Shulkes, A., Kriketos, A. and Proietto, J. (2011) Long-term persistence of hormonal adaptations to weight loss. *New England Journal of Medicine* 365: 1597–604.

Swift, D.L., Johannsen, N.M., Lavie, C.J., Earnest, C.P. and Church, T.S. (2014) The role of exercise and physical activity in weight loss and maintenance. *Progress in Cardiovascular Diseases* 56: 441–7.

Swinburn, B.A., Sacks, G., Hall, K.D., McPherson, K., Finegood, D.T., Moodie, M.L. and Gortmaker, S.L. (2011) The global obesity pandemic: shaped by global drivers and local environments. *The Lancet* 378: 804–14.

Swinburn, B., Sacks, G. and Ravussin, E. (2009) Increased food energy supply is more than sufficient to explain the US epidemic of obesity. *American Journal of Clinical Nutrition* 90: 1453–6.

Szabo, A.N., Washburn, R.A., Sullivan, D.K. and Honas, J.J. (2013) The Midwest exercise trial for the prevention of weight regain: MET POWeR. *Contemporary Clinical Trials* 36: 470–8.

Taylor, H.A., Coady, S.A., Levy, D., Walker, E.R., Vasan, R.S., Liu, J. et al. (2010) Relationship of BMI to cardiovascular risk factors differ by ethnicity. *Obesity* 18: 1638–45.

Thomas, E.L. and Bell, J.D. (2014) Body fat: our own Janus. *Physiology News* Issue 96: 24–27. doi: 10.36866/pn.96.24.

Thomas, J.G., Bond, D.S., Phelan, S., Hill, J.O. and Wing, R.R. (2014) Weight loss maintenance for 10 years in the National Weight Control Registry. *American Journal of Preventive Medicine* 46: 17–23.

Thompson, D., Karpe, F., Lafontan, M. and Frayn, K. (2012) Physical activity and exercise in the regulation of human adipose tissue physiology. *Physiology Reviews* 92: 157–91.

Tillin, T., Sattar, N., Godsland, I.F., Hughes, A.D., Chaturvedi, N. and Forouhi, N.G. (2015) Ethnicity-specific obesity cut-points in the development of type 2 diabetes – a prospective study including three groups in the United Kingdom. *Diabetes Medicine* 32: 226–34.

Vague, J. (1956) The degree of masculine differentiation of obesities: a factor determining predisposition to diabetes, atherosclerosis, gout, and uric calculous disease. *American Journal of Clinical Nutrition* 4: 20–34.

Van Dyck, D., Cerin, E., De Bourdeaudhuij, I., Hinkson, E., Reis, R.S., Davey, R., et al. (2015) International study of objectively measured physical activity and sedentary time with body mass index and obesity: IPEN adult study. *International Journal of Obesity* 39: 199–207.

Van Loon, L.J.C., Greenhaff, P.L., Constantin-Teodosiu, D., Saris, W.H.M. and Wagenmakers, A.J.M. (2001) The effects of increasing exercise intensity on muscle fuel utilisation in humans. *The Journal of Physiology* 536: 295–304.

Villareal, D.T., Aguirre, L., Gurney, A.B., Waters, D.L., Sinacore, D.R., Colombo, E. et al. (2017) Aerobic or resistance exercise, or both, in dieting obese older adults. *New England Journal of Medicine* 376: 1943–55.

Villareal, D.T., Chode, S., Parimi, N., Sinacore, D.R., Hilton, T., Armamento-Villareal, R. et al. (2011) Weight loss, exercise, or both and physical function in obese older adults. *New England Journal of Medicine* 364: 1218–29.

Villareal, D.T., Fontana, L., Weiss, E.P., Racette, S.B., Steger-May, K., Schechtman, K.B. et al. (2006) Bone mineral density response to caloric restriction-induced weight loss or exercise-induced weight loss: a randomized controlled trial. *Archives of Internal Medicine* 166: 11–25.

Waalen, J. (2014) The genetics of human obesity. *Translation Research* 164: 293–301.

Wadden, T.A. (1993) Treatment of obesity by moderate and severe caloric restriction: results of clinical research trials. *Annals of Internal Medicine* 119: 688–93.

Wang, T., Huang, T., Heianza, Y., Sun, D., Zheng, Y., Ma, W. et al. (2017) Genetic susceptibility, change in physical activity, and long-term weight gain. *Diabetes* 66: 2704–12.

Wang, T., Heianza, Y., Sun, D., Huang, T., Ma, W., Rimm et al. (2018) Improving adherence to healthy dietary patterns, genetic risk, and long-term weight gain: gene–diet interaction analysis in two prospective cohort studies. *British Medical Journal* 360: j5644. doi: 10.1136/bmj.j5644.

Wang, Z., Ying, Z., Bosy-Westphal, A., Zhang, J., Heller, M., Later, W. et al. (2011) Evaluation of specific metabolic rates of major organs and tissues: comparison between men and women. *American Journal of Human Biology* 23: 333–8.

Weiss, E.P., Jordan, R.C., Frese, E.M., Albert, S.G. and Villareal, D.T. (2017) Effect of weight loss on lean mass, strength, bone, and aerobic capacity. *Medicine and Science in Sports and Exercise* 49: 206–17.

Westerterp, K.R. (2004) Diet-induced thermogenesis. *Nutrition and Metabolism* 1: 5. doi: 10.1186/1743-7075-1-5.

Weyer, C., Walford, R.L., Harper, I.T., Milner, M., MacCallum, T., Tataranni, P.A. and Ravussin, E. (2000) Energy metabolism after 2 y of energy restriction: the biosphere 2 experiment. *American Journal of Clinical Nutrition* 72: 946–53.

Willet, W., Hu, F.B. and Thun, M. (2013) Overweight, obesity and all-cause mortality. *Journal of the American Medical Association* 309: 1618–82.

World Health Organization. (1998) Obesity: preventing and managing the global epidemic [online], available at: http://apps.who.int/iris/handle/10665/63854 (accessed 29 June 2017).

World Health Organization. (2016) Obesity and overweight fact sheet [online], available at: http://www.who.int/topics/obesity/en/ (accessed 29 June 2017).

7 Cardio-metabolic risk factors

Kevin Deighton

INTRODUCTION

Evidence collected over many decades has identified a number of major risk factors for cardio-metabolic disease. The concept of risk factors is useful when examining the role of physical activity in disease prevention because intervention studies can be conducted to examine the effects of exercise on known risk factors. As highlighted previously, randomised controlled trials examining the effect of exercise on disease endpoints (heart attack, stroke) are generally not feasible due to the very large sample sizes and long durations of follow-up needed to detect statistically significant effects on these outcomes (although a small number of these trials have now been performed, see Chapter 4). However, if it can be demonstrated that exercise positively influences cardio-metabolic risk factors in intervention trials, this would provide strong evidence that the associations between inactivity/low fitness and cardio-metabolic disease, established through epidemiological studies, are likely to be causal. This concept was illustrated in Figure 2.7, in Chapter 2. Furthermore, this would also provide strong evidence that cardio-metabolic disease could be prevented through physical activity because studies have demonstrated that favourable changes in the major risk factors reduce the subsequent risk of disease.

Table 7.1 lists the major risk factors for cardiovascular disease (CVD) and Figure 7.1 displays the prevalence of some of these risk factors in England. Other, newer risk factors not listed in Table 7.1 include apolipoprotein B, small low-density lipoproteins, markers for inflammation (e.g. C-reactive protein, interleukin-6), chronic infections, aortic stiffness, thrombogenic (blood clotting) factors such as fibrinogen, homocysteine and coronary-artery calcium content. These are omitted from Table 7.1 because at present none of these factors add substantially to the prediction of CVD risk above that indicated by the 'classic' risk factors, and they do not have a clearly defined role

Table 7.1 Major risk factors for cardiovascular disease.	
MODIFIABLE RISK FACTORS	NON-MODIFIABLE RISK FACTORS
• Dyslipidaemia: elevated total cholesterol or low-density lipoprotein cholesterol concentrations, depressed high-density lipoprotein cholesterol concentrations, elevated triglyceride concentrations • Hypertension • Cigarette smoking • Obesity (particularly central/abdominal obesity) • Hyperglycaemia or type 2 diabetes	• Family history: risk is increased in first-degree relatives (parents, siblings and offspring) of people with premature atherosclerotic disease (<60 years) • Age: higher risk in older individuals • Sex: higher risk in men than women • Ethnicity: higher risk in individuals with South Asian ethnicity • Socio-economic status: higher risk with greater deprivation • Existing diseases/conditions: higher risk in individuals with type 1 diabetes, chronic kidney disease, rheumatoid arthritis, atrial fibrillation or familial hypercholesterolaemia

Note: For further information on CVD risk factors and prediction models for CVD, the reader is referred to the JBS3 (2014) guidelines.

Figure 7.1 Prevalence of several major CVD risk factors in adult men and women in England.

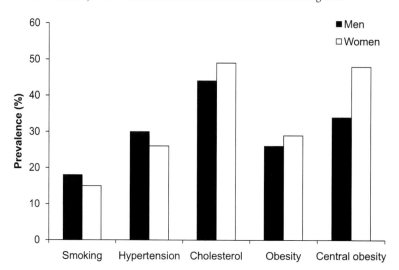

Source: Data are from the Health Survey for England 2018 courtesy of the National Centre for Social Research (NatCen), University College London, Department of Epidemiology and Public Health (2019).

Notes: Risk factor definitions: hypertension, systolic blood pressure $\geq$140 mm Hg and/or diastolic blood pressure $\geq$90 mm Hg; high cholesterol, total cholesterol $\geq$5 mmol l^{-1}; obesity, BMI $\geq$30 kg m^{-2}; central obesity, waist circumference >102 cm for men and >88 cm for women.

in the clinical management of patients (JBS3 2014). However, this does not mean that these factors are unimportant for CVD risk or that intervening to alter them would not provide benefit. Note also that physical inactivity and low physical fitness are not listed in Table 7.1. It could be argued that they should be since the evidence discussed previously indicates that low levels of physical activity and physical fitness are independently related to CVD risk. In view of this there is an argument for including activity and/ or fitness assessments routinely in clinical practice. Indeed, a recent paper using the UK Biobank cohort showed that the addition of grip strength to a traditional CVD risk score which already included age, sex, body mass index, systolic blood pressure, smoking and presence of diabetes, significantly improved prediction of all-cause and CVD mortality, suggesting that inclusion of grip strength may have clinical utility in disease risk prediction models (Celis-Morales et al. 2018). In the discussion which follows we will examine the evidence that physical activity favourably influences some of the major risk factors for CVD.

PHYSICAL ACTIVITY AND RISK FACTORS FOR CARDIO-METABOLIC DISEASE

Figure 7.2 provides a summary of the mechanisms by which physical activity is likely to influence cardio-metabolic disease risk. In summary, physical activity, either directly, or via effects on fitness or adiposity, has been shown to positively affect a number of risk

Figure 7.2 Mechanisms by which physical activity is likely to influence cardio-metabolic disease risk.

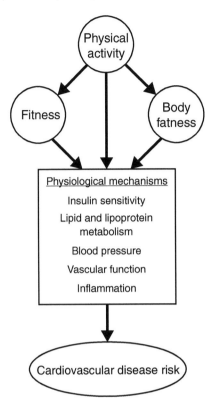

Source: Reprinted with permission from Gill, J.M.R. and Malkova, D. (2006) 'Physical activity, fitness and cardiovascular disease risk in adults: interactions with insulin resistance and obesity', *Clinical Science* 110: 409–25. Available at: https://doi.org/10.1042/CS20050207.

factors on the causal pathway for cardiovascular and metabolic disease. The evidence for each of these mechanisms is described in the sections below.

LIPIDS AND LIPOPROTEINS

One of the major mechanisms by which physical activity may lead to a reduced risk of CVD is via an effect on lipid and lipoprotein metabolism. The major lipoproteins are displayed in Figure 7.3. The main role of chylomicrons is to transport exogenous (dietary) triglyceride, whereas very low-density lipoproteins (VLDL) transport endogenous triglyceride (i.e. triglyceride which is synthesised within the liver). Together, chylomicrons and VLDL are sometimes referred to as triglyceride-rich lipoproteins since they are largely composed of triglyceride. Low-density lipoproteins (LDL) are the main carriers of cholesterol in the plasma. Elevated concentrations of all three of these lipoproteins (chylomicrons, VLDL and LDL) are atherogenic. In contrast, high

Figure 7.3 Composition of the four major lipoproteins.

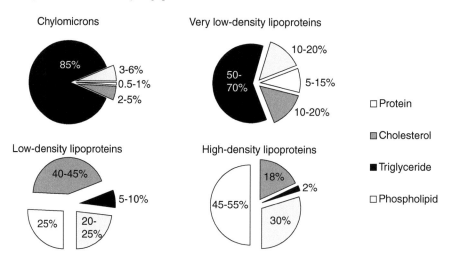

Source: McArdle et al. (2010).

concentrations of high-density lipoproteins (HDL) protect from CVD because HDL assists in the transfer of excess cholesterol from the tissues to the liver from where it can be excreted as cholesterol and as bile salts body in a process termed 'reverse cholesterol transport'. A detailed explanation of lipid and lipoprotein metabolism is beyond the scope of this book, and the interested reader is referred to the chapter on lipoprotein metabolism in Frayn (2010).

Triglyceride-rich lipoproteins are hydrolysed within the capillary beds of adipose tissue and skeletal muscle by the actions of the enzyme lipoprotein lipase (LPL). The hydrolysis of the triglyceride portion of these lipoproteins releases non-esterified fatty acids (NEFA) for uptake into the adipose tissue (for esterification and storage) and skeletal muscle (for oxidation and/or storage). Due to the reduction in triglyceride content (and therefore size) of the lipoproteins, this process also causes the release of un-esterified cholesterol and phospholipid surface material which is transferred to HDL. Consequently, high levels of LPL activity can increase HDL concentration by rapidly hydrolysing triglyceride-rich lipoproteins and stimulating the transfer of surface material to HDL particles. Alternatively, if triglyceride clearance is slow then high plasma concentrations stimulate neutral lipid exchange between triglyceride-rich lipoproteins and HDL. This process involves the reciprocal transfer of triglyceride to HDL, and cholesterol ester from HDL to triglyceride-rich lipoproteins due to the concentration gradient of these substances between particles. Consequently, after the triglyceride portion of the lipoproteins is eventually hydrolysed, smaller cholesterol ester-depleted HDL particles will remain, while the triglyceride-rich lipoprotein remnants will be larger due to the additional cholesterol ester gained from the HDL. These processes are thought to be responsible for the inverse relationship observed between plasma triglyceride and HDL concentrations.

Considering the role of HDL in reverse cholesterol transport, it is not surprising that low HDL concentrations are a risk factor for CVD. Equally, low HDL concentrations may be a marker for defective metabolism of triglyceride-rich lipoproteins. Importantly, the combination of low HDL and elevated triglyceride concentrations is also associated with circulating LDL particles that are smaller and more dense than normal. As with the process described for HDL above, high levels of triglyceride-rich lipoproteins will stimulate neutral lipid exchange with LDL due to the increased concentration gradient between particles. The depletion of cholesterol ester from LDL through this process results in smaller and denser LDL particles which may be particularly likely to penetrate the endothelial lining, thereby entering the sub-endothelial space to initiate the formation of atherosclerotic lesions. The combination of low HDL, elevated triglyceride concentrations and smaller denser LDL particles is termed the 'atherogenic lipoprotein phenotype'.

In accordance with the central role of elevated triglyceride concentrations in the development of the atherogenic lipoprotein phenotype, the ability of the body to clear triglycerides from the circulation after feeding represents a major predictor of CVD risk. This is commonly tested using meal tolerance tests whereby a mixed-macronutrient or high-fat test meal is consumed by participants and their plasma triglyceride responses are assessed during the postprandial period. This is a valuable diagnostic test but also reflects a situation that occurs several times a day as most humans spend the majority of their day in a postprandial (fed) state. Consequently, atherosclerosis may be regarded as a postprandial phenomenon.

Indirect observational evidence supports the concept that physical activity may be able to modify lipids and lipoproteins and hence atherosclerosis. An example of such evidence has recently been provided from the study of indigenous Tsimane of the Bolivian Amazon (Kaplan et al. 2017). This population have the lowest reported levels of coronary artery disease of any population recorded to date, which is associated with low levels of fasting total cholesterol, LDL, triglyceride and glucose throughout adult life. These effects are associated with their subsistence lifestyle, which results in high levels of physical activity and a diet very low in saturated fat, simple sugars and trans fats. The likely benefits of physical activity result from estimates that men and women engage in physical activity for an average of six to seven hours and four to six hours per day, respectively. Furthermore, less than 10% of daylight hours are spent completing sedentary activities, compared with more than 54% in industrial populations. Interestingly, the availability of small gasoline motors for canoes beginning around 2011 has coincided with an average increase in total cholesterol (TC) and LDL of 0.12 mmol l^{-1} (4.8 mg dl^{-1}) and 0.15 mmol l^{-1} (5.9 mg dl^{-1}) per year, respectively, while HDL has decreased by an average of 0.02 mmol l^{-1} (0.76 mg dl^{-1}) per year. These figures are based on yearly assessments between 2011 and 2015 after controlling for age, sex and community of residence. The precise reason for these changes cannot be inferred but it may be related to the reduced need for manual canoeing or rafting for river travel, an increased availability of non-subsistence food in the local market town, or other unknown factors.

Many studies have investigated the effects of exercise more directly and demonstrated favourable improvements in lipid and lipoprotein metabolism. The most consistent findings are of an increase in the concentration of protective HDL and reduced concentrations of plasma triglycerides and the triglyceride-rich lipoproteins chylomicrons and VLDL. Less consistently, reductions in total cholesterol and LDL have been observed. One unique study examined HDL cholesterol in several groups of men with widely differing levels of physical activity, ranging from almost complete inactivity in those with recent spinal cord injuries to 80 miles per week of running in individuals training for the Boston marathon. The findings revealed a clear gradient in HDL, ranging from a mean of 0.7 mmol l^{-1} (27 mg dl^{-1}) for new spinal cord injured patients to 1.6 mmol l^{-1} (61 mg dl^{-1}) for the marathon runners (LaPorte et al. 1983) (Figure 7.4). Moreover, HDL concentration was below the fifth percentile of the normal population in all of the new spinal cord injured patients (who were presumably the least active group). These findings were confirmed in a study of over 1,800 female runners and a study of over 8,000 male runners which both demonstrated a positive dose–response association between running mileage and HDL concentration (Williams 1996, 1997).

Well-designed randomised controlled intervention trials have shown that exercise training causes reductions in VLDL triglyceride and increases in HDL. Relevant here is the Studies of a Targeted Risk Reduction Intervention through Defined Exercise (STRRIDE) project (Huffman et al. 2012; Kraus et al. 2002; Slentz et al. 2007). In addition to demonstrating reductions in VLDL triglyceride and increases in HDL with eight months of exercise training in previously inactive, overweight men and women, these studies also found reductions in small LDL particles which are particularly atherogenic (as discussed earlier in the chapter). The amount of exercise was found to be more important than its intensity for changing lipoprotein concentrations, and some of the changes were maintained during a 15-day period of detraining (Kraus et al. 2002; Slentz et al. 2007). Participants were instructed not to change their diets during these intervention studies and the changes in lipoprotein profile occurred in the absence of major weight loss. However, other studies have shown that exercise-induced changes to lipoprotein metabolism are enhanced if accompanied by reductions in fat mass (Wood et al. 1988). The dose–response relationship between weekly volume of

Figure 7.4 High-density lipoprotein (HDL) cholesterol concentrations (mmol l^{-1}) in seven groups of individuals characterised by widely different habitual physical activity levels.

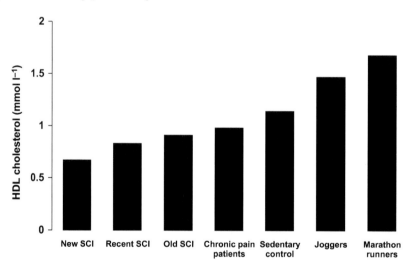

Source: LaPorte et al. (1983).
Note: SCI: spinal cord injury. Concentrations displayed are 50th percentile values for each group.

exercise and change in HDL concentrations shown in STRRIDE has been confirmed in a meta-analysis of 25 randomised controlled trials of exercise training interventions of 11–52 weeks in duration, which included a total of 1,404 adults aged 23–75 years (Kodama et al. 2007). In this analysis, intensity of exercise did not significantly affect the extent of change in HDL concentration in response to training, but a threshold of exercise energy expenditure of 900 kcal per week or overall exercise duration of at least 120 minutes per week appeared to be required to significantly increase HDL concentrations.

Do exercise-induced changes in lipoprotein metabolism result in a reduction in coronary atherosclerosis? This question is difficult to answer with certainty because few studies have addressed this issue. A study in monkeys, however, suggests that changes in blood lipids as a result of exercise training can reduce atherosclerosis. This study examined two groups of monkeys consuming atherogenic (atherosclerosis-inducing) diets over a two-year period. One group was maintained in a sedentary state throughout the study while the other group was trained to 'run' on a non-motorised treadmill wheel for one hour, three times per week. By the end of the study, total cholesterol was substantially elevated in both groups of monkeys and did not differ significantly between groups (mean values were approximately 15.5 mmol l^{-1} in both groups, compared with normal values of around 2 mmol l^{-1}). However, HDL was significantly higher and triglycerides significantly lower in the trained compared with the sedentary monkeys. Moreover, assessments of the degree of coronary artery narrowing revealed that this was much greater in the sedentary monkeys than in those who exercised (Figure 7.5). The authors concluded that 'the benefits derived from such moderate exercise for one hour three times per week in the presence of hypercholesterolaemia were less atherosclerosis in wider coronary arteries supplying a larger heart that functioned at a slower rate' (Kramsch et al. 1981, p. 1488). Whether such findings apply to humans is not

Figure 7.5 The percentage narrowing (reduction in cross-sectional area) in the coronary arteries of sedentary and physically active monkeys consuming an atherogenic diet.

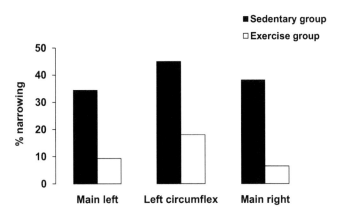

Source: Kramsch et al. (1981).
Note: Atherogenic diet consumed for two years. Active monkeys exercised for one hour, three times per week. Percentage narrowing was determined by histology post-mortem.

known with certainty. The findings are consistent, however, with those of more recent observational studies indicating an association between high cardiorespiratory fitness levels and slower progression of carotid atherosclerosis in middle-aged men (Lakka et al. 2001; Sandrock et al. 2008).

Physical activity and postprandial lipaemia

As explained earlier in the chapter, many of the abnormalities in metabolism related to CVD risk can be linked to the impairment of events during the postprandial period. Repeated exaggerated episodes of postprandial lipaemia lead to low HDL and a preponderance of small dense LDL. Additionally, when triglycerides are high, blood has an increased propensity to clot, there are detrimental effects on endothelial function and systemic inflammation is increased (these factors are discussed in later sections of this chapter), which contributes towards the formation of atherosclerotic plaque. Therefore, the influence of exercise on postprandial events is a topic of significant research interest.

Early studies found that endurance-trained athletes show a lower postprandial rise in triglycerides after a high-fat meal than do sedentary controls (Merrill et al. 1989) (Figure 7.6). However, if trained people go just 2.5 days without training, they experience a marked increase in postprandial triglycerides. Therefore, their characteristically low response to dietary fat is due, at least in part, to the fact that they have always exercised recently.

Figure 7.6 Plasma triglyceride responses to a meal containing fat (approx. 70 g) and carbohydrate in endurance-trained and untrained men who were matched for age, height and weight.

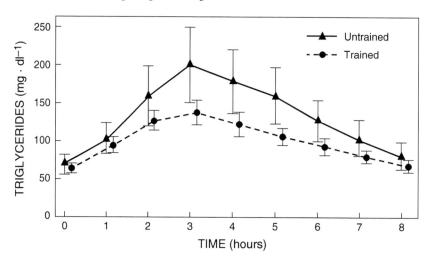

Source: Reprinted with permission from Wolters Kluwer Health, Inc.: Merrill, J.R. et al. (1989) 'Hyperlipidemic response of young trained and untrained men after a high fat meal', *Arteriosclerosis* 9: 217–23. Available at: https://doi.org/10.1161/01.ATV.9.2.217.

Figure 7.7 Influence of prior exercise on postprandial responses of plasma triglycerides (top panel) and insulin (bottom panel) in lean men (left panel) and centrally obese men (right panel).

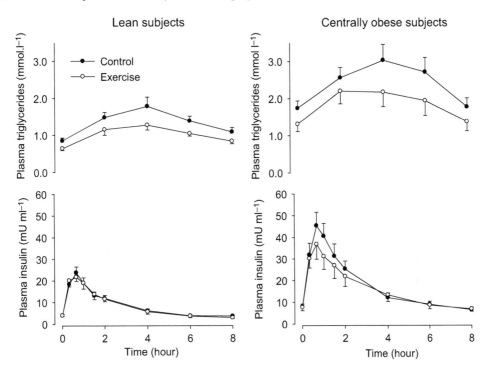

Source: Reprinted from the *Journal of the American College of Cardiology*, 44: 2375–82, Gill, J.M.R. et al., 'Effects of prior moderate exercise on postprandial metabolism and vascular function in lean and centrally obese men', page 2378, copyright © 2004, with permission from Elsevier.
Note: Middle-aged men walked for 90 mins at ~50% $\dot{V}O_2$max during the afternoon before the exercise trial.

Consistent with this hypothesis, a single session of aerobic exercise has been shown to attenuate postprandial hypertriglyceridaemia. Figure 7.7 presents data from a repeated measures laboratory study in lean middle-aged men and in men with central obesity (Gill et al. 2004). On one occasion the men walked briskly for 90 minutes at 50% of $\dot{V}O_2$max in the afternoon before eating the test meal for breakfast the following morning (exercise); in the control situation they refrained from all exercise the day before the test meal (control). Postprandial triglycerides were reduced by about 25% with prior exercise, while postprandial hyperinsulinaemia was significantly reduced only in the obese men.

The benefits of a single bout of aerobic exercise in participants with an increased risk of CVD has also been demonstrated in individuals of South Asian ethnicity, who have been shown to have an increased risk of coronary heart disease both in South Asia and after migration to Western nations (Ghaffar et al. 2004; Wild et al. 2007). Using a similar study design to that described above, the completion of 60 minutes of running at 70% of $\dot{V}O_2$max in the afternoon before consuming standardised high fat meals for breakfast and lunch reduced postprandial triglycerides by approximately 22% in

Figure 7.8 Prior exercise attenuates increases in plasma triglycerides after high fat feeding in participants of South Asian (SA) and white European (EU) descent.

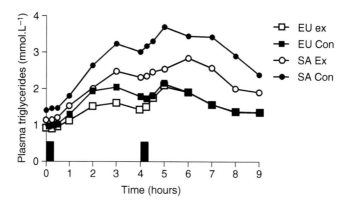

Source: Reprinted with permission from Wolters Kluwer Health, Inc.: Arjunan, S.P. et al. (2013) 'Exercise and coronary heart disease risk markers in South Asian and European men', *Medicine and Science in Sports and Exercise*, 45: 1261–8. Available at: https://doi.org/10.1249/MSS.0b013e3182853ecf.
Notes: Participants ran for 60 mins at ~70% of $\dot{V}O_2$max during the afternoon before the exercise trial. Note that exercise reduced postprandial lipaemia by a greater extent in South Asian participants but that their values remained higher than the control (no exercise) trial for white European participants.

South Asian participants and 10% in European participants, respectively (Arjunan et al. 2013) (Figure 7.8). However, despite the effectiveness of exercise in the South Asian participants, it is important to note that their postprandial triglycerides values still remained 33% higher after exercise than the control trial values exhibited by the European participants. This difference in postprandial metabolism may contribute to the elevated CVD risk in South Asian populations. The higher baseline triglyceride values may have also contributed to the greater reductions observed in response to exercise (i.e. higher values provide a greater potential for reductions). Nevertheless, this supports the effectiveness of exercise to reduce excursions in postprandial triglycerides even in participants with impaired metabolic control.

The energy expenditure of an exercise session is an important determinant of its effects on postprandial lipaemia, as shown by a study in which exercise intensity was 'traded' for duration (Tsetsonis and Hardman 1996). Postprandial lipaemia was measured on three mornings, again in a repeated measures design. These were: after two days with minimal activity (control); after a 90-minute walk at 60% of $\dot{V}O_2$max the previous afternoon; and after walking for twice as long at half the intensity (Figure 7.9). Prior exercise reduced postprandial lipaemia by nearly one-third, irrespective of its intensity. The importance of energy expenditure has been further substantiated by evidence that the reduction in postprandial lipaemia after two hours of brisk walking is approximately twice as large as that achieved with one hour of brisk walking (Gill et al. 2002). This is consistent with the evidence from randomised controlled trials investigating the effects of longer-term exercise training described above, where a clear dose–response relationship between exercise energy expenditure and increases in HDL concentrations has been observed.

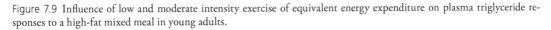

Figure 7.9 Influence of low and moderate intensity exercise of equivalent energy expenditure on plasma triglyceride responses to a high-fat mixed meal in young adults.

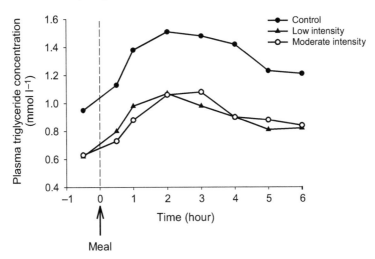

Source: Reprinted with permission from Wolters Kluwer Health, Inc.: Tsetsonis, N.V. and Hardman, A.E. (1996) 'Reduction in postprandial lipemia after walking: influence of exercise intensity', *Medicine and Science in Sports and Exercise*, 28: 1235–42. Available at: https://doi.org/10.1097/00005768-199610000-00005.

The reduction in postprandial lipaemia as a result of exercise is substantially larger than that observed in response to dietary-induced energy deficit of similar magnitude; in other words, expending 400 kcal through exercise has a greater effect on postprandial lipid metabolism than reducing energy intake by 400 kcal (Gill and Hardman 2000). However, if the energy expended during exercise is replaced by increasing subsequent energy intake, the effect on postprandial triglyceride concentrations is markedly attenuated (Burton et al. 2008), suggesting that the size of the exercise-induced energy deficit is an important mediator of the triglyceride-lowering effect, at least in response to aerobic exercise sessions. Resistance exercise (Peddie et al. 2012) and short-duration high-intensity interval exercise (Freese et al. 2011) are also both effective in lowering postprandial triglyceride concentrations. For these forms of exercise, the reductions in postprandial lipaemia occur despite relatively low levels of exercise energy expenditure, suggesting that for exercise modes involving intense muscle contractions factors other than energy expenditure are likely to contribute to the triglyceride-lowering effect. This is an area where further research is required.

Mechanisms for improvements in lipid metabolism after physical activity

Prior exercise appears to reduce postprandial lipaemia by increasing triglyceride clearance from the circulation, rather than reducing hepatic triglyceride production. There are several factors that may contribute to this improvement in triglyceride clearance, including: a) increased muscle LPL activity as the rate-limiting step in triglyceride

251

clearance, and b) increased blood perfusion towards skeletal muscle after exercise thereby increasing the exposure of triglyceride-rich lipoproteins to LPL for the stimulation of lipolysis and consequent reductions in plasma triglycerides. Although these factors may often be involved in the observed improvements in circulating triglyceride concentrations after exercise, beneficial effects have been observed even in the absence of any increases in muscle LPL activity. Indeed, recent evidence suggests that the dominant mechanism underlying the improvements in postprandial lipaemia is a specific beneficial effect of exercise on VLDL packaging (in the liver) and subsequent breakdown (at the muscle).

These changes in VLDL 'packaging' are demonstrated by the release of larger, more triglyceride-enriched VLDL particles by the liver after prior exercise. The mechanisms responsible for changes to the composition of VLDL particles are not fully understood but these alterations increase the affinity of LPL to bind with the VLDL and hydrolyse the triglyceride content. This change is considered to be the dominant mechanism for improvements in postprandial lipaemia because the affinity of LPL to hydrolyse chylomicrons and small VLDL particles does not change in response to exercise (Ghafouri et al. 2015). It seems likely that the biggest improvements in postprandial lipaemia will involve an interaction between improved VLDL packaging, increased LPL activity and increased muscle blood flow. However, ongoing research seeks to further understand the mechanisms for these improvements in response to different types of exercise.

BLOOD PRESSURE

Hypertension is another major risk factor for CVD which is influenced by exercise. According to Messerli and colleagues (2007) the risk of becoming hypertensive (blood pressure >140/90 mm Hg; Table 7.2) during a lifetime exceeds 90% in industrialised countries. The fact that the prevalence of hypertension increases dramatically with age suggests that high blood pressure is an inevitable consequence of ageing. This is not the case, however, and there are reports from several groups around the world demonstrating that blood pressure does not always increase with age. This includes the indigenous Tsimane of the Bolivian Amazon who were described earlier in the chapter, and previous evidence from the Kung Bushmen of Northern Botswana who also live as hunter-gatherers all year round. In contrast to the situation in developed

Table 7.2 Blood pressure classification for adults aged 18 and older.

BLOOD PRESSURE CATEGORY	SYSTOLIC BLOOD PRESSURE (mm Hg)		DIASTOLIC BLOOD PRESSURE (mm Hg)
Normal	<120	and	<80
Prehypertension	120–139	or	80–89
Stage 1 hypertension	140–159	or	90–99
Stage 2 hypertension	≥160	or	≥100

Source: Joint National Committee on Prevention, Detection, Evaluation, and Treatment of High Blood Pressure (2004).

Figure 7.10 Systolic blood pressures for Kung Bushmen and women of Northern Botswana and for men and women living in England.

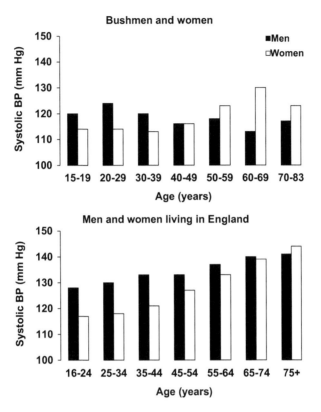

Source: Data for the Kung tribe are from Truswell et al. (1972). Data for English men and women are for the year 2005 courtesy of the British Heart Foundation (2007).

countries, systolic and diastolic blood pressures remain low throughout life in male and female Kung Bushmen (Truswell et al. 1972) (Figure 7.10). Several factors may explain their low blood pressure values, including a low salt intake, freedom from the stresses of civilisation and the high levels of physical activity which are characteristic of a hunter-gatherer lifestyle.

The question 'Are people who are physically active and fit less likely to develop hypertension than their inactive, unfit peers?' was addressed by landmark cohort studies in the 1980s. Among the Harvard alumni studied by Paffenbarger and colleagues (1983), men who did not report engaging in vigorous sports were 35% more likely to develop hypertension during the 6–10-year follow-up than those who did. Among men and women in the Aerobics Center Longitudinal Study, individuals with low fitness (least-fit quintile) were 52% more likely than those with high fitness (most-fit quintile) to develop hypertension (Blair et al. 1984).

The inverse relationship between fitness and hypertension risk is supported by the more recent Coronary Artery Risk Development in Young Adults (CARDIA) study

(Carnethon et al. 2003). The fitness of 4,392 participants aged 18–30 years was assessed during an incremental exercise test in 1985–6 and the incidence rate of hypertension was then monitored for 15 years. The findings revealed that those classified as having low baseline fitness (below the 20th percentile of the study cohort) had approximately double the risk for developing hypertension as those with the highest baseline fitness (above the 60th percentile of the study cohort). This increased risk was calculated after adjustment for other risk factors (age, race, sex, smoking status, BMI, and family history of diabetes, hypertension or premature myocardial infarction), which demonstrates the independent benefits of aerobic fitness to reduce hypertension risk.

The benefits of aerobic fitness also extend to populations that have developed 'prehypertension'. In a study of 2,303 prehypertensive middle-aged and older male veterans, a lower baseline exercise capacity was associated with an increased risk of developing hypertension over a median follow-up period of 7.8 years (Faselis et al. 2012). The hazard ratios for this relationship are displayed in Figure 7.11, which demonstrates the marked protective effects of fitness when exercise capacity exceeded 8.5 METs.

Intervention studies have confirmed the blood pressure lowering effect of exercise. A meta-analysis of 54 randomised controlled trials whose intervention and control groups differed only in aerobic exercise, reported average reductions in systolic and diastolic blood pressure of 3.8 and 2.6 mm Hg, respectively. Reductions were noted in hypertensive and normotensive participants and in overweight as well as in normal weight participants (Whelton et al. 2002). This is further supported by a recent meta-analysis

Figure 7.11 Higher baseline exercise capacity is associated with a reduced risk of developing hypertension in prehypertensive middle-aged and older males.

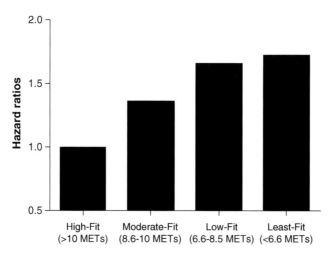

Source: Adapted with permission from Wolters Kluwer Health, Inc.: Faselis, C. et al. (2012) 'Exercise capacity and progression from prehypertension to hypertension', *Hypertension*, 60: 333–8. Available at: https://doi.org/10.1161/HYPERTENSIONAHA.112.196493.

Notes: The hazard ratios are based on a median follow-up period of 7.8 years. Note the marked protective effects of fitness when exercise capacity exceeded 8.5 METs. Hazard ratios were adjusted for age, body mass index, resting systolic blood pressure, diabetes mellitus and smoking.

which reported reductions in systolic and diastolic blood pressure of 11.4 and 6.5 mm Hg, respectively, after physical activity interventions in a total of 1,014 hypertensive participants (Baena et al. 2014).

The beneficial effects of exercise extend to patients with resistant hypertension. This is defined by either: being unable to reach target blood pressure readings despite receiving three or more anti-hypertension medications (one of which being a diuretic); or a blood pressure controlled by >4 antihypertensive agents. In this population, Dimeo and colleagues (2012) revealed that walking at an intensity slightly above the aerobic threshold, three times per week for 8 to 12 weeks, reduced daytime systolic and diastolic ambulatory blood pressure by an average of 5.9 and 3.3 mm Hg, respectively. Hence, a low responsiveness to antihypertensive drug therapy does not inevitably mean a low responsiveness to exercise.

Exercise has both acute and chronic effects on blood pressure, and it is now well documented that a single session of aerobic exercise causes a transient lowering of blood pressure. This has been termed post-exercise hypotension and the effect has been shown to last for up to 22 hours in elderly hypertensive patients (Rondon et al. 2002). These benefits can also be achieved by accumulating smaller bouts of physical activity throughout the day. This has been shown by Bhammar and colleagues (2012) who completed a randomised cross-over trial with 11 prehypertensive participants. On one occasion the participants walked for 10 minutes in the morning, at midday and in the evening (accumulated exercise); on another occasion the participants walked continuously for 30 minutes at midday (continuous exercise); and in the control situation did not perform any exercise during the day (control). Although both exercise regimens reduced 24-hour ambulatory blood pressure compared with the control trial, this effect was greater and lasted for longer in the accumulated exercise trial (Figure 7.12). Additionally, the fractionising of exercise bouts to be accumulated throughout the day may be particularly beneficial for very inactive and/or unfit participants who are likely to better tolerate smaller exercise doses.

The effects of resistance exercise on blood pressure responses are less clear. This is highlighted through the conflicting findings of two recent meta-analyses investigating the acute and repeated effects of resistance exercise. The meta-analysis of 28 randomised controlled trials (each of which lasted for a minimum of four weeks) and included a total of 1,012 participants, demonstrated a significant decrease in blood pressure for normotensive and prehypertensive subgroups after resistance exercise training but no significant changes for the five interventions performed in hypertensive participants (Cornelissen et al. 2011). By contrast, a meta-analysis of 30 acute studies involving 646 participants revealed a reduction in blood pressure for up to 24 hours after a single bout of resistance exercise, with a more pronounced effect in hypertensive than in normotensive participants (Casonatto et al. 2016). Further investigations into the effects of resistance exercise training on blood pressure responses in hypertensive participants are required before its potential utility as an antihypertensive exercise mode can be assessed.

Aerobic exercise is an established nonpharmacological therapy for hypertension, along with salt and alcohol restriction. Whether exercise can reduce hypertensive blood pressure values to normotensive values depends on the severity of hypertension and the amount of exercise performed. For those with mild hypertension, exercise may be sufficient to reduce blood pressure below hypertensive cut-off points, although not

Figure 7.12 Percentage of normal, prehypertensive and hypertensive range systolic blood pressure readings for 24 hours with fractionised (3 x 10 min) exercise, a single bout of exercise (1 x 30 min) or no exercise (control).

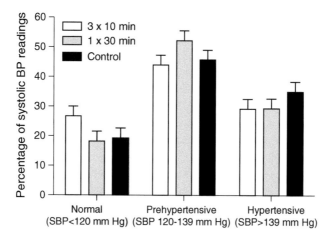

Source: Adapted with permission from Wolters Kluwer Health, Inc.: Bhammar, D.M. et al. (2012) 'Effects of fractionized and continuous exercise on 24-h ambulatory blood pressure', *Medicine and Science in Sports and Exercise*, 44: 2270–6. Available at: https://doi.org/10.1249/MSS.0b013e3182663117.

Notes: Exercise consisted of walking on a treadmill at 60–65% of $\dot{V}O_2$max. Blood pressure was assessed as 24-hour ambulatory blood pressure. The percentage of systolic blood pressure values <120 mm Hg was significantly higher with the fractionised exercise compared with the other trials ($P < 0.001$).

necessarily to normal or optimal levels. Nevertheless, the hypotensive effects of exercise described in this chapter are of clinical relevance based on data from large, prospective intervention studies investigating morbidity and mortality outcomes. For example, a meta-analysis of data for one million adults in 61 prospective studies revealed that a 2 mm Hg lower usual systolic blood pressure would reduce the risk of stroke mortality by approximately 10% and reduce the risk of mortality from ischaemic heart disease or other vascular causes by approximately 7%, in middle age (Lewington et al. 2002).

Several mechanisms have been proposed to explain the blood pressure lowering effect of exercise, and these include reductions in total peripheral resistance due to reduced sympathetic nerve activity and increased responsiveness to vasodilators such as nitric oxide. Exercise may also invoke structural changes to arteries and veins, leading to increases in cross-sectional area and hence less resistance to blood flow. The stimulation of sustained vasodilation from acute aerobic exercise appears to be primarily due to increases in the vasodilator histamine and resetting of the baroreceptor reflex and sympathetic withdrawal after exercise. In contrast, resistance exercise may reduce systemic vascular conductance; subsequently the hypotension experienced after resistance exercise is more likely the result of central mechanisms such as reductions in cardiac output. These mechanisms have been recently reviewed in detail by Romero and colleagues (2017) and the interested reader is directed to their publication. Several of these mechanisms also relate to improvements in endothelial function, which will be discussed next.

ENDOTHELIAL FUNCTION

Endothelial function refers to the ability of the endothelium (the thin layer of cells lining blood vessels) to interact with vascular smooth muscle to influence blood flow. Endothelial cells exert their effects by secreting various agents that diffuse to the adjacent vascular smooth muscle and induce either vasodilation or vasoconstriction. One important vasodilator released by endothelial cells is nitric oxide. This is released continuously in the basal state, but its secretion can be rapidly increased in response to chemical stimulants such as those released during exercise. Nitric oxide secretion is also elevated in response to increases in shear stress – that is, the force exerted on the endothelium by blood flow. This would result in flow-induced arterial vasodilation, thereby allowing the blood to flow freely and preventing undue increases in blood pressure. This is also an important mechanism for increasing blood flow when required, such as increasing blood flow to the working muscles during exercise.

Endothelial dysfunction is thought to contribute towards all stages of atherosclerosis. Endothelial injury or dysfunction increases permeability to lipoproteins and promotes the adhesion of monocytes to the endothelium to progress the initial stages of atherosclerosis. Once atherosclerotic plaques are formed within blood vessels, endothelial dysfunction is also associated with these plaques becoming particularly vulnerable to rupture which increases the risk of adverse cardiovascular events. Vulnerable plaques are characterised by the presence of a large lipid pool inside the plaque, a thin fibrous cap, increased macrophage infiltration and apoptosis (cell death) within the cap which results in the growth of a necrotic core. The rupture of coronary atherosclerotic plaques is the major mechanism of coronary thrombosis (the formation of a blood clot within a blood vessel of the heart) which can restrict blood flow within the heart and cause myocardial infarction. These consequences highlight the importance of maintaining endothelial function to minimise the initiation and development of vulnerable plaques throughout all stages of atherosclerosis (Matsuzawa and Lerman 2014). Figure 7.13 provides an illustration of vulnerable atherosclerotic plaque rupture.

Prolonged improvements in endothelial function as a result of exercise training appear to stimulate additional adaptations in the form of arterial remodelling (increased arterial size). Indeed, prolonged exercise training in various animal models enlarges the diameter of arteries and it is well established that exercise training induces structural enlargement of conduit vessels (large blood vessels that conduct blood from the heart to the systemic circulation) in humans. This is supported by observational evidence in the form of autopsy studies. An example is the case study of Clarence DeMar ('Mr Marathon'). DeMar was a prolific marathon runner who competed throughout his adult life. He died of cancer at the age of 70. The autopsy of his coronary arteries revealed that they were two or three times the normal diameter (Currens and White 1961) (Figure 7.14). Although there was some evidence of atherosclerosis in DeMar's arteries, no impairment of blood supply was apparent because of their large size. The question this study cannot answer is whether these large coronary arteries were the result of genetic inheritance, regular vigorous exercise or a combination of the two.

Cross-sectional studies have demonstrated that the coronary arteries of endurance-trained athletes have a significantly greater dilating capacity than those of inactive men

Figure 7.13 Schematic of vulnerable atherosclerotic plaque rupture.

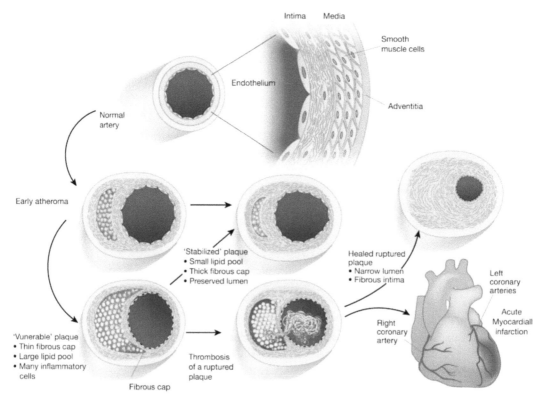

Source: Reprinted by permission from Springer Nature Customer Service Centre GmbH: Springer Nature, *Nature*, 'Inflammation in atherosclerosis', Libby, P., copyright © 2002.

(Haskell et al. 1993). Moreover, exercise training improves endothelium-dependent vasodilation; an effect which was elegantly and comprehensively demonstrated by Hambrecht and colleagues in 2003. In this study, 17 patients with stable coronary artery disease completed four weeks of aerobic exercise training while a matched control group of 18 participants remained sedentary throughout this period. Participants were assessed for *in vivo* measures of endothelial function before and after the intervention period by measuring the vasodilatory response to acetylcholine infusion (an endothelium-dependent vasodilator) and adenosine-mediated increases in blood flow in the left internal mammary artery. All participants underwent prescheduled coronary bypass surgery at the end of the four weeks which enabled tissue sampling of the left internal mammary artery for molecular analysis. Exercise training improved vasodilation in response to acetylcholine infusion and increased blood flow in the left internal mammary artery after adenosine infusion (Figure 7.15). These findings were supported by significantly greater *in vitro* endothelium-dependent vasodilation and approximately double the levels of endothelial nitric oxide synthase mRNA and protein content in the trained group compared with the control group. The rise in endothelial nitric oxide synthase expression is most likely

Figure 7.14 Cross-section of the left and right coronary arteries of Clarence DeMar 'Mr Marathon'.

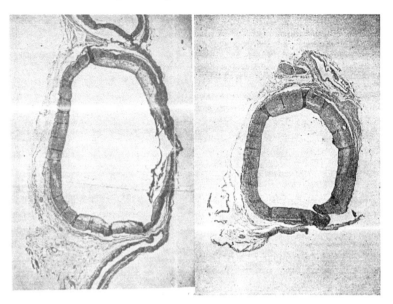

Left coronary artery   **Right coronary artery**

Source: From the *New England Journal of Medicine*, Currens, J.H. and White, P.D., 'Half a century of running: clinical, physiologic and autopsy findings in the case of Clarence DeMar ("Mr. Marathon")', 16: 988–93. Copyright © 1961 Massachusetts Medical Society. Reprinted with permission from Massachusetts Medical Society.
Note: DeMar was a prolific marathon runner and following his death an autopsy of his heart revealed that his coronary arteries were two to three times the normal diameter. Note the large lumens and minimal atherosclerosis.

mediated by increases in sheer stress during exercise training and this is thought to be largely responsible for the associated *in vivo* improvements in vasodilatory responsiveness.

Although the 'gold-standard' measure of vascular function is to assess the change in coronary artery diameter in response to acetylcholine infusion, the invasive nature of this procedure has precluded many investigations and resulted in the introduction of an alternative technique involving the examination of flow-mediated dilation of a peripheral conduit artery (Box 7.1) This method is based on the principle that an increase in blood flow due to reactive hyperaemia can enhance shear stress-induced nitric oxide production, and this approach has been shown to correlate well with results acquired from more invasive tests (for a review of techniques, see Barac et al. (2007)). Improvements in flow-mediated dilatation in response to exercise training have recently been highlighted in a meta-analysis of 51 randomised controlled trials including a total of 2,260 participants (Ashor et al. 2015). The results revealed a mean improvement of 2–2.8% units in response to ≥ 4 weeks of exercise training, with further analysis revealing a dose–response relationship between aerobic exercise intensity and improvements in endothelial function. In this regard, although exercise of all intensities was deemed to be beneficial (ranging from light to vigorous exercise), an increase in absolute exercise intensity of two metabolic equivalents (METs), or a 10% increase in relative

Figure 7.15 The percentage change in diameter of the left internal mammary artery in response to acetylcholine (left panel) and adenosine (right panel) infusion before and after four weeks of exercise training or sedentary activity.

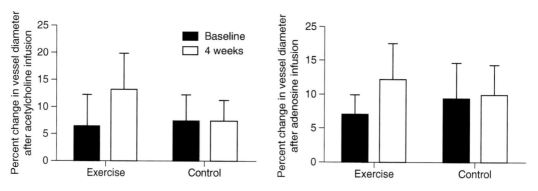

Source: Hambrecht et al. (2003).

Notes: Acetylcholine stimulates endothelium-dependent vasodilatory responses, adenosine infusion stimulates increases in blood flow and subsequently assesses flow-dependent vasodilation. Participants were patients with stable coronary artery disease. Note the improvements after exercise training but no changes in the sedentary control group. Acetylcholine infusion was 7.2 μg min^{-1}, adenosine infusion was 2.4 mg min^{-1}.

exercise intensity, resulted in a 1% unit improvement in flow-mediated dilatation. Such an effect may be caused by higher levels of shear stress on the endothelium during higher intensity exercise, and subsequently greater production and release of nitric oxide. Regardless of intensity, the magnitude of improvement in flow-mediated dilatation as a result of exercise training appears to be clinically relevant based on reports from prospective cohort studies that a 1% unit increase is associated with a 13% reduction in the risk of cardiovascular events (Inaba et al. 2010).

In order to more directly assess the impact of exercise training on vascular function and remodelling in humans, Tinken and colleagues (2008) investigated changes in brachial and popliteal arteries every two weeks during an eight week aerobic training programme in healthy young men. The results demonstrated an increase in flow-mediated dilatation within two weeks of exercise training but a return towards baseline levels after eight weeks of training. Brachial and popliteal artery dilator capacity (a surrogate marker for arterial remodelling) gradually increased across the eight-week training period as functional measures returned to baseline levels (Figure 7.16). The time course of these responses provides further support for the concept that exercise-induced functional changes in conduit arteries precede structural adaptations. Indeed, this response may be expected as the improvements in vascular function due to repeated sheer stress from exercise drive arterial remodelling to reduce the shear stress induced by similar stimuli in the future. This time course of events should also be considered when interpreting the effects of exercise training on flow-mediated responses because structural changes may partly supersede and replace the need for vasodilator mechanisms if the exercise stimulus is not increased.

In addition to increases in nitric oxide production as described above, other potential mechanisms responsible for exercise-induced improvements in endothelial function include a decrease in oxidative stress and an increased production of extracellular superoxide dismutase (an antioxidant enzyme which prevents the premature breakdown

BOX 7.1 METHODS FOR ASSESSING FLOW-MEDIATED DILATION (FMD). ▮

Flow-mediated dilation measures changes in the diameter of a conduit artery in response to an increase in shear stress induced by a surge in blood flow. This is most commonly measured using the brachial artery (located close to the inside of the elbow).

A surge in blood flow is stimulated by reactive hyperaemia whereby a cuff is inflated either above or below the conduit artery to induce ischemia of the distal tissues. The rapid release of the inflated pressure cuff then stimulates an increase in blood flow to these distal tissues, with the increase in shear stress stimulating flow-mediated vasodilation of the conduit artery. The change in artery diameter is measured using ultrasound.

Flow-mediated dilation has been used in a number of large-sized studies to investigate vascular function due to the simplicity and non-invasive nature of this measure. However, it is important to note that this technique is highly dependent on the skill of the examiner to produce high-quality ultrasound images for accurate analysis.

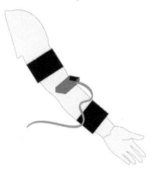

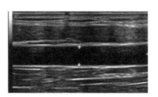

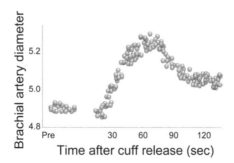

Source: Figures reprinted with permission from Wolters Kluwer Health, Inc.: Matsuzawa, Y. and Lerman, A., (2014) 'Endothelial dysfunction and coronary artery disease: assessment, prognosis, and treatment', *Coronary Artery Disease*, 25: 713–24. Available at: https://doi.org/10.1097/MCA.0000000000000178.

Figure 7.16 Changes in flow-mediated dilatation and dilator capacity of the brachial artery during eight weeks of aerobic exercise training.

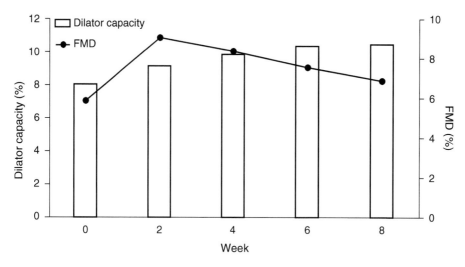

Source: Tinken et al. (2008).
Notes: Dilator capacity is a surrogate marker for arterial remodelling. Flow-mediated dilation improved after two weeks of exercise which indicates improved endothelial function. Continuous improvements in dilator capacity during the eight weeks may partly supersede and replace the need for vasodilator mechanisms, resulting in values for flow-mediated dilatation returning towards baseline values.

of nitric oxide). These improvements in vascular function and structure allow for an appropriate distribution of blood to cardiac muscle at all times and represent a direct means by which exercise may aid in the prevention of CVD.

INSULIN RESISTANCE AND GLUCOSE TOLERANCE

The beneficial effects of exercise on glucose tolerance and type 2 diabetes incidence have been explained in Chapter 5. The following section complements this evidence by discussing the acute enhancements to insulin sensitivity and glucose tolerance observed in response to physical activity and the mechanisms underlying this effect.

The level of glucose within the circulation is ultimately determined by the balance between glucose entry and removal. Glucose enters the circulation from the absorption of exogenous carbohydrate across the small intestine after a meal, and from the liver as a result of liver glycogen breakdown and/or gluconeogenesis. It leaves the blood by uptake into various tissues, including the brain, liver and muscle. The disposal of glucose into skeletal muscle after a meal is particularly important to prevent excessive increases in blood glucose. This process is stimulated by insulin and skeletal muscle is the body's largest insulin-sensitive tissue and the major influence on whole-body responsiveness to insulin.

Although insulin resistance can occur and limit glucose clearance from the blood at rest, it is well established that skeletal muscle contractions during exercise stimulate an increase in glucose uptake independently of insulin signalling. This effect can be large, with evidence in rodent studies demonstrating that muscle contraction during exercise can be a more potent physiological stimulus of skeletal muscle glucose uptake than even maximal insulin stimulation (James et al. 1985). Exercise-induced increases in glucose uptake are achieved by an increase in glucose delivery, glucose transport and glucose metabolism, which all work together during exercise to increase muscle glucose uptake. The increase in glucose delivery to the muscle is achieved by an increase in muscle blood flow during exercise which is proportional with exercise intensity. Increases in glucose transport into the muscle occur as a result of GLUT-4 translocation to the cell membrane which is stimulated by muscle contraction independently of insulin signalling (Figure 7.17). This is further supported by the utilisation and depletion of muscle glycogen concentrations during exercise, which reduce the accumulation of intramuscular glucose-6-phosphate and subsequently increase the use of intramuscular glucose for energy production. Consequently, free glucose concentrations in the muscle are reduced, which increases the concentration gradient for glucose uptake from the bloodstream. For an extensive review of these processes, see Sylow et al. (2017).

An example of the insulin-independent effects of exercise for increasing glucose uptake can be demonstrated in participants with type 2 diabetes. Despite being resistant to the effects of insulin, these individuals do not show impairments in glucose uptake during exercise when compared with healthy, matched control participants. This was shown in a sophisticated experiment by Martin and colleagues (1995) through the measurement of glucose concentrations in the femoral artery and femoral vein during 40 minutes of cycling at 60% of $\dot{V}O_2$max. The difference in glucose concentrations

Figure 7.17 Stimulation of glucose transporter 4 (GLUT-4) translocation to the cell membrane by the actions of insulin and muscle contraction.

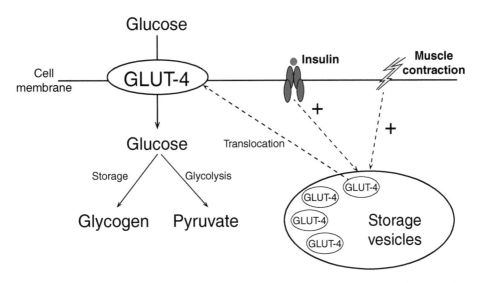

Note: Muscle contraction and/or the binding of insulin to its receptor signals for the translocation of GLUT-4 from storage vesicles inside the cell towards the cell membrane. Once GLUT-4 is located at the cell membrane, glucose can enter the cell down the concentration gradient.

between these blood samples (termed the arteriovenous difference) was multiplied by blood flow across the working muscle during exercise to determine total glucose uptake by the quadriceps during exercise. Rather than being impaired, leg glucose uptake was actually enhanced in the participants with type 2 diabetes compared with the control group, which is most likely to have been mediated by an enhanced concentration gradient for glucose transport across the muscle cell membrane due to elevated plasma glucose concentrations (Figure 7.18). These insulin-independent increases in muscle glucose uptake during exercise demonstrate the potential benefits of physical activity as a nonpharmacological method by which to decrease hyperglycaemia in insulin-resistant states.

In addition to increases in glucose uptake during exercise, the completion of an exercise bout is associated with improvements in insulin sensitivity and responsiveness (assessed by glucose clamp techniques – see Box 7.2) in the hours and days after exercise. One elegant study demonstrating that exercise improves glucose transport into muscle and muscle glycogen synthesis employed phosphorus-31 and carbon-13 nuclear magnetic resonance spectroscopy and a hyperglycaemic-hyperinsulinaemic clamp technique (Perseghin et al. 1996). Nuclear magnetic resonance enables identification of organic molecules within skeletal muscle (and other targeted tissues), with phosphorus-31 used to identify glucose-6-phosphate concentrations within the muscle,

Figure 7.18 Glucose uptake by the working muscles is not impaired during exercise in patients with non-insulin-dependent diabetes mellitus (NIDDM; the earlier term for type 2 diabetes) compared with healthy control participants.

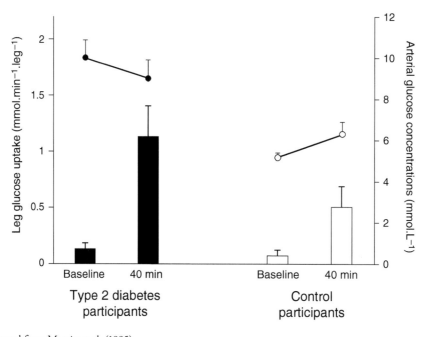

Source: Adapted from Martin et al. (1995).
Notes: Single leg glucose uptake is displayed by the bars, arterial glucose concentrations are displayed by the lines and associated data points. Exercise consisted of 40 minutes of cycling at 60% of V̇O₂max and glucose uptake was estimated from arteriovenous differences.

BOX 7.2 GLUCOSE CLAMP TECHNIQUES.

The most accurate (gold-standard) method for determining the blood glucose response to insulin is the euglycaemic clamp technique. This involves intravenous (via a vein) infusion of insulin to produce the same plasma insulin concentration in all individuals. Simultaneously, glucose is infused intravenously to obtain euglycaemia (equal blood glucose concentration). The greater the quantity of glucose required to produce euglycaemia, the more insulin sensitive (less insulin resistant) the individual.

An alternative glucose clamp technique is the hyperglycaemic clamp which involves continuous intravenous glucose infusion to maintain a stable level of elevated blood glucose concentrations (hyperglycaemia). The measurement of insulin secretion in response to the glucose infusion provides a measure of beta-cell function, while the requirement of a greater quantity of glucose to maintain a constant level of hyperglycaemia indicates higher levels of glucose metabolism by the body's tissues.

---

and carbon-13 used to identify the incorporation of infused glucose into muscle glycogen (the infused glucose was 'labelled' with carbon-13 to identify incorporation, whereas the body's natural glucose contains only carbon-12). The simultaneous hyperglycaemic-hyperinsulinaemic clamp technique was used to maximise glucose transport into skeletal muscle by elevating circulating concentrations of both glucose and insulin.

Ten adult children of parents with type 2 diabetes and a control group of eight adult children of parents who did not have type 2 diabetes were studied before starting an exercise programme, after one session of exercise, and after six weeks of exercise training four times per week. At baseline, muscle glycogen synthesis (indicated by carbon-13 concentration in the gastrocnemius muscle) was 63% lower in the offspring of diabetic parents than in control participants. Glycogen synthesis increased 69% and 62% after the first exercise session and 102% and 97% after six weeks of exercise training in the offspring and control participants, respectively. The increment in glucose-6-phosphate during hyperglycaemic-hyperinsulinaemic clamping was lower in the offspring than in control subjects at baseline (reflecting impaired glucose transport into muscle because glucose is converted into glucose-6-phosphate once entering muscle cells) but this increment was normalised in the offspring after one exercise session and after exercise training (Figure 7.19). These findings indicate that exercise increases insulin sensitivity in both healthy participants and in insulin-resistant participants.

Improvements in glucose tolerance after an acute bout of exercise have been elegantly demonstrated in recent years by a series of studies involving single leg exercise, led by Eric Richter at the University of Copenhagen. The use of single leg exercise protocols provides a direct investigation into the effects of skeletal muscle contractions on glucose tolerance by making comparisons with the non-exercising muscle of the opposite leg, while ensuring that all other central and peripheral metabolism is matched. Using this design, single leg knee extensions have been shown to enhance the effects of circulating insulin on glucose uptake and glycogen synthase activity in the exercised quadriceps compared with the rested quadriceps three to four hours after the completion of exercise (Wojtaszewski et al. 2000). The mechanisms underlying this effect are not fully elucidated but current evidence suggests that this is not mediated by increases

Figure 7.19 Increased glucose transport and glycogen synthesis in control subjects and in offspring of parents with type 2 diabetes after a single session of exercise and after six weeks of exercise training.

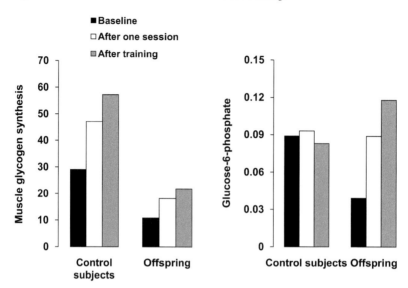

Source: Perseghin et al. (1996).

Notes: Glucose transport into muscle was estimated from phosphorus-31 concentrations, glycogen synthesis was estimated from carbon-13 concentrations. These were determined using nuclear magnetic resonance spectroscopy during a hyperglycaemic-hyperinsulinaemic clamp test. Units for muscle glycogen are mg per litre of muscle per min., units for glucose-6-phosphate are mmol l^{-1}.

in proximal insulin signalling (i.e. increased insulin receptor and IRS1/2 phosphorylation). Instead, a prior bout of exercise seems to enhance the activation of more distal insulin-signalling components in response to insulin stimulation, which may enhance GLUT4 translocation and fusion to the membrane for glucose entry into muscle cells (see Figure 7.17). The enhanced glycogen synthase activity after exercise may further facilitate glucose transport by reducing the accumulation of free glucose in the muscle and thereby maintaining the concentration gradient for glucose uptake from the bloodstream via GLUT4.

The beneficial effects of physical activity for postprandial glucose control has also been demonstrated in participants that have developed type 2 diabetes. This can be viewed as being particularly important as the progression of insulin resistance and development of type 2 diabetes results in repeated episodes of hyperglycaemia and hyperinsulinaemia after feeding, which indefinitely contributes to the health consequences of diabetes. Exercise performed in the postprandial period appears to be particularly effective for reducing glycaemic excursions after a meal. An early study to demonstrate this effect was conducted by Larsen and colleagues (1997) who found that 45 minutes of cycling at a moderate intensity attenuated postprandial hyperglycaemia and hyperinsulinaemia in patients with mild type 2 diabetes when performed 45 minutes after feeding (Figure 7.20). The timing of exercise to coincide with the increases in blood glucose that occur after food consumption stimulates an interactive effect between the

Figure 7.20 Exercise performed during the postprandial period attenuates postprandial hyperglycaemia and hyperinsuli-naemia in patients with mild non-insulin-dependent diabetes mellitus (NIDDM; the older term for type 2 diabetes).

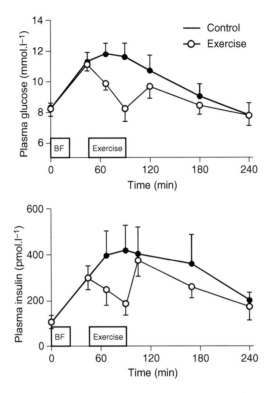

Source: Adapted by permission from Springer Nature Customer Service Centre GmbH: Springer Nature, *Diabetologia*, 'The effect of moderate exercise on postprandial glucose homeostasis in NIDDM patients', Larsen, J.J.S. et al., copyright © 1997.
Notes: BF denotes the consumption of a breakfast meal. Exercise consisted of 45 minutes of cycling at approximately 50% of $\dot{V}O_2$max and commenced 45 minutes after the first bite of the breakfast meal.

insulin-stimulated glucose uptake induced from feeding and the non-insulin stimulated glucose uptake induced by the muscular contractions. This combined effect appears to be optimal for the control of postprandial glycaemic excursions and is supported by the within-subjects comparison of preprandial and postprandial exercise by Colberg and colleagues (2009). Twelve participants with type 2 diabetes completed three trials on separate days which included a resting control trial, and two exercise trials involving 20 minutes of low to moderate intensity walking exercise either immediately before or 15–20 minutes after a 400–450 kcal evening meal. The findings demonstrated a significantly lower peak glucose concentration in response to feeding when the exercise bout was completed after the meal than when exercise was completed before the meal.

The acute benefits of performing exercise in the postprandial period intuitively suggests that the completion of regular physical activity (i.e. after each meal) is important to maximise glycaemic control in populations that either have type 2 diabetes or are at risk of developing insulin resistance. Accordingly, the promotion of an 'exercise snacking' approach has developed, which involves the completion of multiple smaller bouts of exercise throughout the day rather than a single larger bout of exercise. The benefits of an exercise snacking approach for glycaemic control was demonstrated by DiPietro and colleagues in 2013 in a group of obese older adults with a mean age of 69 years and BMI of 30 kg m^{-2}, and who were at risk of developing impaired glucose tolerance. In a randomised cross-over design, this study investigated the effects of completing 15 minutes of treadmill walking 30 minutes after the consumption of breakfast, lunch and dinner meals, compared with performing a single 45-minute bout of treadmill walking in either the mid-morning or mid-afternoon (i.e. between meals). All walks were completed at an absolute intensity of 3.0 METs, which corresponded to an average walking speed of three miles per hour. The results of the study revealed similar improvements in 24-hour glycaemic control after the intermittent walking and morning walking protocols but that the intermittent walking exercise was the only intervention to lower blood glucose excursions during the three-hour period after the evening meal was consumed. This suggests that a smaller exercise dose repeated several times per day may provide greater overall benefits than a single larger dose performed once per day.

The beneficial effects of physical activity for glycaemic control are further supported by improvements in glucose tolerance after the completion of exercise training programmes, as well as the long-standing observation that aerobic fitness is positively associated with insulin signalling in skeletal muscle (Kirwan et al. 2000). The benefits of exercise training have been nicely demonstrated in a recent experiment by Consitt and colleagues (2013). This study assessed insulin sensitivity using a euglycaemic-hyperinsulinaemic clamp and performed muscle biopsies to investigate insulin signalling before and after 12 weeks of endurance- or strength-orientated training in previously sedentary young (~24 years old) and older (~69 years old) participants. Fasting plasma glucose and insulin concentrations were reduced in response to both training regimens for both age groups. Peripheral insulin sensitivity was also improved in all groups as demonstrated by a higher M-value (representing the amount of glucose infused (M) in order to maintain basal plasma glucose concentration) during the euglycaemic-hyperinsulinaemic clamp. Accordingly, the analysis of muscle biopsies from the vastus lateralis revealed that both the endurance- and strength-orientated training improved insulin signalling within skeletal muscle. This demonstrates the importance of skeletal muscle for whole body glucose tolerance and shows that regular exercise can reverse the impairments developed from sedentary behaviour even in older age (Figure 7.21).

The plasticity of the human body to positively adapt in response to exercise training is matched by the reversal of these adaptations during periods of detraining. This is demonstrated by the transient nature of exercise training benefits on glucose tolerance which emphasises the importance of regular physical activity to maintain metabolic health. One of the landmark studies to show this effect was completed by Lipman and colleagues in 1972 by employing prolonged periods of bed rest to prevent physical activity and investigate the subsequent effects on glucose tolerance. This study found impairments in glucose tolerance in eight healthy young men following five weeks of bed rest but that this impairment was less severe in those permitted one hour of vigorous (70% of $\dot{V}O_2$max) supine exercise each day. Additionally, a notable study investigating masters' athletes demonstrated a loss of insulin sensitivity and glucose tolerance

Figure 7.21 Improved insulin action in younger and older adults after 12 weeks of endurance or strength training.

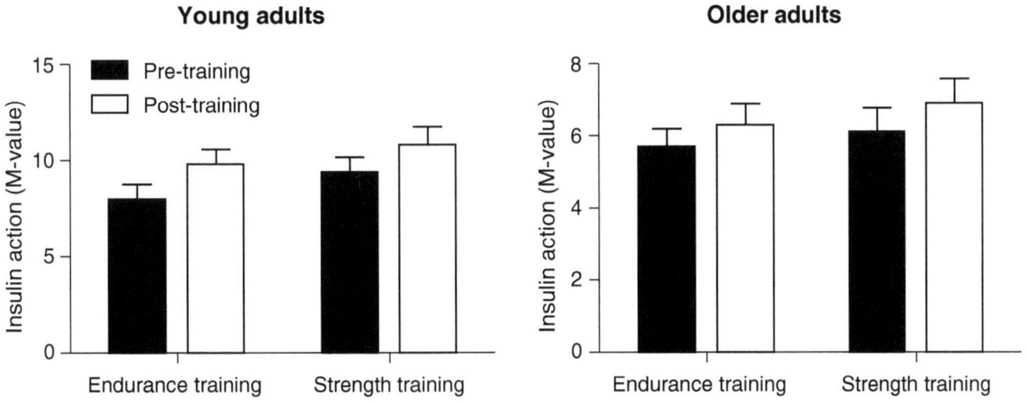

Source: Consitt et al. (2013).

Notes: Insulin action was quantified as an M-value which represents the amount of glucose infused (M) in order to maintain basal plasma glucose concentration during the euglycaemic-hyperinsulinaemic clamp. The unit of measurement is $mg\,kg^{-1}\,min^{-1}$.

after a ten-day detraining period (Rogers et al. 1990). This response concords with the rapid decline in skeletal muscle GLUT4 content observed with the cessation of exercise training and periods of inactivity (McCoy et al. 1994).

The inclusion of resistance exercise within a training programme appears to confer additional benefits for glucose tolerance. This is perhaps not surprising when considering that skeletal muscle is responsible for approximately 80% of insulin-mediated glucose uptake after a meal and that resistance training is often associated with increases in muscle mass. Such increases in muscle mass can increase the area in which glucose disposal occurs, or expressed another way – it can increase the size of the 'sink' available for the removal of glucose from the bloodstream.

The benefits of resistance exercise for glucose disposal have been demonstrated through a randomised controlled trial of 251 adults with type 2 diabetes (Sigal et al. 2007). This study evaluated the effects of three training programmes on glycated haemoglobin (HbA1c) levels, in which exercise was performed three times per week for 22 weeks. The training programmes consisted of either an aerobic exercise programme, a resistance training programme, or a combination of the two. Although HbA1c levels were reduced in all exercise groups (−0.4% and −0.5% for the resistance and aerobic training groups, respectively), the improvement was significantly greater in the participants who completed the combined aerobic and resistance training (−1.0%). As discussed in Chapter 5, HbA1c represents a form of haemoglobin which is covalently bound to glucose and provides a marker of average blood glucose concentrations from the previous two to three months. Therefore, the improvements in HbA1c in this study are indicative of medium-term improvements in blood glucose concentrations.

One important limitation of the study above is that the combined aerobic and resistance exercise group completed the full volume of the training programmes for each exercise mode and therefore completed a greater total exercise volume than the partici-pants completing training programmes for either exercise mode in isolation (270 mins per week versus 135 mins per week). In order to clarify whether the observed improve-ments were a result of the combined exercise modes or additional training volume, Church and colleagues (2010) performed a similar study but during which all exercise training programmes comprised a comparable volume of exercise. This randomised controlled trial assigned 262 sedentary men and women with type 2 diabetes to a non-exercise control group, a resistance training group, an aerobic training group, or a training group involving a combination of resistance and aerobic training. The findings followed a similar pattern to the previous study, with the combined training group demonstrating the greatest reduction in HbA1c levels. This suggests that a combination of resistance and aerobic exercise training can produce synergistic benefits, even when the total exercise volume is matched.

Although increases in muscle mass may drive some of the improvements in glucose disposal with the combination of resistance and aerobic exercise training, this is un-likely to explain the beneficial effects compared with resistance training alone. It seems most likely that the mechanisms of improvements from aerobic exercise discussed above are present with resistance exercise and/or combine with the increases in muscle mass to increase glucose disposal. Both resistance and aerobic exercise are also capable of increasing skeletal muscle mitochondrial content and oxidative capacity which may also help to prevent and reduce insulin resistance by increasing the capacity to match rates of fatty acid uptake with oxidation. This would, in turn, prevent an accumulation of lipid intermediates such as diglycerides and ceramides within skeletal muscle which is thought to impair insulin signalling and be implicated in the pathophysiology of insulin resistance. Other training adaptations which may facilitate improved glucose and NEFA delivery and metabolism include increased capillary density and blood flow, increased muscle GLUT4 content, and increased activity of the enzymes involved in glucose (hexokinase, glycogen synthase) and oxidative metabolism (citrate synthase, succinate dehydrogenase). Similarly, reductions in body fat with exercise training may improve glucose tolerance as a result of reduced NEFA flux to the liver and muscles. These concepts are discussed further towards the end of this chapter when considering the clustering of cardio-metabolic risk factors.

THROMBOTIC RISK

As discussed in Chapter 4, regular physical activity contributes to a lower risk of thrombotic cardiovascular events. In addition to the improvements in risk factors demonstrated so far in the present chapter, exercise training may also function by di-rectly reducing the risk of thrombosis (i.e. the formation of blood clots). The potential mechanisms underlying an anti-thrombotic effect of exercise training include a reduc-tion in platelet activation (a trigger for the formation of clots), lower circulating levels of procoagulant (or clotting) factors and increased fibrinolysis activity (the enzymatic breakdown of blood clots). These mechanisms have been comprehensively reviewed by Chen and colleagues (2014) and the interested reader is referred to this source for further information.

The potential benefits of exercise to reduce the risk of thrombosis are particularly relevant considering that the only available clinical approach to managing an increased risk for arterial thrombosis is currently low-dose aspirin or other antiplatelet drugs. These medications are associated with side effects such as increased bleeding risk and, in addition, resistance towards their protective effects may develop (Colwell 2004). Consequently, any reductions in thrombotic risk as a result of exercise represent an attractive proposition. Preliminary evidence in support of this approach has been demonstrated in postmenopausal women, a population of relevance due to the increased risk of thrombosis with advancing age. In one study, twenty sedentary healthy participants were randomly separated into either an exercise training group or a control group. The exercise group completed 35 minutes of aerobic cycling exercise three times per week for a total of ten sessions, while the control group remained sedentary. The findings from the study revealed improvements in fibrinolytic function in the exercise training group, which were associated with reductions in fibrinogen (a key coagulation factor) and plasminogen activator inhibitor-1 (PAI-1) activity (a factor which inhibits the degradation of blood clots). No changes were observed in the sedentary control group which suggests that aerobic exercise training may be effective for improving fibrinolytic function in populations with an elevated risk of thrombosis (Jahangard et al. 2009). Further research is required to fully understand the effects of exercise on thrombosis risk, with a particular need for large-scale randomised controlled trials to examine the effects of different exercise protocols and the consistency of outcomes in populations with varying risks of encountering thrombotic events.

Although some evidence suggests that chronic exercise may provide an anti-thrombotic effect, an acute bout of vigorous exercise has been shown to *increase* the risk of thrombotic events. This will be discussed further in Chapter 13, but it is worth stating for now that the absolute risk of encountering a thrombotic event during exercise is very low. Current evidence suggests that light and moderate intensity exercise do not acutely increase the risk of thrombosis but that strenuous exercise ($\geq$75% of $\dot{V}O_2$max) in sedentary participants may increase platelet reactivity and thrombosis. The completion of long-term moderate exercise training has been shown to limit the risk of thrombosis evoked by strenuous exercise which further supports the benefits of regular physical activity throughout the lifespan (Wang 2006).

SYSTEMIC INFLAMMATION

Another possible pathway of physical activity benefits may be ascribed to its anti-inflammatory effects. This is supported by cross-sectional evidence from 3,042 seemingly healthy participants living in the Attica province in Greece which demonstrates an inverse association between self-reported leisure time physical activity and several inflammatory markers (Panagiotakos et al. 2005). Participants in the highest quartile for physical activity had lower levels of circulating pro-inflammatory markers, i.e. C-reactive protein (CRP) (29%), tumour necrosis factor α (TNF-α) (20%), interleukin 6 (IL-6) (32%) and fibrinogen (11%), than the participants who did not complete any leisure-time physical activity. These findings suggest that there may be a beneficial effect of physical activity on systemic inflammation even in apparently healthy individuals.

However, although cross-sectional studies provide valuable insight into the associations between physical activity levels and such markers, they cannot establish causality.

A long-term randomised controlled trial of particular note is provided from the STRRIDE project which was mentioned earlier in the chapter. In a subgroup of 139 participants who experienced an average reduction in body fat of 2.5 kg (9%) in response to the eight-month exercise interventions, there were no significant changes in any of the three commonly measured *pro*-inflammatory cytokines (CRP, TNF-α and IL-6) or in the *anti*-inflammatory cytokine interleukin-10 (Huffman et al. 2008). These results are important because several pro-inflammatory cytokines are derived from adipose tissue. Thus, it would be expected that any benefits of exercise training on systemic inflammation would be enhanced by concomitant reductions in fat mass. This suggests that the metabolic changes induced by exercise training occur independently of sustained alterations in the systemic levels of inflammatory mediators.

The contradictory findings provided from the studies described above demonstrate the importance of experimental studies to determine whether observational associations are causative, correlative or chance observations. However, there is currently insufficient research available to fully elucidate the effects of exercise training on systemic inflammation. Greater clarity is required in the future in relation to the effects of different exercise protocols (e.g. mode, intensity and frequency), observation timings (e.g. during the exercise period or in the recovery phase), and populations studied (e.g. age, gender, health conditions).

CLUSTERING OF CARDIO-METABOLIC RISK FACTORS

Although risk factors for cardio-metabolic disease may occur in isolation, some risk factors tend to cluster together. These include dyslipidaemia (specifically, high triglycerides and low HDL), insulin resistance, impaired glucose regulation or diabetes, obesity (particularly visceral obesity), hypertension and systemic low-grade inflammation. The phrase 'cluster together' means that these risk factors co-exist more commonly than would be expected by chance. For example, diabetes and obesity are twice as common among people with hypertension as among those with normal blood pressure.

The common 'cause' of the clustering of risk factors has been a subject of controversy but it seems that this is likely due to a combination of abdominal (particularly visceral) adiposity, insulin resistance and chronic low-grade inflammation. The constellation of disturbances associated with these factors has been termed the 'metabolic syndrome', which is clinically defined as a combination of three or more of the following factors: elevated waist circumference, raised triglycerides, low HDL, raised blood pressure and raised fasting glucose. Although central obesity was previously identified as an essential requirement for the metabolic syndrome by some organisations, it has now been agreed that this should not be a prerequisite for diagnosis (Alberti et al. 2009). This has provided greater clarity in the criteria required to define the metabolic syndrome but there remains considerable debate regarding whether this is a useful tool for clinicians to assess patients and improve their treatment. The main points of the debate regarding whether the metabolic syndrome is a useful concept are provided in Box 7.3.

BOX 7.3 IS THE METABOLIC SYNDROME A USEFUL CONCEPT? ▉

SUPPORT FOR THE CONCEPT OF THE
METABOLIC SYNDROME

- It provides a framework for research exploring a possible unifying pathophysiological basis for the observed cluster of risk factors.
- It quantifies chronic disease risk within populations and facilitates between-country comparisons.
- It can guide relative risk prediction and clinical management decisions.
- It provides an easily comprehensible public health message.
- It reminds health professionals of the need to assess related risk factors when one risk factor is detected.

CRITICISMS OF THE CONCEPT OF THE METABOLIC
SYNDROME

- No single pathophysiological mechanism has been agreed.
- There is no clear basis for including or excluding other CVD risk factors.
- The CVD risk is variable and dependent on the specific risk factors present.
- The equivalence of the risk factors and their cut-off points across different populations has not been established.
- The CVD risk associated with the metabolic syndrome appears to be no greater than the sum of its parts.
- The treatment of the syndrome as a whole is no different from that of each of its components.
- The metabolic syndrome criteria are outperformed by traditional CVD risk prediction algorithms such as the Framingham risk score.

Notes: This information is taken from the WHO Expert Consultation that evaluated the utility of the metabolic syndrome (Simmons et al. 2010). For further information, please refer to this consultation and the accompanying commentary by Borch-Johnsen and Wareham (2010).

The relationship between obesity and insulin resistance has already been briefly discussed in Chapter 5. The mechanisms underlying this relationship will be discussed in more detail below, in addition to the role of insulin resistance in the clustering of other cardio-metabolic risk factors (see Figure 7.22).

The relationship between obesity and insulin resistance appears to be determined by an expansion of fat stores and a subsequent 'fullness' of adipocytes resulting in metabolic dysfunction. As levels of body fat increase, this causes adipocytes to become 'fuller' which limits their ability to take up and buffer increases in circulating fat after consuming a meal. The consequence of this effect is that circulating NEFA and triglycerides remain in the circulation for longer, enhancing uptake by other tissues (e.g. skeletal muscle and liver). The excessive uptake and storage of fat in the liver and skeletal muscle can result in the accumulation of the lipid intermediates diglycerides and ceramides which decrease insulin signalling (and therefore increase insulin resistance). An increase in NEFA supply to the muscle will also promote their use as a fuel for oxidation. This reduces the need for carbohydrate oxidation to meet energy demands in the muscle and reduces glycolytic flux by downregulating phosphofructokinase and pyruvate dehydrogenase activity (two key regulating enzymes for glucose breakdown). The consequent increase in free glucose concentration in the cell then reduces glucose uptake due to a decreased glucose gradient across the sarcolemma, which means that

Figure 7.22 Schematic of the relationships between central obesity, insulin resistance and cardio-metabolic disease risk factors.

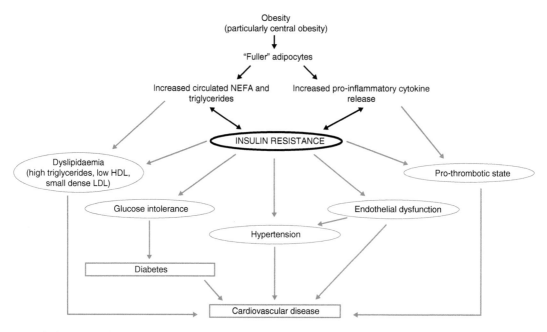

Note: Black arrows indicate the development of insulin resistance. Grey arrows indicate the influence of insulin resistance on the development of cardio-metabolic disease risk factors and subsequent cardio-metabolic disease.

glucose uptake is lower than expected for a given insulin concentration (i.e. sensitivity to insulin is reduced).

The accumulation of adipose tissue in the abdominal cavity (visceral depot) is particularly potent for the development of insulin resistance and CVD. Differences in patterns of body fat distribution may help to explain why some obese populations are at higher risk of insulin resistance than others. However, it is important to appreciate that people with severe obesity usually have high levels of adiposity in all regions and associated insulin resistance. Enlarged and 'full' adipocytes in the visceral depots have a particularly potent role in the development of insulin resistance because this location means that NEFA and triglycerides can 'overflow' directly into the portal vein towards the liver. This promotes the storage of fat within the liver, which is strongly associated with insulin resistance. The importance of abdominal adiposity is well established, with exaggerated plasma glucose and insulin responses to oral glucose challenges in men with high levels of visceral adipose tissue. Moreover, these responses remain exaggerated even when compared against men with similar levels of overall obesity but lower levels of visceral adipose tissue (Couillard et al. 1998; Pouliot et al. 1992).

A final mechanism linking obesity with insulin resistance is the development of chronic low-grade inflammation in adipose and other tissues. When adipocytes become too 'full', it becomes more difficult for oxygen to perfuse throughout the adipocyte, increasing the risk of hypoxia and cell death. Consequently, adipose tissue in the obese has a greater infiltration of macrophages to remove damaged areas of the adipocyte. It is thought that these macrophages secrete pro-inflammatory cytokines which act locally as well as systemically to increase insulin resistance and advance other cardio-metabolic risk factors. Macrophage infiltration and pro-inflammatory cytokine production is particularly prominent in visceral adipose tissue compared with subcutaneous adipose tissue, which may also contribute to explaining why fat accumulation in this area is particularly problematic for the development of insulin resistance. Increases in systemic pro-inflammatory cytokines are also thought to directly stimulate insulin resistance in the liver and muscle, thereby creating a vicious cycle between insulin resistance and inflammation. The diverse pathways by which insulin resistance and chronic low-grade inflammation increase the risk of developing cardio-metabolic disease are presented in Box 7.4, with the main aspects discussed further below.

As discussed in Chapter 5, maintaining insulin sensitivity is important for enabling glucose uptake into the muscle and adipose tissue, as well as for suppressing glucose release from the liver after feeding. Consequently, when insulin resistance develops, blood glucose concentration rises and insulin is released in greater quantities from the pancreas. Some people can maintain this and avoid becoming diabetic, exhibiting higher than normal responses of both glucose and insulin to a standard oral glucose test. In others, the ability of the islets of Langerhans to sustain high rates of insulin production begins to fail and type 2 diabetes develops.

Insulin also exerts multiple influences on lipid metabolism that affect plasma lipoprotein variables. Collectively, they promote the uptake and storage of fatty acids in adipose tissue, inhibit their mobilisation from adipose tissue and decrease secretion of VLDL from the liver. When insulin resistance develops, its normal effects are impaired, leading to high plasma concentrations of triglycerides. As discussed earlier in the chapter, exaggerated and prolonged increases in triglycerides after feeding are

---

BOX 7.4 ABNORMALITIES ASSOCIATED WITH INSULIN RESISTANCE AND CHRONIC LOW-GRADE INFLAMMATION.

- Diabetes or impaired fasting glucose/impaired glucose tolerance.
- Hyperinsulinaemia.
- Raised blood pressure.
- Atherogenic dyslipidaemia, e.g. raised triglycerides, low HDL-cholesterol, high levels of apolipoprotein B and C-III, small dense LDLs.
- High levels of postprandial lipaemia.
- Endothelial dysfunction.
- Pro-thrombotic factors, e.g. high fibrinogen and plasminogen activator inhibitor-1 (PAI-1), high viscosity.
- Microalbinuria*.
- High uric acid[†].
- Non-alcoholic fatty liver disease.

* Abnormally high albumin in urine indicative of vascular damage to glomeruli of kidney.

[†] Abnormally high uric acid in blood resulting from defects in insulin action on renal tubular reabsorption of uric acid.

thought to be causally implicated in the development of the atherogenic lipoprotein phenotype and increased CVD risk.

Insulin-resistant states are consistently associated with hypertension. Current evidence suggests that elevations in circulating insulin concentrations may have a direct influence on blood pressure by increasing sodium reabsorption in the distal tubules of the kidney. Plasma volume expands, leading to an increase in blood pressure. Insulin resistant states also promote endothelial dysfunction through inhibited production of nitric oxide and increased conversion of nitric oxide to other compounds, such as peroxynitrite. Consequently, the reduced bioavailability of nitric oxide impairs vasodilatory capacity.

Insulin resistance and chronic low-grade inflammation are also associated with increased fibrinogen production by the liver, and increased production of PAI-1 by the liver and adipose tissue. As discussed earlier in the chapter, fibrinogen is a key coagulation factor, while PAI-1 inhibits the degradation of blood clots. Subsequently, these changes result in a pro-thrombotic state (i.e. an increased risk of blood clots in blood vessels) and an increased risk of cardiovascular events. Several inflammatory cytokines may act directly to increase coagulation, while increased insulin and triglyceride concentrations also appear to play a role.

SYNERGISTIC EFFECTS OF EXERCISE ON MULTIPLE CARDIO-METABOLIC RISK FACTORS

This chapter has presented evidence which provides strong support for a causal relationship between physical activity and favourable changes in the major CVD risk factors. These benefits of physical activity are most pronounced when high levels of energy are expended on several days of the week, with the frequency of exercise being particularly important for the maintenance of low plasma triglyceride and blood glucose concentrations and to maximise the hypotensive effects of exercise.

The benefits of physical activity for different cardio-metabolic risk factors are mediated by a variety of mechanisms, as demonstrated by differences in the time course of improvements in response to acute and chronic exercise. Nevertheless, beneficial effects of exercise have been demonstrated for each of the 'clustered' risk factors displayed in Figure 7.22. This suggests that even when the effects of exercise on individual factors in isolation are fairly modest, the fact that beneficial changes are being exerted on multiple risk factors at the same time means that the benefits in terms of disease risk are likely to be substantially larger. Furthermore, this chapter has demonstrated improvements in insulin resistance with physical activity, which suggests that beneficial effects may be mediated to some extent by improvements in this key orchestrating mechanism of risk factor clustering. This can be further supported by reductions in body fat (especially central adiposity) with increases in physical activity, as discussed in Chapter 6.

The beneficial effects of physical activity on CVD risk factors are particularly relevant considering the increasing global prevalence of cardio-metabolic disease. This is further enhanced by the evidence that exercise benefits multiple risk factors that cluster together to increase the risk of CVD (i.e. glucose intolerance, dyslipidaemia and hypertension). Subsequently, exercise represents an attractive alternative to pharmacological therapy which may benefit individual pathologies but have a neutral or even negative effect on other cardio-metabolic risk factors. For example, treatment with diuretics reduces blood pressure, but also increases total cholesterol; treatment with beta-blockers reduces blood pressure but leads to a decrease in HDL. Thus, the overall benefit for CVD risk is not always clear and multiple drug regimens are often prescribed which are difficult to adhere to, particularly for older people. Finally, all drugs have side effects that have to be set against their benefits.

INDEPENDENT EFFECTS OF PHYSICAL ACTIVITY NOT EXPLAINED BY KNOWN RISK FACTORS

The protective effects of exercise against CVD appears to be much greater than the combined beneficial effects on cardio-metabolic risk factors. This observation has been referred to as the 'risk factor gap' and was comprehensively demonstrated by Mora and colleagues in 2007. This prospective study of 27,055 apparently healthy female health-care professionals investigated the relationship between baseline CVD risk factors and physical activity levels on CVD incidence over a mean follow-up duration of approximately 11 years. In accordance with previous evidence, an inverse relationship was established between baseline physical activity levels and the risk of incident CVD events during the follow-up period. Although a large proportion of this inverse association was explained by the baseline levels of several CVD risk factors – traditional and novel – 41% of the beneficial effects of exercise on CVD incidence remained unexplained. A similar pattern of results was also observed specifically for incident coronary heart disease with 64.5% of the beneficial effects of exercise remaining unexplained (Figure 7.23).

Figure 7.23 The percentage reduction in CVD and coronary heart disease events associated with physical activity that is explained by the measured risk factors.

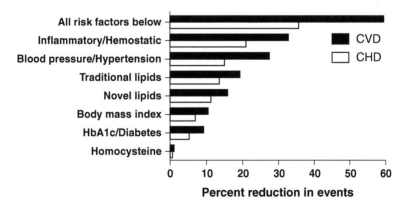

Source: Adapted with permission from Wolters Kluwer Health, Inc.: Mora, S. et al. (2007) 'Physical activity and reduced risk of cardiovascular events: potential mediating mechanisms', *Circulation*, 116: 2110–18. Available at: https://doi.org/10.1161/CIRCULATIONAHA.107.729939.

Notes: The risk reduction is based on the completion of $\geq$1500 kcal week^{-1} compared with the reference group of <200 kcal week^{-1}.

It is important to note that not all CVD risk factors discussed in this chapter were included in the analysis by Mora and colleagues (2007). Consequently, measures of insulin sensitivity and endothelial function may have contributed towards some of the unexplained benefits of physical activity, as well as levels of central adiposity (as discussed in Chapter 6). Autonomic dysfunction represents another risk factor that may be improved by physical activity but current issues with sampling difficulties and agreement over a range of markers used to assess this outcome need to be resolved before these effects can be fully elucidated (for a detailed review, see Joyner and Green 2009). Although the inclusion of these factors is likely to explain a greater proportion of the benefits of exercise, it remains probable that additional risk factors for CVD exist which are yet to be elucidated. An improved understanding of additional novel risk factors for CVD and the effects of physical activity on these measures will likely develop in the future.

SUMMARY

- Changes in risk factors provide causal inferences for the associations between physical activity levels and cardio-metabolic disease observed in epidemiological studies.
- Acute bouts of physical activity improve postprandial lipid metabolism which may contribute to the improvements in lipoprotein profile observed with exercise training.
- Increasing physical activity can reduce blood pressure in populations with normal blood pressure, hypertension or resistant hypertension.
- Improvements in endothelial function in response to physical activity may stimulate arterial remodelling (increased arterial size).
- Physical activity can improve glucose tolerance through insulin-dependent and insulin-independent mechanisms.
- Our understanding of the effects of physical activity on thrombotic risk and levels of systemic inflammation has increased in recent years but further research is required before firm conclusions can be drawn.
- Interactions between visceral obesity, insulin resistance and chronic low-grade inflammation can cause a 'clustering' of cardio-metabolic risk factors, including: glucose intolerance, dyslipidaemia, high blood pressure, endothelial dysfunction and thrombosis.
- Physical activity has a preventive and therapeutic role in ameliorating multiple cardio-metabolic disease risk factors.
- The protective effects of physical activity against CVD are not fully explained by the improvements in established risk factors, which suggests that other mediating influences also exist.

STUDY TASKS

1 Explain why it is important to understand the effects of physical activity on cardio-metabolic risk factors.

2 What are the effects of a single exercise session on postprandial lipaemia? How is this affected by the duration and intensity of exercise?

3 How does accumulating exercise throughout a day affect blood pressure compared with a single bout of exercise? Consider which populations may particularly benefit from this 'exercise snacking' approach.

4 Explain the time course of changes in endothelial function and arterial remodelling in response to exercise training. How do these adaptations help to reduce the risk of CVD?

5 Explain why glucose uptake by the working muscle during exercise is not impaired in patients with type 2 diabetes.

6 Provide an overview of the debate regarding whether the 'metabolic syndrome' is a useful concept.

7 Explain the mechanisms by which over-fatness can induce insulin resistance.

8 Provide an overview of the potential reasons why the benefits of physical activity for reducing CVD are not fully explained by improvements in known risk factors.

9 Explain why increasing physical activity is a particularly attractive approach for improving cardio-metabolic risk factors. Consider why this may be preferable to pharmacological therapy.

▌ FURTHER READING

Barac, A., Campia, U. and Panza, J.A. (2007) Methods for evaluating endothelial function in humans. *Hypertension* 49: 748–60.

Chen, Y.W., Apostolakis, S. and Lip, G.Y.H. (2014) Exercise-induced changes in inflammatory processes: implications for thrombogenesis in cardiovascular disease. *Annals of Medicine* 46: 439–55.

Eckel, R.H., Grundy, S.M. and Zimmet, P.Z. (2005) The metabolic syndrome. *The Lancet* 365: 1415–28.

Frayn, K.N. (2010) *Metabolic regulation: a human perspective*. 3rd edn, Oxford: Wiley-Blackwell.

Green, D.J. (2009) Exercise training as vascular medicine: direct impacts on the vasculature in humans. *Exercise and Sport Sciences Reviews* 37: 196–202.

Joyner, M.J. and Green, D.J. (2009) Exercise protects the cardiovascular system: effects beyond traditional risk factors. *Journal of Physiology* 587 (Pt 23): 5551–8.

Kaplan, H., Thompson, R.C., Trumble, B.C., Wann, L.S., Allam, A.H., Beheim, B. et al. (2017) Coronary atherosclerosis in indigenous South American Tsimane: a cross-sectional cohort study. *The Lancet* 389: 1730–9.

Romero, S.A., Minson, C.T. and Halliwill, J.R. (2017) The cardiovascular system after exercise. *Journal of Applied Physiology* 122: 925–32.

Simmons, R.K., Alberti, K.G.M.M., Gale, A.M., Colagiuri, S., Tuomilehto, J., Qiao, Q. et al. (2010) The metabolic syndrome: useful concept or clinical tool? Report of a WHO Expert Consultation. *Diabetologia* 53: 600–5.

Sylow, L., Kleinert, M., Richter, E.A. and Jensen, T.E. (2017) Exercise-stimulated glucose uptake – regulation and implications for glycaemic control. *Nature Reviews Endocrinology* 13: 133–48.

REFERENCES

Alberti, K.G.M.M., Eckel, R.H., Grundy, S.M., Zimmet, P.Z., Cleeman, J.I., Donato, K.A. et al. (2009) Harmonizing the metabolic syndrome: a joint interim statement of the International Diabetes Federation Task Force on Epidemiology and Prevention; National Heart, Lung, and Blood Institute; American Heart Association; World Heart Federation; International Atherosclerosis Society; and International Association for the Study of Obesity. *Circulation* 120: 1640–5.

Arjunan, S.P., Bishop, N.C., Reischak-Oliveira, A. and Stensel, D.J. (2013) Exercise and coronary heart disease risk markers in South Asian and European men. *Medicine and Science in Sports and Exercise* 45: 1261–8.

Ashor, A.W., Lara, J., Siervo, M., Celis-Morales, C., Oggioni, C., Jakovljevic, D.G. and Mathers, J.C. (2015) Exercise modalities and endothelial function: a systematic review and dose–response meta-analysis of randomized controlled trials. *Sports Medicine* 45: 279–96.

Baena, C.P., Olandoski, M., Younge, J.O., Buitrago-Lopez, A., Darweesh, S.K., Campos, N. et al. (2014) Effects of lifestyle-related interventions on blood pressure in low and middle-income countries: systematic review and meta-analysis. *Journal of Hypertension* 32: 961–73.

Barac, A., Campia, U. and Panza, J.A. (2007) Methods for evaluating endothelial function in humans. *Hypertension* 49: 748–60.

Bhammar, D.M., Angadi, S.S. and Gaesser, G.A. (2012) Effects of fractionized and continuous exercise on 24-h ambulatory blood pressure. *Medicine and Science in Sports and Exercise* 44: 2270–6.

Blair, S.N., Goodyear, N.N., Gibbons, L.W. and Cooper, K.H. (1984) Physical fitness and incidence of hypertension in healthy normotensive men and women. *Journal of the American Medical Association* 252: 487–90.

Borch-Johnsen, K. and Wareham, N. (2010) The rise and fall of the metabolic syndrome. *Diabetologia* 53: 597–9.

British Heart Foundation. (2007) Coronary heart disease statistics 2007 [online], available at: www.bhf.org.uk/what-we-do/our-research/heart-statistics (accessed 14 March 2019).

Burton, F.L., Malkova, D., Caslake, M.J. and Gill, J.M.R. (2008) Energy replacement attenuates the effects of prior moderate exercise on postprandial metabolism in overweight/obese men. *International Journal of Obesity* 32: 481–9.

Carnethon, M.R., Gidding, S.S., Nehgme, R., Sidney, S., Jacobs, D.R. and Liu, K. (2003) Cardiorespiratory fitness in young adulthood and the development of cardiovascular disease risk factors. *Journal of the American Medical Association* 290: 3092–100.

Casonatto, J., Goessler, K.F., Cornelissen, V.A., Cardoso, J.R. and Polito, M.D. (2016) The blood pressure-lowering effect of a single bout of resistance exercise: a systematic review and meta-analysis of randomised controlled trials. *European Journal of Preventive Cardiology* 23: 1700–14.

Celis-Morales, C.A., Welsh, P., Lyall, D.M., Steell, L., Petermann, F., Anderson, J. et al. (2018) Associations of grip strength with cardiovascular, respiratory, and cancer outcomes and all cause mortality: prospective cohort study of half a million UK Biobank participants. *British Medical Journal* 361: k1651. doi: 10.1136/bmj.k1651.

Chen, Y.W., Apostolakis, S. and Lip, G.Y.H. (2014) Exercise-induced changes in inflammatory processes: implications for thrombogenesis in cardiovascular disease. *Annals of Medicine* 46: 439–55.

Church, T.S., Blair, S.N., Cocreham, S., Johannsen, N., Johnson, W., Kramer et al. (2010) Effects of aerobic and resistance training on hemoglobin A1c levels in patients with type 2 diabetes: a randomized controlled trial. *Journal of the American Medical Association* 304: 2253–62.

Colberg, S.R., Zarrabi, L., Bennington, L., Nakave, A., Somma, T, Swain, D.P. and Sechrist, S.R. (2009) Postprandial walking is better for lowering the glycemic effect of dinner than pre-dinner exercise in type 2 diabetic individuals. *Journal of the American Medical Directors Association* 10: 394–7.

Colwell, J.A. (2004) Antiplatelet agents for the prevention of cardiovascular disease in diabetes mellitus. *American Journal of Cardiovascular Drugs* 4: 87–106.

Consitt, L.A., Van Meter, J., Newton, C.A., Collier, D.N., Dar, M.S., Wojtaszewski, J.F.P. et al. (2013) Impairments in site-specific AS160 phosphorylation and effects of exercise training. *Diabetes* 62: 3437–47.

Cornelissen, V.A., Fagard, R.H., Coeckelberghs, E. and Vanhees, L. (2011) Impact of resistance training on blood pressure and other cardiovascular risk factors: a meta-analysis of randomized, controlled trials. *Hypertension* 58: 950–8.

Couillard, C., Bergeron, N., Prud'homme, D., Bergeron J., Tremblay, A., Bouchard, C. et al. (1998) Postprandial triglyceride response in visceral obesity in men. *Diabetes* 47: 953–60.

Currens, J.H. and White, P.D. (1961) Half a century of running: clinical, physiologic and autopsy findings in the case of Clarence DeMar ("Mr. Marathon"). *New England Journal of Medicine* 16: 988–93.

Dimeo, F., Pagonas, N., Seibert, F., Arndt, R., Zidek, W. and Westhoff, T.H. (2012) Aerobic exercise reduces blood pressure in resistant hypertension. *Hypertension* 60: 653–8.

DiPietro, L., Gribok, A., Stevens, M.S., Hamm, L.F. and Rumpler, W. (2013) Three 15-min bouts of moderate postmeal walking significantly improves 24-h glycemic control in older people at risk for impaired glucose tolerance. *Diabetes Care* 36: 3262–8.

Faselis, C., Doumas, M., Kokkinos, J.P., Panagiotakos, D., Kheirbek, R., Sheriff et al. (2012) Exercise capacity and progression from prehypertension to hypertension. *Hypertension* 60: 333–8.

Frayn, K.N. (2010) *Metabolic regulation: a human perspective.* 3rd edn, Oxford: Wiley-Blackwell.

Freese, E.C., Levine, A.S., Chapman, D.P., Hausman, D.B. and Cureton, K.J. (2011) Effects of acute sprint interval cycling and energy replacement on postprandial lipemia. *Journal of Applied Physiology* 111: 1584–9.

Ghaffar, A., Reddy, K.S. and Singhi, M. (2004) Burden of non-communicable diseases in South Asia. *British Medical Journal* 328: 807–10.

Ghafouri, K., Cooney, J., Bedford, D.K., Wilson, J., Caslake, M.J. and Gill, J.M.R. (2015) Moderate exercise increases affinity of large very low-density lipoproteins for hydrolysis by lipoprotein lipase. *Journal of Clinical Endocrinology and Metabolism* 100: 2205–13.

Gill, J.M.R., Al-Mamari, A., Ferrell, W.R., Cleland, S.J., Packard, C.J., Sattar, N. et al. (2004) Effects of prior moderate exercise on postprandial metabolism and vascular function in lean and centrally obese men. *Journal of the American College of Cardiology* 44: 2375–82.

Gill, J.M.R. and Hardman, A.E. (2000) Postprandial lipemia: effects of exercise and restriction of energy intake compared. *American Journal of Clinical Nutrition* 71: 465–71.

Gill, J.M.R., Herd, S.L. and Hardman, A.E. (2002) Moderate exercise and post-prandial metabolism: issues of dose–response. *Journal of Sports Sciences* 20: 961–7.

Gill, J.M.R. and Malkova, D. (2006) Physical activity, fitness and cardiovascular disease risk in adults: interactions with insulin resistance and obesity. *Clinical Science* 110: 409–25.

Hambrecht, R., Adams, V., Erbs, S., Linke, A., Krankel, N., Shu, Y. et al. (2003) Regular physical activity improves endothelial function in patients with coronary artery disease by increasing phosphorylation of endothelial nitric oxide synthase. *Circulation* 107: 3152–8.

Haskell, W.L., Sims, C., Myll, J., Bortz, W.M., Goar, F.G. and Alderman, E.L. (1993) Coronary artery size and dilating capacity in ultradistance runners. *Circulation* 87: 1076–82.

Huffman, K.M., Hawk, V.H., Henes, S.T., Ocampo, C.I., Orenduff, M.C., Slentz, C.A. et al. (2012) Exercise effects on lipids in persons with varying dietary patterns – does diet matter if they exercise? Responses in studies of a targeted risk reduction intervention through defined exercise I. *American Heart Journal* 164: 117–24.

Huffman, K.M., Slentz, C.A., Bales, C.W., Houmard, J.A. and Kraus, W.E. (2008) Relationships between adipose tissue and cytokine responses to a randomized controlled exercise training intervention. *Metabolism* 57: 577–83.

Inaba, Y., Chen, J.A. and Bergmann, S.R. (2010) Prediction of future cardiovascular outcomes by flow-mediated vasodilatation of brachial artery: a meta-analysis. *International Journal of Cardiovascular Imaging* 26: 631–40.

Jahangard, T., Torkaman, G., Ghoosheh, B., Hedayati, M. and Dibaj, A. (2009) The effect of short-term aerobic training on coagulation and fibrinolytic factors in sedentary healthy postmenopausal women. *Maturitas* 64: 223–7.

James, D.E., Kraegen, E.W. and Chisholm, D.J. (1985) Muscle glucose metabolism in exercising rats: comparison with insulin stimulation. *American Journal of Physiology, Endocrinology and Metabolism* 11: E575–80.

JBS3 Board. (2014) Joint British Societies' consensus recommendations for the prevention of cardiovascular disease (JBS3). *Heart* 100 Suppl 2: ii1–ii67. doi: 10.1136/heartjnl-2014–305693.

Joint National Committee on Detection, Evaluation and Treatment of High Blood Pressure. (2004) *The 7th report of the Joint National Committee on Detection, Evaluation and Treatment of High Blood Pressure, National Centre for Biotechnology Information (US), Bethesda (MD)* [online], available at: https://www.ncbi.nlm.nih.gov/books/NBK9633/table/A32/?report=objectonly (accessed 6 June 2017).

Joyner, M.J. and Green, D.J. (2009) Exercise protects the cardiovascular system: effects beyond traditional risk factors. *Journal of Physiology* 587(Pt 23): 5551–8.

Kaplan, H., Thompson, R.C., Trumble, B.C., Wann, L.S., Allam, A.H., Beheim, B. et al. (2017) Coronary atherosclerosis in indigenous South American Tsimane: a cross-sectional cohort study. *The Lancet* 389: 1730–9.

Kirwan, J.P., Del Aguila, L.F., Hernandez, J.M., Williamson, D.L., O'Gorman, D.J., Lewis, R. and Krishnan, R.K. (2000) Regular exercise enhances insulin activation of IRS-1-associated PI3-kinase in human skeletal muscle. *Journal of Applied Physiology* 88: 797–803.

Kodama, S., Tanaka, S., Saito, K., Shu, M., Sone, Y., Onitake, F. et al. (2007) Effect of aerobic exercise training on serum levels of high-density lipoprotein cholesterol: a meta-analysis. *Archives of Internal Medicine* 167: 999–1008.

Kramsch, D.M., Aspen, A.J., Abramowitz, B.M., Kreimendahl, T. and Hood, W.B. (1981) Reduction of coronary atherosclerosis by moderate conditioning exercise in monkeys on an atherogenic diet. *New England Journal of Medicine* 305: 1483–9.

Kraus, W.E., Houmard, J.A., Duscha, B.D., Knetzger, K.J., Wharton, M.B., McCartney, J.S. et al. (2002) Effects of the amount and intensity of exercise on plasma lipoproteins. *New England Journal of Medicine* 347: 1483–92.

Lakka, T.A., Laukkanen, J.A., Rauramaa, R., Salonen, R., Lakka, H.-M., Kaplan, G.A. and Salonen, J.T. (2001) Cardiorespiratory fitness and the progression of carotid atherosclerosis in middle-aged men. *Annals of Internal Medicine* 134: 12–20.

LaPorte, R.E., Brenes, G., Dearwater, S., Murphy, M.A., Cauley, J.A., Dietrick, R. and Robertson, R. (1983) HDL cholesterol across a spectrum of physical activity from quadriplegia to marathon running. *The Lancet* 1: 1212–13.

Larsen, J.J.S., Dela, F., Kjaer, M. and Galbo, H. (1997) The effect of moderate exercise on postprandial glucose homeostasis in NIDDM patients. *Diabetologia* 40: 447–53.

Lewington, S., Clarke, R., Qizilbash, N., Peto, R. and Collins, R. (Prospective Studies Collaboration). (2002) Age-specific relevance of usual blood pressure to vascular mortality: a meta-analysis of individual data for one million adults in 61 prospective studies. *The Lancet* 360: 1903–13.

Libby, P. (2002) Inflammation in atherosclerosis. *Nature* 420: 868–74.

Lipman, R.L., Raskin, P., Love, T., Triebwasser, J., Lecocq, F.R. and Schnure, J.J. (1972) Glucose intolerance during decreased physical activity in man. *Diabetes* 21: 101–7.

Martin, I.K., Katz, A. and Wahren, J. (1995) Splanchnic and muscle metabolism during exercise in NIDDM patients. *American Journal of Physiology* 269: E583–90.

Matsuzawa, Y. and Lerman, A. (2014). Endothelial dysfunction and coronary artery disease: assessment, prognosis and treatment. *Coronary Artery Disease* 25: 713–24.

McArdle, W.D., Katch, F.I. and Katch, V.L. (2010) *Exercise physiology: nutrition, energy, and human performance*. Philadelphia: Lippincott Williams & Wilkins.

McCoy, M., Proietto, J. and Hargreaves, M. (1994) Effect of detraining on GLUT-4 protein content in human skeletal muscle. *Journal of Applied Physiology* 77: 1532–6.

Merrill, J.R., Holly, R.G., Anderson, R.L., Rifai, N., King, M.E. and DeMeersman, R. (1989) Hyperlipidemic response of young trained and untrained men after a high fat meal. *Arteriosclerosis* 9: 217–23.

Messerli, F.H., Williams, B. and Ritz, E. (2007) Essential hypertension. *The Lancet* 370: 591–603.

Mora, S., Cook, N., Buring, J.E., Ridker, P.M. and Lee, I.-M. (2007) Physical activity and reduced risk of cardiovascular events: potential mediating mechanisms. *Circulation* 116: 2110–8.

National Centre for Social Research (NatCen), University College London, Department of Epidemiology and Public Health. (2019) Health Survey for England, 2018 [online], available at: http://digital.nhs.uk/pubs/hse2018 (accessed 20 July 2020).

Paffenbarger, R.S., Wing, A.L., Hyde, R.T. and Jung, D.L. (1983) Physical activity and incidence of hypertension in college alumni. *American Journal of Epidemiology* 117: 245–57.

Panagiotakos, D.B., Pitsavos, C., Chrysohoou, C., Kavouras, S. and Stefanadis, C. (2005) The associations between leisure-time physical activity and inflammatory and coagulation markers related to cardiovascular disease: the ATTICA Study. *Preventive Medicine* 40: 432–7.

Peddie, M.C., Rehrer, N.J. and Perry, T.L. (2012) Physical activity and postprandial lipidemia: are energy expenditure and lipoprotein lipase activity the real modulators of the positive effect? *Progress in Lipid Research* 51: 11–22.

Perseghin, G., Price, T.B., Petersen, K.F., Roden, M., Cline, G.W., Gerow, K. et al. (1996) Increased glucose transport-phosphorylation and muscle glycogen synthesis after exercise training in insulin-resistant subjects. *New England Journal of Medicine* 335: 1357–62.

Pouliot, M.C., Després, J.P., Nadeau, A., Moorjani, S., Prud'Homme, D., Lupien, P.J. et al. (1992) Visceral obesity in men: associations with glucose tolerance, plasma insulin, and lipoprotein levels. *Diabetes* 41: 826–34.

Rogers, M.A., King, D.S., Hagberg, J.M., Ehsani, A.A. and Holloszy, J.O. (1990) Effect of 10 days of physical inactivity on glucose tolerance in master athletes. *Journal of Applied Physiology* 68: 1833–7.

Romero, S.A., Minson, C.T. and Halliwill, J.R. (2017) The cardiovascular system after exercise. *Journal of Applied Physiology* 122: 925–32.

Rondon, M.U.P.B., Alves, M.J.N.N., Braga, A.M.F.W., Teixeira, O.T.U.N., Barretto, A.C.P., Krieger, E.M. and Negrão, C.E. (2002) Postexercise blood pressure reduction in elderly hypertensive patients. *Journal of the American College of Cardiology* 39: 676–82.

Sandrock, M., Schulze, C., Schmitz, D., Dickhuth, H.H. and Schmidt-Trucksaess, A. (2008) Physical activity throughout life reduces the atherosclerotic wall process in the carotid artery. *British Journal of Sports Medicine* 42: 839–44.

Sigal, R.J., Kenny, G.P., Boulé, N.G., Wells, G.A., Prud'homme, D., Fortier, M. et al. (2007) Effects of aerobic training, resistance training, or both on glycemic control in type 2 diabetes: a randomized trial. *Annals of Internal Medicine* 147: 357–69.

Simmons, R.K., Alberti, K.G.M.M., Gale, A.M., Colagiuri, S., Tuomilehto, J., Qiao, Q. et al. (2010) The metabolic syndrome: useful concept or clinical tool? Report of a WHO Expert Consultation. *Diabetologia* 53: 600–5.

Slentz, C.A., Houmard, J.A., Johnson, J.L., Bateman, L.A., Tanner, C.J., McCartney, J.S. et al. (2007) Inactivity, exercise training and detraining, and plasma lipoproteins: STRRIDE: a randomized, controlled study of exercise intensity and amount. *Journal of Applied Physiology* 103: 432–42.

Sylow, L., Kleinert, M., Richter, E.A. and Jensen, T.E. (2017) Exercise-stimulated glucose uptake: regulation and implications for glycaemic control. *Nature Reviews Endocrinology* 13: 133–48.

Tinken, T.M., Thijssen, D.H.J., Black, M.A., Cable, T. and Green, D.J. (2008) Time course of change in vasodilator function and capacity in response to exercise training in humans. *Journal of Physiology* 586(Pt 20): 5003–12.

Truswell, A.S., Kennelly, B.M., Hansen, J.D.L. and Lee, R.B. (1972) Blood pressure of Kung Bushmen in northern Botswana. *American Heart Journal* 84: 5–12.

Tsetsonis, N.V. and Hardman, A.E. (1996) Reduction in postprandial lipemia after walking: influence of exercise intensity. *Medicine and Science in Sports and Exercise* 28: 1235–42.

Wang, J.S. (2006) Exercise prescription and thrombogenesis. *Journal of Biomedical Science* 13: 753–61.

Whelton, S.P., Chin, A., Xin, X. and He, J. (2002) Effect of aerobic exercise on blood pressure: a meta-analysis of randomized, controlled trials. *Annals of Internal Medicine* 136: 493–503.

Wild, S.H., Fischbacher, C., Brock, A., Griffiths, C. and Bhopal, R. (2007) Mortality from all causes and circulatory disease by country of birth in England and Wales 2001–2003. *Journal of Public Health* 29: 191–8.

Williams, P.T. (1996) High-density lipoprotein cholesterol and other risk factors for coronary heart disease in female runners. *New England Journal of Medicine* 334: 1298–303.

Williams, P.T. (1997) Relationship of distance run per week to coronary heart disease risk factors in 8283 male runners: the national runners' health study. *Archives of Internal Medicine* 157: 191–8.

Wojtaszewski, J.F.P., Hansen, B.F., Gade, J., Kiens, B., Markuns, J.F., Goodyear, L.J. and Richter, E.A. (2000) Insulin signaling and insulin sensitivity after exercise in human skeletal muscle. *Diabetes* 49: 325–31.

Wood, P.D., Stefanick, M.L., Dreon, D.M. and Frey-Hewitt, M.S. (1988) Changes in plasma lipids and lipoproteins in overweight men during weight loss through dieting as compared with exercise. *New England Journal of Medicine* 319: 1173–9.

8 Cancer

Adrianne E. Hardman and Fehmidah Munir

INTRODUCTION

Cancer has afflicted humans throughout recorded history. The origin of the word cancer has been credited to Hippocrates (460–370 BC) who used the terms 'carcinos' and 'carcinoma' to describe tumours. In Greek these words refer to a crab, most likely because the finger-like spreading projections from a cancer called to mind the shape of a crab. Carcinoma is the most common type of cancer (Figure 8.1).

Cancer is not one disease but a set of diseases characterised by unregulated cell growth leading to invasion of surrounding tissues and, often, spread to other parts of the body. It is a leading cause of morbidity and mortality, accounting for around a quarter of all deaths in developed countries where the lifetime risk of developing cancer is of the order of one in three. Moreover, cancer is an increasingly important factor in the global burden of disease. The World Health Organization estimates that the number of new cases annually will rise from 18 million in 2018 to nearly 30 million by 2040, with around 80% of the increase occurring in low- and middle-income countries.

Figure 8.1 Main types of cancer – cancer can originate almost anywhere in the body.

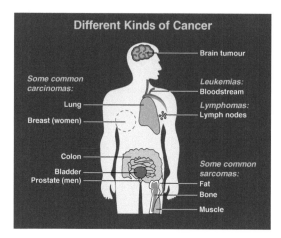

Different Kinds of Cancer

Some common carcinomas:
- Lung
- Breast (women)
- Colon
- Bladder
- Prostate (men)

- Brain tumour
- Leukemias: Bloodstream
- Lymphomas: Lymph nodes

Some common sarcomas:
- Fat
- Bone
- Muscle

Carcinomas, the most common types of cancer, arise from the cells that cover external and internal body surfaces. Lung, breast, and colon are the most frequent cancers of this type.

Sarcomas are cancers arising from cells found in the supporting tissues of the body such as bone, cartilage, fat, connective tissue, and muscle.

Lymphomas are cancers that arise in the lymph nodes and tissues of the body's immune system.

Leukemias are cancers of the immature blood cells that grow in the bone marrow and tend to accumulate in large numbers in the bloodstream

Brain and central nervous system cancers are categorised according to histopathology and molecular characteristics.

Source: US National Cancer Institute (https://www.cancer.gov).

The role of environmental factors in cancer causation is illustrated by the enormous geographical differences in incidence worldwide. For example, Australia has an incidence of skin cancer more than a hundred times higher than that in Japan. These differences cannot be explained fully by genetic factors, as classic studies of migrants have shown. The incidence of stomach cancer is much higher in Japan than in Hawaii, for instance, whilst the incidence of breast cancer is lower. When Japanese people migrate to Hawaii, however, their incidence rates for these two cancers move towards the rates in the indigenous population. Second-generation migrants experience rates even closer to those of the host country, presumably because they have been exposed for longer than their parents to the environmental factors that prevail in the host country. Contrary to public perception, therefore, some risk factors for cancer can be changed and some cancers prevented. For instance, of the 607,000 deaths from cancer expected in the US in 2019, an estimated 45% can be related to potentially modifiable risk factors (Goding Sauer et al. 2019).

Although a role for energy balance in cancer causation was advanced almost three centuries ago, it was not until the mid-1980s that researchers began to ask whether physical activity – the main contributor to inter-individual differences in energy expenditure – influences the risk of cancer. The extent, consistency, strengths and limitations of the available evidence will be discussed later but first it is necessary to understand a little more about how cancer develops.

HOW CANCER DEVELOPS

The fundamental abnormality resulting in the development of cancer is the unregulated proliferation of cancer cells. Rather than responding appropriately to the signals that control normal cell behaviour, cancer cells grow and divide in an uncontrolled

---

BOX 8.1 DIFFERENCES BETWEEN NORMAL CELLS AND CANCER CELLS.

NORMAL CELLS	CANCER CELLS
• Stop reproducing at the right time • Become specialised or mature (differentiation) • Reproduce themselves exactly • Stick together in the right place (cell adhesion) • Self-destruct if they are damaged (apoptosis)	• Carry on reproducing • Do not become specialised but stay immature • Do not obey signals from neighbouring cells • Can become detached from the primary tumour and travel to other parts of the body (metastasis) • Do not die if they move to another part of the body

---

manner, invading normal tissues and organs and eventually spreading throughout the body. The generalised loss of growth control is the result of accumulated abnormalities in cell regulatory systems and is reflected in several aspects of cell behaviour that distinguish cancer cells from their normal counterparts (Box 8.1).

The development of cancer is a multistep process in which cells gradually become malignant through a progressive series of alterations. Carcinogenesis occurs when there is damage to a cell's DNA – the nucleic acid that is the basis of the genetic code. Genes direct the activities of every cell but when mutations (damage to a gene or loss of a gene) occur, vital control systems are lost and cancer cells proliferate abnormally.

Abnormalities of three different types of genes are important in carcinogenesis:

- Genes that encourage the cell to multiply. If these genes, called oncogenes, become abnormal they programme the cell to multiply all the time.
- Genes that stop the cell multiplying and act as a brake to the oncogene's accelerator. If one of these genes becomes damaged, the cell may carry on multiplying – it becomes 'immortal'.
- Genes that repair other damaged genes. If these genes are damaged, other mutations are not repaired but replicated during the process of cell division and inherited by all subsequent daughter cells.

Damage to DNA leads to abnormalities of multiple cell regulatory mechanisms. Normal body cells grow, divide and die in an orderly fashion. After the early years of life, most cells reproduce only to replace those that have died, through injury or illness for example. Cells somehow know (through intercellular signalling) when there are enough new cells and they then stop reproducing. Moreover, they have a natural ability to stick together in the right place forming an orderly array; this property, called cell adhesion, is derived from molecules on the surface of the cell and ensures the integrity of tissues and organs. A normal cell becomes detached from its proper place if it becomes too old and, if its genes are badly damaged, it will 'commit suicide' so that these faults are not passed on to daughter cells. This property is called programmed cell death or apoptosis. Normal cells have a lifespan of about 40 generations (cell doublings) by which time the build-up of errors results in senescence and death.

Figure 8.2 How cancer grows and spreads.

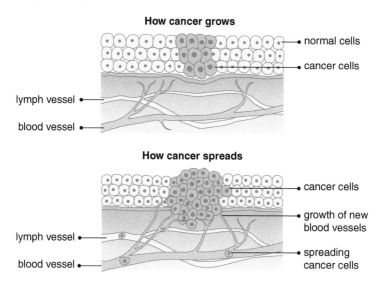

Source: Canadian Cancer Society (2020) How cancer starts, grows and spreads [online], available at: https://www.cancer.ca/en/cancer-information/cancer-101/what-is-cancer/how-cancer-starts-grows-and-spreads/?region=on (accessed 6 May 2020).

By contrast, cancer cells grow in disordered, multi-layered patterns. They progressively increase their capacity for proliferation and survival; they do not stop reproducing and, instead of dying in an orderly way, self-destruct more slowly than they reproduce, so their numbers continue to increase until a lump called a tumour is formed. As it grows, a tumour invades and destroys surrounding tissues (progression). Its centre gets further and further from blood vessels in the area. By secreting growth factors, the cancerous cells promote the development of new blood vessels (angiogenesis) thereby ensuring an adequate supply of oxygen and nutrients and promoting further tumour growth (Figure 8.2).

One of the most troublesome characteristics of cancer cells is that they travel to other sites in the body, where they begin to grow and replace normal tissue. This process, called metastasis, occurs because cancer cells can lose the molecules on their surface that keep normal cells in the right place. The formation of new blood vessels is also important. Actively growing new capillaries are easily penetrated by the tumour cells, providing a ready opportunity for cancer cells to enter the circulatory system and begin the metastatic process. Cancer cells travel in the bloodstream or lymph vessels (Figure 8.2) and stop at the first place they get stuck. In the bloodstream, this is the next capillary bed they encounter – often in the lungs because venous blood from most organs goes next through these capillaries.

How do mutations arise?

Fortunately, it is not easy for a normal cell to turn into a cancer cell. Although DNA is continuously exposed to damaging agents from within as well as outside the body, damage to DNA is normally repaired efficiently so that mutations are not inherited by daughter cells. In cancer cells, the damaged DNA is not repaired.

Mutations can happen by chance when a cell is reproducing but this often leads the cell to self-destruct. Or, cells carrying a mutation may be recognised as abnormal by the immune system and killed. Thus, most pre-cancerous cells die before they can cause disease and only a few develop into a cancer. Carcinogenesis results from the accumulation of errors in the genetic code and it can take a long time before enough mutations happen for a cell to become cancerous. (This is why cancers are so much more common in older people.)

Something that damages the genetic machinery of a cell and makes it more likely to become cancerous is called a carcinogen. People can inherit damaged DNA but fewer than 15% of all cancers are familial. Most often, a person's DNA becomes damaged by exposure to some environmental factor – chemicals, radiation or viruses. For some cancers, initiating agents have been clearly identified. These include lung cancer (tobacco smoke) and leukaemia (ionising radiation) but it is difficult to define initiating agents in cancers of the colon, prostate and breast. Natural events such as free radical generation may play a part.

Once carcinogenesis has been initiated, proliferative signals derive from exogenous factors such as diet, viral infection or hormones (contraceptive pill, hormone replacement therapy) or endogenous factors such as hormonal changes. Cancer is therefore a multi-factorial disease. There is no single cause for any one cancer. For example, tobacco smoke contains potent carcinogens – smoking 20–30 cigarettes a day increases the risk of lung cancer 40-fold – but not everyone who smokes gets lung cancer, so other factors must be at work. Over many years, epidemiology has provided evidence as to factors that increase the risk of developing some cancers (Box 8.2).

BOX 8.2 RISK FACTORS FOR CANCER.

- Age – the single most important factor.
- Diet – diets high in fruit and vegetables are protective against several common cancers. Diets high in fat, meat and salt increase the risk of some cancers.
- Tobacco – the most important human carcinogen.
- Radiation – natural and manmade.
- Occupational exposure – asbestos, some chemicals.
- Genetic susceptibility – for example, genes named BRCA1 and BRCA2 have been identified for breast cancer.
- Heavy alcohol drinking.
- Impaired immune function – those with impaired immune function, for example HIV, are more likely to get some types of cancer.
- Viruses – viruses can cause changes to cells that make them more likely to become cancerous, either directly or by creating chronic inflammation. Examples include hepatitis B virus (liver cancer) and human papilloma virus (cancer of cervix).
- Physical inactivity – now recognised by many agencies worldwide as a risk factor based on evidence explained in the following pages.

WHY MIGHT PHYSICAL ACTIVITY INFLUENCE CANCER RISK?

Several broad categories of mechanisms have been proposed to explain why physically active individuals may be at lower risk of developing cancer. Collectively, these affect the endogenous systemic environment in a manner that influences cellular processes and tumour growth, comprising plausible biological mechanisms which provide justification for epidemiological study.

First, sex hormones may play a role. These hormones have powerful mitogenic and proliferative effects and are important in the aetiology of reproductive cancers. Cancers of the breast, prostate, testes and endometrium are all related to lifetime exposure to endogenous sex steroid hormones. Thus measures that reflect a high level of exposure to oestrogens, for example early menarche, late menopause or an increased number of ovulatory cycles, increase a woman's risk for breast cancer. By contrast, women with irregular menses (thus reduced progesterone and oestradiol) have only half the risk of breast cancer as women with regular cycles. In men, a strong linear trend of increasing risk of prostate cancer with increasing plasma concentrations of testosterone has been observed. Participation in exercise may therefore reduce the risk of hormone-related cancers by lowering concentrations of sex hormones.

Young women who participate at a high level in vigorous sports such as gymnastics, ballet and endurance running have late menarche and exhibit a high incidence of primary and secondary amenorrhoea. Many have irregular, often anovulatory, menstrual cycles, the prevalence of which increases with the volume of training. The majority of the physical activity recorded in observational studies of cancer is not, however, vigorous. Ovarian steroids have been measured in university/college-age women who engaged in moderate leisure-time exercise. Like participants in vigorous sports, these recreational athletes also have low concentrations of oestrogens. Thus it is not only high-intensity, high-volume training that disrupts menstrual function.

Observational studies are supported by randomly controlled intervention trials of the influence of physical activity on oestrogens. For example, in 320 previously sedentary, postmenopausal women aged between 50 and 74 who followed a programme of aerobic exercise for 12 months levels of total and free oestradiol were all reduced, compared with controls who remained sedentary (Friedenreich et al. 2010). Subsequent systematic review and meta-analysis of 18 such trials (pre- *and* post-menopausal women) confirmed this finding; the overall effect of physical activity was a modest but statistically significant decrease in both total and free oestradiol (Ennour-Idrissi et al. 2015).

In men, reduction of androgen levels by physical activity could explain a lower risk of prostate cancer. Some studies have found lower circulating concentrations of androgens in endurance-trained men, elite marathon runners for example, than in sedentary controls. There is no evidence, however, that regular activity at a more moderate intensity leads to lower androgens.

The influence of exercise in reducing concentrations of sex steroid hormones may be enhanced through decreased bioavailability. These hormones are carried in the blood bound to a plasma protein, sex hormone binding globulin. It is the free (unbound) hormone that binds to receptors within the cytoplasm of the target cell. In both sexes, physical activity is associated with an increase in sex hormone binding globulin, thereby decreasing unbound levels of oestrogens/androgens and reducing endogenous exposure to the active hormones.

Obesity is associated with an increased risk of developing as many as 13 types of cancer so physical activity may decrease cancer risk through improved weight regulation. Men and women who are physically active have only slightly higher energy intake than their sedentary peers but are leaner, suggesting that net available energy is lower in active people. This would fit with findings in animals that energy intake restriction inhibits carcinogenesis. In humans, reduction in the highly metabolically active abdominal fat mass – particularly visceral fat – may be of particular importance because rather small (<2 kg) decreases in visceral fat have important beneficial effects on insulin sensitivity.

Insulin is, of course, one of the most important metabolic hormones and exhibits a general anabolic role, stimulating net protein synthesis. Thus hyperinsulinaemia constitutes a growth-promoting milieu that may facilitate carcinogenesis. Elevated concentrations of insulin and insulin-like growth factors have been associated with increased risk of breast, prostate and colon cancers. As discussed in Chapter 5, exercise enhances insulin sensitivity and may therefore contribute to its protective effect against cancers. One pooled analysis of seven exercise trials in breast cancer survivors, average of 16 weeks, found a significant decrease in fasting insulin in those participants who lost weight (Kang et al. 2016).

Another systemic factor that may play a role is inflammation. Over time, chronic inflammation can cause damage to DNA and lead to cancer. For example, people with inflammatory bowel diseases have an increased risk of colon cancer. Regular physical activity has been associated prospectively with lower levels of pro-inflammatory markers. For example, researchers used a composite score based on biomarkers to examine the influence of a 12-month intervention on the inflammatory profile of older, overweight or obese adults. Increases in total, moderate and moderate-to-vigorous physical activity were all associated with a decrease in the inflammatory profile (Fuentes et al. 2020).

The body's innate immune system has the potential to destroy tumour cells and prevent tumour growth. So, if immune surveillance is enhanced, malignant cells are less likely to survive and the risk of cancer would be reduced. There are reports that moderate physical activity enhances immune function by increasing the number and/or activity of macrophages and natural killer cells. Such changes may aid early recognition of tumour cells and/or defence against tumour spread. Prolonged, intense exercise may, however, have the opposite effect, leading to a period (days to two weeks) of immunosuppression (Chapter 13).

One mechanism that has been invoked to explain the lower incidence of colon cancer in physically active people involves intestinal transit time. Physical activity may speed up transit time within the colon, decreasing exposure of bowel mucosa to carcinogens (Sternfeld and Lee 2009). This would fit with findings that physical activity protects against cancer of the colon but not the rectum – which is only intermittently in contact with carcinogens in faecal matter. The evidence for an effect on colonic motility is limited, however, and mostly relates to running – an activity that may have unique effects associated with repeated regular impacts. A further limitation is that, although stool bulk is a good (inverse) correlate of colorectal cancer risk, transit time is not a well-established risk factor.

The molecular basis of the effect of exercise on cancer is – and will continue to be – a topic of intense research interest. Studies in rodents show that exercise training slows tumour development and progression. Speculatively, mechanisms may include direct effects on intrinsic tumour factors, including metabolism and immunogenicity, as well as through interplay with systemic factors such as catecholamines, increased blood flow, shear stress and increased temperature (Hojman et al. 2018).

EPIDEMIOLOGY OF PHYSICAL ACTIVITY AND CANCER

Since the second edition of this book was published three important additional aspects of the epidemiological evidence are evident. First, systematic reviews and meta-analyses have been employed to provide a comprehensive picture of the relationship of physical activity with cancer risk. These pooled analyses help to define the relationship with cancer sub-types and allow dose–response issues to be addressed. Second, the potential role of sedentary behaviours in cancer prevention has been examined. And, third, researchers have begun to describe in cancer patients the relationship of physical activity with cancer mortality, cancer recurrence and quality of life.

Table 8.1, from the 2019 ACSM Roundtable Report, contrasts the level of available epidemiological evidence for 16 cancer types in 2008 with that available ten years later.

Table 8.1 Differences in the level of evidence for lower risk in physically active people of 16 types of cancer between 2008 and 2018.

CANCER TYPE	PHYSICAL ACTIVITY AND LOWER RISK IN 2008	PHYSICAL ACTIVITY AND LOWER RISK IN 2018
Colon	Strong	Strong
Breast	Strong	Strong
Kidney	–	Strong
Endometrial	Limited	Strong
Bladder	–	Strong
Oesophageal	–	Strong
Stomach	–	Strong
Lung	Limited	Moderate
Haematologic	–	Limited
Head and neck	–	Limited
Pancreatic	–	Limited
Prostate	No effect (limited)	Limited
Ovarian	Limited	Limited
Brain	–	Not assignable
Thyroid	–	No effect (limited)
Rectal	No effect (limited)	No effect (limited)

Source: Reprinted with permission from Wolters Kluwer Health, Inc.: Patel, A.V. et al. (2019) 'American College of Sports Medicine Roundtable report on physical activity, sedentary behaviour, and cancer prevention and control', *Medicine and Science in Sports and Exercise*, 51: 2391–402. Available at: https://doi.org/10.1249/MSS.0000000000002117.

Note: Based on 2008 and 2018 Reports of the Physical Activity Guidelines Advisory Committee, US Department of Health and Human Services.

The difference is striking and the evidence that physical activity lowers the risk of a number of cancers has clearly been greatly strengthened over this period. An essential rider is that the studies from which these assessments are derived are all observational and overwhelmingly in Caucasian populations.

One pooled analysis that contributed important data to the ACSM Report is that of Moore and colleagues (Moore et al. 2016). These researchers reported findings from 12 cohorts (eight from USA, four from Europe) with, collectively, 1.44 million participants to evaluate the association of leisure-time physical activity with cancer incidence. Overall, people with high levels of activity (90th percentile) had a 7% lower risk than those with low levels (10th percentile).

This figure masks clear differences between sites, however. Figure 8.3 shows, for ten cancer types, the hazard ratios (high versus low levels of leisure time physical activity) reported by Moore and colleagues, alongside those from subsequent meta-analyses.

Figure 8.3 Multivariate hazard ratios (HR) and 95% confidence intervals (CI) for ten types of cancer comparing high with low levels of physical activity. The HRs from meta-analyses are shown by black dots and the HRs from the pooled analysis by Moore et al. (2016) are shown by open triangles. Where confidence intervals are narrower than 1, the risk difference is significant.

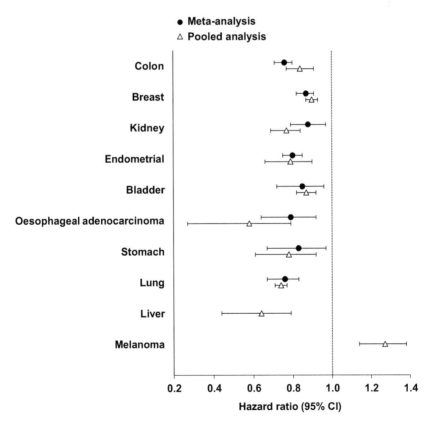

Source: Adapted with permission from Wolters Kluwer Health, Inc.: Patel, A.V. et al. (2019) 'American College of Sports Medicine Roundtable report on physical activity, sedentary behaviour, and cancer prevention and control', *Medicine and Science in Sports and Exercise*, 51: 2391–402. Available at: https://doi.org/10.1249/MSS.0000000000002117.

The magnitude of associations ranged from 10% to 24% lower risks (hazard ratios 0.76–0.90) for the seven cancers for which evidence was deemed to be 'strong' (Table 8.1), with great consistency between estimates from meta-analyses and the pooled analysis. By contrast, findings for malignant melanoma, a serious type of skin cancer and prone to metastasis, stand out; high levels of physical activity are associated with a *higher* risk of this cancer. One likely reason is greater exposure to sun – and perhaps sunburn – in physically active people.

Findings summarised in the ACSM Roundtable (Patel et al. 2019) are bolstered by pooled analyses which reported a significant, inverse association between total physical activity and all-cancer incidence (Barberio et al. 2018) and a lower risk of seven types of cancer, with the most consistent evidence for colon and breast cancer (de Renzende et al. 2018). Evidence related to these two common cancers are discussed in the following sections.

Physical activity and colorectal cancer

The colon or large intestine forms a rectangle in the abdominal cavity that frames the tightly packed small intestine. Its main function is to store waste material until this is eliminated from the body. By contrast, the rectum, which links the colon to the anus, is empty except when the urge to defaecate is initiated. Modifiable lifestyle factors for colorectal cancer that are widely recognised include high body mass index (BMI), high consumption of red or processed meat, smoking and physical inactivity.

Colorectal cancer is the most commonly investigated cancer in relation to physical activity. Some studies present data describing cancers of the colon and rectum collectively, others report data separately. Findings differ according to site so combining data in a single outcome measure may obscure real relationships and the following discussion therefore deals with colon and rectal cancer separately.

At least 60 cohort and case-control[1] studies have investigated whether physical activity is associated with the risk of colon cancer. These have been conducted in many countries – North America, Europe, Asia, Australia and New Zealand – but overwhelmingly in white people. The majority have reported a large and statistically significantly lower risk among the most physically active men and women, compared with the least active. The consistency of these findings across occupational and leisure-time activity and different study designs is all the more remarkable because methods of assessing physical activity have often been quite crude, especially in the earlier literature.

In marked contrast to findings for colon cancer, there is general agreement that there is no association between physical activity and the risk of cancer of the rectum. A few large studies have reported data for cancers of the proximal and distal colon separately and there are indications that the relationship with physical activity level may be stronger for distal rather than proximal tumours (Boyle et al. 2012).

The initial associations between physical activity and colon cancer were derived from observations that people who were physically active in their occupations were less likely to develop colon cancer than those in sedentary occupations. These studies, published in the mid-1980s, stimulated further investigations, predominantly of leisure-time and total physical activity.

One long prospective cohort study referred to in earlier chapters is a good example. Women in the Nurses' Health Study, which began in 1976, completed a comprehensive leisure-time physical activity questionnaire in 1986 and at four-year intervals thereafter. By 2002, 547 cases of colon cancer had been identified and researchers were able to quantify the risk in active versus less active women (Wolin et al. 2007). Women who expended more than 21.5 MET-h week^{-1} in all physical activity had a 23% lower risk of colon cancer than those who expended less than 2 MET-h week^{-1}. Participating in more than four hours per week of moderate or vigorous activity was associated with a 40% lower risk than participating in less than one hour per week (Figure 8.4).

High levels of physical activity maintained over a long period may confer the strongest protection. By 2004, when the surviving women in this cohort were aged about 70, over 700 cases of colon cancer had been observed. Women who engaged in physical activity at a level of 21 MET-h week^{-1} over 40 years had around half the risk of women who reported only 2 MET-h week^{-1} over this same period (Wei et al. 2009) (Figure 8.5).

How do we know that it is physical activity *per se* that is protecting people against colon cancer? The issue of confounding is an important one because physically active people tend to eat healthily (e.g. less red meat, more fibre), be non-smokers and are less prone to overweight than their sedentary peers. Well-planned studies adjust statistically for known confounding factors and have invariably found that this does not materially alter the relationship between colon cancer risk and level of physical activity. For example, in the Health Professionals Follow-up Study, physically active men were more

Figure 8.4 Multivariate relative risk of colon cancer for women in the Nurses' Health Study, 1986–2002. (a) Level of total physical activity and (b) hours per week of moderate and vigorous activity.

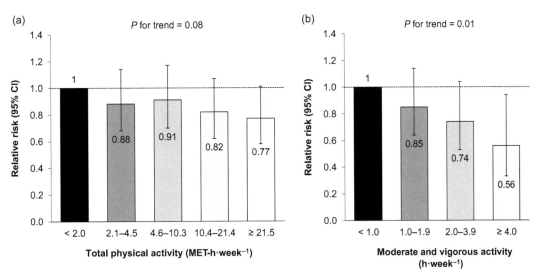

Source: Wolin et al. (2007).
Note: Reference category for total activity <2 MET-h week^{-1}, reference category for moderate and vigorous activity <1 hour week^{-1}.

Figure 8.5 Age-specific incidence of colon cancer per 100,000 person-years for a woman with 2 MET hours per week of physical activity (solid line) and a woman who reported 21 MET hours per week (dashed line) from age 30 to age 70 years.

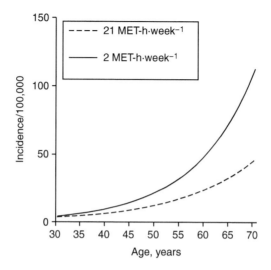

Source: Wei, E.K. et al., 'Cumulative risk of colon cancer up to age 70 years by risk factor status using data from the Nurses' Health Study', *American Journal of Epidemiology*, 2009, 170: 863–72, by permission of Oxford University Press.

likely to use multivitamins than inactive men and had lower intake of saturated fat, higher intakes of fibre, lower prevalence of smoking and lower BMI. After controlling for all these risk factors, as well as for aspirin use (which decreases risk) and family history, the protection associated with physical activity was reduced somewhat but only from 56% to 47% (Giovannucci et al. 1995). Subsequent studies report a similar level of attenuation so it can be concluded that activity is probably not merely a marker of a healthier lifestyle, but exerts an independent protective effect against colon cancer.

Energy balance as a whole seems to be associated with the risk of cancer. This may be illustrated from the findings of a large US case-control study (Slattery et al. 1997). In addition to estimating energy expenditure in physical activity, researchers measured BMI (a crude measure of energy storage) and energy intake. Either a high BMI or a high energy intake was associated with a significant increase in the risk of colon cancer (by 94% and 74%, respectively). The most interesting finding, however, emerged when the interactions between physical activity, energy intake and BMI were examined (Table 8.2). At high levels of physical activity, the risk of colon cancer was not significantly influenced by BMI or energy intake. Among people with low levels of physical activity, two things changed: (a) BMI became a more important indicator of risk and (b) the risk associated with a high energy intake increased. (This is an example of 'effect modification'; that is, the effect of one exposure differs according to the level of another.) This finding suggests that the influence of physical activity on the risk of colon cancer may be mediated through systemic metabolic effects related to energy balance, as discussed earlier.

A consensus is developing concerning the magnitude of the protective effect of physical activity on colon cancer. Meta-analysis of 52 studies (cohort and case-control)

ACTIVITY STATUS	ODDS RATIO	95% CI
Low physical activity	3.35	2.09–5.35
High physical activity	1.28	0.81–2.03

Table 8.2 Risk of colon cancer in people with high energy intake and high BMI.

Source: Slattery et al. (1997).

Note: Risk estimates were adjusted for confounding factors. Referent group: people who were active, consumed low levels of energy and had low BMI.

found a 24% lower risk in the most active men and women (Wolin et al. 2009). Subsequent systematic review and meta-analysis reached a similar conclusion; risk was 27% lower in the most active people (Boyle et al. 2012). Thus, in line with the level of evidence presented in Table 8.1, there is extensive, strong and consistent evidence that physical activity is associated with a materially lower risk of colon cancer.

Physical activity and breast cancer

Collectively, primary studies provide 'strong' evidence for an inverse association between level of physical activity and the risk for female breast cancer. One meta-analysis, restricted to prospective studies which are probably less prone to recall and selection bias than case-control studies, found a summary relative risk of 0.88 (CI 0.85–0.90) for women with the highest vs the lowest level of physical activity, suggesting a 12% risk reduction (Pizot et al. 2016).

What type of activity is associated with reduction of the risk of breast cancer? More than half the studies that measured only occupational activity and 70% of those that measured only leisure-time activity have found risk decreases in the most active women. However, when total activity (i.e. occupational, leisure time and household activity) has been measured, a lower risk in the most active women is consistently reported, suggesting that total activity – regardless of context – is what matters. Two primary studies are described as examples.

One prospective study in more than 15,000 postmenopausal women from five different areas of Italy is the EPIC[2] study (Masala et al. 2017). Physical activity was measured in occupational, leisure time and household domains using an interview and questionnaire protocol and expressed as MET-h week^{-1}. The median follow-up was nearly 15 years. Inverse associations were reported for increasing level of activity in each domain, as well as in total activity (Figure 8.6). The authors commented that, in this cohort, non-work time was mainly dedicated to housework!

Another large prospective study examined breast cancer incidence in 47,456 premenopausal and 126,704 postmenopausal women enrolled in the UK Biobank cohort (Guo et al. 2020). A total of 3,189 cases were diagnosed during a mean follow-up of 5.7 years. Compared with women in the bottom quartile for self-reported physical activity (measured via touch screen questionnaire), women in the top quartile had a lower risk of both premenopausal (RR = 0.77, CI 0.60–0.93) and postmenopausal breast cancer (RR 0.87, CI 0.78–0.96), after adjusting for adiposity. For all women

Figure 8.6 Associations between different domains of physical activity and the risk of breast cancer in 15,010 postmenopausal Italian women in the EPIC study. Hazard ratios and 95% confidence intervals.

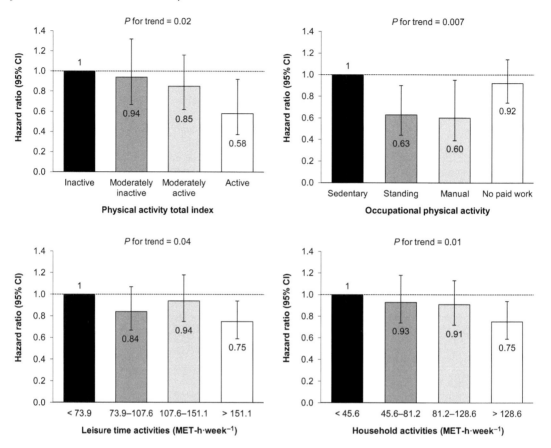

Source: Masala et al. (2017).

combined there was a clear inverse dose–response relationship between level of activity and risk of breast cancer (Figure 8.7). In a sign that advances in technology facilitate more objective measurements, this study measured adiposity using bioimpedance and accelerometry (in a sub-set of participants) to examine bias and misclassification in self-reports of physical activity.

Could confounding explain the findings that physical activity reduces the risk of breast cancer? Besides age, important risk factors include: family history, benign breast disease, variables which reflect exposure to oestrogens, high energy intake, alcohol intake, high intake of fat and – for postmenopausal breast cancer but not pre-menopausal – obesity or adult weight gain. Several of these could distort the estimated effect of physical activity. All the major studies take pains to control statistically for potentially confounding factors, however, and this does not materially alter the risk reduction associated with high levels of physical activity.

Risk has often been examined separately in premenopausal and postmenopausal women, the rationale being that body fatness is related differently to breast cancer risk

Figure 8.7 Association between physical activity and risk of invasive breast cancer in UK Biobank prospective cohort. Point estimates of self-reported physical activity and 95% confidence intervals for premenopausal and postmenopausal women combined.

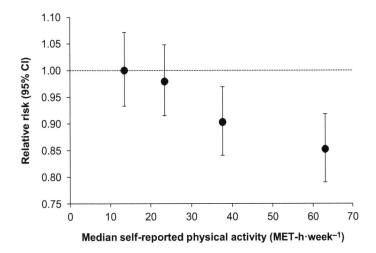

Source: Reprinted with no modifications from 'Physical activity and breast cancer risk: results from the UK Biobank prospective study', Guo, W. et al., *British Journal of Cancer*, 2020, 122: 726–32. Article distributed under the terms of the Creative Commons Attribution 4.0 International Licence (https://creativecommons.org/licenses/by/4.0/).

Note: Data adjusted for a wide range of potential confounders.

in these groups and that physical activity influences body fatness. Adipose tissue is the predominant source of oestrogens after the menopause so overweight and obese postmenopausal women have higher oestrogen concentrations than their normal-weight peers, which probably explains their higher risk of breast cancer. As summarised in pooled analyses, however, there is a lower risk in active women, irrespective of menopausal status (Hardefeldt et al. 2018; Neil-Sztramko et al. 2017).

The relationship between physical activity and breast cancer risk continues to be a topic of active research interest and the adoption of more objective methodology, as in the study of Guo and colleagues (2020) may help in clarification.

Physical activity and other cancers

In addition to breast and colon cancer, the relationship of physical activity with a number of other common cancers has been investigated. For a further five cancer sites – endometrium, kidney, bladder, oesophagus and stomach – evidence for a lower risk among active people has been assessed as 'strong' and that for lung cancer as 'moderate' (Table 8.1). Detailed discussion of evidence related to these sites is beyond the scope of this chapter and the interested reader is referred to the update to the scientific report of the US 2018 Physical Activity Guidelines Advisory Committee (McTiernan et al. 2019). Aspects of the evidence related to endometrial cancer and to lung cancer are, however, presented below to illustrate important generic points.

Worldwide, endometrial cancer is the fifth most common cancer in women, the most important risk factors being postmenopausal unopposed (without progesterone) oestrogen therapy, obesity and never having given birth. Active women tend to be lean so adiposity is an issue for studies of physical activity – it may confound any association but could also mediate an association, i.e. it could be part of a causal pathway.

Overall, epidemiological evidence from around more than 30 studies, cohort and case-control designs suggests a 20% protective effect on the risk of endometrial cancer, comparing the highest level of activity with the lowest (RR 0.80, CI 0.75–0.85) (Schmid et al. 2015). However, when this analysis was stratified according to BMI, there was an inverse relationship between physical activity and risk in over-weight/obese women but not in those of normal weight. One explanation may be that physical activity counterbalances unfavourable effects of obesity on endome-trial cancer risk – in other words that obesity is part of a causal pathway by which physical activity influences the risk for this cancer. This would be consistent with the finding from one pooled analysis that adjustment for BMI resulted in complete attenuation of the endometrial cancer association with physical activity (Matthews et al. 2020).

Meta-analysis of the findings of around 30 studies of the relationship between phys-ical activity and the risk of lung cancer found an inverse association with level of phys-ical activity (Brenner et al. 2016). Nevertheless, evidence overall is not regarded as 'strong' (Table 8.1), largely because cigarette smoking is such a powerful confounder in the causation of lung cancer and people who smoke are less likely to be physically active. Large cohort studies have found that the association of physical activity level with risk for lung cancer differs with smoking status, being absent or weaker in never-smokers (Borch et al. 2019; Patel et al. 2017). Speculatively, physical activity may somehow protect the lungs against the effects of chemical carcinogens and thus de-crease lung cancer risk in current and former smokers. Reverse causality (explained in Chapter 2) may also be an important issue in this field of inquiry because impaired lung function in heavy smokers may result in them being inactive. The extent to which researchers can control adequately for these difficulties is incompletely understood and data for never-smokers is sparse. No study has found increased risk of lung cancer with increasing physical activity, however.

DOSE–RESPONSE ISSUES

This topic is important because it informs decision making for the individual and for public health. Some studies of physical activity and cancer incidence show clear evi-dence of dose–response but others do not. Do meta-analyses and pooled analyses pro-vide an overall picture? What is the shape of the relationship and is there a threshold? Finally, the perennial big public health question – what is the minimum 'dose' of activity likely to reduce the risk of cancer?

This issue is complex because of the inconsistent methods to define and measure physical activity (discussed in detail in Chapter 2). Leisure-time physical activity is the domain most often studied but this may be a relatively small part of total activity (Barberio et al. 2018). The wide range of methods used to assess and categorise physi-cal activity pose fundamental difficulties for meta-analyses. Whilst there is consistent

Figure 8.8 Dose–response relationships of leisure-time physical activity (MET-h week^{-1}) with the risk of cancer at six different sites all of which show strong evidence of association. Mean hazard ratio (HR) and 95% confidence intervals. Shaded areas represent range of weekly physical activity typically recommended by public health agencies.

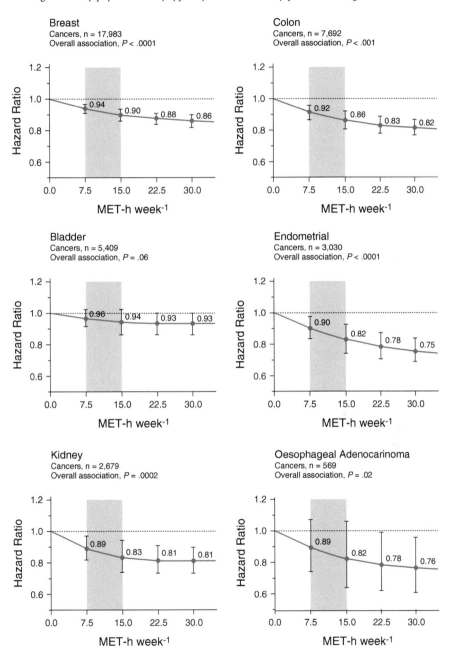

Note: Relationships for breast, colon, endometrial cancers and oesophageal adenocarcinoma are linear. Wide confidence intervals reflect heterogeneity of findings of primary studies and numbers of individuals in each analysis. Adenocarcinoma is cancer that forms in mucus-secreting glands.

evidence for a generalised dose–response relationship for a variety of cancers that indicates lower risk with higher levels of physical activity it is not possible to determine exact levels that provide given levels of effect (McTiernan et al. 2019).

The most informative pooled analysis modelled dose–response relationships from nine prospective cohorts for 15 types of cancer, focusing on the energy cost or total volume of leisure-time activity (MET-h week^{-1}) and the volume of both moderate-intensity (3–5.9 METs) and vigorous-intensity ($\geq$ 6 METs) activity (Matthews et al. 2020). The dose–response relationship was approximately linear for half of the cancer types, including breast, colon and endometrial (Figure 8.8) and curvilinear for others. The different patterns may reflect important differences in the biological mechanisms for different cancer types.

Recommended amounts of physical activity in developed countries, derived mainly from relationships with all-cause and cardiovascular mortality (see Chapter 14 'Public health'), are 7.5 to 15.0 MET-h week^{-1} at a moderate intensity (e.g. brisk walking). This range is represented by the shaded areas in Figure 8.8. Compared with doing no physical activity, engaging in these recommended amounts of leisure-time activity was associated with a significantly lower risk for seven cancer types, i.e. breast, colon, endometrial and kidney cancer (Figure 8.8) and three others not depicted in the figure. On the other hand, exceeding the minimum physical activity guideline may confer additional risk reduction for some cancer types, a conclusion which reinforced that of an earlier systematic review and meta-analysis (Kyu et al. 2016).

SEDENTARY BEHAVIOUR AND CANCER RISK

Over the last two decades, a number of large prospective cohort studies have incorporated measures of sitting time or television viewing time, in order to examine potential relationships with all-cancer or site-specific cancer incidence or mortality. Several have reported higher risk of some cancers in people who spent a longer time sitting. For example, the American Cancer Society Prevention Study found that longer leisure-time sitting was associated with a higher risk of total cancer in women (RR 1.1, CI 1.04–1.17) – although not in men (Patel et al. 2015). Participants in an NIH-funded Diet and Health Study who reported the most television viewing ($\geq$ 7 h day^{-1}) were at 22% higher risk for cancer mortality than those in the lowest viewing category (< 1 h day^{-1}) (Matthews et al. 2012). Cancers reported to be at higher risk in those with the highest levels of sitting or television viewing include those of endometrium, lung and colon (Schmid and Leitzmann 2014a).

This body of literature is now sufficiently extensive for meta-analyses to contribute summary estimates of findings. In one systematic review and meta-analysis television viewing time (but not total daily sitting time) was found to have a linear relationship with total cancer mortality (RR 1.03, CI 1.02–1.04) (Patterson et al. 2018). Analysis of 43 observational studies brought together findings for TV viewing, occupational sitting and total sitting. Comparing the highest levels of sedentary behaviour with the lowest, summary relative risks were between 1.24 and 1.54 for colon cancer, between 1.32 and 1.66 for endometrial cancer and 1.21 for the only available study on lung cancer (Schmid and Leitzmann 2014a). None of these measures of sedentary behaviour was related to any of the other nine cancer types studied. For some cancers, at least, it seems that sedentary behaviour may increase risk.

One important question, however, is whether sedentary behaviour is independent of physical activity. Studies included in these meta-analyses assessed the issue by treating physical activity as a potential confounder and controlling statistically. However, it has been argued that this is insufficient as it ignores the evidence of effect modification – in other words, 'Do the associations between sedentary behaviours and cancer incidence/ mortality differ by levels of physical activity?'

This question has been addressed by examining the associations between sedentary behaviours and cancer mortality in different strata of physical activity (Ekelund et al. 2019). Hazard ratios were identified from eight primary studies which, collectively, recorded more than 458,000 cancer deaths. Sitting time and TV viewing were both categorised in four ordinal groups, as was physical activity level (< 1 h day^{-1} to > 5 h day^{-1}). There was no association between either sitting time (Figure 8.9) or TV-viewing time and cancer mortality in the highest physical activity quartile, although there were indications of increased risk in those who reported more than five hours per day of TV time and were in the two middle quartiles for physical activity. Prolonged sedentary behaviours had adverse effects on cancer mortality but these were not evident in people who reported at least an hour of at least moderate activity per day.

Another methodological issue is relevant. Television viewing time has often been more closely related to cancer outcomes than sitting time so the question is asked: 'Are these comparable behaviours?' The answer is 'probably not'; television viewing time is more likely to be uninterrupted and to be associated with snacking and consuming alcohol – both behaviours that may influence health. Whilst both are regarded as sedentary behaviours (Tremblay et al. 2017), they are probably not interchangeable.

Figure 8.9 Hazard ratios derived from meta-analysis of associations between sitting time and cancer mortality, stratified by daily sitting time for quartiles of physical activity.

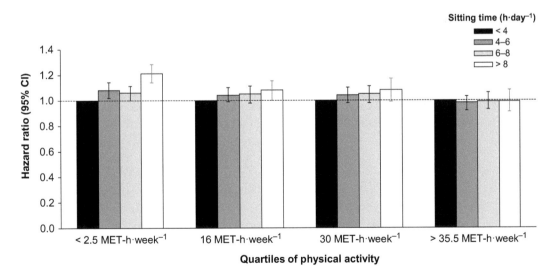

POPULATION-ATTRIBUTABLE RISK

As explained in Chapter 2, the population-attributable risk[3] (PAR) estimates the incidence of a disease that can be attributed to exposure to a particular risk factor, in this case physical inactivity. It reflects not only the strength of the risk associated with inactivity but also its prevalence in a given population. What evidence is available to estimate the health burden of inactivity from cancer?

Based on a definition of inadequate physical activity as 'less than 5 x 30 minutes of moderate exercise per week', PAR estimates for incident cancer cases in 2010 in the UK were 5.3% for colon cancer, 3.4% for breast cancer and 3.8% for endometrial cancer (Parkin 2011). In an Australian study, also based on cancer incidence in 2010, the respective figures were somewhat higher, i.e. 6.5%, 7.8% and 6.0% (Olsen et al. 2015). A study of a nationally representative cohort in Norway concluded that 21.9% of endometrial cancer could be avoided if women with low levels of physical activity (≤ 4 on a 1 to 10 self-reported scale) increased their level to the range 5–10 (Borch et al. 2017).

PARs for each of the cancers for which evidence of an association with physical activity is 'strong' (Table 8.1) have been published for Canada. Based on levels of leisure-time physical activity in a nationally representative, cross-sectional survey, values ranged from 7.8% for kidney cancer to 14.2% for cancer of the oesophagus, with a value for all cancers (which includes types *not* known to be associated with physical activity) of 4.9% (Friedenreich et al. 2019). Projections were then derived to estimate effects on cancer incidence of reductions in the population level of inadequate physical activity; a 50% reduction would be expected to prevent nearly 40,000 cancer cases by 2042 but even a more realistic reduction of 10% would save nearly 8,000 cases (Figure 8.10).

Thus estimates of PAR, despite their heterogeneity, show that increases in physical activity in a population would have a meaningful impact on cancer prevention.

PHYSICAL ACTIVITY IN CANCER SURVIVORS

The term cancer survivor describes someone from the moment of diagnosis through the balance of his or her life. As a result of advances in early detection and improved treatment, their numbers are growing and predicted to continue to grow. Survival has doubled over the last 40 years so that, in the UK for instance, 50% of people diagnosed with cancer now survive for at least ten years. Cancer survivors face unique health issues that result from the disease, its treatment and their consequences for physical and mental wellbeing. The disease causes fatigue, weight loss, loss of appetite, anaemia and weakness. Treatments, often a combination of surgery, chemotherapy and radiotherapy, are debilitating. Fatigue is a common side effect, as are peripheral neuropathies, lymphoedema (excess fluid in tissues from damage to lymph vessels) and sleep disturbances. Most aspects of physical function decline, impairing the quality of life. Some survivors, particularly of breast cancer, experience post-treatment pain which can persist for many years. Depression is common, not least because of the increased risk of cancer recurrence.

Figure 8.10 Projected cumulative preventable cancer cases with reductions of 10%, 20% and 50% in the prevalence of inadequate physical activity in Canada.

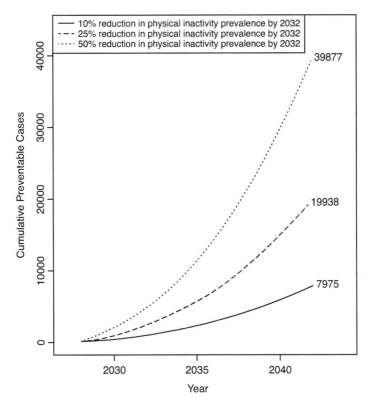

Source: Reprinted from *Preventive Medicine*, 122: 65–72, Friedenreich, C.M. et al., 'Estimates of the current and future burden of cancer attributable to lack of physical activity in Canada', page 71, copyright © 2019, with permission from Elsevier.
Note: A latency period of ten years is assumed, i.e. changes in prevalence of inactivity in 2032 expected to lead to changes in cancer incidence by 2042.

The potential benefits of incorporating exercise into clinical care are two-fold. First, exercise can mitigate the adverse, synergistic effects of cancer treatments – which include deconditioning – and their side-effects. And, second, physical activity is clearly associated with reduced cancer incidence in the general population. Could it also be associated with a reduced risk of cancer recurrence in survivors?

Exercise, quality of life and physical functioning

Around 30 randomised controlled exercise trials in cancer survivors have been published. The majority have been conducted in clinical settings, mainly in patients with early stage breast cancer and prostate cancers. A variety of different exercise modalities have been employed, with interventions during weeks of chemotherapy as well as post-treatment.

Early trials compared the effects of an exercise regimen, typically moderate-intensity aerobic training, with usual care. More recently, the objective has been to compare the effects of different intensities of exercise and different modes of delivery (for example, Brown et al. 2018). Heterogeneity is inevitably a feature of this literature given differences between patients in the aetiology of the disease and treatment regimens. Nevertheless, there is strong evidence that exercise, particularly supervised exercise, improves quality of life – sometimes described as health-related quality of life – and physical functioning (Sweegers et al. 2018). (When 'improvement' is recorded by comparison with usual care this can mean avoidance of a decrease, as is commonly observed for $\dot{V}O_2$max.) Supervised programmes are the most effective for reducing anxiety and symptoms of depression but fatigue is typically reduced in both supervised and unsupervised settings. Recent trials have shown benefits from aerobic exercise, particularly walking, for sleep quality.

In 2017, a systematic review for Cancer Care Ontario concluded that exercise is safe, feasible and improves health-related fitness and quality of life for survivors, whilst they are on active treatment or after treatment (Segal et al. 2017b). These findings were bolstered by the subsequent consensus statement from an ACSM International Multidisciplinary Roundtable (Campbell et al. 2019). An important caveat is the heavy reliance on extrapolation from studies of breast cancer. Box 8.3 summarises exercise recommendations for cancer survivors.

This remains an active research area. The focus is moving away from trials conducted in a clinical setting towards the potential of lifestyle interventions, behaviour change (including decreases in sedentary time) and long-term compliance. Patients with a wider variety of site-specific cancers are subject to study. Effects on bone health are also the subject of research interest because survivors of breast and prostate cancer may have bone fragility as a consequence of hormonal treatments.

BOX 8.3 EXERCISE RECOMMENDATIONS FOR CANCER SURVIVORS.

- Assessment to evaluate any effects of disease, treatments or comorbidities is recommended before starting an exercise intervention.
- 120–150 minutes of moderate-intensity aerobic training per week, spread over three to five days.
- Resistance training using major muscle groups on at least two days per week.
- Where possible, exercise should be in a group or supervised setting.
- An exercise programme should last for at least eight to twelve weeks but thereafter survivors should engage in moderate-intensity exercise on an ongoing basis to maintain benefits.
- At the very least, inactivity should be avoided.

Sources: Adapted from Segal et al. (2017a) and Campbell et al. (2019).

Exercise, cancer mortality and cancer recurrence

Studies on survival are overwhelmingly observational and mostly restricted to breast, colorectal and prostate cancer survivors. For methodological reasons, the outcome measure reported is often all-cause mortality or cancer mortality rather than cancer recurrence.

There is strong and consistent evidence that physical activity is associated with a lower risk of all-cause and cancer mortality in survivors of breast and colorectal cancers (Lahart et al. 2015; Schmid and Leitzmann 2014b). Both these pooled analyses compared cancer mortality in those with the highest level of physical activity with those with the lowest. High post-diagnosis activity level was associated with reductions in the summary risk of breast cancer mortality of 28% and 41%, respectively. For physical activity among colon cancer survivors, a high level of post-diagnosis physical activity was associated with a 39% lower risk (Schmid and Leitzmann 2014b). In both analyses pre-diagnosis physical activity had a protective effect but of a lesser magnitude than post-diagnosis activity, also a feature of a number of other reports.

Fewer studies of prostate cancer survivors are available but they also show a protective effect of physical activity, particularly post-diagnosis. A pooled risk estimate, based on three primary studies, of 0.62 indicates a protective effect of 38%, again based on comparison of high versus low levels of physical activity (Friedenreich et al. 2016).

All the primary studies included in these (and other) meta-analyses relied on self-reported recreational physical activity, with its attendant inaccuracies. Household activity has seldom been measured and, when it has been, findings were mixed (Ammitzbøll et al. 2016; Bonn et al. 2014). Some information is available about dose–response. Figure 8.11 shows differences in the risk of total and cancer mortality in survivors of breast cancer and colorectal cancer with increments (above the lowest level) in post-diagnosis physical activity (Schmid and Leitzmann 2014b). For breast cancer survivors, increments of 5, 10 or 15 MET-h week^{-1} were associated with mean reductions in all-cause mortality of 13%, 24% and 34%, respectively. Corresponding reductions for colorectal cancer survivors were 15%, 28% and 38%. Dose–response analyses for cancer mortality were similar (Figure 8.11). An inverse, non-linear relationship between physical activity and cancer mortality in survivors of breast and colorectal cancer was confirmed in a subsequent meta-analysis; cancer mortality declined by 2% for every increase in MET-h week^{-1} up to 10 MET-h week^{-1} but there was little further decrease above 15 MET-h week^{-1} (Li et al. 2016).

The evidence for cancer recurrence *per se* remains sparse. Rather, benefit is inferred from all-cause mortality or cancer mortality. Future research directions include: more objective measures of physical activity, as in the START trial (Supervised Trial of Aerobic versus Resistance Training) in breast cancer patients; larger numbers of participants through multi-centre collaborations to give more power to look at subgroups; measurements of biomarkers to aid mechanistic research; and randomised, controlled trials. Only the latter design can deal robustly with reverse causation, i.e. the possibility that people are inactive because they are becoming ill. Randomised controlled trials investigating the effect of lifestyle interventions (diet, physical activity and sometimes

Figure 8.11 Dose–response relationships between physical activity and all-cause and cancer mortality among breast and colorectal survivors for an increase of 5, 10 or 15 MET-h week^{-1} in post-diagnosis physical activity.

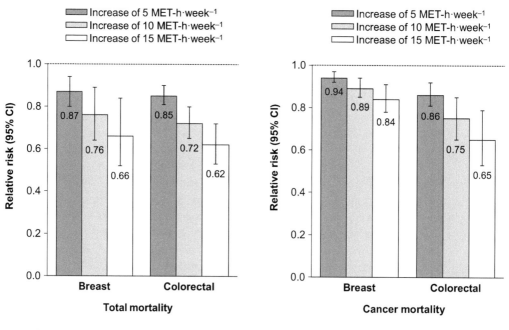

Source: Schmid and Leitzmann (2014b).

vitamin D) on recurrence or disease-free survival are under way and studies have begun to assess sedentary time alongside physical activity (Swain et al. 2020).

The biological mechanisms whereby physical activity could influence recurrence – and thus all-cause or cancer mortality – are poorly understood. Likely candidates include changes in whole-body and visceral fatness, metabolic dysregulation, sex hormones, chronic low-grade inflammation, oxidative stress and impaired immune surveillance (Figure 8.12). Synergistic interactions with cancer treatment which could increase its efficacy are also possible (Hojman et al. 2018). For example, exercise during chemotherapy has been reported to improve adherence to treatment (Courneya et al. 2014) and, speculatively, it could influence the distribution and/or metabolism of drugs. Such interactions could possibly explain why post-diagnosis activity seems to have greater influence on cancer outcomes than pre-diagnosis activity. One further benefit not included in Figure 8.12 is that physical activity may help survivors to avoid comorbidities and this may be particularly important in older people.

Despite the strong body of evidence for benefits, research shows that few cancer survivors maintain the recommended level of physical activity (Yan et al. 2018). Consequently, even if/when exercise programmes are integrated into standard clinical practice, better understanding of the factors which influence adherence to physical activity 'prescriptions' will be needed before its potential to improve survival and quality of life can be widely realised.

Figure 8.12 Commonly proposed mechanisms relating physical activity to cancer recurrence and/or survival. Potential additive or synergistic effects between physical activity and cancer treatment are possible.

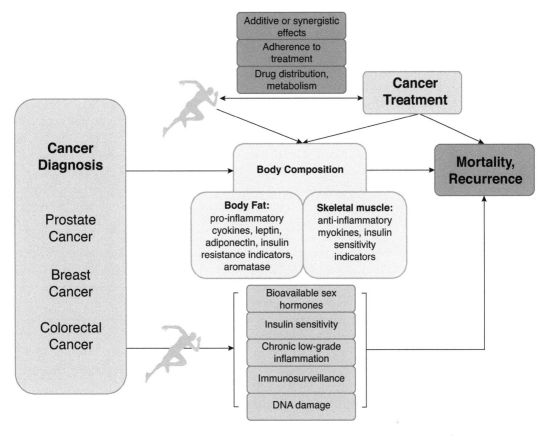

SUMMARY

- Cancer is a major cause of morbidity and mortality. Over half of cancer deaths are accounted for by cancers of the lung, breast, large bowel and prostate. Risk factors vary by tumour site.
- Carcinogenesis involves disruption of the orderly fashion in which normal body cells grow, divide and die.
- Potential systemic mechanisms which might influence the risk of cancer include: changes to metabolic factors, in particular insulin; avoidance of weight gain; reducing inflammation; and improved immune surveillance.
- Hypothesised site-specific mechanisms include: for cancers of the reproductive system, a decrease in exposure to sex steroid hormones; for colon cancer, a decrease in bowel transit time.

- Epidemiological research shows that increasing levels of physical activity are associated with reductions in the risk of a number of cancers. Evidence, predominantly in Caucasians, is strong for seven types of cancer.
- There is some evidence for dose–response relationships between level of activity and risk of several cancers but these are not well described. There does not appear to be a lower threshold below which no effect is evident so some physical activity is better than none for cancer risk.
- The risk for many common cancers is reduced by engaging in the amounts (2.5 to 5.0 hours per week) of moderate-intensity physical activity typically recommended for health benefits, although more may be needed for optimal cancer risk reduction.
- In cancer survivors, physical activity lowers the risk of cancer mortality and improves physical functioning. Deleterious effects of the disease and its treatment are reduced, improving quality of life.

STUDY TASKS

1 What are the possible explanations for the wide differences between countries in the incidence rates for specific cancers? Which seem most tenable and why?
2 How do cancer cells differ from normal cells? Explain how these characteristics lead to the development of a tumour.
3 Briefly describe the mechanisms by which high levels of physical activity may influence the risk of breast cancer.
4 Outline the benefits of physical activity for cancer survivors.
5 Why is confounding an important problem for researchers conducting epidemiological studies of colon cancer? How do researchers tackle this problem?
6 Discuss the evidence for a dose–response relationship between level of physical activity and cancer risk. Does this constitute an adequate basis for recommendations for cancer prevention in the general population?

NOTES

1 Case-control studies comprise a greater proportion of this literature (and that on other cancers) than of literature on coronary heart disease (CHD) and diabetes; the reason is that the incidence of site-specific cancers is much lower than CHD so it is more difficult with a cohort study to obtain sufficient cancer cases to obtain sufficient statistical power to detect effects.
2 EPIC is the abbreviation for the European Prospective Investigation into Cancer.
3 See Chapter 2 for definition and calculation of this statistic.

FURTHER READING

Campbell, K.L., Winters-Stone, K.M., Wiskemann, J., May, A.M., Schwartz, A.L., Courneya, K.S. et al. (2019) Exercise guidelines for cancer survivors: consensus statement from international multidisciplinary roundtable. *Medicine and Science in Sports and Exercise* 51: 2375–90.

Friedenreich, C.M., Shaw, E., Neilson, H.K. and Brenner, D.R. (2017) Epidemiology and biology of physical activity and cancer recurrence. *Journal of Molecular Medicine* 95: 1029–41.

Hojman, P., Gehl, J., Christensen, J.F. and Pedersen, B. (2018) Molecular mechanisms linking exercise to cancer prevention and treatment. *Cell Metabolism* 27: 10–21.

Lee, I.-M. (2012) Physical activity, fitness and cancer: the evidence, the issues, and the challenges. In C. Bouchard, S.N. Blair and W.L. Haskell (eds) *Physical activity and health.* 2nd edn, Champaign, IL: Human Kinetics.

McTiernan, A., Friedenreich, C.M., Katzmarzyk, P.T., Powell, K.E., Macko, R., Buchner, D. et al. for the 2018 Physical Activity Guidelines Advisory Committee. (2019) Physical activity in cancer prevention and survival: a systematic review. *Medicine and Science in Sports and Exercise* 51: 1252–61.

Patel, A.V., Friedenreich, C.M., Moore, S.C., Hayes, S.C., Silver, J.K., Campbell, K.L. et al. (2019) American College of Sports Medicine Roundtable report on physical activity, sedentary behaviour, and cancer prevention and control. *Medicine and Science in Sports and Exercise* 51: 2391–402.

▎ REFERENCES

Ammitzbøll, G., Søgaard, K., Karlsen, R.V., Tjønneland, G., Johansen, C., Frederiksen, K. and Bidstrup, P. (2016) Physical activity and survival in breast cancer. *European Journal of Cancer* 66: 67–74.

Barberio, A.M., Friedenreich, C.M., Lynch, B.M., Campbell, K.L., Arora, P. and Brenner, D.R. (2018) Physical activity and cancer incidence in Alberta's Tomorrow Project; results from a prospective cohort of 26,538 participants. *Cancer Epidemiology Biomarkers and Prevention* 27: 945–54.

Bonn, S.E., Sjölander, A., Trolle Lagerros, Y., Wiklund, F., Stattin, P., Holmberg, E. et al. (2014) Physical activity and survival among men diagnosed with prostate cancer. *Cancer Epidemiology Biomarkers and Prevention* 24: 57–64.

Borch, K.B., Weiderpass, E., Braaten, T., Hansen, M.S. and Licaj, I. (2019) Risk of lung cancer and physical activity by smoking status and body mass index, the Norwegian Women and Cancer Study. *European Journal of Epidemiology* 34: 489–98.

Borch, K.B., Weiderpass, E., Braaten, T., Jareid, M., Gavrilyuk, O.A. and Licaj, I. (2017) Physical activity and risk of endometrial cancer in the Norwegian Women and Cancer (NOWAC) study. *International Journal of Cancer* 140: 1809–18.

Boyle, T., Keegel, T., Bull, F., Heyworth, J. and Fritschi, L. (2012) Physical activity and risks of proximal and distal colon cancers: a systematic review and meta-analysis. *Journal of the National Cancer Institute* 104: 1548–61.

Brenner, D.R., Yannitsos, D.H., Farris, M.S., Johansson, M. and Friedenreich, C.M. (2016) Leisure-time physical activity and lung cancer risk: a systematic review and meta-analysis. *Lung Cancer* 95: 17–27.

Brown, J.C., Troxel, A.B., Ky, B., Damjanov, N., Zemel, B.S., Rickels, M.R. et al. (2018) Dose–response effects of aerobic exercise among colon cancer survivors; a randomized Phase II trial. *Clinical Colorectal Cancer* 17: 32–40.

Campbell, K.L., Winters-Stone, K.M., Wiskemann, J., May, A.M., Schwartz, A.L., Courneya et al. (2019) Exercise guidelines for cancer survivors: consensus statement from international multidisciplinary roundtable. *Medicine and Science in Sports and Exercise* 51: 2375–90.

Canadian Cancer Society (2020) How cancer starts, grows and spreads [online], available at: https://www.cancer.ca/en/cancer-information/cancer-101/what-is-cancer/how-cancer-starts-grows-and-spreads/?region=on (accessed 6 May 2020).

Courneya, K.S., Segal, R.J., McKenzie, D.C., Dong, H., Gelmon, K., Friedenreich, C.M. et al. (2014) Effects of exercise during adjuvant chemotherapy on breast cancer outcomes. *Medicine and Science in Sports and Exercise* 46: 1744–51.

De Rezende, L.F.M., Sá, T.H., Markozannes, G., Rey-López, J.P., Lee, I.-M., Tsilidis, K.K. et al. (2018) Physical activity and cancer: an umbrella review of the literature including 22 major anatomical sites and 770 000 cancer cases. *British Journal of Sports Medicine* 52: 826–33.

Ekelund, U., Brown, W.J., Steene-Johannessen, J., Fagerland, M.W., Owen, N., Powell, K.E. et al. (2019) Do the associations of sedentary behaviour with cardiovascular disease mortality and cancer mortality differ by physical activity level? A systematic review and harmonised meta-analysis of data from 850 060 participants. *British Journal of Sports Medicine* 53: 886–94.

Ennour-Idrissi, K., Maunsell, E. and Diorio, C. (2015) Effect of physical activity on sex hormones in women: a systematic review and meta-analysis. *Breast Cancer Research* 17: 139–48.

Friedenreich, C.M., Barberio, A.M., Pader, J., Poirier, A.E., Ruan, Y., Grevers, X. et al. on behalf of the ComPARe Study Team. (2019) Estimates of the current and future burden of cancer attributable to lack of physical activity in Canada. *Preventive Medicine* 122: 65–72.

Friedenreich, C.M., Shaw, E., Neilson, H.K. and Brenner, D.R. (2017) Epidemiology and biology of physical activity and cancer recurrence. *Journal of Molecular Medicine* 95: 1029–41.

Friedenreich, C.M., Wang, Q., Neilson, H.K., Kopciuk, K.A., McGregor, S.E. and Courneya, K.S. (2016) Physical activity and survival after prostate cancer. *European Journal of Urology* 70: 576–85.

Friedenreich, C.M., Woolcott, C.G., McTiernan, A., Ballard-Barbash, R., Brant, R.F., Stanczy, F.Z. et al. (2010) Alberta physical activity and breast cancer prevention trial: sex hormone changes in a year-long exercise intervention among postmenopausal women. *Journal of Clinical Oncology* 28: 1458–65.

Fuentes, G.C., Castañer, O., Warnberg, J., Subirana, I., Buil-Cosiales, P., Salas-Salvadó, J. et al. (2020) Prospective association of physical activity and inflammatory biomarkers in older adults from the PREDIMED-Plus study with overweight or obesity and metabolic syndrome. *Clinical Nutrition* 39: 3092–8.

Giovannucci, E., Ascherio, A., Rimm, E.B., Colditz, G.A., Stampfer, M.J. and Willett, W.C. (1995) Physical activity, obesity, and risk for colon cancer and adenoma in men. *Annals of Internal Medicine* 122: 327–34.

Goding Sauer, A., Siegel, R.L., Jemal, A. and Fedewa, S.A. (2019) Current prevalence of major cancer risk factors and screening test use in the United States: disparities by education and race/ethnicity. *Cancer Epidemiology, Biomarkers and Prevention* 28: 629–42.

Guo, W., Fensom, G.K., Reeves, G.K. and Key, T.J. (2020) Physical activity and breast cancer risk: results from the UK Biobank prospective study. *British Journal of Cancer* 122: 726–32.

Hardefeldt, P.J., Penninkilampi, R., Edirimanne, S. and Eslick, G.D. (2018) Physical activity and weight loss reduce the risk of breast cancer: a meta-analysis of 139 prospective and retrospective studies. *Clinical Breast Cancer* 18: e601–12.

Hojman, P., Gehl, J., Christensen, J.F. and Pedersen, B. (2018) Molecular mechanisms linking exercise to cancer prevention and treatment. *Cell Metabolism* 27: 10–21.

Kang, D.-W., Lee, J., Suh, S.-H., Ligibel, J., Courneya, K.S. and Jeon, J.Y. (2016) Effects of exercise on insulin, IGF axis, adipocytokines, and inflammatory markers in breast cancer survivors: a systematic review and meta-analysis. *Cancer Epidemiology, Biomarkers and Prevention* 26: 355–65.

Kyu, H.H., Bachman, V.F., Alexander, L.T., Everett Mumford, J., Afshin, A., Estep, K. et al. (2016) Physical activity and risk of breast cancer, colon cancer, diabetes, ischemic heart disease, and ischemic stroke events: systematic review and dose-response meta-analysis for the Global Burden of Disease Study 2013. *British Medical Journal* 354: i3857. doi: 10.1136/bmj.i3857.

Lahart, I.M., Metsios, G.S., Nevill, A.M. and Carmichael, A.R. (2015) Physical activity, risk of death and recurrence in breast cancer survivors: a systematic review and meta-analysis of epidemiological studies. *Acta Oncologica* 54: 635–45.

Li, T., Wei, S., Shi, Y., Pang, S., Qin, Q., Yin, J. et al. (2016) The dose–response effect of physical activity on cancer mortality: findings from 71 prospective cohort studies. *British Journal of Sports Medicine* 50: 339–45.

Masala, G., Bendinelli, B., Assedi, M., Occhini, D., Zanna, I., Sieri, S. et al. (2017) Up to one-third of breast cancer cases in post-menopausal Mediterranean women might be avoided by modifying lifestyle habits: the EPIC Italy study. *Breast Cancer Research and Treatment* 161: 311–20.

Matthews, C.E., George, S.M., Moore, S.C., Bowles, H.R., Blair, A., Park, Y. et al. (2012) Amount of time spent in sedentary behaviors and cause-specific mortality in US adults. *The American Journal of Clinical Nutrition* 95: 437–45.

Matthews, C.E., Moore, S.C., Arem, H., Cook, M.B., Trabert, B., Håkansson, N. et al. (2020) Amount and intensity of leisure-time physical activity and lower cancer risk. *Journal of Clinical Oncology* 38: 686–97.

McTiernan, A., Friedenreich, C.M., Katzmarzyk, P.T., Powell, K.E., Macko, R., Buchner, D. et al. for the 2018 Physical Activity Guidelines Advisory Committee. (2019) Physical activity in cancer prevention and survival: a systematic review. *Medicine and Science in Sports and Exercise* 51: 1252–61.

Moore, S.C., Lee, I.-M., Weiderpass, E., Campbell, T.T., Sampson, J.N., Kitahara, C.M. et al. (2016) Association of leisure-time physical activity with risk of 26 types of cancer in 1.44 million adults. *Journal of the American Medical Association* 176: 816–25.

Neil-Sztramko, S.E., Boyle, T., Milosevic, E., Nugent, S.F., Gotay, C.C. and Campbell, K.L. (2017) Does obesity modify the relationship between physical activity and breast cancer risk? *Breast Cancer Research and Treatment* 166: 367–81.

Olsen, C.M., Wilson, L.F., Nagle, C.M., Kendall, B.J., Bain, C.J., Pandeya, N. et al. (2015) Cancers in Australia in 2010 attributable to insufficient physical activity. *Australian and New Zealand Journal of Public Health* 39: 458–63.

Parkin, D.M. (2011) Cancers attributable to inadequate physical exercise in the UK in 2010. *British Journal of Cancer* 105: S38–S41.

Patel, A.V., Carter, B.D., Stevens, V.L., Gaudet, M.M., Campbell, P.T. and Gapstur, S.M. (2017) The relationship between physical activity, obesity, and lung cancer risk by smoking status in a large prospective cohort of US adults. *Cancer Causes and Control* 28: 1357–68.

Patel, A.V., Friedenreich, C.M., Moore, S.C., Hayes, S.C., Silver, J.K., Campbell, K.L. et al. (2019) American College of Sports Medicine Roundtable report on physical activity, sedentary behaviour, and cancer prevention and control. *Medicine and Science in Sports and Exercise* 51: 2391–402.

Patel, A.V., Hidebrand, J.S., Campbell, P.T., Teras, L.R., Craft, L.L., McCullough, M.L. and Gapstur, S.M. (2015) Leisure-time spent sitting and site-specific cancer incidence in a large U.S. cohort. *Cancer Biomarkers and Prevention* 24: 1350–9.

Patterson, R., McNamara, E., Tainio, M., de Sá, T.H., Smith, A.D., Sharp, S.J. et al. (2018) Sedentary behaviour and risk of all-cause, cardiovascular and cancer mortality, and incident type 2 diabetes: a systematic review and dose response meta-analysis. *European Journal of Epidemiology* 33: 811–29.

Pizot, C., Boniol, M., Mullie, P., Koechlin, A., Boniol, M., Boyle, P. and Autier, P. (2016) Physical activity, hormone replacement therapy and breast cancer risk: a meta-analysis of prospective studies. *European Journal of Cancer* 52: 138–54.

Schmid, D., Behrens, G., Keimling, M., Jochem, C., Ricci, C. and Leitzmann, M. (2015) A systematic review and meta-analysis of physical activity and endometrial cancer risk. *European Journal of Epidemiology* 30: 397–412.

Schmid, D. and Leitzmann, M.G. (2014a) Television viewing and time spent sedentary in relation to cancer risk: a meta-analysis. *Journal of the National Cancer Institute* 106: dju098. doi: 10.1093/jnci/dju098.

Schmid, D. and Leitzmann, M.F. (2014b) Association between physical activity and mortality among breast cancer and colorectal cancer survivors: a systematic review and meta-analysis. *Annals of Oncology* 25: 1293–1311.

Segal, R., Zwaal, C., Green, E., Tomasone, J.R., Loblaw, A. and Petrella, T. and the Exercise for People with Cancer Guidelines Development Group. (2017a) Exercise for people with cancer: a clinical practice guide. *Current Oncology* 24: 40–6.

Segal, R., Zwaal, C., Green, E., Tomasone, J.R., Loblaw, A. and Petrella, T. and the Exercise for People with Cancer Guidelines Development Group. (2017b) Exercise for people with cancer: a systematic review. *Current Oncology* 24: e290–315.

Slattery, M.L., Edwards, S.L., Ma, K.N., Friedman, G.D. and Potter, J.D. (1997) Physical activity and colon cancer: a public health perspective. *Annals Epidemiology* 7: 137–45.

Sternfeld, B. and Lee, I.-M. (2009) Physical activity and cancer: the evidence, the issues, and the challenges. In I.-M. Lee, S.N. Blair, J.E. Manson and R.S. Paffenbarger (eds) *Epidemiologic methods in physical activity studies.* New York: Oxford University Press.

Swain, C.T.V., Nguyen, N.H., Eagles, T., Vallance, J.K., Boyle, T., Lahart, I.M. and Lynch, B.M. (2020) Postdiagnosis sedentary behavior and health outcomes in cancer survivors: a systematic review and meta-analysis. *Cancer* 126: 861–9.

Sweegers, M.G., Altenburg, T.M., Chinapaw, M.J., Kalter, J., Verdonck-de Leeuw, I.M., Courneya, K.S. et al. (2018) Which exercise prescriptions improve quality of life and physical function in patients with cancer during and following treatment? A systematic review and meta-analysis of randomised controlled trials. *British Journal of Sports Medicine* 52: 505–13.

Tremblay, M.S., Aubert, S., Barnes, J.D., Saunders, T.J., Carson, V., Latimer-Cheung, A.E. et al. on behalf of SBRN Terminology Consensus Project Participants. (2017) Sedentary behaviour research network (SBRN): terminology consensus project process and outcome. *International Journal of Behavioural Science and Physical Activity* 14: 75. doi: 10.1186/s12966-017-0525–8.

Wei, E.K., Colditz, G.A., Giovannucci, E.L., Fuchs, C.S. and Rosner, B.A. (2009) Cumulative risk of colon cancer up to age 70 years by risk factor status using data from the Nurses' Health Study. *American Journal of Epidemiology* 170: 863–72.

Wolin, K.Y., Lee, I.-M., Colditz, C.A., Glynn, R.J., Fuchs, C. and Giovannucci, E. (2007) Leisure-time physical activity patterns and risk of colon cancer in women. *International Journal of Cancer* 121: 2776–81.

Wolin, K.Y., Yan, Y., Colditz, G.A. and Lee, I.-M. (2009) Physical activity and colon cancer prevention: a meta-analysis. *British Journal of Cancer* 100: 611–16.

Yan., A.F., Wang, Y. and Ng, A.V. (2018) Physical activity and annual medical outlay in U.S. colorectal, breast and prostate cancer survivors. *Preventive Medicine Reports* 9: 118–23.

9 Skeletal health

Katherine Brooke-Wavell and
Adrianne E. Hardman

INTRODUCTION

The skeleton provides physical support and protection for internal organs and, through the actions of muscles, enables movement. It also acts as a reservoir for minerals, particularly calcium. The structure of bone confers 'strength with lightness', so that transporting the skeleton around is not a metabolic burden. As people age, bone strength decreases and bones become more fragile, with an increased propensity to fracture. Low muscle strength and poor balance in elderly people compound this problem by increasing the likelihood of a fall that may precipitate a fracture.

This chapter reviews the evidence concerning the role of physical activity in skeletal health. Knowledge of the anatomy of bone – as an organ and as a tissue – helps us to understand how different types of activity affect its load-bearing competence. The first section, therefore, provides revision of the basic anatomy of bone and some aspects of its physiology.

BIOLOGY OF BONE

An adult has 10–12 kg of bone, a dynamic tissue with high metabolic activity. It comprises organic material, an inorganic matrix and a small amount of water. The organic component is mainly collagen. The inorganic component is almost all hydroxyapatite, a mineral composed of calcium and phosphate that is hard and brittle like eggshell. Bone is not a homogeneous tissue, however, and these components are organised in different ways in cortical and trabecular bone.

Cortical bone is dense and 'ivory-like', properties well suited to its functions of support and protection. It forms the external part of the long bones and is thickest in the shaft, where it encloses a cavity filled with yellow, fatty marrow (Figure 9.1). Towards the ends of a long bone this cavity is replaced by trabecular bone – also called cancellous or 'spongy' bone. Trabecular bone is much less dense than cortical bone and is made up of a lattice of thin, calcified struts (trabeculae) that form along the lines of greatest stress. Different types of bone predominate at different skeletal sites, according to functional requirements. For example, trabecular bone makes up 40% of vertebrae but only 1% of the mid-radius.

The outer membrane covering cortical bone, facing the soft tissue, is the periosteum. Facing the medullary cavity in a long bone – and covering the trabeculae of trabecular bone – is the endosteum. In both types of bone, cells lining the endosteum are metabolically active and much involved in bone formation and resorption. Trabecular bone has a particularly high metabolic rate as its open structure allows bone marrow, blood vessels and connective tissue to be in contact with the endosteum.

Bone cells regulate bone metabolism and confer adaptive potential by responding to various environmental signals. There are three types of cells: osteocytes, osteoblasts and osteoclasts. Osteocytes are mature cells embedded within small cavities in bone. Their main role is to activate bone turnover and regulate extracellular calcium concentration. Osteoblasts produce bone matrix and build new bone, whilst osteoclasts remove old bone. The activities of osteoblasts and osteoclasts are closely coupled during bone remodelling. Even after growth has ended, the skeleton is in a continuous state of remodelling and between 1% and 10% of skeletal mass is remodelled each year. This process, which takes place in cycles lasting three to five months, enables the maintenance of serum calcium levels, the repair of the microfractures and fatigue damage that bone sustains daily, and confers its adaptive potential.

The events of the remodelling cycle are shown schematically in Figure 9.2. Osteoclasts are abundant at the surfaces of bone undergoing erosion and secrete enzymes that create an acid environment to resorb (digest) old bone, creating a cavity. After a delay, osteoblasts fill this cavity with a volume of new bone which then undergoes remineralisation. Bone resorption initiates bone formation and, under most circumstances, restores lost bone. However, as age advances, less new bone is formed than is resorbed in each remodelling cycle, leading to bone loss and structural damage. It follows that, in older people, increased turnover enhances age-related bone loss.

The remodelling process is influenced by hormones that regulate plasma calcium, i.e. parathyroid hormone, vitamin D and, to a lesser extent, calcitonin. Parathyroid hormone acts to raise plasma calcium levels by stimulating bone resorption, enhancing

Figure 9.1 Structure of a long bone.

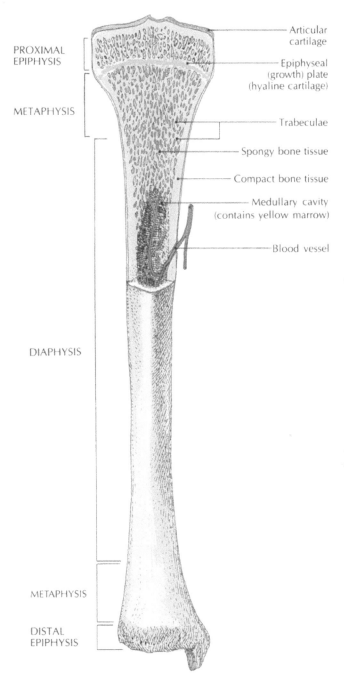

Source: Republished with permission of McGraw-Hill from *Human anatomy*, Carola, R. et al., copyright © 1992; permission conveyed through Copyright Clearance Center, Inc.

Figure 9.2 Remodelling occurs within bone remodelling compartments on trabecular bone surface, surrounded by a canopy of lining cells with a nearby capillary (top). In cortical bone remodelling takes place along a central canal (bottom). Osteoclast precursor cells migrate and differentiate into mature osteoclasts (OC) which resorb bone. Subsequently osteoblasts (derived from their precursors) secrete osteoid (organic component) that is mineralised to form new bone.

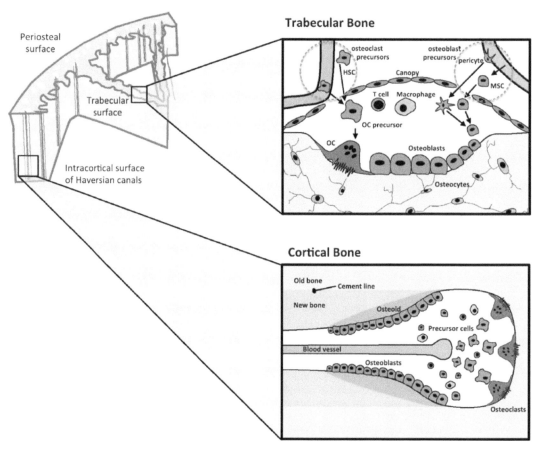

Source: Reprinted by permission from Springer Nature Customer Service Centre GmbH: Springer Nature, *BoneKEy Reports*, 'Coupling the activities of bone formation and resorption: a multitude of signals within the basic multicellular unit', Sims, N.A. and Martin, T.J., copyright © 2014.

calcium absorption from the gut and reducing urinary calcium excretion. Vitamin D is converted in the skin from a precursor in response to exposure to ultraviolet radiation in sunlight. The main action of its metabolites, which behave as hormones, is to stimulate the absorption of ingested calcium. It must also be concerned with calcification of the bone matrix, because vitamin D deficiency gives rise to rickets in children and osteomalacia in adults. Secretion of calcitonin increases when plasma calcium is elevated. Its main effect is to inhibit the activity of osteoclasts, reducing resorption so that less calcium is released into the plasma.

Other hormones influence calcium metabolism although they are not involved in the regulation of plasma calcium. The most important of these is oestrogen which helps to conserve bone mass by limiting bone resorption and turnover. It also increases intestinal calcium absorption and reduces urinary calcium excretion – both bone-conserving effects. Oestrogen withdrawal therefore results in an increase in the intensity of remodelling, accelerating bone loss.

It is now accepted that bone has an unconventional role as an endocrine organ that regulates energy metabolism (Karsenty and Oury 2012). For example, leptin (the adipocyte-derived hormone that plays an important part in energy metabolism) is a powerful inhibitor of bone mass accrual. Thus, bone is highly sensitive to energy availability – a link that makes evolutionary sense because bone remodelling consumes a large amount of energy. Osteocalcin (a protein derived from osteoblasts and a marker for bone formation) favours pancreatic insulin secretion and alters insulin sensitivity in liver, muscle and white adipose tissue.

Bone strength

The strength of bone reflects the integration of two main features: bone mineral density and quality. Quality may include architecture (e.g. mineral distribution, cortical thickness and/or trabecular structure), organic content, turnover and damage accumulation (e.g. microfractures). Bone mineral density is the mass of mineral per unit area or volume. It is measured by imaging techniques, the most common of which is dual energy X-ray absorptiometry (DXA). The principles of these techniques are explained in Box 9.1. DXA measurements of bone density explain 70% of the variance in the breaking strength of bone and, at a group level, are quite good at predicting fracture risk. Ultrasound measurements at the calcaneus are predictive of fracture risk in older women, but there is insufficient standardisation of instruments and reference ranges to allow widely accepted diagnostic thresholds. The introduction of 3D bone imaging techniques, such as quantitative computed tomography (QCT), permits assessment of bone structure and geometry. Recognition of the major role of these determinants of bone strength has created a surge of interest in this technology from researchers interested in exercise.

BOX 9.1 MEASURING THE STRUCTURAL PROPERTIES OF BONE.

Dual energy X-ray absorptiometry

DXA uses X-ray beams of two distinct energy levels to distinguish the relative composition of bone and non-bone compartments of the body. The measurements are based on the degree to which the X-ray beam is attenuated by the tissues. Two measures are derived: bone mineral content – the total grams of bone mineral within a measured region of bone; and bone mineral density (BMD) – the grams of bone mineral per unit of bone area scanned. Note that this is an *areal** density. Bone mineral content is highly dependent on bone size so a larger person will have a greater value than a smaller person. When bone strength is increased through changes in size as well as in mineral content (as might be the case for physical activity during growth), BMD alone may not detect this, so bone mineral content and BMD are complementary measures.

- The main limitation of DXA is that, although it measures all bone within a given area, it does not assess bone architecture, nor does it differentiate between trabecular and cortical bone.
- Advantages of DXA include the low level of radiation exposure and its accuracy and precision. Scans take as little as five minutes and can measure bone at clinically relevant sites.

Quantitative computed tomography

This technique uses X-rays to create an image of specific thin layers through the body that are built up to provide a measure of the density of bone. It measures bone mineral content, volumetric BMD and axial cross-sectional area.

- This technique can measure bone size, shape and mass and discriminate cortical and trabecular bone. It can measure cortical thickness, trabecular bone density and some estimates of strength that take account of both bone mineral content and distribution.
- Limitations include that the resolution is not high enough to isolate thin structures: each volume (voxel) measured may include only partly bone, generating *partial volume effects*. Axial CT scanners involve higher exposure to radiation than DXA and are more expensive. Peripheral QCT (pQCT) has a lower radiation dose and is cheaper, but can only measure sites such as lower leg and forearm.

High resolution peripheral quantitative computed tomography

A purpose-built scanner is used to measure bone mineral content and BMD of the peripheral skeleton, using an X-ray source. It has a resolution that is close to trabecular thickness and generates data that can visualise microarchitecture and quantify microarchitectural parameters.

- Its main advantage is the high resolution that allows assessment of microarchitectural parameters.
- It can only measure the distal forearm and distal part of the lower leg.

Quantitative ultrasound

Ultrasound transducers are positioned on the skeletal site to be measured (most often the calcaneus). Measurements reflect the nature and extent of the distortion of a short burst of variable-frequency ultrasound pulses as they pass through bone.

- Limitations include that measurements are not comparable between different models and that there is not the quantity of reference data or consensus on diagnostic thresholds that are available for DXA.
- Advantages are that ultrasound measurements reflect bone microarchitecture as well as bone density. The technique is cheaper than DXA, can be used outside the laboratory and does not involve exposure to ionising radiation.

* The DXA scan is a two-dimensional scan, so BMD is the ratio of bone mineral content to area rather than volume.

Figure 9.3 Schematic representation of changes in bone mass with age. Peak bone mass, attained in early adulthood, is 30–40% higher in men than in women.

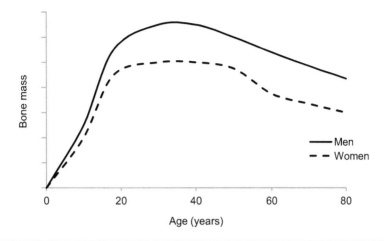

Total skeletal mass increases during growth and reaches a peak during the third decade. Peak rates of bone accrual are about 20% greater in boys than in girls so that, from puberty onwards, bone mass is greater in men than in women. At about 30 years of age, progressive loss of bone begins (Figure 9.3). In women, the rate of bone loss accelerates sharply after the menopause to about 10% per decade, levelling off to about 3% per decade after age 75. Some women lose as much as 30% of bone mass by age 70. Twin and family studies show that differences in bone size, shape and BMD are largely (50–85%) heritable. However, lifestyle factors are also important determinants of adult bone structure. For example, inadequate intake of calcium impairs bone accrual during growth resulting in low bone mass in adults. The potential of the mechanical loading of bone during physical activity to influence its structure will be of particular interest to the reader.

Adaptation to load bearing

Bone is deposited in relation to the load it must bear. It is this principle that makes it biologically plausible that exercise strengthens bone and attenuates bone loss; with greater loading, the load-bearing capacity of bone increases – and vice versa. The strains (deformations) produced during loading stimulate an adaptive response in bone that derives from osteocytes in the region where the strains are experienced and is thus described as a 'local response to local loading'. The mechanisms involved are still being unravelled but it seems that osteocytes coordinate the activity of osteoclasts and osteoblasts through locally acting signalling pathways, to achieve the modelling or remodelling necessary to adjust bone strength to the loads it must bear. Disuse results in an increase in remodelling activity that is dominated by resorption and the consequent loss of bone. Bed rest and space flight, for example, both lead rapidly to net bone loss.

Male astronauts typically lose as much bone mass in the proximal femur in one month as postmenopausal women on Earth lose in one year. Osteoclastic activity increases within a day or two of immobilisation, disturbing the balance between bone resorption and formation.

The general principles governing the response of bone to load bearing have been examined through *in vivo* experiments. Research published in the 1980s using the turkey ulna emphasised the importance of peak skeletal strains for bone adaptation. The reasoning is that, when loading-induced strain exceeds 'normal' strains at a particular skeletal site, new bone is added, increasing bone strength. Bone mass and morphology are thus closely linked to the intensity of loading. It was shown that any unusual distribution of strain enhances the osteogenic response at a given strain magnitude and that bone's response to an overload in the number of strain cycles to which it is exposed appears to 'saturate' quickly. This suggests that many repetitions of a given strain stimulus confer no additional advantage over that achieved by a few.

OSTEOPOROSIS: DEFINITION, PREVALENCE AND CONSEQUENCES

Osteoporosis (literally meaning 'porous bones') is a skeletal disorder characterised by low bone mass and microarchitectural deterioration of bone tissue (Figure 9.4), with a consequent increase in fragility and susceptibility to fracture. Diagnosis relies on measurements of BMD at the hip as a proxy measure of bone strength. The World Health Organization (WHO) operationally defines osteoporosis as bone density at the femoral neck 2.5 standard deviations below the mean (T-score of –2.5) for young white adult women, based on DXA scan results. BMD is also used alongside clinical risk factors in fracture risk prediction algorithms such as the widely used fracture-risk assessment tool FRAX (Kanis et al. 2008).

The major problem for public health is primary osteoporosis, attributable to bone loss associated with ageing. (Secondary osteoporosis is a result of medical conditions, diseases or medications.) Age-related bone loss is, however, not the only contributing factor to primary osteoporosis. Sub-optimal bone growth during childhood and adolescence (see Chapter 11) is as important to its development as bone loss in middle and old age.

Osteoporosis is second only to cardiovascular disease as a leading health-care problem worldwide. The WHO estimates that one in three women and one in eight men over age 50 risk having an osteoporotic fracture during their lifetime. These fractures cause disability and losses of independence and quality of life. Their financial, physical and psychosocial consequences significantly affect the family and the community, as well as the individual. Osteoporotic fractures are a major contributor to medical care costs in many regions of the world. Moreover, the associated social burden is bound to increase, especially in industrialised countries, as the population ages (see Chapter 1).

Osteoporotic fractures

Almost all types of fracture are increased in patients with low BMD, but the most vulnerable skeletal sites are those where trabecular bone predominates. The greater metabolic rate of this type of bone means that it responds more quickly than cortical

Figure 9.4 Osteoporotic changes in lumbar vertebrae. The strong vertebral bodies of (a) early adult life lose much of their structure and become prone to crush fractures as weight-bearing capacity diminishes (b).

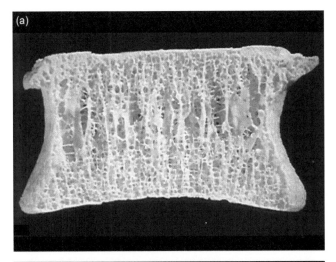

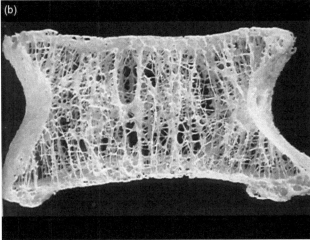

Source: L. Mosekilde MD, DMSci, personal communication.

bone to changes in environmental influences, internal or external. In women, loss of circulating oestrogen (and its bone-conserving effects) around the menopause is the most important cause of bone loss. Box 9.2 shows risk factors for osteoporosis.

The most common sites of osteoporotic fractures are the hip, vertebral bodies and the wrist. Bone loss is an important predisposing factor, but fractures are often the direct result of a fall. The incidence of hip fractures rises exponentially with age. Since women have a lower BMD than men, live longer, experience more bone loss and have more falls, more than three-quarters of these disabling fractures occur in women. Half of the patients who fracture their hip cannot walk independently afterwards and many will move from the community to a nursing home as a consequence. Worldwide, the

> ## BOX 9.2 RISK FACTORS FOR PRIMARY OSTEOPOROSIS.
>
> | STRONGEST RISK FACTORS | OTHER IMPORTANT RISK FACTORS |
> |---|---|
> | • Female sex
• Age greater than 60 years
• Family history of osteoporosis | • White or Asian origin
• Untreated premature menopause
• Low body mass index (BMI)
• History of secondary amenorrhoea for more than one year
• Smoking
• Eating disorder
• Low calcium intake
• Low vitamin D levels (lack of sunlight and/or low dietary intake)
• Inactive lifestyle (particularly during adolescence) or conditions associated with prolonged immobility
• Alcohol abuse
• History of fracture as an adult |

number of hip fractures is expected to increase four-fold (compared with the late 1990s) to more than 6 million in 2050 (WHO 2014).

Vertebral crush fractures result in a loss of weight-bearing competence of the vertebral bodies. Like hip fractures, they occur more often in women than in men and most are precipitated by routine everyday activities. The associated loss of height can be considerable and gives rise to secondary problems because abdominal and thoracic organs are compressed, leading to chronic, disabling pain and deformity.

In perimenopausal women, the wrist is the most common site of fracture. Wrist fractures are usually associated with a fall, typically outdoors and often in icy weather. Few patients are completely disabled by a wrist fracture, but fewer than half experience a satisfactory return to function.

PHYSICAL ACTIVITY AND BONE

As described above, bone mass and structure are sensitive to alterations in its mechanical environment, including forces experienced during exercise. Studies in animals show that growing bone has a substantially greater capacity to add new bone in response to mechanical loading than mature bone. Consequently, childhood and adolescence probably represent a 'window of opportunity' for interventions aimed at reducing the risk of osteoporosis in later life. Evidence on the effects of physical activity and exercise on skeletal health in children is presented in Chapter 11. The present chapter is concerned with the influence of exercise on bone in adults.

Much of the considerable body of research has relied on DXA measurements of BMD. Whilst these have proved a good predictor of fracture risk at a population level, there is increasing recognition that small changes in bone mass distribution, cortical and trabecular structure and bone geometry can lead to large increases in bone strength, independent of BMD (Nikander et al. 2010). Consequently, more recent studies have often employed QCT because it reflects these structural changes better than DXA.

The response to exercise-related bone loading, like other environmental stimuli, may be mediated by individual genetic variability. To date, however, there is no consensus as to the nature of such interactions, or indeed whether or not they exist.

Premenopausal women

Cross-sectional studies have consistently reported that athletes have a higher BMD than inactive controls, especially at the skeletal sites specifically loaded in their sport. Most studies have looked at premenopausal women, although similar findings are available for men, postmenopausal women and children.

For example, researchers in Finland employed peripheral QCT to compare a range of structural variables at different skeletal sites between national-level female athletes and non-athlete controls (Nikander et al. 2006). The athletes were volleyball players, hurdlers, racket games players, soccer players and swimmers. As expected, the athletes' bone mass at the sites loaded in their sports was substantially higher than controls. In addition, the weight-bearing bones of the athletes (swimmers excluded) had larger diaphysis, thicker cortices and somewhat denser trabecular bone than controls. Thus, loading-induced additional bone mass in athletes builds mechanically strong and appropriate bone structures that relate to the nature of the loading.

The same research group compared the geometry of the femoral neck in athletes and controls, using magnetic resonance imaging. Ninety-one athletes were divided into five groups according to the bone-loading demands of their sports on the lower extremities, i.e. high-impact, 'odd-impact', high-magnitude, repetitive low-impact and repetitive non-impact. (Soccer and racquet games were designated 'odd-impact' because they are intense and include rapidly accelerating and decelerating movements, often in different directions than usual walking and running.) High-impact and odd-impact exercise loadings were both associated with a thicker cortex at the femoral neck, suggesting that these exercise regimens are the most effective against hip fragility (Nikander et al. 2009).

Studies comparing athletes with non-athletes are useful indicators of the optimal osteogenic response to mechanical loading, but they cannot control for bias or confounding. Self-selection bias is inevitable (people with strong bones may tend to take up sport). Potential confounding factors include differences in lifestyle (healthy nutrition and avoidance of smoking in athletes) or physical activity history during childhood and adolescence. Alternative experimental designs that take care of some of these factors are: first, side-to-side comparisons in sports where only one limb is exposed to impact; and second, intervention studies where changes in exercisers can be compared with changes in controls.

Using the first of these designs, researchers compared side-to-side differences in indices of bone strength in the humeral shaft of 64 female tennis and squash players and 27 controls matched for age, height and weight (Kontulainen et al. 2003). Players were divided into two groups: 'young starters' had started playing at or before menarche, while 'old starters' had started playing at least one year after menarche. Among old starters, side-to-side differences in indices of bone strength were significantly greater than in controls (Figure 9.5), confirming that loading augments the mature skeleton in a site-specific manner. However, the young starters' side-to-side differences were

Figure 9.5 Side-to-side differences (%) of bone variables at the humeral shaft of female tennis and squash players, according to age of starting training, and age-matched controls.

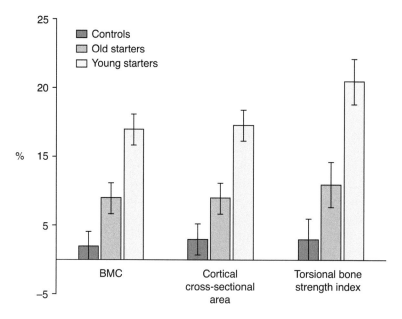

Source: Adapted from Kontulainen et al. (2003).
Note: Values are means and 95% confidence intervals for 36 young starters, 28 old starters and 27 controls. The bone strength index measured the resistance of the humeral shaft to bending and torsional loading.

generally twice as large as those in the old starters, indicating a particularly potent effect on bone during the pubescent years. In both groups of players, the structural adaptation of the humerus was attributable to an enlarged cortical area.

Reviews and meta-analyses of controlled exercise intervention trials in previously inactive premenopausal women have typically found small (1–3%) increases in BMD at the femoral neck, compared with controls (Babatunde et al. 2012; Kelley et al. 2013a). Changes at the lumbar spine are less consistent. Interventions have included jogging, strength training, weightlifting, aerobics and high-impact jumping/hopping activities that can create ground reaction forces up to six times body weight. Strength training, high-impact and odd-impact exercise appear to be an effective osteogenic stimulus but there is no consensus as to the optimal exercise regimen and this may differ according to the skeletal site of interest.

The main findings from one study of high-impact exercise are shown in Figure 9.6 (Bailey and Brooke-Wavell 2010). Healthy, inactive women aged 19–45 were randomly assigned to perform 50 multidirectional hops 0, 2, 4 or 7 days per week for six months. The unilateral design employed decreased the problem of confounding factors. Daily hopping – but not less frequent hopping – increased BMD at the femoral neck by nearly 2%, relative to the control leg.

A handful of studies suggest that exercise-induced benefits for bone start to disappear after cessation of training but there is also evidence to the contrary. For example,

Figure 9.6 Influence of six months of high-impact, unilateral exercise (hopping). Figure shows changes in exercise leg BMD according to exercise frequency, adjusted for change in control leg and baseline BMD. Values are mean and 95% confidence interval for 61 healthy young women. Significant difference between groups, $P = 0.015$ by ANCOVA. Significantly higher in group Ex 7 than in control or Ex 2 groups, $P = 0.003$ and $P = 0.015$, respectively.

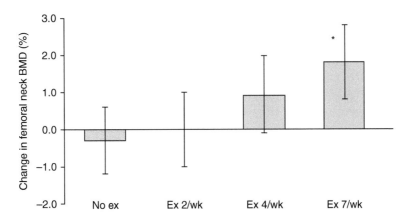

Source: Reprinted from *Bone*, 46: 1043–9, Bailey, C.A. and Brooke-Wavell, K., 'Optimum frequency of exercise for bone health: randomised controlled trial of a high-impact unilateral intervention', page 1047, copyright © 2009, with permission from Elsevier.

3.5 years after the end of an 18-month high-impact exercise intervention, the gains in BMD achieved in exercisers were maintained, relative to controls (Kontulainen et al. 2004). In addition, the greater side-to-side differences in bone mineral content of the humerus of female racquet sport players (compared with controls) persisted after four years of retirement (Kontulainen et al. 1999). Thus, participation in high-impact activities during the premenopausal years may have lasting advantages for skeletal health.

Postmenopausal women

Because bone mass (and thus strength) decrease sharply after menopause, the risk for fracture is high in older women. If exercise has a positive effect on bone in this population, it should influence this risk. What is the evidence?

Prospective studies suggest that a habit of physical activity is associated with a lower risk for hip fracture. For example, in a cohort of more than 60,000 postmenopausal women in the US Nurses' Health Study, women who reported at least 24 MET-h week^{-1} of physical activity had a 55% lower risk than inactive women who reported less than 3 MET-h week^{-1} of activity (Feskanich et al. 2002). There was evidence for a dose–response relationship: the risk for hip fracture was 6% less for each increase in activity of 3 MET-h week^{-1}. Among women who did no other exercise, walking for at least four hours per week was associated with a 41% lower risk for hip fracture than among those who walked for less than one hour per week.

Similar findings were reported by the UK Million Women Study of 2,582 hip fractures over 6.2 years. Women who took any exercise had a 35% lower risk for hip fracture than those who reported none (Armstrong et al. 2011). As in the Nurses' Health

Study, walking was an important part of the total activity. These observations are interesting because they suggest that even a low-impact activity may reduce fracture risk, perhaps through preventing inactivity-related losses.

A handful of prospective studies have examined risk factors for vertebral fractures, including physical inactivity. One reported data from 3.7 years of follow-up of more than 5,800 American women aged 65 or over who had no history of fracture. A low level of physical activity (walking less than one block or doing less than one hour of household chores per day) was associated with a risk of vertebral fracture that was 60% higher than that exhibited by women who were more active (Nevitt et al. 2005). This effect was independent of BMD, showing that exercise-related factors other than bone density are important determinants of fracture risk.

A key question then is: 'Can healthy older women reduce their risk of fracture through increasing their physical activity?' Many controlled intervention trials have addressed this question. The topic is complex, however, not only on account of potential interactions with hormone-replacement therapy (oestrogen may facilitate the osteogenic effect of physical activity) but also because bone loading is a site-specific effect and because such a variety of exercise interventions have been used. The main outcome measure in most studies has been some measure of bone strength, most often BMD. Bone strength is related to fracture risk, but fall-related factors are also important, particularly for fractures of the hip and wrist.

Strength training or high-impact loading has often been the exercise regimen of choice in intervention studies, based on the principles governing the osteogenic response to bone-loading explained earlier. Two well-designed studies of this type are described here as examples. In an 18-month randomised controlled trial, a research group from Germany studied 246 postmenopausal white women aged 65 or over (Kemmler et al. 2010). None was taking hormone-replacement therapy or other medication known to influence bone metabolism. The exercise programme had aerobic and balance training elements but focused primarily on high-intensity strength training. It comprised two 60-minute supervised classes per week as well as two 20-minute sessions at home. Relative to controls, the women who trained increased BMD at both the lumbar spine and the femoral neck. The same group also studied 137 postmenopausal women participating in a similar, but not randomised, intervention over the subsequent 16 years (Kemmler et al. 2016), and the 39 women who continued exercising demonstrated substantially lower bone loss than the women in the control group (Figure 9.7). Even more importantly, the exercise group had only half the incidence of low trauma fractures during the follow-up.

Again, in a randomised, controlled design, researchers compared the effects of three different exercise regimens: resistance training; balance, agility and jumping training; and a combination of these two (Karinkanta et al. 2007). Participants were 149 healthy, community-dwelling women aged 70–78 years and exercise classes were held three times a week for one year. Training, particularly the combination regimen, prevented functional decline in these elderly women. Dynamic balance and lower-limb muscle strength were improved but the only beneficial effect on bone was on 'bending strength' at the femoral neck. In this study also, participants were followed up after the end of the intervention by consulting medical records for falls and fractures (Karinkanta et al. 2015). Despite the limited effect of the intervention on bone, and

Figure 9.7 BMD changes at the lumbar spine (left) and total hip (right) during 16 years of participation in a multipurpose exercise programme in women 65 years or older. Values are mean and SD for 67 women in the exercise group (EG) and 39 in the control group (CG). Significance of change from baseline (within group) is indicated by asterisks adjacent to error bars. Asterisks between curves indicate significance of differences between groups.

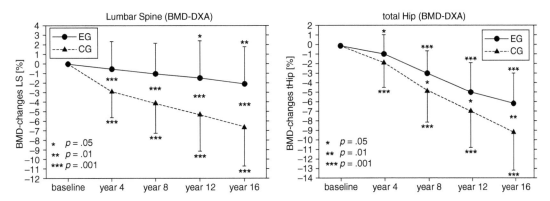

Source: Reprinted from 'Long-term exercise and bone mineral density changes in postmenopausal women – are there periods of reduced effectiveness?', Kemmler, W. et al., *Journal of Bone and Mineral Research* 31: 215–22, page 219, with permission from John Wiley and Sons. Copyright © 2016 American Society for Bone and Mineral Research.

the intervention not having been continued in this study, participants in the combination regimen still had 51% fewer injurious falls and 74% fewer fractures than those who had been in the control group. These exercise interventions including resistance training thus seem to have longer-term benefits to fracture risk that may not entirely be explained through effects on BMD.

Researchers have also examined the potential of simple, everyday aerobic exercise to limit age-related bone loss. For example, in one randomly controlled trial, healthy perimenopausal women aged 52–53 followed a programme of walking, stair climbing, cycling and jogging (55–75% $\dot{V}O_2$max), 3–4 times per week for 18 months (Heinonen et al. 1998). These aerobic exercisers avoided the loss of BMD at the femoral neck that was seen in the control group. On the other hand, a systematic review of intervention trials of walking concluded that this activity has no significant effect on BMD at the hip or lumbar spine (Martyn-St James and Carroll 2008).

By the age of 70 years, the prevalence of low BMD (osteopenia) is 56% in women (and 34% in men) so that it is important to know whether or not exercise can influence the risk for fractures in these elderly people. Very few trials are available but, drawing participants from a birth cohort of 1,690 women aged 70–73 years, researchers in Finland conducted a 30-month, randomly controlled intervention trial of mainly home-based, impact exercise. Bone mineral content and BMD at the hip decreased less in the exercise group (n = 84) than in the control group (n = 76) but these differences were small. However, the exercise group showed clear benefits in terms of fall-related factors, e.g. body sway, leg strength and walking speed (Korpelainen et al. 2006a, 2006b). Participants were followed up for four and a half years after the initial trial. BMD decreased similarly in both groups but exercisers retained their functional improvements and had a lower incidence rate for fractures. So, exercise seemed to have a long-term effect on balance and gait and, speculatively, may have the potential to protect high-risk elderly women from hip fractures (Korpelainen et al. 2010).

Whilst the emphasis in those with low BMD has been on pharmacological treatment and prevention of falls, some recent research suggested that exercise designed to progressively load potential fracture sites can increase BMD. The LIFTMOR study used an eight-month intervention of twice-weekly, 30-minute sessions of high load resistance and impact training. Sessions were supervised and exercises were gradually progressed. Good adherence was seen and there were few adverse events. Most importantly there were more substantial increases in BMD than in some previous studies that used lower loading magnitudes with net benefit around 4% at the spine and 2% at the hip (Watson et al. 2018).

After more than two decades of research on this topic, it can be concluded that exercise has modest but clinically relevant, site-specific effects in postmenopausal women (Kelley et al. 2012; Polidoulis et al. 2012). Whilst these preserve bone or attenuate the rate of loss, they do not affect bone density as much as pharmaceutical treatments. Strength- or odd-impact training or a combination of these appears to be the most effective (Howe et al. 2011). These conclusions are based mainly on studies using DXA to measure BMD and may be revised as the capability of researchers to measure bone architecture and strength increases. In terms of fracture risk, beneficial effects of exercise on fall-related factors may be as – or even more – important than effects on bone tissue.

Men

There is evidence from longitudinal data that exercise is important in optimising peak bone mass in young men (Nilsson et al. 2012), but far fewer exercise intervention studies have been conducted in men than in women.

Cross-sectional comparisons of male athletes with controls have found significantly higher BMD in athletes at skeletal sites loaded in their sports. Side-to-side differences in the bone mineral content of the arm bones have been reported to be 13–25%, depending on the site measured, compared with differences in controls of only 1–5% (Kontulainen et al. 1999). Similarly, Master athletes trained for jumping showed greater side-to-side differences in tibial bone structure than did other Master athletes (Ireland et al. 2011). Among young male military recruits, higher levels of weight-bearing physical activity were associated with higher BMD at the hip and femoral neck (Eleftheriou et al. 2013).

In a unique prospective controlled study, scientists from Lund in Sweden compared BMD in 46 male athletes (in 1968 mean age 22) with measurements made nearly 40 years later when the men had been retired from their sports for an average of 29 years. A cohort of non-athletic men of similar age served as controls. Bone mineral density levels in the femoral condyles were not only higher in athletes than in controls at baseline but also at follow-up. Thus exercise-associated high BMD was maintained three decades after cessation of high-level activity (Tveit et al. 2013).

As regards randomised controlled trials, the paucity of robust data in men is clear from a meta-analysis conducted in 2011 (Kelley et al. 2013b). Only three studies with a total of 275 participants (152 exercisers, 123 controls) met the eligibility criteria and the authors concluded that additional well-designed randomised controlled trials are needed before exercise can be recommending for improving and/or maintaining BMD at the femoral neck or lumbar spine in men.

Several of the small number of controlled exercise intervention studies in men have found small (2–3%), but significant, gains in BMD. For example, one randomised trial examined the influence in elderly men of progressive resistance training with weight-bearing activities (three days per week over 18 months). Exercisers showed a 2% improvement in femoral neck bone geometry and strength, relative to controls (Kukuljian et al. 2011). Allison and co-workers studied 70-year-old men, using a 12-month unilateral intervention (brief daily hopping exercise). There were small but significant increases in BMD, bone mineral content and the cross-sectional area at the femoral neck of the exercised leg, relative to the control leg. QCT scans demonstrated substantially greater localised changes in cortical mass and trabecular density, including at some regions of the femur where localised thinning predisposes to hip fracture (Allison et al. 2015). Such studies demonstrate that by targeting bone areas of structural importance, exercise could increase bone strength to a greater extent than bone density.

Osteoporotic fractures among men are already a major public health problem, worldwide. Some 13% of men will experience an osteoporosis-related fracture at some point during their lifetime (WHO 2014). As the population of elderly men increases, so will research to examine modifiable risk factors, including physical activity. Large prospective cohort studies are under way and are now being complemented by robust intervention studies.

Vibration

Over the last decade there has been an upsurge of interest in the potential of whole-body vibration to benefit bone. The rationale is that high-frequency, low-magnitude strains stimulate an increase in cortical bone in animal models. Vibration is regarded as a surrogate for the spectra of high-frequency, muscle-based signals that are continually evident in bone (Judex and Rubin 2010), but are attenuated with ageing as muscle mass declines. Trials have looked at vibration alone and as an adjunct to traditional resistance regimens. A review and meta-analysis of 14 randomised controlled trials with a total of 1,839 participants concluded that regular whole-body vibration training had no significant effect on BMD or bone architecture, although falls risk was reduced in some studies (Jepsen et al. 2017). It is possible that the ideal vibration characteristics have not yet been identified and vibration training may offer an alternative for those who are otherwise unable to exercise.

PHYSICAL ACTIVITY IN PREVENTION AND MANAGEMENT OF OSTEOPOROSIS

In osteoporosis, prevention has a vital role to play – for the individual and for society. To decrease her lifelong risk of fracture, a woman must maximise peak bone mass as a young adult, maintain this through middle-age and attenuate the rate of loss of bone after menopause. In the later decades of life, she must try to decrease the risk of falls. Intakes of calcium and vitamin D are, of course, also important.

To achieve these aims, a lifelong habit of weight-bearing exercise is clearly important. Its effects are particularly potent during growth but whether bone gain during growth can be maintained during adulthood if the level of activity declines is not clear. The traditional view is that mechanical loading should expose multiple skeletal sites to high and varied strains through high- and odd-impact loading and/or resistance exercises. In practice, two issues limit the implementation of targeted bone-loading exercises as a strategy to reduce fracture risk in older women. These are: (1) poor compliance with high- and odd-impact exercises; and (2) concern about the associated risk of injury and/or falls.

How important, clinically, is a typical exercise-associated ~1% benefit of exercise for BMD at the femoral neck or lumbar spine? Estimates suggest that an increase in BMD of this magnitude could, if maintained, result in a 10% decrease in fracture risk. This is clearly worthwhile, but the overall benefit may be even greater if exercises to improve balance reduce the risk of falls.

Falls

Nearly all hip fractures result from a fall, usually from a standing height or less. Falls also play a role in vertebral fractures, although this is more limited. Intrinsic risk factors include poor levels of muscle strength, range of motion, balance, gait and reaction time – all of which might be improved through regular exercise.

In one large study of falls in 1,090 people over 70, living at home in Australia, researchers examined the potential of three different interventions to reduce falls (Day et al. 2002). These were designed to improve: strength and balance through exercises; home hazard management; and vision. Interventions were implemented singly and in all combinations, allocating participants randomly to one of eight equal-sized groups (one was control, with no intervention). Exercise, either alone or in combination with other interventions, conferred a significant decrease in the risk of a fall. The exercise regimen adopted by these participants was modest: one hour per week of supervised exercises for 15 weeks, supplemented by twice weekly home exercises for the remainder of the 18-month trial.

Systematic reviews of randomised clinical trials that aimed to prevent falls in older adults found that exercise interventions (including balance, leg strength, flexibility and/or endurance training) reduced the rate of falls in community dwelling older people by 21%. A greater reduction of 39% was seen with interventions that challenged balance and involved more than three hours per week of exercise (Sherrington et al. 2017). Such programmes also seem to prevent injuries caused by falls, including the most severe ones (El-Khoury et al. 2013). By increasing confidence and physical function such interventions may increase physical activity participation in frail older people. This could increase exposure to hazards and counter-intuitively increase fall risk, although this is counterbalanced by the potential improvements to quality of life.

Therapy for established osteoporosis

The term 'established osteoporosis' is used for individuals with a history of a fragility fracture as well as low BMD. Pharmacological treatment focuses on agents that reduce bone loss. The first-line treatment is usually one of the bisphosphonates. Other pharmacological agents include peptide hormones (parathyroid hormone and calcitonin) and – for postmenopausal women – oestrogen receptor modulators. With the exception of parathyroid hormone which preferentially stimulates osteoblastic activity over osteoclastic activity, each of these agents acts to prevent bone resorption. A newer therapeutic agent, denosumab, is a monoclonal antibody that inhibits osteoclast formation, function and survival, thus decreasing bone resorption. Oestrogen (in the form of menopausal hormone therapy) reduces the risk of vertebral and hip fractures in postmenopausal women but is now less widely used because of the associated risks for breast cancer, heart disease and thrombotic events.

It is usual clinical practice to ensure that the daily intake of calcium is adequate: recommendations vary in different countries but are generally in the range of 700–1200 mg. Calcium supplementation has been reported to decrease the risk of hip fracture (24% reduction with 1,000 mg day^{-1}). Vitamin D supplementation may also be helpful, as deficiency of this vitamin is not uncommon among the frail elderly living in institutions, probably because of inadequate exposure to sunlight. However, none of these drugs or supplements can restore lost bone.

The therapeutic effectiveness of exercise in women with a clinically defined condition is still being explored. Because of concern that exercise could precipitate fracture in weakened bone, there has been caution about recommending exercise in people with osteoporosis. However, inactivity may exacerbate bone loss and avoiding exercise may increase risk of other adverse health outcomes. Some argue that caution about exercise in people with osteoporosis has meant that there has been reluctance to use sufficient levels of loading to increase bone strength. Recent expert opinion is that exercise guidelines are appropriate for those with osteoporosis, apart from those with vertebral fractures who should modify some activities (Giangregorio et al. 2015).

Vertebral fractures lead to exaggerated kyphosis and this posture not only increases the risk of falling, but also causes severe back pain. Strengthening back extensor muscles and engaging in dynamic posture training can help these patients on both counts. These interventions may also decrease depression and improve the quality of life. Some trials have found that exercise improved outcomes such as pain, performance on the 'Timed Up and Go' test,[1] walking speed, back extensor strength and quality of life but a Cochrane review of all randomised or 'quasi-randomised' controlled trials was not able to draw definitive conclusions because findings were inconsistent and the quality of evidence was low (Giangregorio et al. 2013). Breast cancer survivors[2] are at increased risk for osteoporosis and fractures and, at least in premenopausal women, exercise may be able to offset this risk (Saarto et al. 2012).

For patients who have had a hip fracture, exercise programmes can improve strength and mobility but it is not known whether these improvements are sufficient to prevent falls and further fractures in this high-risk group. Nevertheless, it can be argued that exercise is the only single therapy that can simultaneously ameliorate low BMD, augment muscle mass, promote strength gain, and improve dynamic balance – all of which are independent risk factors for hip fracture.

PHYSICAL ACTIVITY AND OSTEOARTHRITIS

Osteoarthritis – the most common form of arthritis – is a disease entity involving all joint components including cartilage, synovial membrane and bone. Synovial inflammation occurs early in the process and plays a role in the progression of the damage. The joints most frequently affected are fingers, knee, hips and spine. A progressive deterioration of opposing joint surfaces leads to distortion of joint positioning. Osteoarthritis is painful, disabling and impairs the quality of life. It is the most common cause of walking-related disabilities. In many countries the prevalence is increasing rapidly, a trend attributed to the ageing of the population and because of the increasing prevalence of obesity. Obesity is one of the two strongest, modifiable risk factors for osteoarthritis, the other being joint injury.

Two questions may be posed. First, does participation in physical activity and/or exercise (sporting or otherwise) influence the risk of developing osteoarthritis? Second, does physical activity have a therapeutic role for patients with osteoarthritis?

Epidemiological studies have demonstrated that participation in sports that involve high-intensity, acute, direct joint impacts and/or twisting and torsional types of stress appear to increase the risk. Risk correlates with the intensity and duration of exposure and is therefore a particular concern for professional sportsmen and women, particularly in contact sports. In professional or elite sport there is a greater likelihood of joint injury and a greater motivation to continue playing despite pain, potentially adding further injury to the joint (Molloy and Molloy 2011). A systematic review found that overall former athletes had similar prevalence of knee osteoarthritis as controls, although participation in some sports (soccer, elite distance running, competitive weight lifting and wrestling) was associated with increased risk (Driban et al. 2017). However, to put it into perspective, the risk of osteoarthritis associated with sport is less than that associated with a history of trauma or being overweight. Occupational activity can also lead to joint stress and an increased risk.

On the other hand, participation in moderate types and amounts of aerobic activity, including sports that cause minimal joint impact and torsional loading confers little, if any, risk of osteoarthritis of the hip or knee. Indeed, some level of 'ordinary' activity is necessary for joint health – immobilisation is associated not only with loss of muscle and bone, but also with connective tissue stiffness and other effects associated with impairment of joint function. The improved muscle strength and proprioception and reduced body mass index associated with regular physical activity are protective of joints.

The importance of maintaining activity for preventing disability associated with osteoarthritis is demonstrated in a prospective cohort study in 1680 people either with or at risk of arthritis, who had activity measured by accelerometry at baseline and disability measured over the subsequent two years. Those in the lowest quartile for either light or moderate activity were twice as likely to develop disability over the follow-up. Those in the highest quartile for moderate activity had the lowest risk of future disability (Figure 9.8).

Figure 9.8 Risk (hazard ratio) of onset of disability according to accelerometer measured light and moderate activity in people with or at risk of osteoarthritis.

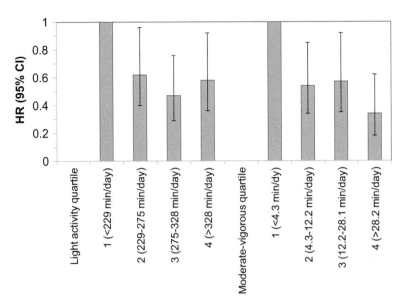

Exercise is increasingly regarded as a key component in the management of osteo-arthritis, for general as well as disease-specific health benefits. Comprehensive interventions that include aerobic exercise (usually walking) and/or resistance exercise to strengthen quadriceps muscles, pain management and education result in moderate improvements in measures of disability, physical performance (e.g. six-minute walking distance, stair-climbing, getting in and out of a car) and perception of pain. Exercise does not worsen the disease, provided that it does not predispose to trauma, and is safe. For example, only 2% of participants had serious musculoskeletal injuries related to exercise in the 18-month-long US Fitness, Arthritis and Seniors Trial (Ettinger et al. 1997).

Systematic review and meta-analysis of 44 randomised controlled trials of knee osteoarthritis and ten trials of hip osteoarthritis demonstrated that exercise reduced joint pain and improved physical function in patients with osteoarthritis, with benefits lasting for several months after the treatment stopped. (Fransen et al. 2014, 2015)

Chronic low back pain – often associated with osteoarthritis – causes a great amount of suffering, loss of productivity and independence, and its prevalence is increasing. Heavy physical work is one of the predisposing factors but, paradoxically, exercise is now regarded as a first-line therapy. Based on a review of randomly controlled trials, exercise is deemed to be 'slightly' effective in decreasing pain and improving function in adults with chronic low back pain, particularly among those whose pain leads them to seek health care (Hayden et al. 2005). On the other hand, exercise therapy appears to be no better than other conservative treatments – or no treatment – for an *acute* episode of back pain. Clearly, more experimental evidence is needed to characterise the influence (beneficial and/or detrimental) of exercise on joint structure and cartilaginous tissue. There is currently no evidence to explain why exercise is effective in reducing pain and improving function in osteoarthritis. A better understanding of the underlying mechanisms may contribute towards more targeted treatment strategies and these are now under debate (Beckwée et al. 2013).

SUMMARY

- Bone is a dynamic tissue that responds to changes in the internal or external environment. Mechanical loading is an important influence on bone remodelling.
- Strain rate and an unusual strain distribution are important determinants of the site-specific osteogenic effects of loading.
- Bone mass increases during growth and reaches a peak towards the end of the second decade. It then remains fairly stable until about 50 years of age when progressive loss begins. Particularly in women, age-related loss of bone can lead to osteoporosis, compromising bone strength and increasing the risk of fracture.
- The potential of exercise to augment bone mineral in the mature skeleton is clear but small. In premenopausal women its effect is mainly conservation of bone, although specific bone-loading exercise can lead to modest bone accrual. In older women its effect is to reduce the rate of loss. Evidence for men is sparse.
- Women with a physically active lifestyle have a lower risk of osteoporotic fracture of the hip and maybe of the spine.
- In established osteoporosis the effects of exercise on BMD are more modest than those of pharmacological treatment and the effects of whole-body vibration therapy are unclear.
- Many fractures are caused by falls. Exercise can decrease the risk of falls through improving balance, strength and maybe neuromuscular coordination.
- Participation in sports involving high-intensity impacts or torsional types of stress increases the risk for osteoarthritis, potentially mediated by joint injury. On the other hand, moderate amounts and intensities of exercise decrease pain and improve function in patients with osteoarthritis of the knee and hip.

STUDY TASKS

1 What features of bone govern its strength? Identify two different types of bone and explain, with examples, why one type may predominate at a particular skeletal site.
2 Describe the basic principles that govern the effect of mechanical loading on bone.
3 Identify the common sites of osteoporotic fracture and suggest specific exercises that might be expected to elicit an osteogenic response at each of these sites.
4 Explain why the age-related rise in hip fractures occurs five to ten years later in men than in women. How might exercise alter the risk of fracture at this skeletal site even if it does not increase BMD?
5 Explain as fully as possible why studies of athletes who play racquet games are so informative in the context of the influence of exercise on BMD.

NOTES

1   The 'Timed Up and Go' test is a simple, quick and widely used clinical performance-based measure of lower extremity function, mobility and fall risk. It measures the time taken by an individual to stand up from a standard armchair, walk a distance of 3 metres, turn, walk back to the chair and sit down.

2   Chemotherapy and hormonal therapies used to treat breast cancer have negative effects on bone, inducing or aggravating low bone mineral density/osteoporosis.

FURTHER READING

Beck, B.R., Daly, R.M., Singh, M.A.F. and Taaffe, D.R. (2017) Exercise and Sports Science Australia (ESSA) position statement on exercise prescription for the prevention and management of osteoporosis. *Journal of Science and Medicine in Sport* 20: 438–45.

Bennell, K.L., Dobson, F. and Hinman, R.S. (2014) Exercise in osteoarthritis: moving from prescription to adherence. *Best Practice and Research Clinical Rheumatology* 28: 93–117.

Driban, J.B., Hootman, J.M., Sitler, M.R., Harris, K.P. and Cattano, N.M. (2017) Is participation in certain sports associated with knee osteoarthritis? A systematic review. *Journal of Athletic Training* 52: 497–506.

Giangregorio, L.M., McGill, S., Wark, J.D., Laprade, J., Heinonen, A., Ashe, M. et al. (2015) Too fit to fracture: a Delphi consensus process on physical activity and exercise recommendations for adults with osteoporosis with or without vertebral fractures. *Osteoporosis International* 26: 891–910.

Hagen, K.B., Dagfinrud, H., Moe, R.H., Østerås, N., Kjeken, I., Grotle, M. and Smedslund, G. (2012) Exercise therapy for bone and muscle health: an overview of systematic reviews. *BMC Medicine* 10: 167. doi: 10.1186/1741-7015-10-167.

Johnson, V.L. and Hunter, D.J. (2014) The epidemiology of osteoarthritis. *Best Practice and Research Clinical Rheumatology* 28: 5–15.

Khan, K., McKay, H., Kannus, R, Bailey, D., Wark, J. and Bennell, K. (2001) *Physical Activity and Bone Health*. Champaign, IL: Human Kinetics.

Nikander, R., Sievänen, H., Heinonen, A., Daly, R.M., Uusi-Rasi, K. and Kannus, P. (2010) Targeted exercise against osteoporosis: a systematic review and meta-analysis for optimizing bone strength throughout life. *BMC Medicine* 8: 47. doi: 10.1186/1741-7015-8-47.

Pedersen, B.K. and Saltin, B. (2006) The evidence for prescribing exercise as therapy in chronic disease. *Scandinavian Journal of Medicine and Science in Sports* 16 (Suppl. 1): 3–63.

Seeman, E. and Delmas, P.D. (2006) Bone quality – the material and structural basis of bone strength and fragility. *New England Journal of Medicine* 354: 2250–61.

Walsh, J. S. (2015) Normal bone physiology, remodelling and its hormonal regulation. *Surgery* 33: 1–6. doi: 10.1016/j.mpsur.2014.10.010.

REFERENCES

Allison, S.J., Poole, K.E.S., Treece, G.M., Gee, A.H., Tonkin, C., Rennie, W.J. et al. (2015) The influence of high-impact exercise on cortical and trabecular bone mineral content and 3D distribution across the proximal femur in older men: a randomised controlled unilateral study. *Journal of Bone and Mineral Research* 30: 1709–16.

Armstrong, M.E.G., Spencer, E.A., Cairns, B.J., Banks, E., Pirie, K., Green, J. et al. (2011) Body mass index and physical activity in relation to the incidence of hip fracture in postmenopausal women. *Journal of Bone and Mineral Research* 26: 1330–8.

Babatunde, O.O., Forsyth, J.J. and Gidlow, C.J. (2012) A meta-analysis of brief high-impact exercises for enhancing bone health in premenopausal women. *Osteoporosis International* 23: 109–19.

Bailey, C.A. and Brooke-Wavell, K. (2010) Optimum frequency of exercise for bone health: randomised controlled trial of a high-impact unilateral intervention. *Bone* 46: 1043–9.

Beckwée, D., Vaes, P., Cnudde, M., Swinnen, E. and Bautmans, I. (2013) Osteoarthritis of the knee: why does exercise work? A qualitative study of the literature. *Ageing Research Reviews* 12: 226–36.

Carola, R., Harley, J.P. and Noback, C.R. (1992) *Human Anatomy*. New York: McGraw-Hill.

Day, L., Fildes, B., Gordon, I., Fitzharris, M., Flamer, H. and Lord, S. (2002) Randomised factorial trial of falls prevention among older people living in their own homes. *British Medical Journal* 325: 128–33.

Driban, J.B., Hootman, J.M., Sitler, M.R., Harris, K.P. and Cattano, N.M. (2017) Is participation in certain sports associated with knee osteoarthritis? A systematic review. *Journal of Athletic Training* 52: 497–506.

Dunlop, D.D., Song, J., Semanik, P.A., Sharma, L., Bathon, J.M., Eaton, C.B. et al. (2014) Relation of physical activity time to incident disability in community dwelling adults with or at risk of knee arthritis: prospective cohort study. *British Medical Journal* 348: g2472. doi: 10.1136/bmj.g2472.

Eleftheriou, K.I., Rawal, J.S., James, L.E., Payne, J.R., Loosemore, M., Pennell, D. J. et al. (2013) Bone structure and geometry in young men: the influence of smoking, alcohol intake and physical activity. *Bone* 52: 17–26.

El-Khoury, F., Cassou, B., Charles, M.-A. and Dargent-Molina, P. (2013) The effect of fall prevention exercise programmes on fall induced injuries in community dwelling older adults: systematic review and meta-analysis of randomised trials. *British Medical Journal* 347: f6234. doi: 10.1136/bmj.f6234.

Ettinger, W.H., Burns, R., Messiear, S.P., Applegate, W., Rejeski, W.J., Morgan, T. et al. (1997) A randomized trial comparing aerobic exercise and resistance exercise with a health education programme in older adults with knee osteoarthritis: the Fitness Arthritis and Seniors Trial (FAST). *Journal of the American Medical Association* 277: 25–31.

Feskanich, D., Willett, W.C. and Colditz, G.A. (2002) Walking and leisure-time activity and risk of hip fracture in postmenopausal women. *Journal of the American Medical Association* 288: 2300–6.

Fransen, M., McConnell, S., Harmer, A.R., Van der Esch, M., Simic, M. and Bennell, K.L. (2015) Exercise for osteoarthritis of the knee. *Cochrane Database of Systematic Reviews* (1): CD004376. doi: 10.1002/14651858.CD004376.pub3.

Fransen, M., McConnell, S., Hernandez-Molina, G. and Reichenbach, S. (2014) Exercise for osteoarthritis of the hip. *Cochrane Database of Systematic Reviews* (4): CD007912. doi: 10.1002/14651858.CD007912.pub2.

Giangregorio, L.M., Macintyre, N.J., Thabane, L., Skidmore, C.J. and Papaioannou, A. (2013) Exercise for improving outcomes after osteoporotic vertebral fractures. *Cochrane Database of Systematic Reviews* (1): CD008618. doi: 10.1002/14651858.CD008618.pub2.

Giangregorio, L.M., McGill, S., Wark, J.D., Laprade, J., Heinonen, A., Ashe, M.C. et al. (2015) Too fit to fracture: a Delphi consensus process on physical activity and exercise recommendations for adults with osteoporosis with or without vertebral fractures. *Osteoporosis International* 26: 891–910.

Hayden, J.A., van Tulder, M.W., Malmivaara, A. and Koes, B.W. (2005) Exercise therapy for treatment of non-specific low back pain. *Cochrane Database of Systematic Reviews* (3): CD000335. doi: 10.1002/14651858.CD000335.pub2.

Heinonen, A., Oja, P., Sievänen, A., Pasanen, M. and Vuori, I. (1998) Effect of two training regimens on bone mineral density in healthy perimenopausal women: a randomized controlled trial. *Journal of Bone and Mineral Research* 13: 483–90.

Howe, T.E., Shea, B., Dawson, L.J., Downie, F., Murray, A., Ross, C. et al. (2011) Exercise for preventing and treating osteoporosis in postmenopausal women. *Cochrane Database of Systematic Reviews* (7): CD000333. doi: 10.1002/14651858.CD000333.pub2.

Ireland, A., Korhonen, M., Heinonen, A., Suominen, H., Baur, G., Stevens, S. et al. (2011) Side-to-side differences in bone strength in master jumpers and sprinters. *Journal of Musculoskeletal and Neuronal Interactions* 11: 298–305.

Jepsen, D.B., Thomsen, K., Hansen, S, Jørgensen, N.R., Masud, T. and Ryg, J. (2017) Effect of whole-body vibration exercise in preventing falls and fractures: a systematic review and meta-analysis. *BMJ Open* 7: e018342. doi: 10.1136/bmjopen-2017–018342.

Judex, S. and Rubin, C.T. (2010) Is bone formation induced by high-frequency mechanical signals modulated by muscle activity? *Journal of Musculoskeletal and Neuronal Interactions* 10: 3–11.

Kanis, J., Johnell, O., Oden, A., Johansson, H. and McCloskey, E. (2008) FRAX and the assessment of fracture probability in men and women from the UK. *Osteoporosis International* 19: 385–97.

Karinkanta, S., Heinonen, A., Sievänen, A., Uusi-Rasi, K., Pasanen, M., Ojala, K. et al. (2007) A multi-component exercise regimen to prevent functional decline and bone fragility in home-dwelling elderly women: randomized, controlled trial. *Osteoporosis International* 18: 453–62.

Karinkanta S., Kannus, P., Uusi-Rasi, K., Heinonen, A. and Seivanen, H. (2015) Combined resistance and balance-jumping exercise reduces older women's injurious falls and fractures: 5-year follow-up study. *Age and Ageing* 44: 784–9.

Karsenty, G. and Oury, F. (2012) Biology without walls: the novel endocrinology of bone. *Annual Review of Physiology* 74: 87–105.

Kelley, G.A., Kelley, K.S. and Kohrt, W.M. (2012) Effects of ground and joint reaction force exercise on lumbar spine and femoral neck bone mineral density in postmenopausal women: a meta-analysis of randomized controlled trials. *BMC Musculoskeletal Disorders* 13: 177. doi: 10.1186/1471-2474-13-177.

Kelley, G.A., Kelley, K.S. and Kohrt, W.M. (2013a) Exercise and bone mineral density in premenopausal women: a meta-analysis of randomized controlled trials. *International Journal of Endocrinology* 2013: Article ID 741639. doi: 10.1155/2013/741639. Correction published in *International Journal of Endocrinology* 2013: Article ID 583217. doi: 10.1155/2013/583217.

Kelley, G.A., Kelly, K.S. and Kohrt, W.M. (2013b) Exercise and bone mineral density in men: a meta-analysis of randomized controlled trials. *Bone* 53: 103–11.

Kemmler, W., Engelke, K. and von Stengel, S. (2016) Long-term exercise and bone mineral density changes in postmenopausal women – are there periods of reduced effectiveness? *Journal of Bone and Mineral Research* 31: 215–22.

Kemmler, W., von Stengel, S., Engelke, K., Häberle, L. and Kalender, W.A. (2010) Exercise effects on bone mineral density, falls, coronary risk factors, and health care costs in older women. The Randomized Controlled Senior Fitness and Prevention (SEFIP) Study. *Archives of Internal Medicine* 170: 179–85.

Kontulainen, S., Heinonen, A., Kannus, P., Pasanen, M., Sievänen, A. and Vuori, I. (2004) Former exercisers of an 18-month intervention display residual aBMD benefits compared with control women 3.5 years post-intervention: a follow-up of a randomized controlled high-impact trial. *Osteoporosis International* 15: 248–51.

Kontulainen, S., Kannus, P., Haapasalo, H., Heinonen, A., Sievänen, A., Oja, P. and Vuori, I. (1999) Changes in bone mineral content with decreased training in competitive young adult tennis players and controls: a prospective 4-yr follow-up. *Medicine and Science in Sports and Exercise* 31: 646–52.

Kontulainen, S., Sievänen, A., Kannus, P., Pasanen, M. and Vuori, I. (2003) Effect of long-term impact loading on mass, size, and estimated strength of humerus and radius of female racquet-sports players: a peripheral quantitative computed tomography study between young and old starters and controls. *Journal of Bone and Mineral Research* 18: 352–9.

Korpelainen, R., Keinänen-Kiukaanniemi, S., Heikkenen, J., Väänänen, K. and Korpelainen, J. (2006a) Effect of impact exercise on bone mineral density in elderly women with low BMD; a population-based randomized controlled 30-month intervention. *Osteoporosis International* 17: 109–18.

Korpelainen, R., Keinänen-Kiukaanniemi, S., Heikkenen, J., Väänänen, K. and Korpelainen, J. (2006b) Effect of exercise on extraskeletal risk factors for hip fractures in elderly women with low BMD: a population-based randomized controlled trial. *Journal of Bone and Mineral Research* 21: 772–9.

Korpelainen, R., Keinänen-Kiukaanniemi, S., Nieminen, P., Heikkenen, J., Väänänen, K. and Korpelainen, J. (2010) Long-term outcomes of exercise: follow-up of a randomized trial in older women with osteopenia. *Archives of Internal Medicine* 170: 1548–56.

Kukuljian, S., Nowson, C.A., Sanders, K.M., Nicholson, G.C., Seibel, M.J., Salmon, J. and Daly, R. (2011) Independent and combined effects of calcium-vitamin D3 and exercise on bone structure and strength in older men: an 18-month factorial design randomized controlled trial. *Journal of Clinical Endocrinology and Metabolism* 96: 955–63.

Martyn-St James, M. and Carroll, S. (2008) Meta-analysis of walking for preservation of bone mineral density in postmenopausal women. *Bone* 43: 521–31.

Molloy, M.G. and Molloy, C.B. (2011) Contact sports and osteoarthritis. *British Journal of Sports Medicine* 45: 275–7.

Nevitt, M.C., Cummings, S.R., Stone, K.L., Palermo, L., Black, D.M., Bauer, H.K. et al. (2005) Risk factors for a first-incident radiographic vertebral fracture in women ≥65 years of age: the study of osteoporotic fractures. *Journal of Bone and Mineral Research* 20: 131–40.

Nikander, R., Kannus, P., Dastidar, P., Hannula, M., Harrison, L., Cervinka, T. et al. (2009) Targeted exercises against hip fragility. *Osteoporosis International* 20: 1321–8.

Nikander, R., Sievänen, A., Daly, R.M., Uusi-Rasi, K. and Kannus, P. (2010) Targeted exercise against osteoporosis: a systematic review and meta-analysis for optimising bone strength throughout life. *BMC Medicine* 8: 47. doi: 10.1186/1741-7015-8-47.

Nikander, R., Sievänen, A., Uusi-Rasi, K., Heinonen, A. and Kannus, P. (2006) Loading modalities and bone structures at non-weight-bearing upper extremity and weight-bearing lower extremity: a pQCT study of adult female athletes. *Bone* 39: 886–94.

Nilsson, M., Ohlsson, C., Odén, Mellström, D. and Lorentzon, M. (2012) Increased physical activity is associated with enhanced development of peak bone mass in men: a five-year longitudinal study. *Journal of Bone and Mineral Research* 27: 1206–14.

Polidoulis, I., Beyene, J. and Cheung, A.M. (2012) The effect of exercise on pQCT parameters of bone structure and strength in postmenopausal women – a systematic review and meta-analysis of randomized, controlled trials. *Osteoporosis International* 23: 39–51.

Saarto, T., Sievänen, A., Kellokumpu-Lehtinen, P., Nikander, R., Vehmanen, L., Huovinen, R. et al. (2012) Effect of supervised and home exercise training on bone mineral density among breast cancer patients: a 12-month randomised controlled trial. *Osteoporosis International* 23: 1601–12.

Sherrington, C., Michaleff, Z.A., Fairhall, N., Paul, S.S., Tiedemann, A., Whitney, J. et al. (2017) Exercise to prevent falls in older adults: an updated systematic review and meta-analysis. *British Journal of Sports Medicine* 51: 1750–8.

Sims, N.A. and Martin, T.J. (2014) Coupling the activities of bone formation and resorption: a multitude of signals within the basic multicellular unit. *BoneKEy Reports* 3: 481. doi: 10.1038/bonekey.2013.215.

Tveit, M., Rosengren, B.E., Jilsson, J.-Å., Ahlborg, H.G. and Karlsson, M.K. (2013) Bone mass following physical activity in young years: a mean 39-year prospective controlled study in men. *Osteoporosis International* 24: 1389–97.

Watson, S.L., Weeks, B.K., Weis, L.J., Harding, A.T., Horan, S.A. and Beck, B.R. (2018) High-intensity resistance and impact training improves bone mineral density and physical function in postmenopausal women with osteopenia and osteoporosis: the LIFTMOR randomized controlled trial. *Journal of Bone and Mineral Research* 33: 211–20.

World Health Organization (2014) Nutrition for older persons. Ageing and nutrition: a growing global challenge. http://www.who.int/nutrition/topics/ageing/en/ (accessed 3 May 2019).

10 Mental health

Clare Stevinson

INTRODUCTION

Mental health is defined by the World Health Organization as 'a state of well-being in which the individual realizes his or her own abilities, can cope with the normal stresses of life, can work productively and fruitfully, and is able to make a contribution to his or her community' (World Health Organization 2004). This definition therefore considers positive mental health to be more than the absence of mental illness, and recognises that there is a spectrum of wellbeing for people with and without mental disorders. Based on the concepts of languishing and flourishing (Keyes 2002), Figure 10.1 illustrates the interacting dimensions of mental illness and mental wellbeing. Even individuals with no mental disorder can experience low wellbeing and, therefore, overall reduced mental health.

AETIOLOGY OF MENTAL DISORDERS

Contributors to mental illness include a range of biological, environmental, social and psychological factors. There is considerable evidence for genetic causation with estimated heritability highest for severe mental disorders such as schizophrenia and bipolar disorder (Rasic et al. 2014). In some cases, it is not the disease that is inherited but the sensitivity to environmental risk factors which may trigger the onset of illness. These include prenatal and childhood exposures, brain injury, substance abuse and serious adverse life events (Uher and Zwicker 2017). In addition, some chronic medical conditions are increasingly recognised as leading to mental disorders. An analysis of nearly two million primary care patients indicated that 19.8% with a chronic physical illness has a comorbid mental disorder (Barnett et al. 2012).

Figure 10.1 Interacting dimensions of mental illness and mental wellbeing that contribute to overall mental health status, based on the concepts of psychological flourishing and languishing.

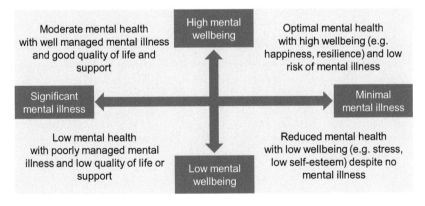

Source: Keyes (2002).

PREVALENCE OF MENTAL DISORDERS

The current edition of the Diagnostic and Statistical Manual for Mental Disorders (DSM-5) includes 21 categories of mental disorder (American Psychiatric Association 2013). A systematic review of population-based prevalence surveys from 63 countries indicated that anxiety and mood disorders are most common (Steel et al. 2014), with female cases outnumbering male by approximately half. Table 10.1 provides the prevalence estimates for specific mood and anxiety disorders based on studies from 30 European nations (Wittchen et al. 2011). All studies used diagnostic interviews to ascertain the prevalence of disorders over the previous 12 months in representative samples of the general population.

BURDEN OF MENTAL DISORDERS

Poor mental health has negative consequences for individuals and for society. These can include psychological distress, strain on personal relationships, experiencing stigma and discrimination, and poor physical health. Obesity, cardiovascular disease, and diabetes are more prevalent among the mentally ill, than in the general population (De Hert et al. 2011). This disparity is attributed to a combination of maladaptive lifestyle choices (e.g. smoking, alcohol, diet), the side effects of psychotropic medication and differences in health-care utilisation.

Collectively, these contribute to significant loss of personal and social functioning. According to the World Health Organization (2016), mental disorders are the leading cause of global disease burden, as measured by years lived with disability (YLD). This is a calculation based on the prevalence of the disorder, and the loss of health associated with it. As shown in Figure 10.2, mental and substance use disorders represent 22% of the total burden, dwarfing all other disease categories. Musculoskeletal problems comprise the next largest category at 14%. A breakdown of the most common individual health problems reveals that depressive disorders are ranked

Table 10.1 Prevalence estimates of mood and anxiety disorders in Europe.

DIAGNOSIS	NUMBER OF STUDIES	MEDIAN ESTIMATE	INTERQUARTILE RANGE
Major depression	25	5.7%	3.2–7.4
Bipolar disorder	11	0.7%	0.7–0.9
Generalised anxiety disorder	14	2.0%	0.6–2.2
Agoraphobia	16	1.2%	0.4–2.0
Panic disorder	18	1.2%	0.4–2.0
Social phobia	15	2.0%	1.1–4.4
Specific phobias	12	4.9%	3.4–7.1
Post-traumatic stress disorder	12	2.3%	0.7–2.5
Obsessive-compulsive disorder	10	0.7%	0.5–1.1

Source: Wittchen et al. (2011).

Figure 10.2 Global estimates of disease burden (years lost to disability) by disease category.

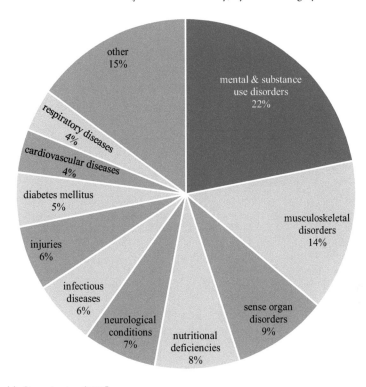

other
15%

mental & substance
use disorders
22%

respiratory diseases
4%

cardiovascular diseases
4%

diabetes mellitus
5%

injuries
6%

infectious
diseases
6%

neurological
conditions
7%

nutritional
deficiencies
8%

sense organ
disorders
9%

musculoskeletal
disorders
14%

Source: World Health Organization (2016).

first or second in every region in the world, and anxiety disorders are also in the top ten in all regions. Even when mortality rates are included in the calculation, mental disorders are ranked third behind cardiovascular disease and cancer as causes of non-communicable global disease burden. The associated economic burden is also considerable, including health-care costs, reduced productivity, absenteeism and welfare payments. The total global cost of mental illness has been estimated at $US2.5 trillion for 2010 and is predicted to rise to $US6.0 trillion by 2030 (Mnookin 2016). In addition, suicide accounts for 1.5% of deaths globally (World Health Organization 2017), and a strong correlation exists between mental illness and attempted and completed suicides (Bertolote et al. 2003).

DIAGNOSTIC CRITERIA

A diagnosis of major depressive disorder, according to DSM-5 criteria (American Psychiatric Association 2013), is based on an individual reporting the presence of at least five out of nine symptoms, for two weeks or longer. These symptoms are not clearly attributable to another medical condition or to substance use, and cause significant distress, or impairment of social, occupational or other important areas of functioning.

At least one of the five diagnostic symptoms has to be either depressed mood, or markedly diminished interest or pleasure in activities, most of the time. Other symptoms are: significant weight gain or loss (when not dieting) or increased or decreased appetite; insomnia or hypersomnia; agitation or retardation; fatigue; a sense of worthlessness or inappropriate guilt; difficulties thinking, concentrating or decision making; and recurrent thoughts of death, suicidal ideation or suicide attempt or plan.

Table 10.2 provides a summary of the symptoms included in diagnostic criteria for five anxiety disorders (DSM-5). As with depression, symptoms should not be attributable to other medical condition, medication or other substance use. Furthermore, the symptoms cause significant distress or impairment of social, occupational or other area of functioning.

Table 10.2 Summary of key diagnostic criteria for five anxiety disorders (DSM-5).

ANXIETY DISORDER	SYMPTOMS
Generalised anxiety disorder	• Excessive anxiety and worry about multiple events or activities for ≥6 months. • Difficulty controlling the worry. • ≥3 of 6 symptoms present for ≥6 months: (1) restlessness; (2) fatigue; (3) difficulty concentrating; (4) irritability; (5) muscle tension; (6) sleep disturbance.
Agoraphobia	• Disproportionate fear or anxiety about ≥2 of 5 situations: (1) public transport; (2) open spaces; (3) enclosed spaces; (4) in crowds; (5) alone outside of home. • Fear of escape being difficult or help unavailable in these situations. • Situations are avoided, require companions or endured with intense anxiety
Social anxiety disorder (social phobia)	• Disproportionate fear or anxiety about ≥1 social or performance situations for ≥6 months. • Fear of being negatively evaluated (i.e. embarrassed, humiliated, being rejected, offending others). • Situations are avoided or endured with intense anxiety.
Panic disorder	• Recurrent unexpected panic attacks involving a sudden surge of intense fear with ≥4 of 13 symptoms: (1) palpitations; (2) sweating; (3) shaking; (4) shortness of breath; (5) choking sensation; (6) chest pain; (7) nausea; (8) dizziness; (9) chills or heat sensation; (10) paraesthesia (numbness or tingling); (11) derealisation or depersonalisation; (12) fear of losing control or 'going crazy'; (13) fear of dying. • Attacks followed for ≥1 month by at least one of: (1) worry about additional panic attack or their consequences (e.g. losing control, heart attack, 'going crazy'); (2) avoidance of situations that might trigger attack.
Specific phobia	• Disproportionate and marked fear or anxiety about a specific object or situation for ≥6 months. • Exposure to the object or situation reliably provokes immediate fear or anxiety. • Object or situation is avoided or endured with intense anxiety.

Source: American Psychiatric Association (2013).

PHYSICAL INACTIVITY AS A RISK FACTOR

Physical activity levels are inversely associated with the prevalence of mental disorders. For example, a large population-based study of 15–54-year-olds in the United States (n = 5877) demonstrated a dose–response relationship between reported regularity of physical activity and prevalence of ten mental disorders (Goodwin 2003). Figure 10.3 displays the association for depressive and anxiety disorders. After adjusting for a range of factors (age, gender, race, marital status, education, income and physical illnesses), the odds of a diagnosis of depression were 0.66 lower among regular exercisers than among those who were occasionally or never active. Similar odds ratios were reported for anxiety disorders.

Interpretation of these data are constrained by the cross-sectional nature of the dataset. The inverse associations may indicate protection from developing mental disorders due to regular physical activity. Equally, they may suggest that those with mental health problems tend to avoid frequent activity (reverse causality). The control of confounding factors strengthens the likelihood of physical activity being an independent predictor. Nonetheless, a clearer insight into the role of physical activity in preventing mental health problems is gained from prospective cohort studies.

DEPRESSIVE DISORDERS

For depression, a sizable body of evidence exists to support a protective effect of regular physical activity. A comprehensive systematic review on this subject included

Figure 10.3 Prevalence of depressive and anxiety disorders by regularity of physical activity. Data are from the National Comorbidity Survey of adults (n = 8098) aged 15–54 years in the United States.

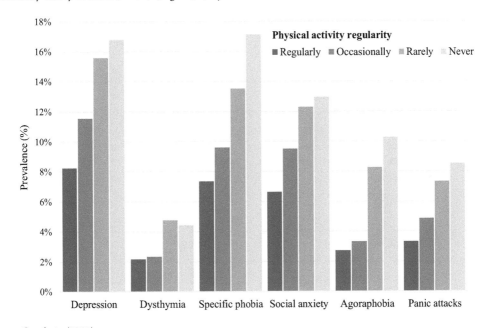

Source: Goodwin (2003).

30 cohort studies all of which involved participants who were free of depression at baseline (Mammen and Faulkner 2013). Self-reported physical activity was measured at the start of each study, and the number of cases of depression were recorded after follow-up, which ranged from one to 27 years. Eleven of the studies also assessed physical activity and depression at intermediate time points during follow-up. Assessment of depression included physician diagnosis, hospital records or meeting a defined threshold on a validated screening tool.

Twenty-five studies reported a significant inverse association between baseline physical activity and risk of developing depression over the follow-up period. The majority of these studies were rated as having high methodological quality. No clear minimum volume or frequency of physical activity emerged in relation to risk, but benefits were demonstrated with even low to moderate levels of activity. For example, in an eight-year study involving 1,481 older men, the odds of depression were nearly halved for those walking at least a quarter of a mile daily, when compared with inactive men. This was after controlling for demographic factors, as well as physical and functional health (Smith et al. 2010).

Eleven of the studies reviewed examined changes in physical activity over time and associations with depression status. Three of these revealed that depression risk was lower after physical activity increased, and two others found that participants who maintained activity over time had lower depression risk than those who were inactive throughout the study. In support of these findings, four studies indicated an increased risk of depression after reducing physical activity levels. One of these studies was an eight-year follow-up of 663 older Finnish adults (Lampinen et al. 2000). Among regular walkers who decreased their physical activity over time, the odds of developing depression were ten times higher than those who maintained or increased their physical activity level after adjusting for potential confounders.

A subsequent large study in Norway provided further evidence of protection from depression through regular physical activity. A cohort of 33,908 healthy adults were followed for 11 years with depression assessed by a validated screening tool (Harvey et al. 2018). For participants reporting no physical activity, the odds of meeting the diagnostic criteria for depression were 1.44 higher than those exercising at least one hour per week after adjustment for demographic factors, body mass index and lifestyle behaviours. The results applied to men and women, and in both younger and older age groups. Further support for a protective relationship of physical activity on depression was provided by a pooled analysis of data from large-scale genomic studies (Choi et al. 2019). Based on a Mendelian randomisation design, a significant causal association was reported for objectively measured physical activity (by accelerometery) although not for self-reported activity.

ANXIETY DISORDERS

The association between physical inactivity and incidence of anxiety disorders has been investigated in fewer studies than depression and results have been less consistent. One German study assessed physical activity via interview in 2,458 healthy young adults (14–24-year-olds) at baseline and monitored them over four years (Ströhle et al. 2007).

Diagnostic interviews determined the incidence of a range of mental disorders. For regularly active participants, the risk of developing any anxiety disorder was almost half that for those who were inactive (odds ratio of 0.52).

Similar results were reported from a Dutch study involving 7,076 healthy adults aged 18 to 64 years (Ten Have et al. 2011). Participants reported the number of hours per week spent exercising and underwent diagnostic interviews. After four years, the odds of an anxiety disorder for those exercising for one to three hours per week were nearly half those for inactive participants (odds ratio of 0.56) with adjustments for demographic factors and health. Significantly lower odds were also evident for five specific anxiety disorders (Figure 10.4). There was no further reduction in risk for participants exercising for four or more hours per week.

Other cohort studies have not produced the same results, however. The Norwegian study referred to above that found a reduced risk of depression in physically active people did not see the same protective effect for anxiety (Harvey et al. 2018). Similarly, in a two-year follow-up of 1,204 Korean older adults (Kang et al. 2016), and an eight-year study of British civil servants (Azevedo Da Silva et al. 2012), level of physical activity was not associated with the development of anxiety symptomology.

McDowell and colleagues undertook a systematic review of 24 prospective studies examining baseline physical activity and the development of anxiety disorders or self-reported anxiety symptoms over a median of 4.75 years (McDowell et al. 2019). Meta-analyses suggested that physical activity was inversely associated with a diagnosis of any anxiety disorder (odds ratio of 0.66), and specifically with generalised anxiety

Figure 10.4 Odds of developing anxiety disorders over three years among adults exercising for one to three hours per week compared with inactive adults. Data are from the Netherlands Mental Health Survey and Incidence Study of Dutch adults (n = 7076) aged 18–64 years.

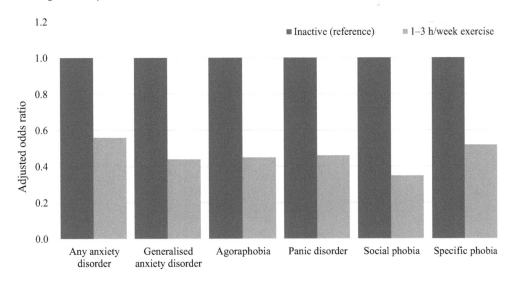

Source: Ten Have et al. (2011).

disorder (odds ratio of 0.54) as well as lower odds (0.87) of self-reported anxiety symptoms. The authors concluded that, despite methodological heterogeneity, the overall evidence was supportive of the proposition that physical activity affords some protection from anxiety.

MECHANISMS OF INTERACTIONS WITH PHYSICAL ACTIVITY

The suggested mechanisms by which physical activity might reduce the risk of mental illness are diverse (Figure 10.5). A range of neurobiological adaptations resulting from exercise are compatible with the pathophysiology of depressive and anxiety disorders. In addition, some of the observed psychological and social benefits of exercise may have a role in protecting mental health.

Animal studies have demonstrated that voluntary exercise helps maintain regulation of the central noradrenergic, serotonergic and dopaminergic systems, which can be disrupted in patients with mental disorders (Remington 2009). Similarly, research in rodent models has shown that exercise can increase synthesis of neurotrophic factors (in particular brain-derived neurotrophic factor), and facilitate neurogenesis, both of which are important for cognition, mood and behaviour (Deslandes et al. 2009).

Exercise also affects the neuroendocrine system and has been shown to modulate stress reactivity in animals and humans (Salmon 2001). Since dysregulation of the hypothalamic-pituitary-adrenal axis is implicated in the development of depression

Figure 10.5 Potential biopsychosocial mechanisms for the role of physical activity in maintaining mental health.

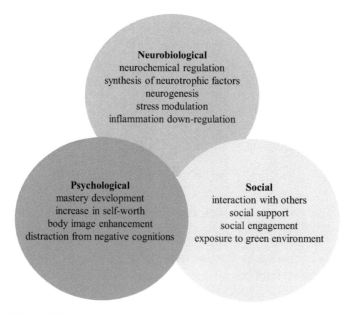

and anxiety disorders (Ströhle and Holsboer 2003), the protective effects of physical activity may partly be attributable to attenuation of the stress response.

Lack of physical activity has been identified as a potential risk factor for depression and other mental disorders through contributing to systemic inflammation (Berk et al. 2013). Other modifiable risk factors for inflammation related to lifestyle include smoking, poor sleep and dietary intake. However, regular exercise has been shown to have an adaptive immunomodulatory effect, leading to down-regulation of inflammatory responses, which may be important for maintaining mental health (Berk et al. 2013).

A physiological explanation for the preventative effects of physical activity is possibly supported by evidence of low cardiorespiratory fitness being a significant predictor of depression or anxiety onset (Baumeister et al. 2017; Becofsky et al. 2015; Dishman et al. 2012; Schuch et al. 2016b). However, fitness may be confounded by health or genetic factors, and studies have not identified a dose–response relationship between either the volume or intensity of physical activity and the degree of protection from mental disorders observed, nor identified a specific threshold of activity or fitness.

Maintaining positive self-perceptions is a significant component of mental health, and physical activity is associated with improvements in physical self-efficacy, self-esteem, physical self-worth and bodily attractiveness among individuals with low mood (White et al. 2009). The self-regulatory skills involved in initiating and sustaining physical activity, and the sense of mastery that can be generated from these accomplishments, contribute to the development and strengthening of self-efficacy and self-worth (Sonstroem et al. 1994). Self-perceptions around body image and attractiveness can be enhanced by exercise due to perceived positive changes in physical characteristics (e.g. muscle tone, fat loss) or competence (Campbell and Hausenblas 2009; Monshouwer et al. 2013).

The social or environmental context of physical activity may be relevant to the positive effects on wellbeing and contribute to maintaining mental health. Social interaction in various forms is associated with mental wellbeing (Sandstrom and Dunn 2014), and social interactions and social support experienced through physical activity predicts lower odds of mental health problems (Monshouwer et al. 2013). Similarly, there is evidence that exposure to nature and green space contributes to reducing stress and fatigue (Hartig et al. 1991; Kaplan 1995; Ulrich 1979) and is associated with lower risk of mental health diagnoses (Maas et al. 2009). Physical activity that takes place in natural environments (known as green exercise) is associated with lower odds of reporting poor mental health than exercise in synthetic settings (Mitchell 2013). A systematic review of 28 trials of green exercise indicated favourable acute effects over indoor exercise for affective states and enjoyment, although the methodological quality of the overall evidence base is limited (Lahart et al. 2019).

The psychological value of physical activity may also relate to its potential for providing distraction from, and reinterpretation of, mood and anxiety symptoms. Negative thinking styles, such as ruminating on depressed or anxious feelings, lead to poorer mental health, while engaging in distraction activities helps break the cycle of negative thoughts (Nolen-Hoeksema et al. 1994). Reduced rumination over time and transient mood-lift after exercise sessions were reported in a study with depressed women (Craft 2005). Similarly, acute exercise bouts reduced state anxiety in healthy volunteers as effectively as other distraction strategies (Bahrke and Morgan 1978; Raglin and Morgan

1987), with exercise having a more sustained anxiolytic (anxiety-relieving) effect (Raglin and Morgan 1987).

Physical activity may be particularly valuable for individuals with high levels of anxiety sensitivity. This refers to the tendency to fear and catastrophise the normal experience of anxiety and is a risk factor for developing anxiety disorders (Korte et al. 2013). An inverse association exists between anxiety sensitivity and exercise frequency, reflecting avoidance of the physical sensations of exercise (e.g. increased heart rate and respiration) that resemble anxiety symptoms (McWilliams and Asmundson 2001). However, exposure to these symptoms within the 'safe' context of exercise allows the individual to learn to reinterpret these symptoms as harmless and increases tolerance to experiencing them (Smits et al. 2008).

Despite the plausible hypotheses and supportive data, the mechanisms whereby physical activity protects mental health are still undetermined. Knowledge of the genes that may influence the relationship between physical activity and mental health is currently limited, but evidence of heritability exists for both (Boomsma et al. 2000; De Moor et al. 2007; Stubbe et al. 2006). An interesting study of the genetic and environmental influences on the association between physical activity and depression or anxiety concluded that this is not a causal effect (De Moor et al. 2008). Using data from 8,558 adult twins, siblings and parents, the cross-sectional and 11-year prospective associations between physical activity and psychological outcomes were best explained by shared genetic factors. The authors suggested that a common genetic susceptibility may underlie an individual's propensity to exercise and predisposition for depression or anxiety symptoms.

MANAGEMENT OF MENTAL HEALTH WITH PHYSICAL ACTIVITY

Consistent with the suggestion of genetic vulnerability, voluntary physical activity tends to decline during episodes of depression or anxiety (Azevedo Da Silva et al. 2012; Hiles et al. 2017; Lindwall et al. 2011). Furthermore, many of the symptoms of poor mental health experienced by individuals can make exercise difficult. For example, depression is characterised by low mood, loss of motivation, social withdrawal and fatigue, all of which deter energetic behaviour. Sleep disturbance and fatigue are common symptoms of anxiety, and for some individuals with agoraphobia or social phobia, exercise in public settings can be daunting. Some of the symptoms of a panic attack resemble the physical sensations of exercise (e.g. breathlessness, palpitations, perspiration), which may lead to avoidance of physical activities.

However, there is a considerable body of evidence suggesting that participants recruited for prescribed exercise programmes can achieve lowered symptomology. Systematic reviews of randomised controlled trials (RCTs) have consistently demonstrated the efficacy of supervised exercise interventions in reducing symptoms of depression (Cooney et al. 2013; Kvam et al. 2016; Schuch et al. 2016a; Silviara et al. 2013). Kvam and colleagues identified a total of 23 RCTs involving adults with clinically diagnosed depression, and subjected the data to meta-analysis (Figure 10.6). The results indicated superior effects for exercise than no treatment or usual care, and

Figure 10.6 Standardised effect sizes of exercise interventions in comparison with other approaches from a meta-analysis of randomised controlled trials in patients with depression.

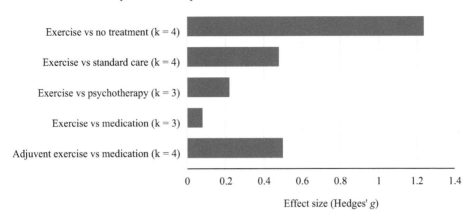

Source: Kvam et al. (2016).

similar outcomes when directly compared with conventional antidepressant medication or psychological therapy. Exercise as an adjunct to medication produced greater benefit than medication alone, but the effect size was not statistically significant (Kvam et al. 2016).

There are fewer trials for anxiety disorders, but evidence is encouraging. In 2015, Stonerock and colleagues drew cautiously positive conclusions about the usefulness of exercise as a treatment approach, based on reviewing 12 RCTs of adults with anxiety disorders or anxiety symptoms, and five previously published meta-analyses (Stonerock et al. 2015). In an earlier meta-analysis of eight RCTs with clinically diagnosed anxiety disorders (Jayakody et al. 2014), results indicated that exercise interventions were superior to no treatment, but less effective than conventional therapy. The authors therefore suggested that exercise may have value as an adjunctive therapy.

Based on the current evidence, supervised group physical activity interventions are recommended by the National Institute of Health and Clinical Excellence (NICE) in the United Kingdom as a first-line therapeutic option for patients with mild to moderate depression (NICE 2009). The guidelines for Generalised Anxiety Disorder and Panic Disorder include advice for health professionals to discuss the benefits of exercise for general health, but not yet as a treatment option. However, they identify physical activity as having potential value, and as a priority for research (NICE 2011). For patients with psychosis and schizophrenia, it is recommended that health-care providers offer a programme of physical activity (and healthy eating) to address physical health (NICE 2014a). The same recommendation is made for patients with bipolar disorder (NICE 2014b). Patients with schizophrenia and other serious mental disorders have low life expectancy related to poor physical health, underlining the importance of improving physical activity and other lifestyle habits for such individuals (McNamee et al. 2013).

SUMMARY

- Mental health is defined as positive wellbeing as well as the absence of mental illness.
- Based on prevalence and morbidity, mental disorders represent 22% of the global burden of years lost to disability.
- Regular physical activity among healthy adults is associated with a lower risk of developing depression.
- For anxiety disorders a similar association exists, but the evidence base is smaller and less consistent.
- The physiological mechanisms through which regular physical activity might help protect mental health include regulation of monoamine function and the sympathetic nervous system, neurogenesis and inflammation.
- Psychosocial mechanisms include changes in self-perceptions, distraction from negative thought patterns, social or environmental interactions, and reductions in anxiety sensitivity.
- Supervised group physical activity programmes are recommended as a treatment option for patients with mild to moderate depressive disorders, and exercise is encouraged for general health in all patients with mental illness.

STUDY TASKS

1 Consider the diagnostic criteria for depression. Aside from the two core symptoms (low mood and loss of interest), identify which of the other seven associated symptoms have the potential to be influenced by physical activity.
2 Describe why people with anxiety sensitivity may avoid physical activity and explain why exercise may be particularly beneficial for these individuals in helping reduce risk of anxiety disorders.
3 Consider the mechanisms by which physical activity may protect mental health. Choose one or more of the neurophysiological or psychological hypotheses and design a study that would test the role of the mechanism(s) in preventing the development of mental disorders.

FURTHER READING

Clow, A. and Edmunds, S. (2014) *Physical activity and mental health*. Champaign, IL: Human Kinetics.
Ekkekakis, P. (2013) *Handbook of physical activity and mental health*. Abingdon: Routledge.
Zschucke, E., Gaudlitz, K. and Ströhle, A. (2013) Exercise and physical activity in mental disorders: clinical and experimental evidence. *Journal of Preventive Medicine and Public Health* 46: S12–21.

REFERENCES

American Psychiatric Association. (2013) *Diagnostic and statistical manual of mental disorders*. 5th edn, Arlington, VA: American Psychiatric Association.

Azevedo Da Silva, M., Singh-Manoux, A., Brunner, E.J., Kaffashian, S., Shipley, M.J., Kivimäki, M. and Nabi, H. (2012) Bidirectional association between physical activity and symptoms of anxiety and depression: the Whitehall II study. *European Journal of Epidemiology* 27: 537–46.

Bahrke, M.S. and Morgan, W.P. (1978) Anxiety reduction following exercise and meditation. *Cognitive Therapy and Research* 2: 323–33.

Barnett, K., Mercer, S.W., Norbury, M., Watt, G., Wyke, S. and Guthrie, B. (2012) Epidemiology of multimorbidity and implications for health care, research, and medical education: a cross-sectional study. *The Lancet* 380: 37–43.

Baumeister, S.E., Leitzmann, M.F., Bahls, M., Dörr, M., Schmid, D., Schomerus, G. et al. (2017) Associations of leisure-time and occupational physical activity and cardiorespiratory fitness with incident and recurrent major depressive disorder, depressive symptoms, and incident anxiety in a general population. *Journal of Clinical Psychiatry* 78: e41–7.

Becofsky, K.M., Sui, X., Lee, D.C., Wilcox, S., Zhang, J. and Blair, S.N. (2015) A prospective study of fitness, fatness, and depressive symptoms. *American Journal of Epidemiology* 181: 311–20.

Berk, M., Williams, L.J., Jacka, F.N., O'Neil, A., Pasco, J.A., Moylan, S. et al. (2013) So depression is an inflammatory disease, but where does the inflammation come from? *BMC Medicine* 11: 200. doi: 10.1186/1741-7015-11-200.

Bertolote, J.M., Fleischmann, A., Leo, D.D. and Wasserman, D. (2003) Suicide and mental disorders: do we know enough? *British Journal of Psychiatry* 183: 382–3.

Boomsma, D.I., Beem, A.L., van den Berg, M., Dolan, C.V., Koopmans, J.R., Vink, J.M. et al. (2000) Netherlands Twin Family Study of Anxious Depression (NETSAD). *Twin Research* 3: 323–34.

Campbell, A. and Hausenblas, H. (2009) Effects of exercise interventions on body image: a meta-analysis. *Journal of Health Psychology* 14: 780–93.

Choi, K.W., Chen, C.Y., Stein, M.B., Klimentidis, Y.C., Wang, M.J., Koenen, K.C. and Smoller, J.W.; Major Depressive Disorder Working Group of the Psychiatric Genomics Consortium. (2019) Assessment of bidirectional relationships between physical activity and depression among adults: a 2-sample Mendelian randomization study. *JAMA Psychiatry* 76: 399–408.

Cooney, G.M., Dwan, K., Greig, C.A., Lawlor, D.A., Rimer, J., Waugh, F.R. et al. (2013) Exercise for depression. *Cochrane Database of Systematic Reviews* 12: CD004366. doi: 10.1002/14651858. CD004366.pub6.

Craft, L.L. (2005) Exercise and clinical depression: examining two psychological mechanisms. *Psychology of Sport and Exercise* 6: 151–71.

De Hert, M., Correll, C.U., Bobes, J., Cetkovich-Bakmas, M., Cohen, D., Asai, I. et al. (2011) Physical illness in patients with severe mental disorders. I. Prevalence, impact of medications and disparities in health care. *World Psychiatry* 10: 52–77.

De Moor, M.H.M., Boomsma, D.I., Stubbe, J.H., Willemsen, G. and de Geus, E.J.C. (2008) Testing causality in the association between regular exercise and symptoms of anxiety and depression. *Archives of General Psychiatry* 65: 897–905.

De Moor, M.H.M., Posthuma, D., Hottenga, J.J., Willemsen, A.H.M., Boomsma, D.I. and de Geus, E.J.C. (2007) Genome-wide linkage scan for exercise participation in Dutch sibling pairs. *European Journal of Human Genetics* 15: 1252–9.

Deslandes, A., Moraes, H., Ferreira, C., Veiga, H., Silveira, H., Mouta, R. et al. (2009) Exercise and mental health: many reasons to move. *Neuropsychobiology* 59: 191–8.

Dishman, R.K., Sui, X., Church, T.S., Hand, G.A., Trivedi, M.H. and Blair, S.N. (2012) Decline in cardiorespiratory fitness and odds of incident depression. *American Journal of Preventive Medicine* 43: 361–8.

Goodwin, R.D. (2003) Association between physical activity and mental disorders among adults in the United States. *Preventive Medicine* 36: 698–703.

Hartig, T., Mang, M. and Evans, G.W. (1991) Restorative effects of natural environment experiences. *Environment and Behavior* 23: 3–26.

Harvey, S.B., Øverland, S., Hatch, S.L., Wessely, S., Mykletun, A. and Hotopf, M. (2018) Exercise and the prevention of depression: results of the HUNT cohort study. *American Journal of Psychiatry* 175: 28–36.

Hiles, S.A., Lamers, F., Milaneschi, Y. and Penninx, B.W.J.H. (2017) Sit, step, sweat: longitudinal associations between physical activity patterns, anxiety and depression. *Psychological Medicine* 47: 1466–77.

Jayakody, K., Gunadasa, S. and Hosker, C. (2014) Exercise for anxiety disorders: systematic review. *British Journal of Sports Medicine* 48: 187–96.

Kang, H.-J., Bae, K.-Y., Kim, S.-W., Shin, I.-S., Yoon, J.-S. and Kim, J.-M. (2016) Anxiety symptoms in Korean elderly individuals: a two-year longitudinal community study. *International Psychogeriatrics* 28: 423–33.

Kaplan, S. (1995) The restorative benefits of nature: toward an integrative framework. *Journal of Environmental Psychology* 15: 169–82.

Keyes, C.L.M. (2002). The mental health continuum: from languishing to flourishing in life. *Journal of Health and Social Research* 43: 207–22.

Korte, K., Brown, M.A.S. and Schmidt, N.B. (2013) Anxiety sensitivity and impairment: evidence for a direct association and partial mediation by subclinical anxiety symptoms. *Journal of Affective Disorders* 151: 875–81.

Kvam, S., Kleppe, C.L., Nordhus, I.H. and Hovland, A. (2016) Exercise as a treatment for depression: a meta-analysis. *Journal of Affective Disorders* 202: 67–86.

Lahart, I., Darcy, P., Gidlow, C. and Calogiuri, G. (2019) The effects of green exercise on physical activity and mental wellbeing: a systematic review. *International Journal of Environmental Research and Public Health* 16: 1352. doi: 10.3390/ijerph16081352.

Lampinen, P., Heikkinen, R.L. and Ruoppila, I. (2000) Changes in intensity of physical exercise as predictors of depressive symptoms among older adults: an eight year follow-up study. *Preventive Medicine* 12: 113–80.

Lindwall, M., Larsman, P. and Hagger, M.S. (2011) The reciprocal relationship between physical activity and depression in older European adults: a prospective cross-lagged panel design using SHARE data. *Health Psychology* 30: 453–62.

Maas, J., Verheij, R.A., de Vries, S., Spreeuwenberg, P., Schellevis, F.G. and Groenewegen, P.P. (2009) Morbidity is related to a green living environment. *Journal of Epidemiology and Community Health* 63: 967–73.

Mammen, G. and Faulkner, G. (2013) Physical activity and the prevention of depression: a systematic review of prospective studies. *American Journal of Preventive Medicine* 45: 649–57.

McDowell, C.P., Dishman, R.K., Gordon, B.R. and Herring, M.P. (2019) Physical activity and anxiety: a systematic review and meta-analysis of prospective cohort studies. *American Journal of Preventive Medicine* 57: 545–56.

McNamee, L., Mead, G., MacGillivray, S. and Lawrie, S.M. (2013). Schizophrenia, poor physical health and physical activity: evidence-based interventions are required to reduce major health inequalities. *The British Journal of Psychiatry* 203: 239–41.

McWilliams, L.A. and Asmundson, G.J.G. (2001) Is there a negative association between anxiety sensitivity and arousal-increasing substances and activities? *Journal of Anxiety Disorders* 15: 161–70.

Mitchell, R. (2013). Is physical activity in natural environments better for mental health than physical activity in other environments? *Social Science and Medicine* 91: 130–4.

Mnookin, S. (2016) *Out of the shadows: making mental health a global development priority*. Washington, DC: World Bank Group and World Health Organization.

Monshouwer, K., ten Have, M., Van Poppel, M., Kemper, H. and Vollebergh, W. (2013) Possible mechanisms explaining the association between physical activity and mental health. *Clinical Psychological Science* 1: 64–74.

National Institute for Health and Clinical Excellence. (2009) *Depression: the treatment and management of depression in adults (NICE clinical guideline 90)*. London: National Institute for Health and Clinical Excellence.

National Institute for Health and Clinical Excellence. (2011) *Generalised anxiety disorder and panic disorder (with or without agoraphobia) in adults: management in primary, secondary and community care. (NICE clinical guideline 113)*. London: National Institute for Health and Clinical Excellence.

National Institute for Health and Clinical Excellence. (2014a) *Psychosis and schizophrenia in adults: treatment and management (NICE clinical guideline 178)*. London: National Institute for Health and Clinical Excellence.

National Institute for Health and Clinical Excellence. (2014b) *Bipolar disorder: assessment and management (NICE clinical guideline 185)*. London: National Institute for Health and Clinical Excellence.

Nolen-Hoeksema, S., Parker, L. and Larson, J. (1994) Ruminative coping with depressed mood following loss. *Journal of Personality and Social Psychology* 67: 92–104.

Raglin, J.S. and Morgan, W.P. (1987) Influence of exercise and quiet rest on state anxiety and blood pressure. *Medicine and Science in Sports and Exercise* 19: 456–63.

Rasic, D., Hajek, T., Alda, M. and Uher, R. (2014) Risk of mental illness in offspring of parents with schizophrenia, bipolar disorder, and major depressive disorder: a meta-analysis of family high-risk studies. *Schizophrenia Bulletin* 40: 28–38.

Remington, G. (2009) From mice to men: what can animal models tell us about the relationship between mental health and physical activity? *Mental Health and Physical Activity* 2: 10–15.

Salmon, P. (2001) Effects of physical exercise on anxiety, depression and sensitivity to stress: a unifying theory. *Clinical Psychology Review* 21: 33–61.

Sandstrom, G.M. and Dunn, E.W. (2014) Social interactions and well-being: the surprising power of weak ties. *Personality and Social Psychology Bulletin* 40: 910–22.

Schuch, F.B., Vancampfort, D., Richards, J., Rosenbaum, S., Ward, P.B. and Stubbs, B. (2016a) Exercise as a treatment for depression: a meta-analysis adjusting for publication bias. *Journal of Psychiatric Research* 77: 42–51.

Schuch, F.B., Vancampfort, D., Sui, X., Rosenbaum, S., Firth, J., Richards, J. et al. (2016b) Are lower levels of cardiorespiratory fitness associated with incident depression? A systematic review of prospective cohort studies. *Preventive Medicine* 93: 159–65.

Silveira, H., Moraes, H., Oliveira, N., Coutinho, E.S., Laks, J. and Deslandes, A. (2013) Physical exercise and clinically depressed patients: a systematic review and meta-analysis. *Neuropsychobiology* 67: 61–8.

Smith, T.L., Masaki, K.H., Fong, K., Abbott, R.D., Ross, G.W., Petrovitch, H. et al. (2010) Effect of walking distance on 8-year incident depressive symptoms in elderly men with and without chronic disease: the Honolulu-Asia aging study. *Journal of American Geriatric Society* 58: 1447–52.

Smits, J.A., Berry, A.C., Rosenfield, D., Powers, M.B., Behar, E. and Otto, M.W. (2008) Reducing anxiety sensitivity with exercise. *Depression and Anxiety* 25: 689–99.

Sonstroem, R.J., Harlow, L.L. and Josephs, L. (1994) Exercise and self-esteem: validity of model expansion and exercise associations. *Journal of Sport and Exercise Psychology* 16: 29–42.

Steel, Z., Marnane, C., Iranpour, C., Chey, T., Jackson, J.W., Patel, V. and Silove, D. (2014) The global prevalence of common mental disorders: a systematic review and meta-analysis 1980–2013. *International Journal of Epidemiology* 43: 476–93.

Stonerock, G.L., Hoffman, B.M., Smith, P.J. and Blumenthal, J.A. (2015) Exercise as treatment for anxiety: systematic review and analysis. *Annals of Behavioral Medicine* 49: 542–56.

Ströhle, A., Höfler, M., Pfister, H., Müller, A.G., Hoyer, J., Wittchen, H.U. and Lieb, R. (2007) Physical activity and prevalence and incidence of mental disorders in adolescents and young adults. *Psychological Medicine* 37: 1657–66.

Ströhle, A. and Holsboer, F. (2003) Stress responsive neurohormones in depression and anxiety. *Pharmacopsychiatry* 36: S207–14.

Stubbe, J.H., Boomsma, D.I., Vink, J.M., Cornes, B.K., Martin, N.G., Skytthe, A. et al. (2006) Genetic influences on exercise participation in 37,051 twin pairs from seven countries. *PLoS One* 1: e22. doi: 10.1371/journal.pone.0000022.

Ten Have, M., de Graaf, R. and Monshouwer, K. (2011) Physical exercise in adults and mental health status findings from the Netherlands mental health survey and incidence study (NEMESIS). *Journal of Psychosomatic Research* 71: 342–8.

Uher, R. and Zwicker, A. (2017) Etiology in psychiatry: embracing the reality of poly-gene-environmental causation of mental illness. *World Psychiatry* 16: 121–9.

Ulrich, R.S. (1979) Visual landscapes and psychological well-being. *Landscape Research* 4: 17–23.

White, K., Kendrick, T. and Yardley, L. (2009) Change in self-esteem, self-efficacy and the mood dimensions of depression as potential mediators of the physical activity and depression relationship: exploring the temporal relation of change. *Mental Health and Physical Activity* 2: 44–52.

Wittchen, H.U., Jacobi, F., Rehm, J., Gustavsson, A., Svensson, M., Jönsson, B. et al. (2011) The size and burden of mental disorders and other disorders of the brain in Europe 2010. *European Neuropsychopharmacology* 21: 655–79.

World Health Organization. (2004) *Promoting mental health: concepts, emerging evidence, practice (summary report)*. Geneva: World Health Organization.

World Health Organization. (2016) *Global health estimates 2015*. Geneva: World Health Organization. Available at http://www.who.int/healthinfo/global_burden_disease/estimates/en/index2.html (accessed 21 November 2017).

World Health Organization. (2017) *Depression and other common mental disorders: global health estimates*. Geneva: World Health Organization.

Part III
Physical activity in youth and old age

11 Child and adolescent health

Alice E. Thackray

INTRODUCTION

There is compelling and irrefutable evidence in adults supporting the promotion of regular physical activity in the prevention and treatment of several chronic diseases. Whilst the clinical manifestations of many chronic diseases are delayed until adulthood, the pathophysiological determinants underlying these diseases can often be traced back to childhood and adolescence. The prospect of establishing physical activity behaviours early in life which may delay precursors of chronic disease and diminish the risk of adverse health outcomes in adulthood is undoubtedly appealing from a primary prevention perspective. There is widespread support advocating the promotion of physical activity in children and adolescents, and the importance of physical activity as a strategy to optimise the current and future health of young people continues to attract significant scientific inquiry across disciplines in paediatric exercise science. The quality of evidence in recent years has been enriched by the increased adoption of robust measurement techniques such as accelerometry to capture physical activity, imaging of body composition, high-resolution ultrasound to assess vascular endothelial health and hyperinsulinaemic-euglycaemic clamps to measure insulin sensitivity. Although considerable progress has been achieved, understanding of many aspects of physical activity and health in children and adolescents remains incomplete.

It is important to note that the first two decades of life from birth to adulthood are characterised by considerable growth, maturation and development. The underlying effects of these processes could influence responses to physical activity and structured exercise making it challenging to derive definitive conclusions on causality. A child becomes taller and heavier, fat and muscle mass are gained, organ size increases and the skeletal system develops with increasing age. These morphological changes occur simultaneously with fluctuations in almost all physiological parameters that underpin exercise performance as children grow, including increases in maximum oxygen uptake, muscular strength, anaerobic capacity, running economy and lung function. Pubertal development is marked by a transient period of insulin resistance, and metabolic responses to exercise in youth also show some features that favour greater lipid utilisation during prolonged exercise in young people than in adulthood. These age-related changes are not uniform across the growing years but vary markedly between individuals, adding a further complexity to the study of paediatric exercise physiology. The growth-related morphological and physiological changes summarised here have been reviewed comprehensively in previous work and the interested reader is directed here for a more detailed insight (Armstrong and van Mechelen 2017).

Despite the challenges of studying exercise physiology in young people, the paediatric years represent an important period of life to understand. This chapter will summarise the current evidence examining the relationship between physical activity, physical fitness or sedentary behaviour and health outcomes in young people. The health outcomes examined are obesity, type 2 diabetes, cardiovascular disease (CVD), bone health and mental health and cognitive function. We will distinguish between studies focusing on physical activity and health in young people and those examining the impact of physical activity in the paediatric years on future health consequences in adulthood. Where possible, in this chapter, a distinction is made between 'childhood', defined as the period before puberty, and 'adolescence', defined as the period from the beginning of puberty until adulthood. The term 'young people' or 'youth' is used to capture the entire period between birth and adulthood.

PHYSICAL ACTIVITY, PHYSICAL FITNESS AND SEDENTARY BEHAVIOUR

There is a prevailing view that physical activity levels are low in young people, and that engagement in physical activity has declined and time spent sedentary has increased in the last two decades. Although the physical activity guidelines for children and adolescents (outlined in Chapter 14) have evolved from a limited evidence base, they provide a useful framework for evaluating current physical activity levels in young people. In this regard, a comprehensive analysis of survey data from 105 countries revealed that

80.3% of 13- to 15-year-old adolescents fall short of the current physical activity recommendations (Hallal et al. 2012). Furthermore, the Active Healthy Kids Global Alliance facilitated a recent synthesis of physical activity report cards for young people aged 5 to 17 years from 49 nations across six continents. Whilst substantial variability was noted both within and between countries, the average grade assigned for overall physical activity was 'D' and sedentary behaviour was 'D+' indicating that only 27–33% and 34–39% of young people are meeting current internationally accepted guidelines for overall physical activity and sedentary behaviour, respectively (Aubert et al. 2018).

Low physical activity levels have also been reported in the International Children's Accelerometry Database. This project involved the consolidation of objective accelerometry data using standardised methods from 27,637 young people aged 2.8 to 18.4 years participating in 20 studies conducted in Europe, North America, Australia and Brazil. Among young people aged 5 to 17 years, only 9.0% of boys and 1.9% of girls achieved the recommended levels of physical activity on all measured days (Cooper et al. 2015). There is also evidence demonstrating that young people spend a considerable proportion of the day sedentary both in and outside of school. For example, longitudinal data from the Gateshead Millennium Study reported that total sedentary behaviour assessed using accelerometry increased, on average, from 347 min day^{-1} (51.5% of wear time) at 7 years to 535 min day^{-1} (73.4% of wear time) at 15 years in boys and girls (Janssen et al. 2019) (Figure 11.1).

Figure 11.1 Mean daily sedentary time, light physical activity (PA), and moderate-to-vigorous physical activity (MVPA) in boys and girls followed from age 7 to 15 years. Data are presented as (a) mean minutes per day and (b) as a percentage of total accelerometer wear time.

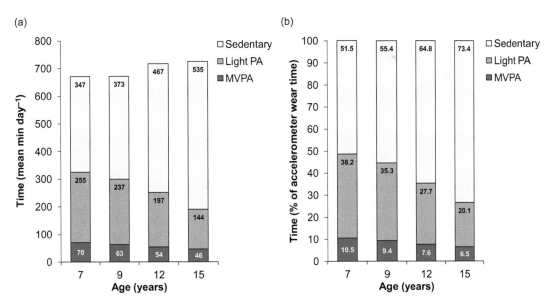

Source: Janssen et al. (2019).
Notes: Data are from participants in the Gateshead Millennium Study in England providing repeated physical activity data using accelerometry at 7 (*n* = 502), 9 (*n* = 506), 12 (*n* = 420) and 15 (*n* = 306) years.

Common and consistent findings in the literature indicate that boys are more active than girls, youth who are overweight or obese are less active than their lean peers, and physical activity levels decline, and sedentary behaviours increase during childhood and adolescence (Cooper et al. 2015; Hallal et al. 2012). The latter finding is highlighted by cross-sectional data from the International Children's Accelerometry Database demonstrating that total physical activity was on average 3.7% and 4.6% lower in boys and girls, respectively, with each additional year of age relative to levels at 5 years of age (Cooper et al. 2015) (Figure 11.2a). The decline in physical activity during childhood and adolescence appears largely attributable to a reduction in light-intensity physical activity and a commensurate increase in time spent sedentary rather than a marked decline in moderate-to-vigorous physical activity (MVPA) (Cooper et al. 2015; Janssen et al. 2019) (Figures 11.1 and 11.2).

Many physical activity strategies targeting young people are based on the assumption that physically active children will remain active in adulthood, which has prompted investigations into the stability or 'tracking' of physical activity over time. The general consensus from these studies is that physical activity and sedentary behaviour are relatively stable in the short term but tracking in the longer term from childhood to adulthood is weak (Biddle et al. 2010; Telama 2009). Although the concept of promoting lifelong participation is appealing, much of the evidence is limited by the inadequate assessment of physical activity behaviours. Furthermore, it is important to recognise that temporal fluctuations in physical activity habits and motives will naturally occur across different transitions in life; for example, changes in education, employment, living arrangements, social relationships and ill health are all factors that could influence an individual's engagement in physical activity. Physical activity behaviours in young people are also fundamentally different from adults and are typically stop-start in nature comprising shorter, intermittent bursts of activity at variable intensities (Baquet et al. 2007).

Studies in adults have consistently observed a positive association between physical activity and physical fitness, and it has been suggested that high physical fitness may confer greater protection from disease than high physical activity. In contrast, the relationship between objective measures of physical activity and physical fitness (most commonly assessed as aerobic fitness using peak oxygen uptake) in children and adolescents is weak to moderate (Dencker and Andersen 2011). This discrepancy is perhaps not surprising considering that the intermittent nature of young people's physical activity habits may limit opportunities to accumulate activity of sufficient intensity and/or duration to enhance aerobic fitness (Armstrong et al. 2011). Nevertheless, peak oxygen uptake (expressed in $l\ min^{-1}$) increases with age and maturation during the paediatric years, and there is little evidence that levels are low or have deteriorated over time in young people (Armstrong et al. 2011). Furthermore, the latest systematic review concluded that a programme of endurance exercise (~12 weeks, 40–60 mins at 85–90% maximum heart rate, 3–4 times $week^{-1}$) will elicit, on average, an 8–9% increase in peak oxygen uptake in young people (Armstrong and Barker 2011).

The well-established health benefits of high physical activity and fitness have stimulated efforts to develop interventions that modulate these outcomes in young people. This body of evidence has been appraised in several systematic reviews with the school environment identified as a key setting to implement interventions targeting physical

Figure 11.2 Mean (a) daily volume of total physical activity and percentage of daily time spent in (b) moderate-to-vigorous physical activity (MVPA), (c) light physical activity (PA) and (d) sedentary time by age group and sex across childhood and adolescence. Boys aged 5 to 6 years are the reference population, and values represent the mean difference (95% confidence interval) adjusted for study population and season.

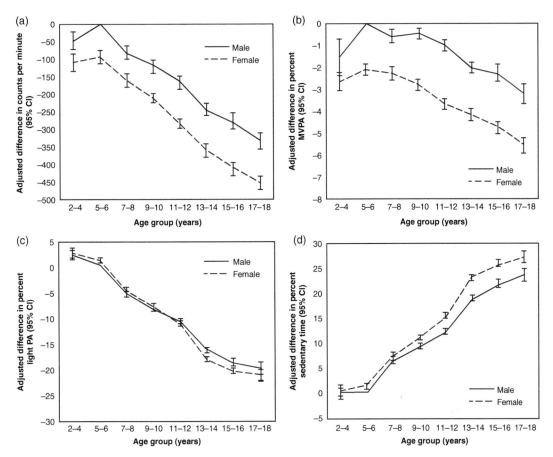

Source: Reprinted with no modifications from 'Objectively measured physical activity and sedentary time in youth: the International Children's Accelerometry Database (ICAD)', Cooper, A.R. et al., *International Journal of Behavioral Nutrition and Physical Activity*, 2015, 12: 113. Article distributed under the terms of the Creative Commons Attribution 4.0 International Licence (http://creativecommons.org/licenses/by/4.0/).

Notes: Data are from 27,637 children and adolescents (11,199 boys, 16,438 girls) aged 2.8 to 18.4 years from 20 studies conducted in Europe, North America, Australia and Brazil collated as part of the International Children's Accelerometry Database. Physical activity was measured using accelerometry and standard cut-points were applied to calculate the daily time spent sedentary (≤ 100 counts min^{-1}) and engaged in light PA (101–2,295 counts min^{-1}) and MVPA ($\geq 2,296$ counts min^{-1}).

activity and fitness. A defining feature of recent reviews is the inclusion of studies that focused exclusively on objectively measured physical activity using accelerometry and, therefore, these are likely to reflect the best indication to date of the efficacy of interventions tailored to promote physical activity in young people. In a systematic review of controlled trials, physical activity interventions were found to elicit a negligible effect on young people's overall physical activity levels (increase of ~4 minutes per day)

(Metcalf et al. 2012). More recently, Love and colleagues (2019) synthesised findings in a meta-analysis from 17 cluster randomised controlled trials (RCTs) implementing school-based physical activity interventions and reported no effect on daily time spent in MVPA. Despite these underwhelming findings, two notable physical activity initiatives targeting MVPA in the school environment – 'The Daily Mile' (The Daily Mile Foundation) and 'Marathon Kids UK' (Kids Run Free) – have gained considerable popularity in recent years. However, until rigorous scientific evidence accrues, and the longevity of implementation is widely established, the efficacy of these initiatives to promote the health and wellbeing of young people cannot be determined.

Previous chapters have highlighted the myriad of physical and mental health benefits of regular physical activity and high physical fitness in adults, as well as the possible detriments of excessive sedentary behaviour. The following sections will scrutinise the evidence investigating the current and future health benefits of physical activity and fitness and the potential adverse effects of sedentary behaviour in children and adolescents.

OBESITY

Over the last four decades, the escalating prevalence of obesity in young people has propelled the prevention and management of childhood obesity to the forefront of the global public health agenda. A recent analysis of obesity trends over 42 years including data from 200 countries estimated that 50 million girls and 74 million boys aged 5 to 19 years old were obese in 2016. The authors also reported that the global age-standardised prevalence of obesity has increased from 0.7% in 1975 to 5.6% in 2016 in girls, and from 0.9% in 1975 to 7.8% in 2016 in boys (NCD Risk Factor Collaboration 2017) (Figure 11.3). Although encouraging findings indicate that the rise in excess weight in paediatric populations may be stabilising and perhaps even declining in high-income countries (NCD Risk Factor Collaboration 2017), the prevalence remains high worldwide and reports of increased rates of severe paediatric obesity are disconcerting (Skinner and Skelton 2014).

Similar to studies in adults, body mass index (BMI) is considered an acceptable, albeit imperfect, tool for diagnosing obesity in young people (Reilly 2006). However, BMI varies considerably with age and sex during childhood and adolescence so weight status must be interpreted using growth charts depicting population reference data. The age- and sex-specific definitions developed by the International Obesity Task Force provide a robust and widely adopted criterion for classifying BMI in young people. The authors derived percentile curves that corresponded to adult BMI cut-offs of 25 (overweight) and 30 (obesity) kg m^{-2} at age 18 based on data from six countries (Cole et al. 2000), and have been revised to include guidelines for thinness and morbid obesity (Cole and Lobstein 2012) (Table 11.1). National level sex-specific BMI-for-age charts have also been developed, and BMI is usually expressed as a z-score (sometimes referred to as a SD score) or percentile relative to children of the same age and sex. Although definitions vary, a BMI z-score of 1.04 and 1.64 SD above the population mean (equivalent to the 85th and 95th BMI-for-age and sex percentile) are often used as thresholds to define overweight and obesity, respectively.

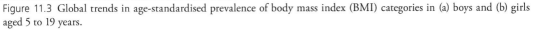

Figure 11.3 Global trends in age-standardised prevalence of body mass index (BMI) categories in (a) boys and (b) girls aged 5 to 19 years.

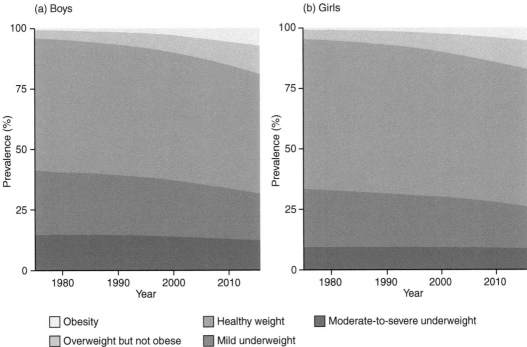

Source: Reprinted with no modifications from 'Worldwide trends in body-mass index, underweight, overweight, and obesity from 1975 to 2016: a pooled analysis of 2416 population-based measurement studies in 128.9 million children, adolescents, and adults', NCD Risk Factor Collaboration, *The Lancet*, 2017, 390: 2627–42. Article distributed under the terms of the Creative Commons Attribution 4.0 International Licence (https://creativecommons.org/licenses/by/4.0/).

Notes: Data are pooled from population-based data collected between 1975 and 2016 from a total of 31.5 million girls and boys aged 5 to 19 years from 200 countries. The following categories were established for BMI prevalence: i) moderate-to-severe underweight: more than 2 SD below the median of the World Health Organization growth reference for children and adolescents; ii) mild underweight: 2 SD to more than 1 SD below the median; iii) healthy weight: 1 SD below to 1 SD above the median; iv) overweight but not obese: more than 1 SD to 2 SD above the median; and v) obesity: more than 2 SD above the median. It is estimated that more children and adolescents worldwide are moderately or severely underweight than obese (192 versus 124 million, respectively). However, the global age-standardised mean BMI has increased from 17.2 to 18.6 kg m^{-2} in girls, and from 16.8 to 18.5 kg m^{-2} in boys between 1975 and 2016, respectively, and paediatric obesity is projected to surpass moderate-to-severe underweight by 2022 if post-2000 trends persist.

As in adults, paediatric obesity is characterised by a chronic energy imbalance and is influenced by complex interactions between genetic, metabolic, behavioural and environmental factors. There is currently no consensus on whether elevated energy intake or reduced energy expenditure is the primary driver of excess weight gain in children and adolescents (Bleich et al. 2011), but in reality, it is likely that synergistic alterations to both sides of the energy balance equation contribute to a positive energy balance over time. The health risks of obesity in adults were discussed in Chapter 6, and many of these complications are also associated with overweight and obesity in young people (Friedemann et al. 2012). One topic of ongoing debate concerns the contribution of paediatric obesity to long-term health outcomes independent of adult weight status. A large study including data for 6,328 individuals from four prospective cohort studies

Table 11.1 Cut-off points for body mass index (BMI) for overweight, obesity and morbid obesity by sex between ages 11 and 18 years, defined to pass through a BMI of 25, 30 and 35 kg m^{-2} at age 18.

Age (years)	BMI 25 kg m^{-2}		BMI 30 kg m^{-2}		BMI 35 kg m^{-2}	
	Males	Females	Males	Females	Males	Females
11	20.5	20.7	25.1	25.3	30.0	30.1
12	21.2	21.6	26.0	26.5	31.2	31.7
13	21.9	22.5	26.9	27.6	32.2	32.9
14	22.6	23.3	27.6	28.4	33.0	33.8
15	23.3	23.9	28.3	29.0	33.6	34.3
16	23.9	24.3	28.9	29.4	34.0	34.6
17	24.5	24.7	29.4	29.7	34.4	34.8
18	25.0	25.0	30.0	30.0	35.0	35.0

Source: Reprinted from 'Extended international (IOTF) body mass index cut-offs for thinness, overweight and obesity', Cole, T.J. and Lobstein, T., *Pediatric Obesity* 7: 284–94, with permission from John Wiley and Sons. Copyright © 2012 The Authors. Pediatric Obesity © 2012 International Association for the Study of Obesity.
Notes: See Cole and Lobstein (2012; Supplementary Table S2) for a more extensive table of BMI cut-off points for thinness, overweight, obesity and morbid obesity in 0.5-year increments from age 2 to 18 years.

demonstrated that those who were obese as adults, irrespective of their adiposity status during youth, had a markedly higher risk of type 2 diabetes, hypertension, dyslipidaemia and high carotid artery intima media thickness (IMT; a marker of endothelial function and subclinical atherosclerosis) in adulthood (Figure 11.4). The risk of these adverse health outcomes was reversed when youth who were overweight or obese became non-obese as adults and were similar to those who were never obese (Juonala et al. 2011) (Figure 11.4). However, it is important to highlight the difficulty of normalising adverse weight status between youth and adulthood. In the study by Juonala and colleagues (2011), for example, 64.6% of youth who were overweight or obese were obese as adults and 82.3% of youth who were obese remained obese as adults. Regardless of whether BMI during youth predicts adult obesity, or is an independent risk factor for future adverse health outcomes, or both, compelling evidence supports heightened morbidity and mortality in adults who have a history of excess weight during the formative years (Reilly and Kelly 2011).

Although there is a strong genetic influence on childhood adiposity (Silventoinen et al. 2010), there is also evidence that physical inactivity plays a role. The weight of evidence from cross-sectional studies supports an inverse association between objectively measured physical activity or cardiorespiratory fitness and markers of adiposity in young people (Jiménez-Pavón et al. 2010; Ortega et al. 2008). This is supported by data from 1,862 UK children aged 9 to 10 years demonstrating that the inverse relationship between physical activity (particularly at higher intensities) and markers of adiposity including BMI and waist circumference appears to be independent of sedentary time and other covariates. In contrast, the positive association between sedentary time and adiposity was completely abolished after adjustment for covariates including MVPA (Steele et al. 2009).

Figure 11.4 Relative risk of obesity-related comorbidities in adulthood according to weight status in youth and adulthood: i) group 1 (*n* = 4,742): individuals with a healthy body mass index (BMI) in youth who were non-obese as adults; ii) group 2 (*n* = 274): individuals who were overweight or obese in youth but non-obese as adults; iii) group 3 (*n* = 812): individuals with a healthy BMI in youth who were obese as adults; and iv) group 4 (*n* = 500): individuals who were overweight or obese in youth and obese as adults.

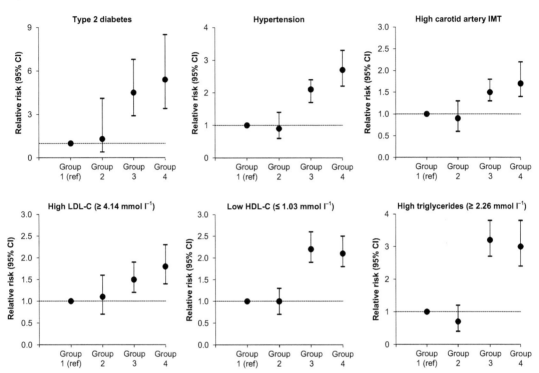

Source: Juonala et al. (2011).
Notes: Data are pooled from four prospective cohort studies – the Bogalusa Heart Study, the Muscatine Study, the Childhood Determinants of Adult Health Study and the Cardiovascular Risk in Young Finns Study. BMI was measured during youth between ages 3 to 19 years and in adulthood after an average follow-up of 23 years. Adiposity status in youth was defined using international age- and sex-specific BMI cut-off points for overweight and obesity (Cole et al. 2000), and a BMI cut-off point of 30 kg m^{-2} was used for adults to define obesity. Type 2 diabetes was defined as a fasting plasma glucose concentration ≥ 7 mmol l^{-1}, use of glucose-lowering medication or taking insulin. Hypertension was defined as a systolic blood pressure ≥ 140 mm Hg, a diastolic blood pressure ≥ 90 mm Hg or use of blood pressure lowering medication. High carotid artery intima media thickness (IMT) was defined as ≥ 90th percentile for age-, sex-, race- and cohort-specific values. All outcomes were higher in group 3 and group 4 compared with group 1 (all *P* ≤ 0.009).

There is also evidence suggesting that the relationship between physical activity and adiposity may be non-linear across the adiposity spectrum throughout childhood and adolescence, with stronger associations emerging at higher adiposity percentiles. A recent example is longitudinal data from the Gateshead Millennium Study where repeated accelerometer and body composition measurements were obtained in boys and girls at 7, 9, 12 and 15 years of age. The authors reported that every additional one hour of daily MVPA was associated with a 1.46 kg m^{-2} and 2.69 kg m^{-2} lower fat mass index (fat mass in kilograms divided by height in metres squared) at the 50th and 90th

Figure 11.5 Longitudinal associations between moderate-to-vigorous physical activity (MVPA) and change in (a) fat mass index (FMI) percentile and (b) body mass index (BMI) percentile from age 7 to 15 years examined using quantile regression. The solid line represents the β coefficients from the quantile regression model. This shows the change in FMI or BMI, at each percentile, for every additional hour spent in MVPA. The shaded area represents the 95% confidence intervals, and the dotted line represents the linear regression coefficient for the change in FMI or BMI percentile per hour of additional MVPA. Models were adjusted for sedentary time and sex.

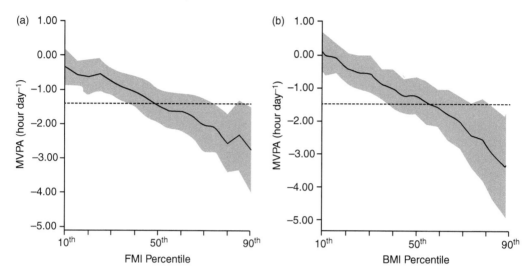

Source: Reprinted with no modifications from 'Non-linear longitudinal associations between moderate-to-vigorous physical activity and adiposity across the adiposity distribution during childhood and adolescence: Gateshead Millennium Study', Janssen, X. et al., *International Journal of Obesity*, 2019, 43: 744–50. Article distributed under the terms of the Creative Commons Attribution 4.0 International Licence (http://creativecommons.org/licenses/by/4.0/).
Notes: Data are from participants in the Gateshead Millennium Study in England providing repeated physical activity data using accelerometry at 7 (*n* = 502), 9 (*n* = 506), 12 (*n* = 420) and 15 (*n* = 306) years.

fat mass index percentiles, respectively (Figure 11.5). The corresponding values for BMI were 1.22 kg m^{-2} and 3.37 kg m^{-2} for the 50th and 90th BMI percentiles, respectively (Figure 11.5). These findings led the authors to conclude that higher engagement in MVPA may help to lower adiposity outcomes particularly in those at the upper extreme of the adiposity distribution (Janssen et al. 2019).

Previous reviews of prospective studies concluded that there is limited evidence that objectively measured physical activity or sedentary behaviour at baseline is predictive of changes in adiposity at follow-up in young people (Tanaka et al. 2014; Wilks et al. 2011). This contrasts with findings from the Avon Longitudinal Study of Parents and Children who examined prospective associations between objective physical activity at 12 years and subsequent fat mass (derived using dual-energy X-ray absorptiometry (DXA)) at 14 years in 4,150 boys and girls. The authors reported that an additional 15 minutes of daily MVPA at 12 years was associated with 11.9% and 9.8% lower fat mass in boys and girls, respectively, at 14 years (Riddoch et al. 2009). Similarly, in a cohort of 554 US boys and girls studied over 7 years (8 to 15 years), higher levels of MVPA were related to lower fat mass independent of sedentary time, whereas sedentary time was not independently related to fat mass after adjustment for MVPA (Kwon et al. 2013). Although this suggests that time spent sedentary may be unrelated to changes in adiposity, a more recent study demonstrated that age-related increases in sedentary behaviour from 7 to 15 years were associated with higher adiposity after adjustment for MVPA (Mann et al. 2017).

The notion that low levels of physical activity may predispose young people to obesity has been challenged by recent evidence suggesting that the direction of association may be reverse or bidirectional. One study supporting the concept of reverse causality (i.e. excess fatness predisposes to inactivity) used accelerometry and DXA to examine prospective associations between physical activity and body fat measured annually in 202 UK children from age 7 to 10 years. Baseline body fat was predictive of a decline in physical activity over three years, but baseline physical activity was not related to changes in body fat at follow-up (Metcalf et al. 2011). Furthermore, a prospective analysis of 6,413 young people from the International Children's Accelerometry Database reported that baseline MVPA and sedentary time were not related to waist circumference after two years, whereas a higher baseline waist circumference was associated with greater sedentary time (but not time in MVPA) at follow-up (Ekelund et al. 2012). Whilst these findings suggest that physical inactivity or sedentary behaviour may be a consequence of excess weight gain in young people, there is typically greater measurement error in behavioural (e.g. physical activity) compared with anthropometric variables which can attenuate associations when the imprecise variable represents the exposure (Hutcheon et al. 2010). Future well-controlled longitudinal studies with precise measurements of the exposure and outcome variables are required to improve understanding of this issue.

As the global challenge of obesity has evolved, a plethora of interventions targeting the prevention and management of obesity in young people have been developed with varying degrees of success. The latest Cochrane review on obesity prevention synthesised evidence from 153 RCTs of physical activity, diet or combined interventions and reported either modest reductions or no change in BMI and BMI z-scores in young people aged 0 to 5 years, 6 to 12 years and 13 to 18 years (Brown et al. 2019). A recent example of an obesity prevention cluster RCT involved a comprehensive 12-month school-based intervention promoting physical activity and healthy eating in UK children aged 5 to 6 years at baseline. The intervention included the opportunity to engage in an additional 30 minutes of physical activity on school days, a six-week nutrition and physical activity programme delivered in conjunction with a professional football (soccer) club, signposting to local physical activity opportunities and school-led family workshops on healthy cooking skills. The authors observed no effect of the intervention on adiposity (BMI z-score, waist circumference z-score, sum of four skinfolds and body fat percentage), dietary intake or objectively measured physical activity at 15 and 30 months after the start of the intervention (Adab et al. 2018). Whilst the school environment remains an important setting for health promotion in young people, novel strategies that simultaneously target the wider society (for example, home, family, community, media, food industry) may be required for the prevention of paediatric obesity.

Evidence has also examined the role of exercise in promoting weight loss and improving adiposity outcomes in young people who are overweight or obese. Although findings are often conflicting, the general consensus from the current evidence base suggests that exercise training (either alone or in combination with dietary therapy) can promote small improvements in adiposity outcomes. For example, a recent meta-analysis pooling data from 15 RCTs involving 556 children and adolescents aged 10 to 19 years (BMI $\geq$ 85th age- and sex-specific percentile) reported an overall pooled reduction in BMI of 2.0 kg m^{-2}, body mass of 3.7 kg, body fat percentage of 3.1% and waist circumference of 3.0 cm after exercise training (Stoner et al. 2016). The efficacy of combined physical activity, diet and behavioural interventions to treat overweight and obesity has been appraised in two recent Cochrane reviews in children aged 6 to 11 years (70 RCTs, 8,461 participants; Mead et al. 2017) and adolescents aged 12 to 17 years (44 RCTs, 4,781 participants; Al-Khudairy et al. 2017). These reviews both concluded that, despite the low quality of evidence, multidisciplinary interventions promote overall small but important reductions in BMI (–0.53 and –1.18 kg m^{-2} in children and adolescents, respectively), BMI z-score (–0.06 and –0.13 units, respectively) and body mass (–1.45 and –3.67 kg, respectively).

One weight-management programme adopting a multi-component strategy which combined physical activity, diet modification and behaviour therapy is the 'Bright Bodies' programme conducted at the Yale Paediatric Obesity Clinic in New Haven, Connecticut. A RCT examining the programme in young people aged 8 to 16 years with obesity (BMI $\geq$ 95th age- and sex-specific percentile) revealed beneficial effects on body weight, BMI and body fat percentage, after 6 and 12 months (Savoye et al. 2007), and the effects were sustained at follow-up 12 months after the intervention ended (Savoye et al. 2011) (Figure 11.6). Whilst the nature of such multi-component approaches makes it difficult to isolate the individual contribution of each component, it is likely that holistic strategies to reduce energy intake and increase energy expenditure are required to combat paediatric obesity.

Recent studies have also harnessed imaging techniques such as magnetic resonance imaging (MRI) and proton magnetic resonance spectroscopy (^{1}H-MRS) to investigate the effect of short-term exercise training on regional body fat distribution in young

Figure 11.6 Change from baseline in body composition and insulin resistance at 6 months, at the end of the intervention (12 months), and one year after the end of the intervention (24 months) in young people with obesity aged 8 to 16 years assigned to a weight management intervention or control group. Values for body mass index (BMI) z score and body fat percentage are mean (95% confidence interval) and values for homeostasis model assessment of insulin resistance (HOMA) are geometric mean (95% confidence interval).

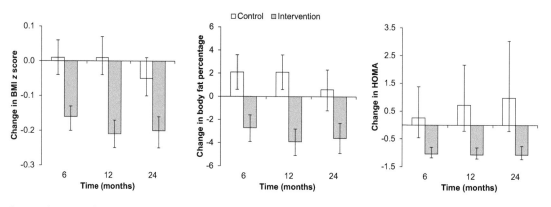

Source: Savoye et al. (2011).

Notes: The 12-month weight-management programme involved a family-based exercise, nutrition and behaviour therapy intervention. Between-group differences for all parameters were identified at 6, 12 and 24 months (all $P \leq 0.0002$).

people. This is important as, similar to adults (Chapter 6), the accumulation of fat in ectopic depots (for example, in the abdominal cavity and liver) is more closely associated with obesity-related comorbidities in youth than global indicators of adiposity such as BMI (Caprio et al. 1996). In one example, Davis and colleagues (2012) used DXA and MRI to accurately quantify changes in total body fat and visceral adipose tissue, respectively, after 13 weeks of 20 or 40 min day^{-1} of aerobic exercise performed five days week^{-1} in children aged 7 to 11 years who were overweight or obese (BMI $\geq$ 85th age- and sex-specific percentile). Both exercise training groups exhibited similar reductions in total body fat and visceral adipose tissue which coincided with improvements in peak oxygen uptake. These findings suggest that regular exercise may represent a viable strategy for reducing abdominal fat in young people.

The evidence appraised here highlights a role for physical activity as a weight-management strategy in young people, but unlike adults, evidence-based guidelines for the prevention and treatment of excess weight gain have yet to be developed in this age group. Achieving successful adiposity outcomes is undoubtedly challenging for young people, but it is also important to recognise the multitude of physical and mental health benefits arising from physical activity even in the absence of adiposity outcomes. Some of these health benefits will be explored in the following sections.

TYPE 2 DIABETES

Before the 1990s, type 2 diabetes was seldom diagnosed in young people, but a marked rise in prevalence has since been observed concurrent with the increasing rates of paediatric obesity (Pinhas-Hamiel and Zeitler 2005). Despite the consensus that paediatric type 2 diabetes is increasing, data concerning the global prevalence and incidence is relatively sparse and varies considerably across countries. The most recent data on the incidence of youth-onset type 2 diabetes in the United States is provided by the SEARCH for Diabetes in Youth study, which analysed data from five clinical centres. Among young people aged 10 to 19 years, the incidence rate of type 2 diabetes increased by 4.8% annually from 9.0 cases per 100,000 youths per year in 2002–2003 to 12.5 cases per 100,000 youths per year in 2011–2012 after adjustment for age, sex and race or ethnic group (Figure 11.7). Furthermore, the annual rate of increase was considerably higher among all other racial and ethnic groups (Hispanic 3.1%, non-Hispanic black 6.3%, Asian or Pacific Islander 8.5%, Native American 8.9%) than in non-Hispanic whites (0.6%) (Mayer-Davis et al. 2017) (Figure 11.7). This supports the findings of others suggesting that the prevalence of type 2 diabetes in young people disproportionally affects certain minority ethnic and racial groups such as the Pima Indians in the United States and those of Pakistani, Indian or Arabic origin in the UK (Pinhas-Hamiel and Zeitler 2005).

Although rates of type 2 diabetes in young people are increasing, the overall frequency remains low and the majority of paediatric diabetes cases are type 1 (Mayer-Davis et al. 2017) (Figure 11.7). Despite this, paediatric type 2 diabetes is associated with accelerated development of diabetes-related complications and comorbidities as well as an increased risk of premature mortality in adulthood compared with early onset type 1 diabetes (Dabelea et al. 2017). A defining feature of youth onset type 2

Figure 11.7 Incidence rates of (a) type 1 and (b) type 2 diabetes in young people from five clinical centres in the United States between 2002 and 2012. The incidence of type 1 diabetes was assessed among young people aged 0 to 19 years and the incidence of type 2 diabetes was assessed among young people aged 10 to 19 years.

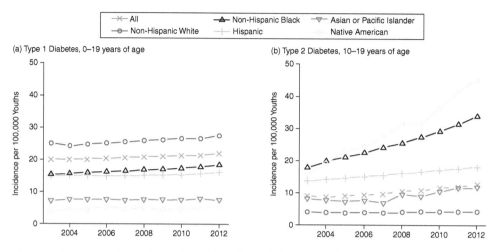

Source: From the *New England Journal of Medicine*, Mayer-Davis, E.J. et al., 'Incidence trends of type 1 and type 2 diabetes among youths, 2002–2012', 376: 1419–29. Copyright © 2017 Massachusetts Medical Society. Reprinted with permission from Massachusetts Medical Society.

diabetes is the presence of obesity or severe obesity (Dabelea et al. 2017), and above average BMI during childhood and adolescence also increases the risk of adult type 2 diabetes (Zimmermann et al. 2017).

The pathophysiology of paediatric type 2 diabetes involves peripheral and hepatic insulin resistance combined with a rapid decline in β-cell function (Bacha et al. 2010), with the deterioration in β-cell function (~15–20% decline per year on average) typically more aggressive compared with adults. Considering the frequency of type 2 diabetes in young people is relatively low, most therapeutic interventions target improvements in these underlying pathophysiological processes. Observational evidence from the paediatric exercise literature suggests that higher levels of physical activity and cardiorespiratory fitness are related to superior insulin sensitivity in children and adolescents. One example involving 630 Canadian children reported that every additional ten minutes of MVPA at 8 to 10 years predicted a 4.8% increase in insulin sensitivity after two years, determined using the Matsuda insulin sensitivity index (an estimate of insulin sensitivity derived from glucose and insulin concentrations during an oral glucose tolerance test (OGTT)). However, this effect was attenuated to 1.8% after adjustment for body fat percentage highlighting a central role of adiposity in determining insulin resistance in youth (Henderson et al. 2016).

The transient decline in insulin resistance of 25–30% that naturally occurs during puberty represents a vulnerable time for the emergence of paediatric type 2 diabetes (Moran et al. 1999). Puberty-related insulin resistance is usually offset by a concurrent increase in insulin secretion in healthy individuals, but inadequate compensation due to impaired β-cell function may predispose susceptible youth to hyperglycaemia (Bacha et al. 2010). As part of the EarlyBird study, Metcalf and colleagues (2015) measured physical activity (accelerometry) and insulin resistance annually in 151 boys and 149 girls from age 9 to 16 years. Insulin resistance was determined using the homeostasis model assessment (HOMA) which represents an estimate of insulin resistance derived from fasting glucose and insulin concentrations. The natural peak in insulin resistance at age 12 to 13 years was attenuated by 17% in boys and girls with higher levels of MVPA (boys ≥ 50 min day^{-1}; girls ≥ 35 min day^{-1}), independent of body fat percentage and pubertal status (Figure 11.8). This difference diminished progressively over the next three years and was abolished completely by 16 years of age (Figure 11.8). These findings suggest that physical activity may be particularly efficacious in ameliorating insulin resistance during the puberty-related peak in insulin resistance.

The potential acute benefits of physical activity on insulin sensitivity and glucose tolerance in young people is supported by studies examining metabolic responses to repeated sit-to-activity transitions. Interrupting continuous sitting with short, three-minute bouts of moderate-intensity walking performed every 30 minutes during a three-hour OGTT reduced insulin concentrations by 32% and glucose concentrations by 7% in 7- to 11-year-old children with healthy weight and normoglycaemia (mean BMI 16.2 kg m^{-2}, BMI z-score 0.3) (Belcher et al. 2015) (Figure 11.9). Favourable reductions in insulinaemia of 21% have since been reported in response to the same intermittent exercise stimulus in similarly aged children who were overweight or obese (mean BMI 24.5 kg m^{-2}, BMI z-score 1.8) and at elevated risk of adverse excursions

Figure 11.8 Changes in insulin resistance from age 9 to 16 years in (a) boys and (b) girls according to the level of physical activity. Black line: more active group (time spent in moderate-to-vigorous physical activity above the median of 50 and 35 min day^{-1} for boys and girls, respectively); grey line: less active group (below the median). Values are unadjusted age-related coefficients predicted by a longitudinal multi-level model with 95% confidence intervals.

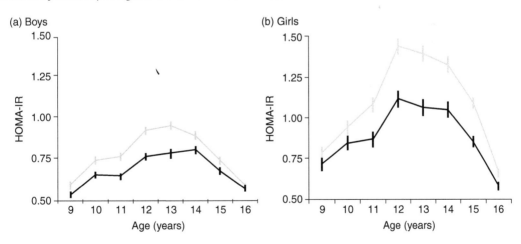

Source: Reprinted by permission from Springer Nature Customer Service Centre GmbH: Springer Nature, *Diabetologia*, 'Physical activity attenuates the mid-adolescent peak in insulin resistance but by late adolescence the effect is lost: a longitudinal study with annual measures from 9–16 years (EarlyBird 66)', Metcalf, B.S. et al., copyright © 2015.
Notes: Abbreviations: HOMA-IR, homeostasis model assessment of insulin resistance.

Figure 11.9 Serum concentrations of (a) insulin and (b) glucose quantified using an oral glucose tolerance test during uninterrupted sitting ('sitting') and sitting interrupted with three minutes of moderate-intensity walking every 30 minutes ('sitting plus walking'). Values are mean (SEM) in 28 children aged 7 to 11 years who were lean and normoglycaemic.

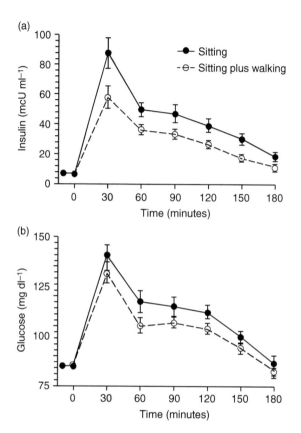

Source: Belcher, B.R. et al., 'Effects of interrupting children's sedentary behaviors with activity on metabolic function: a randomized trial', *Journal of Clinical Endocrinology and Metabolism*, 2015, 100: 3735–43, by permission of Oxford University Press.

in glucose homeostasis (Broadney et al. 2018). Such findings are encouraging given increasing concerns surrounding the detrimental effects of prolonged sitting early in life and suggest benefits in glucose homeostasis can be achieved from a relatively low exercise commitment in children with healthy or excess weight. This pattern of activity could also be more conducive to adherence as it may be easier for young individuals to accumulate activity in short bouts throughout a typical day, but further work is required to determine the implications of these findings in the longer term. The mechanisms underlying these findings were also not explored and are often precluded in investigations during the formative years due to the invasive nature of the techniques required. The interested reader is directed to Chapter 7 for an overview of the insulin-dependent and insulin-independent pathways proposed to enhance glucose tolerance in adults after acute and chronic exercise stimuli which may also apply earlier in life.

A meta-analysis of 24 RCTs involving 1,599 young people concluded that exercise training elicits small to moderate reductions in fasting insulin concentrations and insulin resistance (assessed using HOMA) (Fedewa et al. 2014). However, chronic exercise-induced improvements in markers of type 2 diabetes risk are not reported consistently. A notable three-month RCT in adolescent boys with obesity (BMI ≥ 95th age- and sex-specific percentile) examined the effect of three 60-minute sessions of supervised aerobic or whole-body resistance exercise per week on insulin sensitivity, insulin secretion and intra-abdominal fat content. The primary strength of this RCT was the inclusion of hyperinsulinaemic-euglycaemic and hyperglycaemic clamps to determine insulin sensitivity and secretion, respectively (see Box 7.2 for description), and advanced imaging techniques (MRI and ^{1}H-MRS) to quantify body composition. The authors reported reductions in total adiposity, visceral adipose tissue and intrahepatic lipid content after both aerobic and resistance exercise interventions. Insulin secretion was unchanged in response to exercise training, and only the resistance exercise intervention improved insulin sensitivity during the hyperinsulinaemic-euglycaemic clamp (Lee et al. 2012). The latter finding likely reflects the propensity of this exercise mode to augment skeletal muscle mass which may contribute to enhanced insulin-mediated glucose uptake with exercise. When the study was replicated in adolescent girls with obesity, both exercise protocols reduced total body fat, but only aerobic exercise reduced abdominal adiposity and liver fat and enhanced insulin sensitivity (Lee et al. 2013b). The reasons for the disparate findings for boys and girls reported here, and the contrasting findings reported generally in the wider paediatric literature, are unclear. Future well-controlled RCTs with robust measurement techniques are required to fully establish the efficacy of exercise as a strategy to curtail risk factors for type 2 diabetes early in life.

Several studies adopting multi-component approaches to health promotion in young people have measured markers of type 2 diabetes risk. One example tailored to type 2 diabetes risk reduction is the HEALTHY study involving a three-year cluster RCT across 42 schools in the United States. The study sample included a total of 4,603 sixth-graders (age 11 to 12 years) at high risk of obesity and type 2 diabetes who were followed up at the end of eighth grade (age 13 to 14 years). A multi-component intervention combining physical activity, nutrition and behavioural components reduced the prevalence of overweight and obesity to a similar extent as the control group, but elicited greater reductions in other indices of adiposity and metabolic risk, including BMI z-score, waist circumference ≥ 90th percentile and fasting insulin (The HEALTHY Study Group 2010). In the Bright Bodies programme involving youth without diabetes (BMI ≥ 95th age- and sex-specific percentile), the previously reported favourably changes in adiposity outcomes occurred in parallel with improved insulin sensitivity (determined using HOMA) (Savoye et al. 2007, 2011) (Figure 11.6). An extension to these findings also revealed greater reductions in 2 h glucose and insulin concentrations during an OGTT in adolescents with pre-diabetes and obesity receiving the Bright Bodies programme for six months compared with usual care (Savoye et al. 2014).

The evidence for lifestyle intervention effects among youth diagnosed with type 2 diabetes are restricted to the Treatment Options for type 2 Diabetes in Adolescents and Youth (TODAY) study. Specifically, a lifestyle-intervention (diet and physical activity) combined with metformin (an oral antidiabetic drug) treatment was no more effective than metformin monotherapy for preventing loss of glycaemic control over an average follow-up of 3.86 years, despite greater improvements in adiposity status (TODAY Study Group 2012). The TODAY study defined loss of glycaemic control as a glycated haemoglobin level (HbA1c) of at least 8% for six months or persistent metabolic complications of diabetes requiring insulin and reported failure rates of 51.7% and 46.6% in the metformin alone and metformin plus lifestyle treatment groups, respectively. Furthermore, metformin alone or in combination with a lifestyle intervention did not promote favourable changes in insulin sensitivity or β-cell function measured during an OGTT in young people who were overweight and had type 2 diabetes over four years of follow-up (TODAY Study Group 2013).

Despite recent progress, future work is required to expand the evidence base in this field of paediatric exercise science. It is likely that intensified efforts will be required in the future to curtail current worldwide trends in paediatric type 2 diabetes, particularly if projections that the number of young people with type 2 diabetes will increase substantially from 2010 to 2050 (Imperatore et al. 2012) prove correct.

CARDIOVASCULAR DISEASE

Although the clinical expression of CVD is typically delayed until mid-adulthood (discussed in Chapter 4), the paediatric origins of atherosclerosis are well established (McGill et al. 2000). Accumulating evidence from a variety of cohort studies suggest that CVD risk markers in youth predict later preclinical CVD outcomes in adulthood. Relevant studies in this regard include the Muscatine Study (Davis et al. 2001), the Bogalusa Heart Study (Li et al. 2003), the Amsterdam Growth and Health Longitudinal Study (Ferreira et al. 2012), and the Cardiovascular Risk in Young Finns Study (Raitakari et al. 2003). Evidence linking early life CVD risk factors to premature adult mortality is sparse (Franks et al. 2010) but will start to accrue in the future as the youth-to-adult cohort studies capture data on clinical CVD outcomes.

The health implications of long-term exposure to precursors of CVD and the upward trajectory in paediatric obesity have driven efforts to target cardio-metabolic health outcomes early in life in the hope of delaying the premature progression of atherosclerosis. Studies examining the effect of exercise in youth on clinical CVD endpoints, such as myocardial infarction and stroke, emerging > 30 years later in mid-adulthood are unrealistic. However, the influence of physical activity, physical fitness and/or sedentary behaviour during the formative years on risk factors for CVD (e.g. blood pressure and blood lipids) evident during youth or emerging in later life have been examined. These findings are now reviewed.

A burgeoning body of observational research supports the association between low levels of objectively measured physical activity or fitness and an adverse CVD risk factor profile in children and adolescents. These observations tend to be stronger in studies measuring the clustering of multiple CVD risk factors rather than individual markers of CVD risk, and time spent in higher intensity physical activity irrespective of bout duration appears important for promoting a more favourable CVD risk factor profile in young people (Tarp et al. 2018).

Pooled data from the International Children's Accelerometry Database comprising 20,871 youth aged 4 to 18 years reported inverse associations between MVPA and a variety of CVD risk markers (waist circumference, systolic blood pressure, fasting insulin, fasting triglyceride and fasting high-density lipoprotein cholesterol). These associations were independent of sedentary time and other confounders, but time spent sedentary was not related to cardio-metabolic health outcomes after adjustment for MVPA (Ekelund et al. 2012). Similarly, higher levels of objectively measured physical activity, but not sedentary time, have been prospectively associated with a healthier CVD risk factor profile at follow-up in the Active Smarter Kids Study (Skrede et al. 2017) and the Avon Longitudinal Study of Parents and Children (Stamatakis et al. 2015). However, certain sedentary pursuits, most notably television viewing, may prompt deleterious CVD health outcomes early in life. Specifically, high television use (≥ 4 hours per day) emerged as a strong determinant of clustered CVD risk independent of MVPA and other confounders in 2,527 youth aged 6 to 19 years from the 2003–2004 and 2005–2006 National Health and Nutrition Examination Survey (Carson and Janssen 2011) (Figure 11.10).

Low levels of cardiorespiratory fitness in youth have also been related to antecedents of future CVD including obesity, dyslipidaemia, elevated blood pressure and inflammatory markers during the paediatric years (Carnethon et al. 2005; Ruiz et al. 2007) (Figure 11.11) and a greater risk of all-cause mortality in later life (Högström et al.

Figure 11.10 Odds ratio for high cardio-metabolic risk score (CRS) according to quartiles of (a) total sedentary behaviour and (b) mean hours of daily television viewing in children and adolescents aged 6 to 19 years.

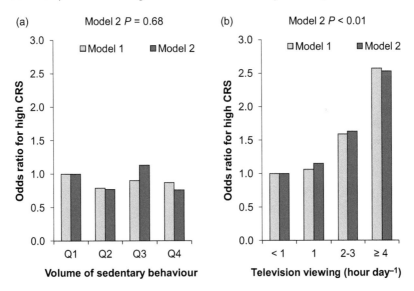

Source: Carson and Janssen (2011).
Notes: A CRS was calculated based on age- and sex-adjusted waist circumference, systolic blood pressure, non-high-density lipoprotein cholesterol and C-reactive protein. High CRS is defined as the highest quartile of CRS. Volume of sedentary behaviour was measured using accelerometry. Information on television viewing was obtained by questionnaire. Between ages 6 and 11 years, parents were asked, 'Over the past 30 days, on average how many hours per day did your child sit and watch TV or video?' At ages 12 to 19 years, the participants provided the information for themselves. Model 1: adjusted for age, sex, race, socioeconomic status, smoking, total fat, saturated fat, cholesterol and sodium. Model 2: adjusted for the covariates in Model 1 and moderate-to-vigorous physical activity.

Figure 11.11 Age- and race-adjusted odds of having cardiovascular disease risk factors in male and female US adolescents aged 12 to 19 years with low (versus moderate or high) fitness status.

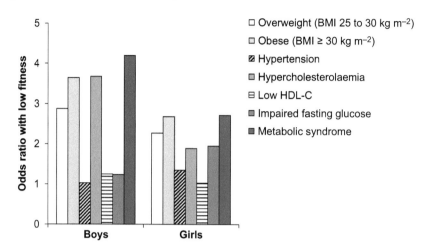

Source: Carnethon et al. (2005).

Notes: Abbreviations: BMI, body mass index, HDL-C, high-density lipoprotein cholesterol. The participants were 3,110 adolescents participating in the 1999–2000 and 2001–2002 National Health and Nutrition Examination Survey (NHANES). Low fitness was defined as < 20th percentile of estimated peak oxygen uptake. Hypercholesterolaemia was defined as a total cholesterol level > 5.2 mmol l^{-1} (200 mg dl^{-1}). Impaired fasting glucose was defined as a glucose level > 5.6 mmol l^{-1} (100 mg dl^{-1}). The metabolic syndrome was identified in adolescents with three or more of the following: triglycerides ≥ 1.4 mmol l^{-1} (110 mg dl^{-1}), HDL-C ≤ 1.0 mmol l^{-1} (40 mg dl^{-1}), waist circumference ≥ the sex-specific 90th percentile, fasting glucose level > 5.6 mmol l^{-1} (100 mg dl^{-1}), or hypertension > 90th percentile of systolic or diastolic blood pressure by age, sex and height.

2016; see Figure 3.10). However, it has been suggested that body fat partly mediates the relationship between cardiorespiratory fitness (adjusted for fat-free mass) and clustered CVD risk in young people. In contrast, the association of objectively measured physical activity with clustered CVD risk markers appears independent of adiposity (Ekelund et al. 2007). Although unravelling the complex interactions between physical activity, physical fitness and body fatness is challenging, the potential mediating or confounding role of adiposity on these relationships reaffirms the importance of identifying successful strategies targeting the reversal of paediatric obesity and other detrimental CVD risk factors.

Several prospective cohort studies have examined the relationship between physical activity and/or fitness in the paediatric years and long-lasting CVD health outcomes in adulthood. In the Oslo Youth Study, cardiorespiratory fitness (predicted peak oxygen uptake), but not self-reported physical activity, at 13 years was inversely associated with adiposity and blood pressure at ages 15, 25 and 33 years. However, the strength of these relationships diminished over time and was eliminated by age 40 years (Kvaavik et al. 2009). Findings from the Amsterdam Growth and Health Longitudinal Study have also indicated that peak oxygen uptake during adolescence (13 to 16 years), but not self-reported physical activity, was associated with a healthier CVD risk factor profile in adulthood at 32 years (Twisk et al. 2002). Although this may suggest that paediatric physical fitness is a stronger determinant of adult CVD risk than physical activity, studies to date have relied upon self-reported measures of physical activity, and the positive effect of adolescent fitness on adult cardio-metabolic health is not supported universally. Specifically, the Aerobics Centre Longitudinal Study failed to detect a relationship between adolescent cardiorespiratory fitness (mean age of 15.8 years) and adult cholesterol, blood pressure and glucose levels (mean age of 26.6 years) (Eisenmann et al. 2005).

Some ongoing cohort studies have capitalised on non-invasive ultrasound imaging of vascular endothelial function to derive surrogate indicators of early atherosclerosis such as carotid artery IMT, carotid artery elasticity and flow-mediated dilation (FMD) (these vascular measurements are described in Fernhall and Agiovlasitis (2008); see also Box 7.1 for the underlying principle of FMD). This is important as endothelial dysfunction is considered a prerequisite of the early atherosclerotic processes initiated in the first two decades of life. In the Cardiovascular Risk in Young Finns study, higher levels of self-reported leisure-time physical activity in 698 boys aged 9 to 15 years was associated with better carotid artery elasticity 21 years later in adulthood (Pälve et al. 2014). This finding has been replicated in the Danish arm of the European Youth Heart Study whereby higher levels of objectively measured physical activity at age 15 years were related to lower arterial stiffness 6 to 12 years later (Ried-Larsen et al. 2015). A further cohort study of more than 1 million Swedish men found that low muscular strength in adolescence (age 16 to 19 years) was associated with a greater risk of premature all-cause and cardiovascular mortality before the age of 55 years (median follow-up period 24.2 years) (Ortega et al. 2012).

Many of the favourable modifications in CVD risk can be derived from both acute and chronic exercise exposures. An expanding evidence base in young people supports the acquisition of transient health-related changes in CVD risk factors after single bouts of exercise. Acute moderate- to high-intensity exercise has been shown consistently to diminish postprandial triglyceride concentrations in young people and appears particularly amenable to reduction in those with elevated visceral adiposity (Lee et al. 2013a) (Figure 11.12). Other proposed benefits of prior acute exercise in children and adolescents include transient reductions in postprandial glucose and systolic blood pressure and increased resting fat oxidation (Bond et al. 2015). A single bout of exercise has also been shown in adolescent boys to negate the postprandial decline in FMD that is usually apparent after ingesting high-fat meals (Sedgwick et al. 2013). Although the mechanistic underpinnings of these effects have not been elucidated directly in this age group, the exercise-induced reduction in postprandial triglyceride concentrations may result from augmented clearance of circulating triglyceride mediated by an increase in the activity of lipoprotein lipase in the capillary beds of skeletal muscle. Furthermore, the secretion of fewer triglyceride-rich very low-density lipoproteins from the liver may also contribute to the triglyceride lowering effect of exercise (see Chapter 7 for a more detailed explanation of these mechanisms). The post-exercise shift in whole-body substrate oxidation in favour of fat may also be linked to mechanistic pathways facilitating the restoration of depleted skeletal muscle and/or hepatic glycogen stores (Kiens and Richter 1998). Regardless of the mechanisms responsible, evidence accrued thus far advocates the promotion of interventions targeting postprandial metabolic health outcomes which if commenced early in life may preserve cardio-metabolic health in the longer term.

Figure 11.12 Influence of prior acute moderate-intensity exercise on postprandial plasma triglyceride concentrations in 17 adolescent boys and girls aged 12 to 18 years (BMI ≥ 85th age- and sex-specific percentile) with low or high levels of visceral adipose tissue (VAT). Values are mean (SEM).

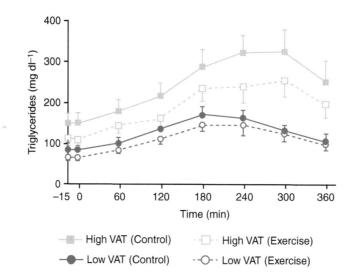

Source: Adapted by permission from Springer Nature Customer Service Centre GmbH: Springer Nature, *International Journal of Obesity*, 'Effects of acute exercise on postprandial triglyceride response after a high-fat meal in overweight black and white adolescents', Lee, S. et al., copyright © 2013.
Notes: Participants cycled for 60 minutes at 50% of peak oxygen uptake in the exercise trial or rested for an equivalent duration in the control trial approximately 14 hours before a high-fat breakfast meal was provided at 0 minutes (~08:00). A single axial image of the abdomen was taken using computed tomography to quantify visceral adipose tissue. The lower two tertiles were combined and comprised the low visceral adipose tissue group (≤ 75.6 cm^2) and the top tertile was categorised as high visceral adipose tissue (> 75.6 cm^2). Note that exercise reduced postprandial triglyceride concentrations to a greater extent in adolescents with high visceral adipose tissue, but the mean concentrations remained above the control values for the low visceral adipose tissue group.

Regular application of the acute exercise stimuli is required to maintain optimum health outcomes over the long term and, therefore, a variety of intervention studies have been conducted in young people with the aim of modifying CVD risk. Emergent from this body of work is the consensus that a structured exercise training intervention elicits modest improvements in CVD risk factors in young people who display adverse levels at baseline. Meyer and colleagues (2006), for example, randomised 67 youth aged 11 to 16 years who were obese (BMI > 97th population-specific percentile) to a six-month supervised aerobic exercise training (three 60–90 minute sessions per week) or non-exercise protocol. The young participants with obesity exhibited impaired endothelial function and a myriad of adverse CVD risk markers at baseline compared with 35 controls aged 12 to 16 years who were lean (Figure 11.13). However, the exercise training intervention improved carotid artery IMT and FMD (Figure 11.13), with the latter likely mediated by endothelium-dependent vasodilation through increased production of nitric oxide facilitated by upregulation of the enzyme endothelial nitric oxide synthase (Fernhall and Agiovlasitis 2008). These vascular changes occurred

Figure 11.13 Values for selected cardiovascular disease risk markers at baseline in the lean comparator group (*n* = 35; mean age 14.7 years, body mass index (BMI) *z*-score –0.08), and at baseline and the end of the six-month intervention in adolescents with obesity randomly allocated to the non-exercise control group (*n* = 34; mean age 14.1 years, BMI *z*-score 2.58) or exercise training intervention group (*n* = 33; mean age 13.7 years, BMI *z*-score 2.33).

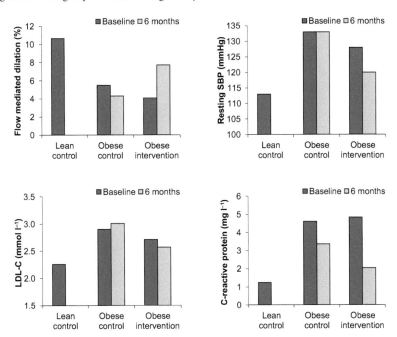

Source: Reprinted from the *Journal of the American College of Cardiology*, 48: 1865–70, Meyer, A.A. et al., 'Improvement of early vascular changes and cardiovascular risk factors in obese children after a six-month exercise program', page 1867–8, copyright © 2006, with permission from Elsevier.

Notes: Abbreviations: SBP, systolic blood pressure; LDL-C, low-density lipoprotein cholesterol. Obesity was defined as a BMI > 97th population-specific percentile. The six-month exercise training intervention involved a combination of swimming and aqua aerobic training, sports games and walking performed in three sessions per week. Pre-to-post changes for flow mediated dilation, resting SBP, LDL-C and C-reactive protein were statistically significant for intervention participants (all *P* ≤ 0.048). The only statistically significant pre-to-post change in obese control participants was for a reduction in flow mediated dilation (*P* = 0.044).

concomitantly with favourable reductions in other CVD risk factors including BMI *z*-score, resting systolic blood pressure, fasting insulin, low-density lipoprotein cholesterol and markers of low-grade inflammation (C-reactive protein, fibrinogen) (Figure 11.13). However, findings are not consistent across studies and the optimum exercise characteristics (intensity and duration) required to favourably modify CVD risk factors in young people remains elusive. Furthermore, the potential for exercise training to elicit salutary changes in antecedents of future CVD risk independent of concurrent effects on body fat continues to be debated. Whilst exercise may ameliorate CVD risk in young people who exhibit unhealthy profiles, regular physical activity exerts minimal effects in healthy individuals but may help to maintain the constellation of CVD risk factors within a healthy range throughout the paediatric years.

BONE HEALTH

Considering the antecedents of osteoporosis are purported to reside in youth, the role of physical activity in enhancing skeletal development in young people continues to attract scientific attention. Two notable reviews have been published on this topic and the interested reader is directed to these for a more comprehensive insight (Gunter et al. 2012; Weaver et al. 2016). An important determinant of skeletal health during the life course is peak bone mass which is typically achieved by the end of the second or early in the third decade of life (see Figure 9.3). It is acknowledged that the rapid accrual of bone mineral that occurs during puberty and the adolescent growth spurt may represent a critical period for maximising peak bone mass in response to physical activity (Weaver et al. 2016). One notable cross-sectional study compared the dominant-to-non-dominant arm differences in areal bone mineral density (BMD) (defined as bone mineral content (BMC) per unit area) using DXA in 91, 7- to 17-year-old Finnish female tennis players and 58 female controls. The authors identified side-to-side differences in areal BMD at all stages of sexual maturation in tennis players (range 1.6% to 15.7%), whereas the control participants displayed much smaller differences (range −0.2% to 4.6%). Furthermore, bilateral arm areal BMD differences between the players and controls became accentuated at sexual maturation stage 3 (mean age 12.6 years) coinciding with the adolescent growth spurt (Haapasalo et al. 1998).

A recent scientific statement by the National Osteoporosis Foundation presents compelling evidence highlighting the importance of weight-bearing exercise to promote and maintain skeletal health during childhood and adolescence (Weaver et al. 2016). Observational studies using accelerometry have suggested that higher levels of habitual physical activity, particularly of vigorous intensity, are related to higher DXA-based measures of areal BMD, BMC and bone strength in young people (Sardinha et al. 2008; Tobias et al. 2007). The osteogenic effect of physical activity early in life is further supported by school-based exercise interventions demonstrating greater areal BMD and/or BMC accrual at loaded sites in boys and girls randomised to the intervention arm (for example, Meyer et al. 2011). Whilst the optimum exercise prescription for promoting bone growth has yet to be determined, these studies indicate that exercise must be high impact and weight bearing with short bursts of plyometric-based activities such as jumping, hopping and skipping appearing particularly efficacious (Figure 11.14). Combining exercise with calcium supplementation also appears a more potent stimulus for promoting bone accretion in children than either intervention alone (Bass et al. 2007).

Recent advances in three-dimensional bone-imaging techniques, most notably peripheral quantitative computed tomography (pQCT) and MRI, have enabled parameters of bone geometry and strength to be characterised more precisely in young people. Specifically, cross-sectional findings from the Avon Longitudinal Study of Parents and Children reported that objectively measured vigorous, but not light-to-moderate, physical activity was positively associated with pQCT derived cortical BMC of the mid-tibia in 1,748 boys and girls (mean age 15.5 years) (Sayers et al. 2011). Controlled intervention trials of bone-loading exercise and structural outcomes have thus far yielded inconsistent findings, which may partly reflect the multitude of bone structural

Figure 11.14 Sports and activities involving impact forces such as gymnastics and jumping are particularly beneficial for bone health in children and adolescents.

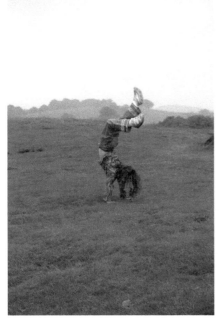 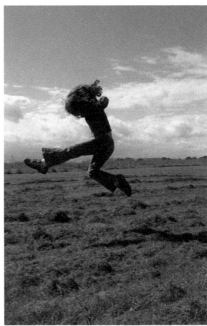

Source: Photos courtesy of Mr James Smith.

indices employed across the paediatric literature. For example, the Action Schools! BC programme involved a 16-month school-based jumping and physical activity intervention in Canadian boys and girls aged 10 years at baseline. Whilst the authors reported greater exercise-induced gains in some localised parameters of tibial bone strength and geometry, the beneficial changes were generally small and other structural outcomes were not different (Macdonald et al. 2007, 2009). This supports other well-controlled exercise interventions that have induced modest or negligible structural bone adaptations beyond those observed with natural growth and maturation (reviewed by Weaver et al. 2016).

A key question concerns whether the bone health benefits induced by regular physical activity in youth confers reduced propensity for osteoarthritis and/or fragility fracture in later life. Such evidence is, unfortunately, sparse but a few studies have highlighted the potential longevity of bone outcomes accrued with exercise in youth. The Iowa Bone Development Study, for example, demonstrated that boys and girls accumulating the greatest amount of objectively measured MVPA from age 5 through to age 17 years had higher bone strength indices (assessed using DXA and pQCT) at age 17 years (Janz et al. 2014). In another study, Gunter and colleagues (2008) observed sustained bone health effects of a seven-month high-impact jumping intervention conducted in pre-pubertal boys and girls (mean baseline age 7.6 years). The intervention

Figure 11.15 Influence of a seven-month school-based jumping intervention on the change in total hip bone mineral content (BMC) over eight years in boys and girls. Values represent the percent change from baseline in jumpers (*n* = 33; mean age at baseline 7.6 years) above that of a stretching control group (*n* = 24; mean age at baseline 7.9 years) at the end of the intervention (7 months), after one year of detraining (19 months) and after three to seven years of detraining (43–91 months).

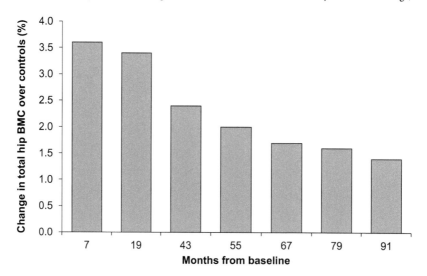

Source: Reprinted from 'Impact exercise increases BMC during growth: an 8-year longitudinal study', Gunter, K. et al., *Journal of Bone and Mineral Research* 23: 986–93, page 990, with permission from John Wiley and Sons. Copyright © 2008 American Society for Bone and Mineral Research.
Notes: The jumping (intervention) and stretching (control) programmes involved three 20-minute sessions per week performed on separate days to scheduled physical education classes. BMC was measured using dual-energy X-ray absorptiometry. Results are adjusted for baseline age, change in height, change in body mass, maturity status and sports participation, and are statistically significant at each of the seven measurement periods ($P < 0.05$).

participants had a 3.6% greater gain in total hip BMC (measured using DXA) than controls immediately after the intervention, which was maintained, albeit attenuated to 1.4%, approximately seven years after the intervention (Figure 11.15).

Beyond the formative years, the Saskatchewan Pediatric Bone Mineral Accrual Study reported that those who were physically active during adolescence exhibited enhanced pQCT bone traits at the tibial diaphysis as young adults (aged 24 to 34 years) compared with their less active peers. Specifically, bone strength and total bone area were higher in men and cortical bone area and content were higher in women classified in the top quartile of self-reported physical activity during adolescence (after adjustment for adult physical activity) (Duckham et al. 2014). Skeletal health benefits of physical activity completed during youth (9 to 18 years) have also been shown to persist into adulthood (31 to 46 years) in the Cardiovascular Risk in Young Finns study. These benefits, however, did not translate into an altered risk of fracture during the 28-year follow-up (Tolonen et al. 2015).

The lifelong osteogenic effect of physical activity accumulated early in life has been examined in a cross-sectional study comparing throwing-to-non-throwing arm properties of the humeral diaphysis of professional baseball players at various stages of their career with age-matched controls. The authors demonstrated accelerated age-related declines in cortical bone mass, area and thickness with the cessation of activity

Figure 11.16 Mean difference (95% confidence interval) in humeral diaphysis bone properties between the throwing-to-non-throwing arm of nine active and 84 former professional baseball players normalised to differences between the dominant-to-non-dominant arms of 94 age-matched controls.

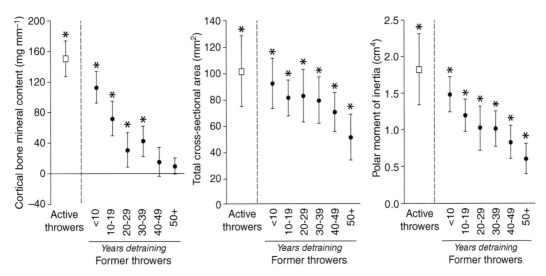

Source: Reprinted with permission from Warden, S.J. et al. (2014) 'Physical activity when young provides lifelong benefits to cortical bone size and strength in men'. *Proceedings of the National Academy of Sciences of the United States of America* 111: 5337–42.

Notes: Bone properties were assessed using peripheral quantitative computed tomography. Polar moment of inertia is an estimate of torsional (bending) bone strength. Asterisks indicate the side-to-side differences in throwers (throwing minus non-throwing arm) was different from the side-to-side differences in controls (dominant minus non-dominant arm) ($P < 0.01$).

(Warden et al. 2014) (Figure 11.16). This supports previous findings in male soccer players indicating that those who had been retired for 35 or more years had no residual benefit in DXA-derived BMD or altered fracture risk in old age compared with age-matched controls (Karlsson et al. 2000). However, Warden and colleagues (2014) also reported that former baseball players in the ninth decade of life retained half of the bone size (total cross-sectional area) and one-third of the bone strength (polar moment of inertia) benefits of throwing-related activity achieved early in life (Figure 11.16). Furthermore, greater maintenance of the cortical bone mass and strength benefits induced by previous physical activity was apparent when throwing activity was continued during ageing. Collectively, these findings suggest that although exercise in youth has undoubted benefits for bone health, continuity of exercise in adulthood may be necessary to optimise these benefits.

MENTAL HEALTH AND COGNITIVE FUNCTION

A physically active lifestyle exerts a plethora of mental health benefits in adults (reviewed in Chapter 10), and accumulating evidence indicates that some of these favourable effects may extend to young people. One important caveat is the paucity of high-quality RCTs on this topic in young people, with the majority of evidence derived

387

from cross-sectional studies and, therefore, limited by the inability to establish causality. Furthermore, the lack of consistency in assessment tools utilised to measure the various mental health and cognitive outcomes will inevitably introduce variability when scrutinising the evidence. Current research in young people has primarily focused on the effect of physical activity on depression, anxiety, self-esteem, cognitive function and academic achievement. Consequently, this section is restricted to discussions on these aspects of mental health and cognitive performance in young people.

The weight of cross-sectional evidence supports an inverse association between overall physical activity levels and depressive symptoms in children and adolescents (Rodriguez-Ayllon et al. 2019). However, evidence is far from consistent and ambiguity remains on whether physical activity is associated with lower anxiety and enhanced self-esteem in young people (Rodriguez-Ayllon et al. 2019). One of the few studies to utilise accelerometry to measure physical activity is the Avon Longitudinal Study of Parents and Children. This cross-sectional analysis indicated that higher levels of overall, but not moderate-to-vigorous, physical activity were related to lower levels of depressive symptoms in 2,951 adolescents (mean age 13.8 years) (Wiles et al. 2012). Conversely, longitudinal evidence has thus far yielded equivocal findings but much of this evidence has relied upon self-reported physical activity. A notable exception reported that objectively measured physical activity at baseline in 736 adolescents (mean age 14.5 years) was not predictive of depressive symptoms or diagnosed major depressive disorder after three years of follow-up (Toseeb et al. 2014). Beyond the observational evidence outlined thus far, the impact of physical activity and structured exercise interventions on mental health outcomes in children and adolescents has been synthesised in meta-analyses with favourable, albeit modest, effects emerging for depressive symptoms (Brown et al. 2013) and overall mental health (Rodriguez-Ayllon et al. 2019).

There is also increasing awareness that sedentary behaviour may be linked with deleterious mental health outcomes in children and adolescents. Specifically, a meta-analysis of observational studies concluded that screen time was associated with depressive symptoms in a non-linear dose-response manner, with a higher risk emerging when screen time exceeds 2 hours day^{-1} (Liu et al. 2016). However, the existing evidence base in young people linking sedentary behaviour to facets of mental health, including depression, anxiety and self-esteem, is inconclusive and limited by considerable methodological shortcomings (Carson et al. 2016). Future high-quality experimental studies with standardised exposure and outcome measures are essential to better elucidate the effects of physical activity and sedentary behaviour on mental health outcomes in children and adolescents.

A recent position stand has comprehensively reviewed the existing literature focusing on cognitive function and academic achievement in school-aged youth (Donnelly et al. 2016). Despite a lack of uniformity in findings and a dearth of high-quality evidence, the authors concluded that physical activity and fitness has an overall positive effect on aspects of cognitive function and academic achievement in young people. In one example, the FITKids RCT investigated the impact of a nine-month extra-curricular physical activity intervention in children aged 7 to 9 years on selected aspects of executive function (a set of cognitive processes underlying perception, memory and action). The intervention was delivered on 90% of school days during the academic year and aimed to provide children with at least 70 minutes of MVPA per session integrated with health education lessons. Children receiving the intervention exhibited greater improvements in peak oxygen uptake along with selective indices of executive control and brain function compared with a 'wait-list' control group (who would be offered the intervention later) (Hillman et al. 2014). Several potential mechanisms may be responsible for exercise-induced changes in cognitive function including increases in brain-derived neurotrophic factor, catecholamines and growth hormones such as insulin-like growth factor and vascular endothelial growth factor (see Chapter 12 for further discussion of these mechanisms), but confirmation of these pathways are required in young people (Donnelly et al. 2016).

The purported benefits of physical activity on cognitive function in young people is intuitively appealing if such benefits translate into enhanced academic achievement. This avenue of enquiry has thus far yielded a distinct lack of consensus with high-quality studies few in number and heterogeneity evident in the methods used to assess academic performance (Donnelly et al. 2016). For example, the Active Smarter Kids cluster RCT introduced a seven-month physical activity intervention in 596 children aged 10.2 years at baseline consisting of: (i) 90 min week^{-1} of physically active educational lessons predominantly delivered in the playground; (ii) 5 min day^{-1} of physical activity breaks during classroom lessons; and (iii) 10 min day^{-1} of physical activity homework. The intervention had no effect on academic performance in numeracy, reading or English compared with 533 similarly aged controls (Resaland et al. 2016). In contrast, the Physical Activity Across the Curriculum cluster RCT introduced 90 min week^{-1} of moderate-to-vigorous intensity physically active academic lessons and found greater increases in daily physical activity and academic scores in children exposed to the intervention after three years (Donnelly et al. 2009) (Figure 11.17). Clearly, many questions remain to be answered to elucidate the impact of physical activity on the current and future mental health and cognitive function of young people.

Figure 11.17 Change in academic score from baseline to three years in 117 intervention children and 86 control children aged 7 to 9 years at baseline.

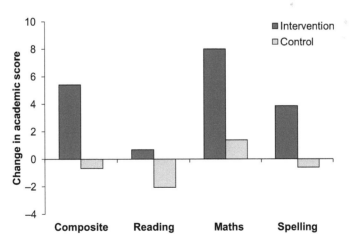

Source: Reprinted from *Preventive Medicine*, 49: 336–41, Donnelly, J.E. et al., 'Physical Activity Across the Curriculum (PAAC): a randomized controlled trial to promote physical activity and diminish overweight and obesity in elementary school children', page 339, copyright © 2009, with permission from Elsevier.
Notes: Intervention children receiving 90 min week^{-1} of moderate-to-vigorous intensity physically active academic lessons demonstrated greater changes in all academic achievement scores than control children (all between-group differences $P \leq 0.01$).

SUMMARY

- Many young people exhibit low levels of physical activity, and there is a marked decline in physical activity and increase in sedentary behaviours during childhood and adolescence.
- Targeted interventions have been largely unsuccessful in increasing objectively measured levels of overall physical activity in children and adolescents.
- The prevalence of overweight and obesity in young people remains high in many countries and increased rates of paediatric type 2 diabetes have emerged in parallel with increasing obesity rates in recent decades.
- The consensus of evidence supports an inverse, albeit modest, association between physical activity or fitness and a variety of health outcomes (adiposity, insulin resistance, CVD risk factors) in young people. Conversely, sedentary time does not appear to be an independent predictor of these outcomes after controlling for physical activity levels.
- Physical activity has a role to play in the prevention and management of obesity in young people, but evidence to support effective interventions is limited.
- Exercise training may lead to favourable changes in CVD risk factors, including insulin resistance, blood pressure and blood lipids, in children and adolescents who exhibit unhealthy profiles.
- Understanding of whether increasing physical activity and decreasing sedentary behaviour in youth promotes future cardiovascular health benefits in adulthood is limited.
- There is good evidence that physical activity, particularly high-impact activity, is effective for promoting bone growth and possibly bone strength in children and adolescents. This effect may last well into adulthood but is unlikely to reduce the risk of fracture in old age unless physical activity is maintained.
- Physical activity may be an effective strategy for enhancing facets of mental health and performance in young people including depression and cognitive function, but existing evidence is low in quality.
- Although technological developments have facilitated considerable progress in this field of study in recent years, further concerted efforts are required to initiate and maintain optimum health behaviours early in life.

STUDY TASKS

1 What is the basis for stating that many young people lead sedentary lives? What factors may influence engagement in physical activity and sedentary behaviours during childhood and adolescence?
2 Give examples of studies observing a relationship between physical inactivity and adiposity in young people. What are the implications of these findings?
3 Design an intervention-based study with the primary aim of reducing the risk of type 2 diabetes in adolescent boys and girls. What study design will you use? What population will you recruit? What will the intervention involve? What outcome measures will you investigate? How will the study advance knowledge?

4 Describe findings from three studies linking physical activity levels during childhood and adolescence with cardiovascular health outcomes in adulthood and highlight the strengths and limitations of these studies.

5 Discuss the research evidence that childhood may provide a unique opportunity for developing bone mass and strength. What exercise prescription would you recommend for optimising bone mineral accrual in young people?

FURTHER READING

Donnelly, J.E., Hillman, C.H., Castelli, D., Etnier, J.L., Lee, S., Tomporowski, P. et al. (2016) Physical activity, fitness, cognitive function, and academic achievement in children: a systematic review. *Medicine and Science in Sports and Exercise* 48: 1197–222.

Ekelund, U., Luan, J., Sherar, L.B., Esliger, D.W., Griew, P. and Cooper, A.; International Children's Accelerometry Database (ICAD) Collaborators. (2012) Moderate to vigorous physical activity and sedentary time and cardiometabolic risk factors in children and adolescents. *Journal of the American Medical Association* 307: 704–12.

Fedewa, M.V., Gist, N.H., Evans, E.M. and Dishman, R.K. (2014) Exercise and insulin resistance in youth: a meta-analysis. *Pediatrics* 133: e163–74.

Fernhall, B. and Agiovlasitis, S. (2008) Arterial function in youth: window into cardiovascular risk. *Journal of Applied Physiology* 105: 325–33.

Gunter, K.B., Almstedt, H.C. and Janz, K.F. (2012) Physical activity in childhood may be the key to optimizing lifespan skeletal health. *Exercise and Sport Sciences Reviews* 40: 13–21.

Janssen, I. and LeBlanc, A.G. (2010). Systematic review of the health benefits of physical activity and fitness in school-aged children and youth. *International Journal of Behavioral Nutrition and Physical Activity* 7: 40. doi: 10.1186/1479-5868-7-40.

Metcalf, B., Henley, W. and Wilkin, T. (2012) Effectiveness of intervention on physical activity of children: systematic review and meta-analysis of controlled trials with objectively measured outcomes (EarlyBird 54). *British Medical Journal* 345: e5888. doi: 10.1136/bmj.e5888.

Ortega, F.B., Ruiz, J.R., Castillo, M.J. and Sjöström, M. (2008) Physical fitness in childhood and adolescence: a powerful marker for health. *International Journal of Obesity* 32: 1–11.

Stoner, L., Rowlands, D., Morrison, A., Credeur, D., Hamlin, M., Gaffney, K. et al. (2016) Efficacy of exercise intervention for weight loss in overweight and obese adolescents: meta-analysis and implications. *Sports Medicine* 46: 1737–51.

Weaver, C.M., Gordon, C.M., Janz, K.F., Kalkwarf, H.J., Lappe, J.M., Lewis, R. et al. (2016) The National Osteoporosis Foundation's position statement on peak bone mass development and lifestyle factors: a systematic review and implementation recommendations. *Osteoporosis International* 27: 1281–386.

REFERENCES

Adab, P., Pallan, M.J., Lancashire, E.R., Hemming, K., Frew, E., Barrett, T. et al. (2018) Effectiveness of a childhood obesity prevention programme delivered through schools, targeting 6 and 7 year olds: cluster randomised controlled trial (WAVES study). *British Medical Journal* 360: k211. doi: 10.1136/bmj.k211.

Al-Khudairy, L., Loveman, E., Colquitt, J.L., Mead, E., Johnson, R.E., Fraser, H. et al. (2017) Diet, physical activity and behavioural interventions for the treatment of overweight or obese adolescents aged 12 to 17 years. *The Cochrane Database of Systematic Reviews* 6: CD012691. doi: 10.1002/14651858.CD012691.

Armstrong, N. and Barker, A.R. (2011) Endurance training and elite young athletes. *Medicine and Sport Science* 56: 59–83.

Armstrong, N., Tomkinson, G. and Ekelund, U. (2011) Aerobic fitness and its relationship to sport, exercise training and habitual physical activity during youth. *British Journal of Sports Medicine* 45: 849–58.

Armstrong, N. and van Mechelen, W. (eds). (2017) *Oxford Textbook of Children's Sport and Exercise Medicine.* 3rd edn, Oxford: Oxford University Press.

Aubert, S., Barnes, J.D., Abdeta, C., Abi Nader, P., Adeniyi, A.F., Aguilar-Farias, N. et al. (2018) Global matrix 3.0 physical activity report card grades for children and youth: results and analysis from 49 countries. *Journal of Physical Activity and Health* 15: S251–73.

Bacha, F., Lee, S., Gungor, N. and Arslanian, S.A. (2010) From pre-diabetes to type 2 diabetes in obese youth: pathophysiological characteristics along the spectrum of glucose dysregulation. *Diabetes Care* 33: 2225–31.

Baquet, G., Stratton, G., Van Praagh, E. and Berthoin, S. (2007) Improving physical activity assessment in prepubertal children with high-frequency accelerometry monitoring: a methodological issue. *Preventive Medicine* 44: 143–7.

Bass, S.L., Naughton, G., Saxon, L., Iuliano-Burns, S., Daly, R., Briganti, E.M. et al. (2007) Exercise and calcium combined results in a greater osteogenic effect than either factor alone: a blinded randomized placebo-controlled trial in boys. *Journal of Bone and Mineral Research* 22: 458–64.

Belcher, B.R., Berrigan, D., Papachristopoulou, A., Brady, S.M., Bernstein, S.B., Brychta, R.J. et al. (2015) Effects of interrupting children's sedentary behaviors with activity on metabolic function: a randomized trial. *Journal of Clinical Endocrinology and Metabolism* 100: 3735–43.

Biddle, S.J., Pearson, N., Ross, G.M. and Braithwaite, R. (2010) Tracking of sedentary behaviours of young people: a systematic review. *Preventive Medicine* 51: 345–51.

Bleich, S.N., Ku, R. and Wang, Y.C. (2011) Relative contribution of energy intake and energy expenditure to childhood obesity: a review of the literature and directions for future research. *International Journal of Obesity* 35: 1–15.

Bond, B., Williams, C.A., Jackman, S.R., Woodward, A., Armstrong, N. and Barker, A.R. (2015) Accumulating exercise and postprandial health in adolescents. *Metabolism: Clinical and Experimental* 64: 1068–76.

Broadney, M.M., Belcher, B.R., Berrigan, D.A., Brychta, R.J., Tigner, I.L., Shareef, F. et al. (2018) Effects of interrupting sedentary behavior with short bouts of moderate physical activity on glucose tolerance in children with overweight and obesity: a randomized crossover trial. *Diabetes Care* 41: 2220–8.

Brown, H.E., Pearson, N., Braithwaite, R.E., Brown, W.J. and Biddle, S.J. (2013) Physical activity interventions and depression in children and adolescents: a systematic review and meta-analysis. *Sports Medicine* 43: 195–206.

Brown, T., Moore, T.H., Hooper, L., Gao, Y., Zayegh, A., Ijaz, S. et al. (2019) Interventions for preventing obesity in children. *The Cochrane Database of Systematic Reviews* 7: CD001871. doi: 10.1002/14651858.CD001871.pub4.

Caprio, S., Hyman, L.D., McCarthy, S., Lange, R., Bronson, M. and Tamborlane, W.V. (1996) Fat distribution and cardiovascular risk factors in obese adolescent girls: importance of the intra-abdominal fat depot. *The American Journal of Clinical Nutrition* 64: 12–17.

Carnethon, M.R., Gulati, M. and Greenland, P. (2005) Prevalence and cardiovascular disease correlates of low cardiorespiratory fitness in adolescents and adults. *Journal of the American Medical Association* 294: 2981–8.

Carson, V., Hunter, S., Kuzik, N., Gray, C.E., Poitras, V.J., Chaput, J.P. et al. (2016) Systematic review of sedentary behaviour and health indicators in school-aged children and youth: an update. *Applied Physiology, Nutrition, and Metabolism* 41(Suppl. 3): S240–65.

Carson, V. and Janssen, I. (2011) Volume, patterns, and types of sedentary behavior and cardiometabolic health in children and adolescents: a cross-sectional study. *BMC Public Health* 11: 274. doi: 10.1186/1471-2458-11-274.

Cole, T.J., Bellizzi, M.C., Flegal, K.M. and Dietz, W.H. (2000) Establishing a standard definition for child overweight and obesity worldwide: international survey. *British Medical Journal* 320: 1240–3.

Cole, T.J. and Lobstein, T. (2012) Extended international (IOTF) body mass index cut-offs for thinness, overweight and obesity. *Pediatric Obesity* 7: 284–94.

Cooper, A.R., Goodman, A., Page, A.S., Sherar, L.B., Esliger, D.W., van Sluijs, E.M. et al. (2015) Objectively measured physical activity and sedentary time in youth: the International Children's Accelerometry Database (ICAD). *International Journal of Behavioral Nutrition and Physical Activity* 12: 113. doi: 10.1186/s12966-015-0274-5.

Dabelea, D., Stafford, J.M., Mayer-Davis, E.J., D'Agostino, R., Dolan, L., Imperatore, G. et al.; for the SEARCH for Diabetes in Youth Research Group. (2017) Association of type 1 diabetes vs type 2 diabetes diagnosed during childhood and adolescence with complications during teenage years and young adulthood. *Journal of the American Medical Association* 317: 825–35.

Davis, C.L., Pollock, N.K., Waller, J.L., Allison, J.D., Dennis, B.A., Bassali, R. et al. (2012) Exercise dose and diabetes risk in overweight and obese children: a randomized controlled trial. *Journal of the American Medical Association* 308: 1103–12.

Davis, P.H., Dawson, J.D., Riley, W.A. and Lauer, R.M. (2001) Carotid intimal-medial thickness is related to cardiovascular risk factors measured from childhood through middle age: The Muscatine Study. *Circulation* 104: 2815–19.

Dencker, M. and Andersen, L.B. (2011) Accelerometer-measured daily physical activity related to aerobic fitness in children and adolescents. *Journal of Sports Sciences* 29: 887–95.

Donnelly, J.E., Greene, J.L., Gibson, C.A., Smith, B.K., Washburn, R.A., Sullivan, D.K. et al. (2009) Physical Activity Across the Curriculum (PAAC): a randomized controlled trial to promote physical activity and diminish overweight and obesity in elementary school children. *Preventive Medicine* 49: 336–41.

Donnelly, J.E., Hillman, C.H., Castelli, D., Etnier, J.L., Lee, S., Tomporowski, P. et al. (2016) Physical activity, fitness, cognitive function, and academic achievement in children: a systematic review. *Medicine and Science in Sports and Exercise* 48: 1197–222.

Duckham, R.L., Baxter-Jones, A.D., Johnston, J.D., Vatanparast, H., Cooper, D. and Kontulainen, S. (2014) Does physical activity in adolescence have site-specific and sex-specific benefits on young adult bone size, content, and estimated strength? *Journal of Bone and Mineral Research* 29: 479–86.

Eisenmann, J.C., Wickel, E.E., Welk, G.J. and Blair, S.N. (2005) Relationship between adolescent fitness and fatness and cardiovascular disease risk factors in adulthood: the Aerobics Center Longitudinal Study (ACLS). *American Heart Journal* 149: 46–53.

Ekelund, U., Anderssen, S.A., Froberg, K., Sardinha, L.B., Andersen, L.B. and Brage, S. (2007) Independent associations of physical activity and cardiorespiratory fitness with metabolic risk factors in children: the European youth heart study. *Diabetologia* 50: 1832–40.

Ekelund, U., Luan, J., Sherar, L.B., Esliger, D.W., Griew, P. and Cooper, A; International Children's Accelerometry Database (ICAD) Collaborators. (2012) Moderate to vigorous physical activity and sedentary time and cardiometabolic risk factors in children and adolescents. *Journal of the American Medical Association* 307: 704–12.

Fedewa, M.V., Gist, N.H., Evans, E.M. and Dishman, R.K. (2014) Exercise and insulin resistance in youth: a meta-analysis. *Pediatrics* 133: e163–74.

Fernhall, B. and Agiovlasitis, S. (2008) Arterial function in youth: window into cardiovascular risk. *Journal of Applied Physiology* 105: 325–33.

Ferreira, I., van de Laar, R.J., Prins, M.H., Twisk, J.W. and Stehouwer, C.D. (2012) Carotid stiffness in young adults: a life-course analysis of its early determinants: the Amsterdam Growth and Health Longitudinal Study. *Hypertension* 59: 54–61.

Franks, P.W., Hanson, R.L., Knowler, W.C., Sievers, M.L., Bennett, P.H. and Looker, H.C. (2010) Childhood obesity, other cardiovascular risk factors, and premature death. *New England Journal of Medicine* 362: 485–93.

Friedemann, C., Heneghan, C., Mahtani, K., Thompson, M., Perera, R. and Ward, A.M. (2012) Cardiovascular disease risk in healthy children and its association with body mass index: systematic review and meta-analysis. *British Medical Journal* 345: e4759. doi: 10.1136/bmj.e4759.

Gunter, K.B., Almstedt, H.C. and Janz, K.F. (2012) Physical activity in childhood may be the key to optimizing lifespan skeletal health. *Exercise and Sport Sciences Reviews* 40: 13–21.

Gunter, K., Baxter-Jones, A.D., Mirwald, R.L., Almstedt, H., Fuchs, R.K., Durski, S. and Snow, C. (2008) Impact exercise increases BMC during growth: an 8-year longitudinal study. *Journal of Bone and Mineral Research* 23: 986–93.

Haapasalo, H., Kannus, P., Sievänen, H., Pasanen, M., Uusi-Rasi, K., Heinonen, A. et al. (1998) Effect of long-term unilateral activity on bone mineral density of female junior tennis players. *Journal of Bone and Mineral Research* 13: 310–19.

Hallal, P.C., Andersen, L.B., Bull, F.C., Guthold, R., Haskell, W. and Ekelund, U. (2012) Global physical activity levels: surveillance progress, pitfalls, and prospects. *The Lancet* 380: 247–57.

Henderson, M., Benedetti, A., Barnett, T.A., Mathieu, M.E., Deladoëy, J. and Gray-Donald, K. (2016) Influence of adiposity, physical activity, fitness, and screen time on insulin dynamics over 2 years in children. *Journal of the American Medical Association Pediatrics* 170: 227–35.

Hillman, C.H., Pontifex, M.B., Castelli, D.M., Khan, N.A., Raine, L.B., Scudder, M.R. et al. (2014) Effects of the FITKids randomized controlled trial on executive control and brain function. *Pediatrics* 134: e1063–71.

Högström, G., Nordström, A. and Nordström, P. (2016) Aerobic fitness in late adolescence and the risk of early death: a prospective cohort study of 1.3 million Swedish men. *International Journal of Epidemiology* 45: 1159–68.

Hutcheon, J.A., Chiolero, A. and Hanley, J.A. (2010) Random measurement error and regression dilution bias. *British Medical Journal* 340: c2289. doi: 10.1136/bmj.c2289.

Imperatore, G., Boyle, J.P., Thompson, T.J., Case, D., Dabelea, D., Hamman, R.F. et al.; SEARCH for Diabetes in Youth Study Group (2012) Projections of type 1 and type 2 diabetes burden in the U.S. population aged <20 years through 2050: dynamic modeling of incidence, mortality, and population growth. *Diabetes Care* 35: 2515–20.

Janssen, X., Basterfield, L., Parkinson, K.N., Pearce, M.S., Reilly, J.K., Adamson, A.J. and Reilly, J.J. (2019) Non-linear longitudinal associations between moderate-to-vigorous physical activity and adiposity across the adiposity distribution during childhood and adolescence: Gateshead Millennium Study. *International Journal of Obesity* 43: 744–50.

Janz, K.F., Letuchy, E.M., Burns, T.L., Eichenberger Gilmore, J.M., Torner, J.C. and Levy, S.M. (2014) Objectively measured physical activity trajectories predict adolescent bone strength: Iowa Bone Development Study. *British Journal of Sports Medicine* 48: 1032–6.

Jiménez-Pavón, D., Kelly, J. and Reilly, J.J. (2010) Associations between objectively measured habitual physical activity and adiposity in children and adolescents: systematic review. *International Journal of Pediatric Obesity* 5: 3–18.

Juonala, M., Magnussen, C.G., Berenson, G.S., Venn, A., Burns, T.L., Sabin, M.A. et al. (2011) Childhood adiposity, adult adiposity, and cardiovascular risk factors. *New England Journal of Medicine* 365: 1876–85.

Karlsson, M.K., Linden, C., Karlsson, C., Johnell, O., Obrant, K. and Seeman, E. (2000) Exercise during growth and bone mineral density and fractures in old age. *The Lancet* 355: 469–70.

Kids Run Free. *Marathon Kids UK* [online], available at: https://www.marathonkids.co.uk/ (accessed 20 September 2019).

Kiens, B. and Richter, E.A. (1998) Utilization of skeletal muscle triacylglycerol during postexercise recovery in humans. *The American Journal of Physiology* 275: E332–7.

Kvaavik, E., Klepp, K.I., Tell, G.S., Meyer, H.E. and Batty, G.D. (2009) Physical fitness and physical activity at age 13 years as predictors of cardiovascular disease risk factors at ages 15, 25, 33, and 40 years: extended follow-up of the Oslo Youth Study. *Pediatrics* 123: e80–6.

Kwon, S., Burns, T.L., Levy, S.M. and Janz, K.F. (2013) Which contributes more to childhood adiposity-high levels of sedentarism or low levels of moderate-through-vigorous physical activity? The Iowa Bone Development Study. *The Journal of Pediatrics* 162: 1169–74.

Lee, S., Bacha, F., Hannon, T., Kuk, J.L., Boesch, C. and Arslanian, S. (2012) Effects of aerobic versus resistance exercise without caloric restriction on abdominal fat, intrahepatic lipid, and insulin sensitivity in obese adolescent boys: a randomized, controlled trial. *Diabetes* 61: 2787–95.

Lee, S., Burns, S.F., White, D., Kuk, J.L. and Arslanian, S. (2013a) Effects of acute exercise on postprandial triglyceride response after a high-fat meal in overweight black and white adolescents. *International Journal of Obesity* 37: 966–71.

Lee, S., Deldin, A.R., White, D., Kim, Y., Libman, I., Rivera-Vega, M. et al. (2013b) Aerobic exercise but not resistance exercise reduces intrahepatic lipid content and visceral fat and improves insulin sensitivity in obese adolescent girls: a randomized controlled trial. *American Journal of Physiology. Endocrinology and Metabolism.* 305: E1222–9.

Li, S., Chen, W., Srinivasan, S.R., Bond, M.G., Tang, R., Urbina, E.M. and Berenson, G.S. (2003) Childhood cardiovascular risk factors and carotid vascular changes in adulthood: the Bogalusa Heart Study. *Journal of the American Medical Association* 290: 2271–6.

Liu, M., Wu, L. and Yao, S. (2016) Dose-response association of screen time-based sedentary behaviour in children and adolescents and depression: a meta-analysis of observational studies. *British Journal of Sports Medicine* 50: 1252–8.

Love, R., Adams, J. and van Sluijs, E.M.F. (2019) Are school-based physical activity interventions effective and equitable? A meta-analysis of cluster randomized controlled trials with accelerometer-assessed activity. *Obesity Reviews* 20: 859–70.

Macdonald, H.M., Cooper, D.M. and McKay, H.A. (2009) Anterior-posterior bending strength at the tibial shaft increases with physical activity in boys: evidence for non-uniform geometric adaptation. *Osteoporosis International* 20: 61–70.

Macdonald, H.M., Kontulainen, S.A., Khan, K.M. and McKay, H.A. (2007) Is a school-based physical activity intervention effective for increasing tibial bone strength in boys and girls? *Journal of Bone and Mineral Research* 22: 434–46.

Mann, K.D., Howe, L.D., Basterfield, L., Parkinson, K.N., Pearce, M.S., Reilly, J.K. et al. (2017) Longitudinal study of the associations between change in sedentary behavior and change in adiposity during childhood and adolescence: Gateshead Millennium Study. *International Journal of Obesity* 41: 1042–7.

Mayer-Davis, E.J., Lawrence, J.M., Dabelea, D., Divers, J., Isom, S., Dolan, L. et al.; SEARCH for Diabetes in Youth Study. (2017) Incidence trends of type 1 and type 2 diabetes among youths, 2002–2012. *New England Journal of Medicine* 376: 1419–29.

McGill, H.C., McMahan, C.A., Herderick, E.E., Malcom, G.T., Tracy, R.E. and Strong, J.P. (2000) Origin of atherosclerosis in childhood and adolescence. *The American Journal of Clinical Nutrition* 72: 1307S–15S.

Mead, E., Brown, T., Rees, K., Azevedo, L.B., Whittaker, V., Jones, D. et al. (2017) Diet, physical activity and behavioural interventions for the treatment of overweight or obese children from the age of 6 to 11 years. *The Cochrane Database of Systematic Reviews* 6: CD012651. doi: 10.1002/14651858.CD012651.

Metcalf, B., Henley, W. and Wilkin, T. (2012) Effectiveness of intervention on physical activity of children: systematic review and meta-analysis of controlled trials with objectively measured outcomes (EarlyBird 54). *British Medical Journal* 345: e5888. doi: 10.1136/bmj.e5888.

Metcalf, B.S., Hosking, J., Henley, W.E., Jeffery, A.N., Mostazir, M., Voss, L.D. and Wilkin, T.J. (2015) Physical activity attenuates the mid-adolescent peak in insulin resistance but by late adolescence the effect is lost: a longitudinal study with annual measures from 9–16 years (EarlyBird 66). *Diabetologia* 58: 2699–708.

Metcalf, B.S., Hosking, J., Jeffery, A.N., Voss, L.D., Henley, W. and Wilkin, T.J. (2011) Fatness leads to inactivity, but inactivity does not lead to fatness: a longitudinal study in children (EarlyBird 45). *Archives of Disease in Childhood* 96: 942–7.

Meyer, A.A., Kundt, G., Lenschow, U., Schuff-Werner, P. and Kienast, W. (2006) Improvement of early vascular changes and cardiovascular risk factors in obese children after a six-month exercise program. *Journal of the American College of Cardiology* 48: 1865–70.

Meyer, U., Romann, M., Zahner, L., Schindler, C., Puder, J.J., Kraenzlin, M. et al. (2011) Effect of a general school-based physical activity intervention on bone mineral content and density: a cluster-randomized controlled trial. *Bone* 48: 792–7.

Moran, A., Jacobs, D.R., Steinberger, J., Hong, C.P., Prineas, R., Luepker, R. and Sinaiko, A.R. (1999) Insulin resistance during puberty: results from clamp studies in 357 children. *Diabetes* 48: 2039–44.

NCD Risk Factor Collaboration (NCD-RisC). (2017) Worldwide trends in body-mass index, underweight, overweight, and obesity from 1975 to 2016: a pooled analysis of 2416 population-based measurement studies in 128.9 million children, adolescents, and adults. *The Lancet* 390: 2627–42.

Ortega, F.B., Ruiz, J.R., Castillo, M.J. and Sjöström, M. (2008) Physical fitness in childhood and adolescence: a powerful marker for health. *International Journal of Obesity* 32: 1–11.

Ortega, F.B., Silventoinen, K., Tynelius, P. and Rasmussen, F. (2012) Muscular strength in male adolescents and premature death: cohort study of one million participants. *British Medical Journal* 345: e7279. doi: 10.1136/bmj.e7279.

Pälve, K.S., Pahkala, K., Magnussen, C.G., Koivistoinen, T., Juonala, M., Kähönen, M. et al. (2014) Association of physical activity in childhood and early adulthood with carotid artery elasticity 21 years later: the Cardiovascular Risk in Young Finns Study. *Journal of the American Heart Association* 3: e000594. doi: 10.1161/JAHA.113.000594.

Pinhas-Hamiel, O. and Zeitler, P. (2005) The global spread of type 2 diabetes mellitus in children and adolescents. *The Journal of Pediatrics* 146: 693–700.

Raitakari, O.T., Juonala, M., Kähönen, M., Taittonen, L., Laitinen, T., Mäki-Torkko, N. et al. (2003) Cardiovascular risk factors in childhood and carotid artery intima-media thickness in adulthood: the Cardiovascular Risk in Young Finns Study. *Journal of the American Medical Association* 290: 2277–83.

Reilly, J.J. (2006) Diagnostic accuracy of the BMI for age in paediatrics. *International Journal of Obesity* 30: 595–7.

Reilly, J.J. and Kelly, J. (2011) Long-term impact of overweight and obesity in childhood and ado-lescence on morbidity and premature mortality in adulthood: systematic review. *International Journal of Obesity* 35: 891–8.

Resaland, G.K., Aadland, E., Moe, V.F., Aadland, K.N., Skrede, T., Stavnsbo, M. et al. (2016) Effects of physical activity on schoolchildren's academic performance: The Active Smarter Kids (ASK) cluster-randomized controlled trial. *Preventive Medicine* 91: 322–8.

Riddoch, C.J., Leary, S.D., Ness, A.R., Blair, S.N., Deere, K., Mattocks, C. et al. (2009) Prospec-tive associations between objective measures of physical activity and fat mass in 12–14 year old children: the Avon Longitudinal Study of Parents and Children (ALSPAC). *British Medical Journal* 339: b4544. doi: 10.1136/bmj.b4544.

Ried-Larsen, M., Grøntved, A., Kristensen, P.L., Froberg, K. and Andersen, L.B. (2015) Moderate-and-vigorous physical activity from adolescence to adulthood and subclinical atherosclerosis in adulthood: prospective observations from the European Youth Heart Study. *British Journal of Sports Medicine* 49: 107–12.

Rodriguez-Ayllon, M., Cadenas-Sánchez, C., Estévez-López, F., Muñoz, N.E., Mora-Gonzalez, J., Migueles, J.H. et al. (2019) Role of physical activity and sedentary behavior in the mental health of preschoolers, children and adolescents: a systematic review and meta-analysis. *Sports Medicine* 49: 1383–410.

Ruiz, J.R., Ortega, F.B., Warnberg, J. and Sjöström, M. (2007) Associations of low-grade inflam-mation with physical activity, fitness and fatness in prepubertal children; the European Youth Heart Study. *International Journal of Obesity* 31: 1545–51.

Sardinha, L.B., Baptista, F. and Ekelund, U. (2008) Objectively measured physical activity and bone strength in 9-year-old boys and girls. *Pediatrics* 122: e728–36.

Savoye, M., Caprio, S., Dziura, J., Camp, A., Germain, G., Summers, C. et al. (2014) Reversal of early abnormalities in glucose metabolism in obese youth: results of an intensive lifestyle rand-omized controlled trial. *Diabetes Care* 37: 317–24.

Savoye, M., Nowicka, P., Shaw, M., Yu, S., Dziura, J., Chavent, G. et al. (2011) Long-term results of an obesity program in an ethnically diverse pediatric population. *Pediatrics* 127: 402–10.

Savoye, M., Shaw, M., Dziura, J., Tamborlane, W.V., Rose, P., Guandalini, C. et al. (2007) Effects of a weight management program on body composition and metabolic parameters in overweight chil-dren: a randomized controlled trial. *Journal of the American Medical Association* 297: 2697–704.

Sayers, A., Mattocks, C., Deere, K., Ness, A., Riddoch, C. and Tobias, J.H. (2011) Habitual levels of vigorous, but not moderate or light, physical activity is positively related to cortical bone mass in adolescents. *Journal of Clinical Endocrinology and Metabolism* 96: E793–802.

Sedgwick, M.J., Morris, J.G., Nevill, M.E., Tolfrey, K., Nevill, A. and Barrett, L.A. (2013) Effect of exercise on postprandial endothelial function in adolescent boys. *British Journal of Nutrition* 110: 301–9.

Silventoinen, K., Rokholm, B., Kaprio, J. and Sørensen, T.I. (2010) The genetic and environmental influences on childhood obesity: a systematic review of twin and adoption studies. *International Journal of Obesity* 34: 29–40.

Skinner, A.C. and Skelton, J.A. (2014) Prevalence and trends in obesity and severe obesity among children in the United States, 1999–2012. *Journal of the American Medical Association Pediatrics* 168: 561–6.

Skrede, T., Stavnsbo, M., Aadland, E., Aadland, K.N., Anderssen, S.A., Resaland, G.K. and Ekelund, U. (2017) Moderate-to-vigorous physical activity, but not sedentary time, predicts changes in cardiometabolic risk factors in 10-y-old children: the Active Smarter Kids Study. *The American Journal of Clinical Nutrition* 105: 1391–8.

Stamatakis, E., Coombs, N., Tiling, K., Mattocks, C., Cooper, A., Hardy, L.L. and Lawlor, D.A. (2015) Sedentary time in late childhood and cardiometabolic risk in adolescence. *Pediatrics* 135: e1432–41.

Steele, R.M., van Sluijs, E.M., Cassidy, A., Griffin, S.J. and Ekelund, U. (2009) Targeting sedentary time or moderate- and vigorous-intensity activity: independent relations with adiposity in a population-based sample of 10-y-old British children. *The American Journal of Clinical Nutrition* 90: 1185–92.

Stoner, L., Rowlands, D., Morrison, A., Credeur, D., Hamlin, M., Gaffney, K. et al. (2016) Efficacy of exercise intervention for weight loss in overweight and obese adolescents: meta-analysis and implications. *Sports Medicine* 46: 1737–51.

Tanaka, C., Reilly, J.J. and Huang, W.Y. (2014) Longitudinal changes in objectively measured sedentary behaviour and their relationship with adiposity in children and adolescents: systematic review and evidence appraisal. *Obesity Reviews* 15: 791–803.

Tarp, J., Child, A., White, T., Westgate, K., Bugge, A., Grøntved, A. et al.; International Children's Accelerometry Database (ICAD) Collaborators. (2018) Physical activity intensity, bout-duration, and cardiometabolic risk markers in children and adolescents. *International Journal of Obesity* 42: 1639–50.

Telama, R. (2009) Tracking of physical activity from childhood to adulthood: a review. *Obesity Facts* 2: 187–95.

The Daily Mile Foundation. The Daily Mile [online], available at: www.thedailymile.co.uk (accessed 20 September 2019).

The HEALTHY Study Group. (2010) A school-based intervention for diabetes risk reduction. *New England Journal of Medicine* 363: 443–53.

Tobias, J.H., Steer, C.D., Mattocks, C.G., Riddoch, C. and Ness, A.R. (2007) Habitual levels of physical activity influence bone mass in 11-year-old children from the United Kingdom: findings from a large population-based cohort. *Journal of Bone and Mineral Research* 22: 101–9.

TODAY Study Group. (2012) A clinical trial to maintain glycemic control in youth with type 2 diabetes. *New England Journal of Medicine* 366: 2247–56.

TODAY Study Group. (2013) Effects of metformin, metformin plus rosiglitazone, and metformin plus lifestyle on insulin sensitivity and β-cell function in TODAY. *Diabetes Care* 36: 1749–57.

Tolonen, S., Sievänen, H., Mikkilä, V., Telama, R., Oikonen, M., Laaksonen, M. et al. (2015) Adolescence physical activity is associated with higher tibial pQCT bone values in adulthood after 28-years of follow-up — the Cardiovascular Risk in Young Finns Study. *Bone* 75: 77–83.

Toseeb, U., Brage, S., Corder, K., Dunn, V.J., Jones, P.B., Owens, M. et al. (2014) Exercise and depressive symptoms in adolescents: a longitudinal cohort study. *Journal of the American Medical Association Pediatrics* 168: 1093–100.

Twisk, J.W., Kemper, H.C. and van Mechelen, W. (2002) The relationship between physical fitness and physical activity during adolescence and cardiovascular disease risk factors at adult age. The Amsterdam Growth and Health Longitudinal Study. *International Journal of Sports Medicine* 23: S8–14.

Warden, S.J., Mantila Roosa, S.M., Kersh, M.E., Hurd, A.L., Fleisig, G.S., Pandy, M.G. and Fuchs, R.K. (2014) Physical activity when young provides lifelong benefits to cortical bone size and strength in men. *Proceedings of the National Academy of Sciences of the United States of America* 111: 5337–42.

Weaver, C.M., Gordon, C.M., Janz, K.F., Kalkwarf, H.J., Lappe, J.M., Lewis, R. et al. (2016) The National Osteoporosis Foundation's position statement on peak bone mass development and lifestyle factors: a systematic review and implementation recommendations. *Osteoporosis International* 27: 1281–386.

Wiles, N.J., Haase, A.M., Lawlor, D.A., Ness, A. and Lewis, G. (2012) Physical activity and depression in adolescents: cross-sectional findings from the ALSPAC cohort. *Social Psychiatry and Psychiatric Epidemiology* 47: 1023–33.

Wilks, D.C., Besson, H., Lindroos, A.K. and Ekelund, U. (2011) Objectively measured physical activity and obesity prevention in children, adolescents and adults: a systematic review of prospective studies. *Obesity Reviews* 12: e119–29.

Zimmermann, E., Bjerregaard, L.G., Gamborg, M., Vaag, A.A., Sørensen, T.I.A. and Baker, J.L. (2017) Childhood body mass index and development of type 2 diabetes throughout adult life – a large-scale Danish cohort study. *Obesity* 25: 965–71.

12 Ageing

David J. Stensel

INTRODUCTION

Chapter 1 highlighted that human life expectancy has increased around the world over the past two centuries and there has been a shift in population demographics leading to an increase in the number of older people worldwide. Debate continues as to where the limit of human lifespan lies (the maximum reported age at death is 122 years according to Dong et al. 2016) but the number of centenarians (those aged 100 years and above) and supercentenarians (those aged 110 years and above) continues to increase worldwide demonstrating that even if lifespan is limited to around 110 to 120 years more people are achieving maximal life expectancy. Although this may be considered a positive trend the prevalence of many diseases (e.g. cancer, chronic kidney disease, dementia, diabetes, heart disease) is closely associated with age. This often leads to a prolonged period of morbidity in older adults impairing the quality of life for them and their families and stretching the resources of health-care systems around the world.

Moreover, lifestyle and the ability to live independently may be compromised even in older adults free from disease due to a reduction in physical capacities (e.g. strength, endurance, flexibility) which limits their ability to perform everyday tasks, such as rising from a chair, getting into and out of a bath, climbing a flight of stairs or crossing a road in the time allotted at a pedestrian crossing.

Aside from declines in physical function and mobility, ageing is also associated with a decline in cognitive function and, in severe cases, dementia. Although equivocal, evidence is accumulating to suggest that regular exercise may help to ameliorate some of the age-related decline in cognitive function and reduce the risk of dementia. This chapter examines how ageing leads to a decline in physical capacities and the extent to which this can be offset by frequent exercise. This chapter also assesses evidence that remaining active into old age reduces the risk of mental infirmity, cognitive decline and disease. Collectively, the evidence surveyed here suggests that regular physical activity helps older adults to maintain their independence and quality of life leading to a compressed end-of-life morbidity. Such evidence has led some to suggest that exercise has 'powerful anti-ageing effects' and the ability to provide the Fountain of Youth (Joyner and Barnes 2013). Although there is very limited evidence that exercise can delay primary ageing (due to an inevitable deterioration in cellular structure and function) there are many mechanisms by which exercise can counter the effects of secondary ageing (due to disease and environmental factors) and the evidence for these mechanisms will be explored in this chapter.

DECLINE IN PHYSICAL FUNCTION

The effect of ageing on physical function is clearly demonstrated by examining World Masters Athletics age group records for events such as the 100 m and the marathon. Beyond age 35–40 years, 100 m time and marathon time increase gradually in men and women until the eighth decade of life (70 to 80 years) after which the decline in performance is more dramatic (as displayed by the exponential increase in performance times after age 80 in Figure 12.1). These observations are consistent with findings from the US Masters Swimming Championships, which also reveal a steep decline in performance beyond age 75 to 80 in both men and women (Tanaka and Seals 1997). These examples are based on the few individuals who maintain heavy training/competition, indicating an effect of age *per se* rather than physical inactivity. Age-related declines in sporting performance are due to declines in various aspects of physiological function and these will be examined here, beginning with maximum oxygen uptake.

Many studies have documented a decline in $\dot{V}O_2$max in ageing humans, and this is the main physiological factor underlying the decrease in endurance performance with age. The approximate rate of decline in $\dot{V}O_2$max is 1% per year or 10% per decade from the third decade of life (mid-20s) onwards, although this varies depending on several factors, including physical activity levels. Continual hard training may be able to prevent any decline in $\dot{V}O_2$max until the mid-to-late 30s, and individuals who continue exercising into old age retain higher $\dot{V}O_2$max values than those who stop training or remain untrained. Figure 12.2 illustrates the decline in $\dot{V}O_2$max with age

Figure 12.1 World Masters Athletics 100 m and marathon age group records for men and women.

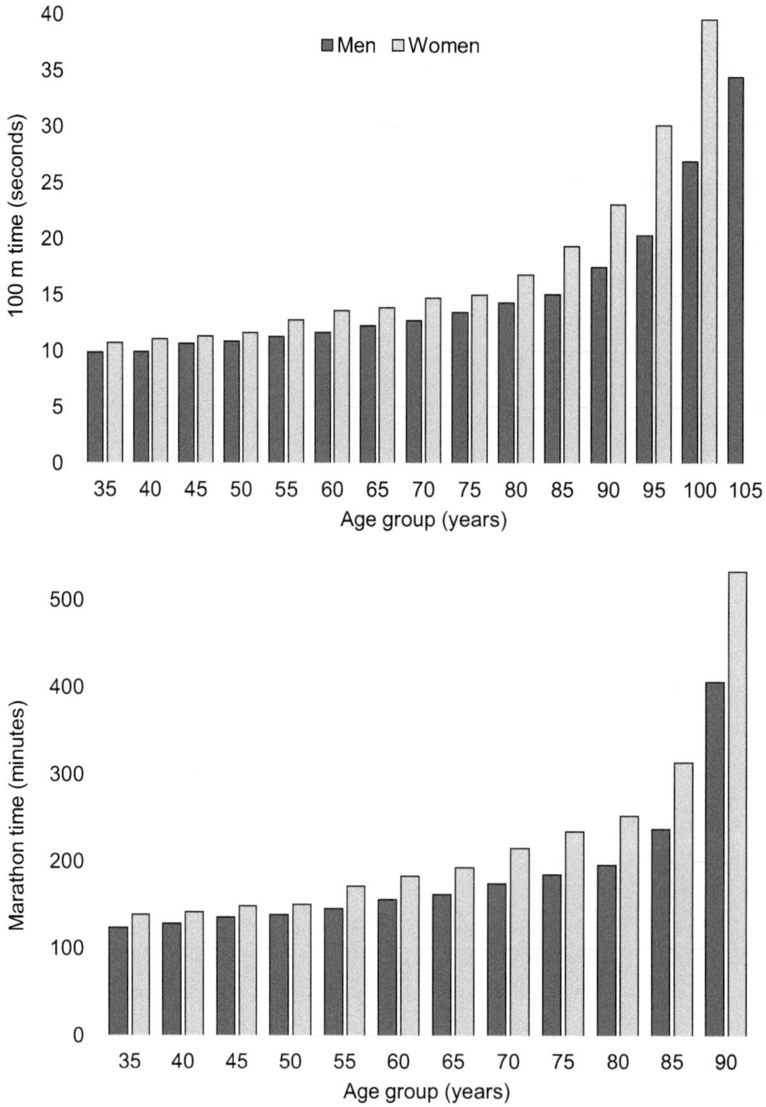

Source: World Masters Athletics records [online], available at: https://world-masters-athletics.com/ (accessed 8 August 2019).
Note: 100 m and marathon times increase gradually in men and women until the eighth decade of life (ages 70 to 80 years), after which times increase exponentially.

using data from the Fitness Registry and the Importance of Exercise National Database (FRIEND). This comprises cross-sectional data from men and women aged 20 to 79 years without cardiovascular disease (Kaminsky et al. 2015). The data were collected from eight laboratories in the US in 2014 and early 2015. A total of 7783 directly

Figure 12.2 Directly measured maximal oxygen uptake ($\dot{V}O_2$max) values for US men and women aged 20 to 79 years from the Fitness Registry and the Importance of Exercise National Database (FRIEND).

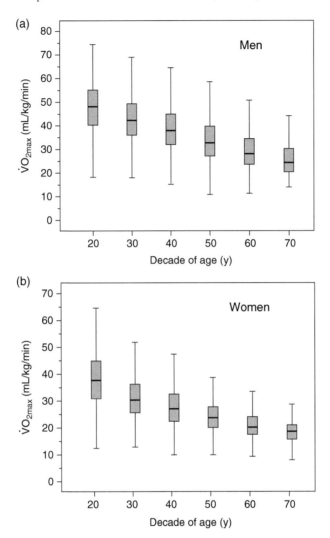

Source: Reprinted from *Mayo Clinic Proceedings*, 90: 1515–23, Kaminsky, L.A. et al., 'Reference standards for cardiorespiratory fitness measured with cardiopulmonary exercise testing: data from the fitness registry and the importance of exercise national database', pages 1518–19, copyright © 2015, with permission from Elsevier.
Note: Box plots display median and interquartile range. Error bars indicate SD. n = 7783.

measured $\dot{V}O_2$max values were obtained and percentile values for men and women were determined for each decade from 20 years of age through to 79 years of age (Table 12.1). In men 50th percentile $\dot{V}O_2$max values decline from 48.0 ml kg^{-1} min^{-1} to 24.4 ml kg^{-1} min^{-1} between the ages of 20–29 and 70–79 years while in women 50th percentile $\dot{V}O_2$max values decline from 37.6 ml kg^{-1} min^{-1} to 18.3 ml kg^{-1} min^{-1} between the ages 20–29 years to 70–79 years. Also evident is the wide range in

Table 12.1 Sex–specific percentiles for directly measured maximum oxygen uptake ($\dot{V}O_2$max, ml kg^{-1} min^{-1}) values (n = 7783) obtained from the Fitness Registry and the Importance of Exercise National Database (FRIEND).

AGE GROUP	PERCENTILES						
	5TH	10TH	25TH	50TH	75TH	90TH	95TH
Men							
20–29	29.0	32.1	40.1	48.0	55.2	61.8	66.3
30–39	27.2	30.2	35.9	42.4	49.2	56.5	59.8
40–49	24.2	26.8	31.9	37.8	45.0	52.1	55.6
50–59	20.9	22.8	27.1	32.6	39.7	45.6	50.7
60–69	17.4	19.8	23.7	28.2	34.5	40.3	43.0
70–79	16.3	17.1	20.4	24.4	30.4	36.6	39.7
Women							
20–29	21.7	23.9	30.5	37.6	44.7	51.3	56.0
30–39	19.0	20.9	25.3	30.2	36.1	41.4	45.8
40–49	17.0	18.8	22.1	26.7	32.4	38.4	41.7
50–59	16.0	17.3	19.9	23.4	27.6	32.0	35.9
60–69	13.4	14.6	17.2	20.0	23.8	27.0	29.4
70–79	13.1	13.6	15.6	18.3	20.8	23.1	24.1

Source: Reprinted from *Mayo Clinic Proceedings*, 90: 1515–23, Kaminsky, L.A. et al., 'Reference standards for cardiorespiratory fitness measured with cardiopulmonary exercise testing: data from the fitness registry and the importance of exercise national database', page 1520, copyright © 2015, with permission from Elsevier.

$\dot{V}O_2$max values for any given age as demonstrated by the 5th and 95th percentile values (Table 12.1).

Although exercise training can help to maintain a high level of aerobic fitness in older adults it cannot prevent values from declining with age and the rate of decline in athletes who continue to train into old age is reported to be similar to that in sedentary individuals (Hawkins and Wiswell 2003) although there may be exceptions. Trappe and colleagues (2013), for example, report $\dot{V}O_2$max values ranging from 34 to 42 ml kg^{-1} min^{-1} in a group of nine lifelong male octogenarian endurance athletes aged 80 to 91 years. According to Trappe and colleagues (2013) these are the highest values ever reported for octogenarians and place them well above the 5 MET (metabolic equivalent) exercise capacity threshold required for maintenance of an independent lifestyle and in the optimal exercise capacity zone for lowering the risk of all-cause mortality (Figure 12.3). The mean $\dot{V}O_2$max value for these octogenarians (38 ml kg^{-1} min^{-1}) are like those of the average 40–49-year-old according to the data collected in the FRIEND study (Kaminsky et al. 2015) (Table 12.1).

The decline in $\dot{V}O_2$max is thought to be largely related to reductions in maximal heart rate and lean body mass (Hawkins and Wiswell 2003) although this may vary depending on the specific age group studied. There is some evidence that the decline in $\dot{V}O_2$max at around age 50 is primarily due to an impaired efficiency of skeletal muscle to extract oxygen. This is indicated by the findings from a follow-up of the classic Dallas Bed Rest and Training Study (McGuire et al. 2001a, 2001b). In the original

Figure 12.3 Individual data from octogenarian lifelong endurance athletes and healthy untrained octogenarians.

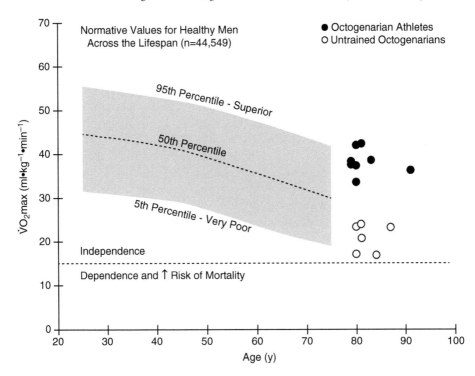

Source: Reproduced from the *Journal of Applied Physiology*, Trappe, S. et al., 114: 3–10, copyright © 2013 with permission from The American Physiological Society.
Note: The dotted line represents the prognostic exercise capacity (5 metabolic equivalents (METs), ml kg^{-1} min^{-1}) generally necessary for an independent lifestyle and associated with an increased risk for mortality as described by Myers et al. (2002). The normative values for healthy men across the lifespan (n = 44,549) were originally obtained from the Cooper Institute in Dallas, Texas, and have been summarised by the American College of Sports Medicine (2010).

study (in 1966), five healthy 20-year-old men were assessed: (1) at baseline; (2) after three weeks of bed rest; and (3) after eight weeks of intensive dynamic exercise training. Follow-up was performed 30 years later (in 1996) when the men were 50 years old. During this 30-year period the men had maintained varying levels of activity. Absolute $\dot{V}O_2$max values were 12% lower (2.9 l min^{-1} versus 3.3 l min^{-1}) and values relative to weight were 28% lower (31 ml kg^{-1} min^{-1} versus 43 ml kg^{-1} min^{-1}) at age 50 compared with age 20. Although maximal heart rate had declined at follow-up, maximal cardiac output remained unchanged due to an increase in maximal stroke volume. Thus, the decline in $\dot{V}O_2$max was entirely due to a 15% reduction in the maximal difference between the oxygen content of arterial and mixed venous blood (arterio-venous oxygen difference). In other words, this study indicates oxygen supply is not compromised with age; rather the ageing process impairs the ability of skeletal muscle to extract and/or utilise oxygen. In contrast, cross-sectional data suggest that a reduced maximum heart rate is the main factor responsible for the decline in $\dot{V}O_2$max in masters athletes compared with young athletes (Heath et al. 1981).

What causes the reduction in oxygen extraction/usage with age? This is not known for certain, but there are several likely causes, the principal one being a loss of muscle mass. Muscle mass is reported to decline by approximately 1% per year from middle age and in severe cases up to 50% of muscle mass may be lost by the eighth to ninth decade of life (Wilkinson et al. 2018). Such losses are due to the combined effects of muscle fibre atrophy and muscle fibre loss (hypoplasia). This is thought to occur due to an imbalance in muscle protein synthesis and muscle protein breakdown due to 'anabolic resistance' which is a desensitisation of aged muscle to anabolic stimuli. There may be several reasons for this anabolic resistance, including an impaired efficiency of the conversion of nutritional/exercise stimuli into signalling impacting mRNA translation and proteolysis. This in turn may be related to oxidative damage cause by factors such as reactive oxygen and nitrogen species, lipid infiltration into muscle, muscle inflammation and physical inactivity. There are also reports of a loss of motor units (determined by imaging electromyography, iEMG) with age (for a review of these factors see Wilkinson et al. 2018). Associated with these factors are declines in mitochondrial respiration and biogenesis possibly linked with age-related insulin resistance (Cartee et al. 2016). Although exercise training cannot completely prevent such changes, cross-sectional studies of lifelong exercisers demonstrate remarkably high levels of muscle capillarisation and oxidative enzymes including citrate synthase, β-hydroxyacyl-CoA dehydrogenase and glycogen phosphorylase (Gries et al. 2018) as well as elevated levels of the peroxisome proliferator-activated receptor-γ coactivator 1a (PGC-1a) and mitochondrial transcription factor A mRNA demonstrating an up-regulation of genes involved in mitochondrial biogenesis (Trappe et al. 2013).

Muscular strength is another key functional capacity which declines with age. According to the American College of Sports Medicine, strength declines occur from around 40 years of age, accelerate after age 65–70 years and occur at a faster rate in the lower body than the upper body (Chodzko-Zajko et al. 2009). An example of the decline in muscle strength with age is illustrated in Figure 12.4. These data are from a cross-sectional study of 45–78-year-old men and women. Muscle strength was determined using an isokinetic dynamometer. Note that ageing is associated with impaired muscle strength in both men and women (Frontera et al. 1991). When the data in Figure 12.4 are expressed per kilogram of muscle mass the differences between the age groups become smaller and there is no significant difference between the strength of males and females. This supports the hypothesis that the decline in muscle strength with age is largely due to a decline in muscle mass (a condition termed 'sarcopenia'). Such declines have been demonstrated in longitudinal studies documenting reductions in muscle cross-sectional area (assessed using computerised tomography) over time (Frontera et al. 2000). Minimising age-related declines in muscular strength is important because reductions in strength are predictive of disability in old age and increased mortality risk.

The reductions in maximum oxygen uptake and muscle strength are among the most notable and possibly the most debilitating effects of ageing, but many other aspects of physiological function decline with age including lung function (vital capacity and forced expiratory volume), resting metabolic rate (largely due to the reduction in fat-free mass), flexibility and joint range of motion. Impaired balance and gait are additional hazards of ageing and these are significant risk factors for limited mobility and

Figure 12.4 Decline in isokinetic muscle strength ($60° \text{ s}^{-1}$) of the knee extensors of the dominant side in men and women.

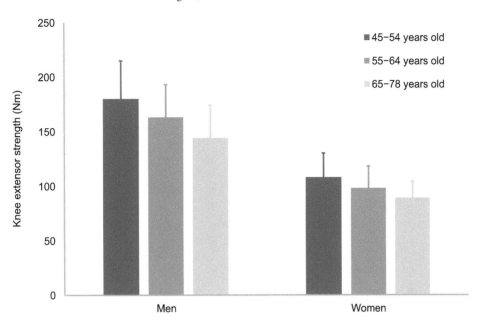

Source: Frontera et al. (1991).

falls in older adults. Many people also gain weight as they age, and this may further impair general mobility (Chodzko-Zajko et al. 2009).

The extent to which the decline in physical characteristics with ageing is a result of ageing *per se* rather than a decline in physical activity is a matter of debate. It is well recognised that physical activity levels decline with age. Using energy expenditure data acquired from the doubly labelled water technique, Westerterp (2015) observed that physical activity levels (calculated as daily energy expenditure divided by resting energy expenditure) are around 1.4 at age 1 and increase to around 1.75 by age 15. Between the ages of 18 and 50 to 55 values average 1.75 in women and 1.84 in men. After age 55 physical activity levels are generally lower and they decrease to a value of around 1.3 for both sexes in participants aged 90 to 100 years (Figure 12.5). This decline is not peculiar to humans and occurs across a wide range of non-human species, including rodents, nematodes (microscopic worms), houseflies, fruit flies, monkeys and dogs (Ingram 2000). Based on these findings it would appear that at least some of the decline in physical activity with age has a biological basis. In humans, however, some of the age-related decline in physical activity is likely due to environmental factors, i.e. modern conveniences (cars, televisions, lifts, escalators, etc.), which limit the requirement to be physically active. Low levels of physical activity in old age are not inevitable. The octogenarian lifelong endurance athletes examined by Trappe and colleagues (2013) recorded an average of 8000 steps per day in comparison with 4300 in an age-matched untrained group. This implies that some of the reductions in physical function with age may be due to disuse rather than ageing *per se*. If this is true, then physical activity

Figure 12.5 Physical activity level for men and women with increasing age.

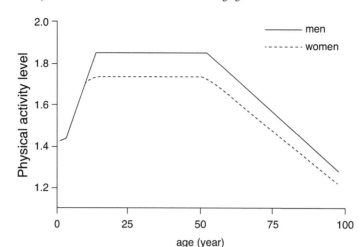

Source: Reprinted with no modifications from 'Daily physical activity as determined by age, body mass and energy balance', Westerterp, K.R., *European Journal of Applied Physiology*, 2015, 115: 1177–84. Article distributed under the terms of the Creative Commons Attribution 4.0 International (CC BY) Licence (https://creativecommons.org/licenses/by/4.0/).
Note: Values are calculated as daily energy expenditure divided by resting energy expenditure. Daily energy expenditure values were calculated using doubly labelled water.

and exercise training may counteract some of the decline in physical function in older adults. The next section examines evidence that aspects of physiological function can be improved in older adults who engage in exercise training.

EXERCISE TRAINING AND PHYSICAL FUNCTION

Exercise training can profoundly influence physical function in older individuals. Again, World Masters Athletics records are informative here. The world record marathon record time for men aged 70–74 is sub-three hours (2:54:48) and for men aged 80–84 it is only just outside three and a quarter hours (3:15:54). For women aged 70–74 the world record marathon time is just over three and a half hours (3:35:29) and for women aged 80–84 it is under four and a quarter hours (4:11:45). Examination of the age group times for 100 m reveals equally impressive accomplishments. World record times for men and women aged 70–74 are 12.77 and 14.73 seconds respectively and for men and women aged 80–84 the times are 14.35 and 16.81 seconds respectively (https://world-masters-athletics.com/, accessed 8 August 2019). These are remarkable performances, and the average 25-year-old male or female would have difficulty matching them. These performances are possible due to a combination of genetic make-up and continual – probably lifelong – hard training. Evidence shows, however, that even untrained older adults can adapt and benefit from exercise training.

Cardiovascular fitness and muscular strength are the two best-studied physical capacities in older adults. A noteworthy study of cardiovascular fitness involved 16 previously untrained men and women aged 70–79 years old (Hagberg et al. 1989). These individuals followed a 26-week endurance-training programme involving walking and slow jogging. Sessions were conducted three times per week. Exercise intensity range was 50–70% of $\dot{V}O_2$max during the first half of the programme and increased to 75–85% of $\dot{V}O_2$max during the second half of the programme. This resulted in an 18% increase in $\dot{V}O_2$max expressed in absolute units (1.88 l min^{-1} versus 1.59 l min^{-1}) and a 20% increase in $\dot{V}O_2$max expressed in relative units (27.1 ml kg^{-1} min^{-1} versus 22.5 ml kg^{-1} min^{-1}). These data demonstrate that men and women retain the ability to respond to exercise training during their eighth decade of life, while another study observed a 15% increase in $\dot{V}O_2$max in women who were in their ninth decade of life (i.e. women aged 79–91) after 24 weeks of exercise training (Malbut et al. 2002).

A further study demonstrating that $\dot{V}O_2$max remains trainable in older individuals is the follow-up to the Dallas Bed Rest and Training Study referred to in the previous section (McGuire et al. 2001a, 2001b). The original study (conducted in 1966) examined aspects of physiological function before and after three weeks of bed rest, and then again after eight weeks of training. In the follow-up study, conducted 30 years later (in 1996), cardiovascular responses to sub-maximal and maximal exercise were examined before and after a six-month endurance-training programme. This programme resulted in a significant improvement in $\dot{V}O_2$max, such that post-training values (l min^{-1}) in 1996 were similar to pre-bed rest values in 1966 (Figure 12.6). The investigators concluded that three weeks of bed rest at age 20 had a more profound effect on $\dot{V}O_2$max

Figure 12.6 Maximum oxygen uptake ($\dot{V}O_2$max) in five male subjects before and after training in 1966 and again in 1996. Subjects were 20 years old in 1966.

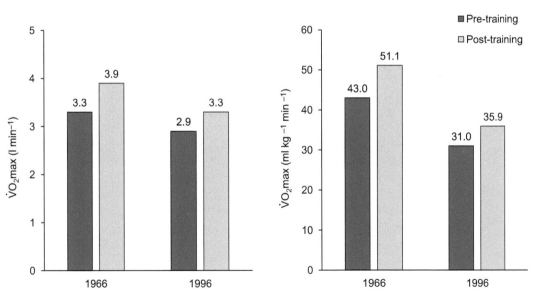

Source: Adapted from McGuire et al. (2001b).
Note: The mean $\dot{V}O_2$max value attained after training in 1996 is the same as the mean pre-training $\dot{V}O_2$max value attained in 1966 when expressed in l min^{-1}. This is not the case when values are expressed in ml kg^{-1} min^{-1} because the participants were 19 kg heavier in 1996 compared with 1966 (96 versus 77 kg).

than did three decades of ageing. Furthermore, 100% of the age-related decline in $\dot{V}O_2$max was reversed by a six-month endurance training programme. However, no subject achieved the same $\dot{V}O_2$max attained after the eight weeks of training undertaken 30 years earlier. This study clearly demonstrates the combined effects of ageing and physical inactivity on $\dot{V}O_2$max.

The increase in $\dot{V}O_2$max after training in the follow-up to the Dallas Bed Rest and Training Study was primarily the result of peripheral adaptation, with no improvement in maximal oxygen delivery. Maximal heart rate was decreased after training compared with before training in 1996, but maximal cardiac output remained unchanged due to an increase in maximal stroke volume. The maximal arteriovenous oxygen increased by 10%, however, and this was the key factor for the increase in $\dot{V}O_2$max in the 50-year-old men (McGuire et al. 2001b). Another study has reported that increases in $\dot{V}O_2$max with endurance exercise are due to increases in both stroke volume and maximal arteriovenous oxygen difference in older men, while in older women oxygen extraction may be more important (Spina et al. 1993).

Several factors could be responsible for an improvement in maximal arteriovenous oxygen difference after endurance training in older individuals. These include increases in skeletal muscle tissue (Figure 12.7), as well as increases in capillary density, mitochondrial content and oxidative enzyme activity. Cross-sectional findings support such mechanisms (Broskey et al. 2014; Coggan et al. 1990; Gries et al. 2018; Trappe et al. 2013) as do training studies. In one study, 60–70-year-old men and women participated in a prolonged period (9–12 months) of endurance training involving walking/jogging at 80% of maximal heart rate for 45 minutes per day, four days per week (Coggan et al. 1992). Needle biopsy samples of the lateral gastrocnemius (calf) muscle obtained before and after training revealed significant increases in capillary density (Figure 12.8) and several enzymes associated with oxidative metabolism, including succinate dehydrogenase, citrate synthase and β-hydroxyacyl-CoA dehydrogenase (Table 12.2). A significant increase in the percentage of type IIa muscle fibres, together with a significant decrease in the percentage of type IIb muscle fibres, was also noted post-training in this study. Another study has documented increases in skeletal muscle mitochondrial content in response to a 16-week, moderate-intensity, aerobic exercise training intervention in previously sedentary adults aged 60 to 80 years (Broskey et al. 2014). These are qualitatively the same changes as those seen in young adults and would enhance stamina/resistance to fatigue. They demonstrate that the skeletal muscle of older men and women retains its ability to adapt to endurance training.

As well as retaining its ability to adapt to endurance training, skeletal muscle also retains its ability to adapt to strength training in older adults. Cross-sectional comparisons demonstrate skeletal muscle hypertrophy in strength trained individuals, and exercise training studies confirm that adaption is possible after relatively brief periods of training. This is demonstrated by a study involving 12 previously untrained men aged 60–72 who completed a 12-week strength-training programme (Frontera et al. 1988). Training was conducted three days per week at an intensity of 80% of one-repetition maximum. Three sets of eight repetitions were completed for the knee extensors and knee flexors on each training day. The findings demonstrated a progressive increase in muscle strength in both the knee flexors and knee extensors over the 12 weeks of the programme (Figure 12.9a). Alongside the increase in strength, there was an increase

Figure 12.7 Typical quadriceps MRI scan of a 40-year-old triathlete, compared with the quadriceps MRI scans of a 70-year-old triathlete and a 74-year-old sedentary man.

40-year-old triathlete

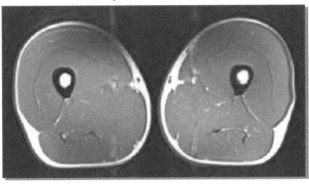

74-year-old sedentary man

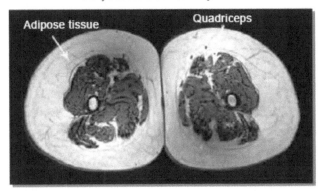

70-year-old triathlete

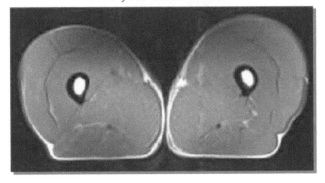

Source: Reprinted by permission of Taylor & Francis Ltd: 'Chronic exercise preserves lean muscle mass in masters athletes', Wroblewski, A.P. et al., *Physician and Sportsmedicine*, 39: 172–8, 2011.
Note: The scan from the sedentary man exhibits a high level of subcutaneous adipose tissue, lower contractile mass and infiltration of fat and connective tissue. Minimal differences are apparent between the images of the younger and older triathlete.

Figure 12.8 Increased capillary density in the gastrocnemius muscles of 60–70-year-old men and women after a 9–12-month period of endurance training.

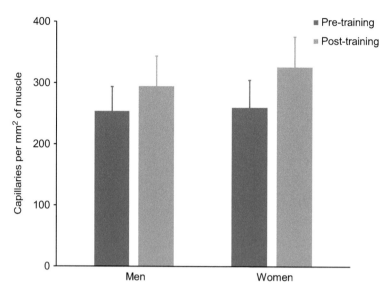

Source: Coggan et al. (1992).
Note: Mean values are displayed. Error bars indicate SD.

Table 12.2 Increased oxidative enzyme activities (mol kg protein^{-1} hour^{-1}) in the gastrocnemius muscles of 60–70-year-old men and women following a 9–12-month period of endurance training.

	MALES		FEMALES	
	PRE-TRAINING	POST-TRAINING	PRE-TRAINING	POST-TRAINING
Succinate dehydrogenase	1.11 ± 0.29	1.83 ± 0.63	0.76 ± 0.29	1.05 ± 0.39
Citrate synthase	2.97 ± 0.71	3.83 ± 1.10	2.21 ± 0.41	2.58 ± 0.55
β-hydroxyacyl-CoA dehydrogenase	5.95 ± 1.03	8.45 ± 2.72	5.29 ± 1.55	7.19 ± 1.54

Source: Coggan et al. (1992).

Note: Values are mean ± SD. The standard unit for enzyme activity is μmoles min^{-1} g wet weight^{-1}. Values in the table should be multiplied by a factor of three to give an approximate conversion to the standard unit. This assumes that muscle contains 20% protein (wet weight).

in quadriceps muscle cross-sectional area as determined by computerised tomography scans (Figure 12.9b). This muscle hypertrophy was in turn due to an increase in both type I and type II muscle fibre area. These findings have been confirmed by several other studies which collectively illustrate that older men and women retain the ability to increase muscular strength with resistance training with increases ranging from less than 25% to greater than 100% (Chodzko-Zajko et al. 2009). Such gains could have

Figure 12.9 Responses to a 12-week strength training programme in men aged 60 to 72 years. Panel a: Improvements in dynamic muscle strength (one-repetition maximum) of the knee extensors and knee flexors. Panel b: Increases in the cross-sectional area of the quadriceps muscles.

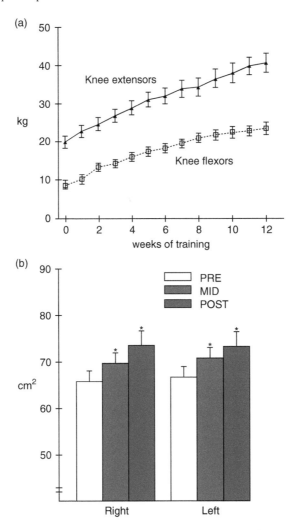

Source: Reproduced from the *Journal of Applied Physiology*, Frontera, W.R. et al., 64: 1038–44, copyright © 1988 with permission from The American Physiological Society.
Note: Mean values are displayed. Error bars are SEM. Muscle cross-sectional area was assessed using computerised tomography.

important implications for the daily living activities of older adults (e.g. the ability to rise from a chair, climb stairs or unscrew the top from a bottle or jar).

Exercise training has been recommended for older individuals for a variety of reasons beyond any effects on $\dot{V}O_2$max and muscle strength. Potential benefits include improvements in body composition (reduced fat mass and increased fat free mass) as well as in postural stability and flexibility. Postural stability refers to the ability of an individual to retain balance which is directly related to the risk of falling among older adults. Flexibility refers to the range of motion of single or multiple joints, and this affects the ability to perform specific tasks. There is evidence supporting the use of exercise as a means of improving balance and flexibility in older individuals (Chodzko-Zajko et al. 2009; Daley and Spinks 2000). Finally, the benefits of exercise described in this section are not limited to older adults who are already fit and healthy; exercise training is effective for improving physical capacities even in frail older people (Chin A Paw et al. 2008).

MOBILITY, DISABILITY AND INDEPENDENT LIVING

The decreases in physical capacities noted above have important implications for the ability to perform many activities of daily living. Unfortunately, decreases in physical capacities (walking speed, quadriceps strength, joint flexibility) often go unnoticed until a threshold is reached when a person has difficulty performing a particular task (e.g. crossing a road in time, getting up from a low chair, climbing stairs, opening the cap on a jar, putting socks on). This results in a loss of independence and an inability to participate fully in life. As might be expected, the number of people reporting that they are unable to perform one or more activities of daily living increases with age (Daley and Spinks 2000).

Longitudinal studies in older adults strongly suggest that physical activity reduces the risk of disability and morbidity. An interesting example is a study involving 538 runners and 423 controls aged 50 and older who were followed for 21 years (Chakravarty et al. 2008). All participants were healthy at baseline. Disability was assessed by the Health Assessment Questionnaire Disability Index which assesses functional ability in eight areas: rising, dressing and grooming, hygiene, eating, walking, reach, grip and routine physical activities. Scores on this index were higher in controls than runners at all time points (indicating greater difficulty in performing certain tasks). Scores increased with age in both groups, but to a lesser degree in runners. After 19 years, 15% of runners had died compared with 34% of controls. Disability and survival curves continued to diverge between runners and controls after the 21 years of follow-up and runners were less likely to suffer from cardiovascular disease, coronary heart disease, stroke, cancer or neurological illness than controls. There are clear limitations to this study, most importantly the potential for self-selection bias (Mackey 2008), but such findings are important for stimulating further research employing randomised controlled trials (RCTs) as discussed later in this section.

Aside from vigorous physical activities like running, the level of proficiency in performing everyday tasks is also related to the risk of disability. This was demonstrated in a four-year follow-up study involving 1122 non-disabled persons (71 years of age or older) living in Iowa. Lower-extremity function was assessed by measuring standing balance, a timed 2.4 m walk at a normal pace and a timed test of five repetitions of rising from a chair and sitting down. Those attaining the lowest performance scores on these tests were found to be between 4.2 and 4.9 times more likely to have a disability at four years as those attaining the highest performance scores. The authors concluded that older persons with a preclinical stage of disability may benefit from interventions to prevent the development of frank disability (Guralnik et al. 1995). Another study involving 3075 community-dwelling adults aged 70–79 observed that long-distance corridor walk performance was inversely related to mobility limitation, mobility disability and CVD risk over a 4.9-year period (Newman et al. 2006).

Although informative, the previous examples are all limited by the observational study designs. Several intervention trials have been conducted to assess the extent to which exercise training can enhance the ability to perform activities of daily living in older adults. Some of these trials have been conducted in individuals living in nursing homes, others have assessed community-dwelling older adults. Although the findings are not unanimous, several intervention studies show that exercise training, particularly resistance/weight training, can help to restore physical function, thus improving quality of life and the ability for independent living.

The importance of leg strength for walking endurance was demonstrated by a randomised intervention trial conducted in healthy men and women aged 65–79 years. Exercise intervention involved a 12-week resistance-training programme. This programme consisted of three sets of eight repetitions of seven exercises on three days per week. Resistance was initially set at 50% of one-repetition maximum and was increased to 80% of one-repetition maximum by week nine. This programme led to a significant improvement in leg strength and walking endurance at 80% of baseline $\dot{V}O_2$max (Figure 12.10). $\dot{V}O_2$max was unaltered by the training programme (Ades et al. 1996).

The potential of resistance training to counteract physical frailty has also been demonstrated in a RCT involving 100 very old people (mean age of 87 years; age range of 72–98 years) resident in a nursing home (Fiatarone et al. 1994). Participants in the

Figure 12.10 A 12-week weight training programme improves leg strength (one-repetition maximum) and walking endurance (time to exhaustion at 80% of $\dot{V}O_2$max) in healthy men and women aged 65 to 79 years.

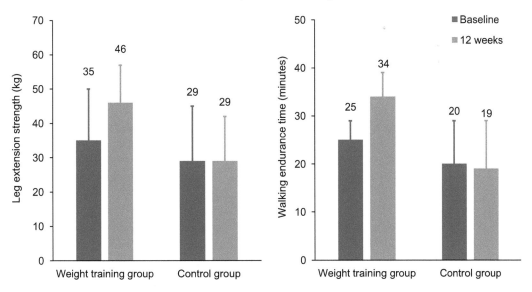

Source: Ades et al. (1996).
Note: Mean values are displayed. Error bars are SD.

	CONTROL GROUP (N = 26)	EXERCISE GROUP (N = 25)
Muscle strength	3 ± 9	113 ± 8
Walking speed	−1 ± 4	12 ± 4
Stair-climbing power	4 ± 7	28 ± 7
Thigh-muscle area	−2 ± 2	3 ± 2

Table 12.3 Percentage change (mean ± SEM) in muscle strength, walking speed, stair-climbing power and thigh-muscle cross-sectional area in frail nursing home residents (mean age 87 years, range 72 to 98 years) after a ten-week resistance exercise training programme.

Source: Fiatarone et al. (1994).

Note: The exercise programme targeted the hip and knee extensors and was conducted at 80% of one-repetition maximum. Three sessions were conducted each week and each session lasted for 45 minutes. Muscle strength of the hip and knee extensors was assessed using a dynamic concentric one-repetition maximum test. Walking speed was measured over a 6.1 m course. Stair climbing power was calculated using a four-riser staircase with banisters. Thigh-muscle cross-sectional area was quantified using computed tomography.

exercise intervention group followed a high-intensity (80% of one-repetition maximum) ten-week progressive-resistance training programme (three sessions per week) targeting the hip and knee extensors. This programme increased muscle strength, walking speed, stair-climbing power and thigh muscle cross-sectional area (Table 12.3). There was also an increase in spontaneous physical activity in the resistance-training group (assessed using activity monitors worn around both ankles). Over the same period there were small but significant reductions in walking speed and thigh muscle cross-sectional area in non-exercising participants. The authors concluded that 'high-intensity resistance exercise training is a feasible and effective means of counteracting muscle weakness and physical frailty in very elderly people' (Fiatarone et al. 1994: p. 1769).

More recently Pahor and colleagues (2014) conducted the Lifestyle Interventions and Independence for Elders (LIFE) study (a multicentre, randomised trial) to test the hypothesis that a long-term structured physical activity programme is more effective than a health education programme in reducing the risk of major mobility disability. This study involved 1635 sedentary men and women aged 70 to 89 years who had physical limitations, defined as a score on the Short Physical Performance Battery of 9 or below, but were able to walk 400 m. Participants were randomised to a structured, moderate-intensity physical activity programme (n = 818) or to a health education programme (n = 817). The physical activity programme was conducted in a centre (twice/week) and at home (three to four times/week) and included aerobic, resistance, and flexibility training activities. The health education programme consisted of workshops on topics relevant to older adults and upper extremity stretching exercises. The primary outcome of the study was major mobility disability objectively defined by loss of ability to walk 400 m. Follow-up duration was 2.6 years. Compared with the health education programme the physical activity intervention significantly reduced major mobility disability (hazard ratio, 0.82; $P = 0.03$), persistent mobility disability (hazard ratio,

0.72; P = 0.006), and the combined outcome of major mobility disability or death (hazard ratio, 0.82; P = 0.02) demonstrating the effectiveness of physical activity for reducing major mobility disability over 2.6 years among older adults at risk for disability (Pahor et al. 2014). These findings have been confirmed by a one-year randomised intervention trial demonstrating that unsupervised walking exercise is effective for preventing mobility loss and improving walking velocity in participants with peripheral artery disease (McDermott et al. 2015).

Another recent study has examined the effect of exercise intervention on functional decline in 'very elderly' patients experiencing acute hospitalisation (Martinez-Velilla et al. 2019). This is an important question to address because muscle and bone loss may occur within days of bed rest such as that experienced during acute hospitalisation. This study was conducted in an acute care unit in a public hospital in Navarra, Spain. A total of 370 patients with a mean age of 87 (SD 5) years (130 nonagenarians) were randomly assigned to an exercise or control (usual care) intervention. On average the patients had nine comorbidities. The usual care group received physical rehabilitation 'when needed' while the in-hospital exercise intervention group performed individualised, moderate-intensity resistance, balance and walking exercises for 20 minutes twice daily (morning and evening) for five to seven consecutive days. The primary end point in this study was change in functional capacity from baseline to hospital discharge, assessed with the Barthel Index of independence and the Short Physical Performance Battery (SPPB). The median length of hospital stay was eight days in both groups and the median duration of the intervention was five days. At discharge, the exercise group showed a mean increase of 2.2 points on the SPPB scale and 6.9 points on the Barthel Index over the usual-care group. Hospitalisation led to an impairment in functional capacity, but the exercise intervention reversed this trend. Significant intervention benefits were also found at the cognitive level (assessed using the Mini-Mental State Examination questionnaire) and no adverse effects were observed with the intervention. The investigators concluded that the exercise intervention was safe and effective to reverse the functional decline associated with acute hospitalisation in very elderly patients (Martinez-Velilla et al. 2019).

The findings from intervention studies such as the ones described here demonstrate that exercise training offers a valuable means of maintaining physical capacities and mobility throughout adult life as well as preventing or minimising disability. Two recent papers (both involving a systematic review and meta-analysis of RCTs) also demonstrate that exercise – either alone or in combination with other interventions – is effective for reducing the risk of falls in older adults (de Souto Barreto et al. 2019; Tricco et al. 2017). Collectively such evidence is strongly supportive of the role of exercise for preserving independence and quality of life in older adults. An area of increasing interest in recent years is the intriguing question of whether regular exercise can assist in preserving cognitive function and lowering the risk of dementia in older adults. These topics will be addressed in the next two sections.

COGNITIVE FUNCTION

As with physical function, cognitive function also declines with age and in severe cases this can lead to dementia. Many studies have demonstrated an association between higher levels of physical activity in middle age/old age and a lower risk of cognitive decline or a reduced rate of cognitive decline although most of this evidence is observational and reverse causation is a possible explanation. Noteworthy examples of observational studies linking low levels of physical activity with cognitive impairment include the Nurses' Health Study, the INVADE (Intervention Project on Cerebrovascular Diseases and Dementia in the Community of Ebersberg, Bavaria) Study, the Health, Aging and Body Composition (Health ABC) Study and the Women's Antioxidant Cardiovascular Study (WACS). A report from the Nurses' Health Study observed that long-term regular physical activity, including walking, was associated with significantly better cognitive function and less cognitive decline in 18,766 US women aged 70 to 81 years (Weuve et al. 2004). These findings were confirmed by the INVADE Study which involved a two-year follow-up of 3903 men and women aged above 55 years living in southern Bavaria, Germany (Etgen et al. 2010). Vercambre and colleagues (2011) studied women with vascular disease or at least three coronary heart disease risk factors in the WACS. A total of 2809 women aged 65 years or older were followed for an average of 5.4 years. Again, regular physical activity, including walking, was associated with better preservation of cognitive function. Finally, the Health ABC Study examined 197 initially healthy men and women (mean age 74.8 years) whose physical activity was assessed at baseline using doubly labelled water and whose cognitive function was assessed at baseline and again two years and five years later. Greater activity energy expenditure at baseline was associated with a lower risk of cognitive impairment in a dose–response manner (Middleton et al. 2011).

The observational findings discussed above are supported by the outcomes of RCTs. Although fewer in number and involving smaller sample sizes the findings from RCTs back up and extend those of observational studies. One example is a six-month exercise intervention RCT involving 16 men and 17 women (mean age 70; range 55 to 85 years) with amnestic (memory loss) mild cognitive impairment. This study examined the effects of aerobic exercise on multiple tests of executive function (a set of cognitive processes necessary for the cognitive control of behaviour). Aerobic exercise was supervised and involved exercise on a treadmill, stationary bicycle or elliptical trainer at an intensity of 75%–85% of heart rate reserve for 45–60 mins per day, four days per week. The control group performed stretching and balance exercises at less than 50% of heart rate reserve. Aerobic exercise was effective for improving executive function in women but not men (despite comparable gains in cardiorespiratory fitness). The reason for this sex difference is not clear but it may be a statistical artefact (due to the small sample size) or it might be related to the observed difference in cortisol response: cortisol decreased in the women in response to the aerobic exercise intervention while increasing slightly in the men (elevated cortisol has been linked to memory impairment) (Baker et al. 2010). A larger RCT conducted in Vancouver involving 155 community-dwelling women aged 65–75 years demonstrated that 12 months of once-weekly or twice-weekly resistance training benefited executive cognitive function (assessed by performance on the Stroop test) compared with twice-weekly balance and tone training (Liu-Ambrose et al. 2010).

To enhance understanding of how exercise affects brain function some studies have sought to assess changes in brain structure and volume in response to exercise. A notable example is the Cardiovascular Health Cognition Study which followed 299 men and women (mean age 78 years) over 13 years. A primary outcome of this study was grey matter – a major component of the central nervous system consisting of neuronal cell bodies (nerve cells), unmyelinated axons, synapses and capillaries. Physical activity was assessed as the number of blocks walked during a one-week period. Grey matter volume was assessed nine years after physical activity assessment using high-resolution, magnetic resonance imaging (MRI) brain scans and cognitive function was assessed 13 years after baseline by clinical adjudication. The study observed greater grey matter volumes in four areas of the brain (left precentral gyrus, supplementary motor area, precuneus and hippocampus) in those in the highest quartile for physical activity (walking 72 blocks or more per week which the investigators estimated was equivalent to 6 to 9 miles per week). Moreover, greater grey matter volume with physical activity was associated with a halving of the risk of cognitive impairment at the end of follow-up (Erickson et al. 2010). These findings have recently been confirmed by those of a cross-sectional study involving 2354 participants in the Framingham Heart Study (Figure 12.11). In this study accelerometer-measured light-intensity physical activity (200–1486 counts per min.) was associated with larger brain volume. The investigators estimated that each additional hour of light-intensity physical activity was associated with 1.1 years less brain ageing and achieving 10,000 steps per day was associated with a higher brain volume compared with those achieving fewer than 5000 steps per day (Spartano et al. 2019). Another recent study has observed an association between slow walking speed in midlife (age 45) and several markers of adverse neurocognitive function and brain health in midlife including smaller brain volume, more cortical thinning and smaller cortical surface area (Rasmussen et al. 2019).

Figure 12.11 Association of physical activity with total cerebral brain volume (TCBV) by age category.

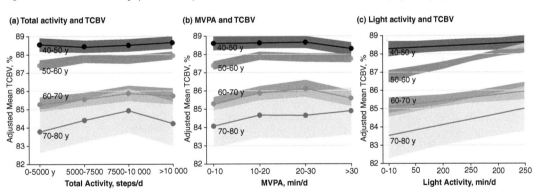

Source: Reprinted with no modifications from 'Association of accelerometer-measured light-intensity physical activity with brain volume: The Framingham Heart Study', Spartano, N.L. et al., *Journal of the American Medical Association Network Open*, 2019, 2: e192745. Article distributed under the terms of the Creative Commons Attribution 4.0 International (CC BY) Licence (https://creativecommons.org/licenses/by/4.0/).

Note: Shaded areas indicate SE bars; MVPA, moderate-to-vigorous physical activity. Physical activity was measured using accelerometers. Brain volume was determined by MRI. Values are adjusted for age, sex, smoking status and other covariates. Light-intensity physical activity 200–1486 counts per min.; MVPA >1486 counts per min. Achieving 10,000 or more steps per day was associated with higher brain volume compared with those achieving fewer than 5000 steps per day. The strongest associations were noted for light-intensity physical activity in those aged 50 years and above. MVPA was not significantly associated with TCBV after adjusting for light-intensity physical activity.

Several RCTs have been conducted to test the hypothesis that high levels of physical activity reduce the shrinkage of brain volume which occurs with ageing. Possibly the most eloquent of these is a study conducted by Erickson and colleagues (2011) published in the Proceedings of the National Academy of Sciences. In this study 120 older adults were randomly assigned to either an aerobic exercise intervention involving walking (n = 60, 73% female, mean age 67.6 years) or a stretching and toning control condition (n = 60; 60% female, mean age 65.5 years). The duration of the intervention was 12 months. The walking intervention resulted in a small but significant increase in $\dot{V}O_2$max (21.4 to 22.6 ml kg^{-1} min^{-1}) which remained unchanged in the control group (21.8 to 21.9 ml kg^{-1} min^{-1}). Assessment of brain volume by MRI revealed significant (2%) increases in left and right hippocampus brain volume in the aerobic exercise group while decreases (1.4%) were noted in the control group (Figure 12.12). Aerobic exercise

Figure 12.12 Increase in left and right hippocampus volume in response to a one-year walking intervention (exercise) in older adults.

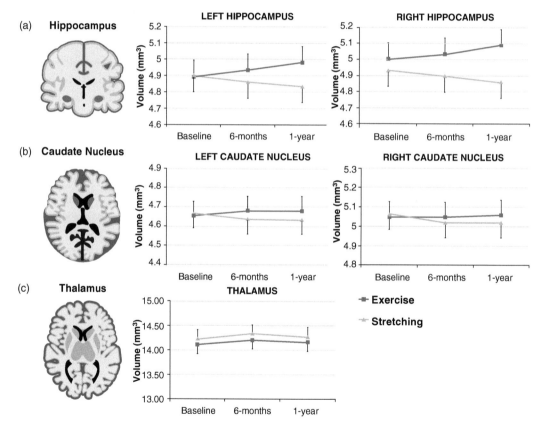

Source: Reprinted with permission from Erickson, K.I. et al. (2011) 'Exercise training increases size of hippocampus and improves memory', *Proceedings of the National Academy of Sciences* 108: 3017–22.
Note: The hippocampus is a part of the brain that is essential for memory but is sensitive to ageing and neurodegeneration. Walking exercise increased hippocampus volume in older adults. In contrast values decreased in the stretching control group. Walking duration was ten minutes per session at the beginning of the intervention, building to 40 minutes per session by week seven and maintained at this level thereafter. Walking frequency was three days per week. Changes in caudate nucleus and thalamus volumes were not significant.

also led to improvements in memory (assessed by a computerised spatial memory task) and significant correlations were observed between changes in left and right hippocampus volume and: a) change in $\dot{V}O_2$max; b) change in brain derived neurotropic factor (BDNF: see below); and c) change in memory performance (Erickson et al. 2011). These findings have since been confirmed by a six-month RCT involving 86 women aged 70 to 80 years with probable mild cognitive impairment. Aerobic exercise was found to increase left and right hippocampus volume by 5.6% and 2.5% respectively although this was not associated with improvements in memory, possibly due to white matter degeneration because of mild cognitive impairment (Ten Brinke et al. 2015).

It should be noted that not all studies support an independent effect of physical activity on cognitive function. In fact there are some notable exceptions, including a report from the Whitehall II cohort study involving 28 years of follow-up. This study involved 10,308 participants aged 35–55 years at study inception (1985–88). Physical activity was assessed seven times between 1985 and 2013 and a battery of cognitive tests was administered up to four times between 1997 and 2013. The study found no association between physical activity and subsequent 15-year cognitive decline. The investigators concluded that there was no evidence from their study of a neuroprotective effect of exercise and that observational studies – with shorter follow-up periods – may be confounded by reverse causation (Sabia et al. 2017). Similarly, a Cochrane Review of RCTs (12 trials including 754 participants) 'found no evidence … that aerobic physical activities, including those which successfully improve cardiorespiratory fitness, have any cognitive benefit in cognitively healthy older adults' (Young et al. 2015). Nevertheless, while acknowledging that no RCT has demonstrated that exercise can reduce the incidence of mild cognitive impairment or dementia, Nagamatsu and colleagues (2014) point out that exercise significantly reduces the key vascular risk factors (e.g. hypertension, type 2 diabetes, hypercholesterolaemia) for Alzheimer's disease and vascular dementia – the two most common types of dementia – and argue that there is sufficient evidence to warrant promotion of exercise and further investigation. This view is endorsed by that of a recent umbrella review on physical activity, cognition and brain outcomes (Erickson et al. 2019).

The mechanisms by which exercise influences the brain and cognition are discussed in insightful reviews by Michael Voss and colleagues (2011) and Pedro Valenzuela and colleagues (2020). They involve neurogenesis (generation of new neurones, e.g. in the hippocampus) and angiogenesis (growth of new blood vessels – outside of the hippocampus – including areas activated by movement such as the cerebellum and primary motor cortex). Brain-derived neurotropic factor is considered critical for exercise-induced improvements in memory. Brain derived neurotropic factor is produced throughout the brain and is important for nerve cell growth. Central (within the brain) and peripheral (outside of the brain) BDNF is increased by both acute and chronic exercise and may reflect increased BDNF production in the brain. Another neurochemical which may mediate the effects of exercise is insulin-like growth factor-1 (IGF-1) which is produced in the central nervous system and is thought to aid in neurogenesis and angiogenesis. Exercise-induced increases in BDNF and IGF-1 may promote growth, differentiation, survival and repair of brain cells. Exercise may also influence other neurotropic factors (a family of biomolecules – nearly all of which are peptides or small proteins – that support the growth, survival and differentiation of both developing and mature neurones). Synaptic plasticity may facilitate the integration of new hippocampal neurones into existing brain networks. Exercise might also influence neurotransmitter systems in the brain increasing circulating dopamine, serotonin and acetylcholine. Much of this evidence comes from animal studies but there is evidence to support some of these mechanisms in human studies also. For example, data from the Harvard Aging Brain Study (HABS) suggests that physical activity can counteract the effects of β-amyloid-related cognitive decline in older adults (β-amyloid is the main component of amyloid plaques found in the brains of Alzheimer patients) (Rabin et al. 2019). This is possibly aided by the preservation of cerebral small vein integrity with exercise in older adults, thus reducing tortuosity (the twisting of small veins which are straight in healthy conditions) and maintaining cerebral blood flow (Shaaban et al. 2019).

DEMENTIA

Dementia is an umbrella term used to describe a range of progressive neurological disorders affecting the brain. According to Dementia UK there are over 200 subtypes of dementia, but the five most common are: Alzheimer's disease, vascular dementia, dementia with Lewy bodies, frontotemporal dementia and mixed dementia. Some people have a combination of different types of dementia and this is referred to as mixed dementia (https://www.dementiauk.org/, accessed 21 August 2019). Dementia damages the nerve cells in the brain interfering with the way they intercommunicate so messages cannot be sent from and to the brain effectively. Dementia is characterised by a deterioration in mental ability resulting in memory loss, confusion and general intellectual decline.

If physical activity is effective in preserving cognitive function, this suggests that it may assist in the prevention of dementia. Observational evidence is available to support this suggestion. One example is the Honolulu–Asia Aging Study (Abbott et al. 2004) which reported that walking <0.25 miles per day was associated with a 1.8-fold excess risk of dementia and Alzheimer's disease compared with walking >2 miles per day. Other observational studies have identified a similar association including the Cardiovascular risk factors, Aging and Incidence of Dementia study in eastern Finland (Kuopio and North Karelia) which observed that people in their late 40s and early 50s who exercised for 20 to 30 minutes at least twice a week had a 50% lower risk of dementia in later life than those who were less active during midlife (Rovio et al. 2005). In addition, the Washington Heights–Inwood Columbia Aging Project observed that both higher physical activity and adherence to a Mediterranean diet were independently related to lower risk of Alzheimer's disease (Scarmeas et al. 2009).

As with studies of cognitive function not all studies support that physical activity reduces the risk of dementia. The Whitehall II cohort study mentioned in the previous section found no evidence that physical activity protects from dementia and the authors speculate that the positive findings in previous studies may be due to reverse causation related to a decline in physical activity levels in the preclinical phase of dementia (Sabia et al. 2017). This is supported by the findings of a meta-analysis of 19 prospective cohort studies which concluded that intervention strategies targeting physical inactivity alone will have limited effectiveness for dementia prevention (Kivimäki et al. 2019). Based on current evidence, therefore, physical activity may be best recommended as part of a lifestyle package for preventing dementia. This was demonstrated by the Caerphilly Cohort Study which examined five healthy lifestyle behaviours (non-smoking, healthy body mass index, fruit and vegetable consumption, regular physical activity, light/moderate drinking) and observed a 60% lower risk of dementia after 30 years of follow-up in those exhibiting any three or more of these healthy lifestyle factors (Elwood et al. 2013). These findings are supported by a subsequent report from the Whitehall II cohort study which examined four behavioural (body mass index, diet, physical activity and smoking) and three biological (fasting glucose, cholesterol and blood pressure) factors. The study found that adherence to the 'Life Simple 7' ideal cardiovascular health recommendations at age 50 was associated with a lower risk of dementia later in life (Sabia et al. 2019). Finally, a report from the UK Biobank nicely demonstrates how lifestyle factors (including physical activity) and genetic risk interact to influence dementia risk (Lourida et al. 2019). This study involved eight years of follow-up and observed the highest risk of dementia in the group with a high genetic risk and an unfavourable lifestyle and the lowest risk of dementia in the group with a low genetic risk and a favourable lifestyle (Figure 12.13).

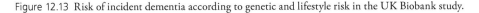

Figure 12.13 Risk of incident dementia according to genetic and lifestyle risk in the UK Biobank study.

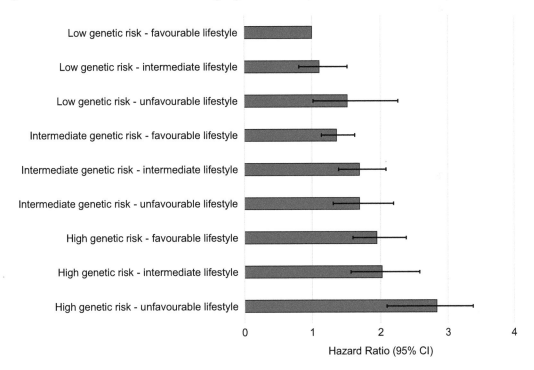

Source: Adapted from Lourida et al. (2019).
Note: This is a retrospective cohort study that included men and women (n = 196,383) of European ancestry aged at least 60 years without cognitive impairment or dementia at baseline. Participants joined the UK Biobank study from 2006 to 2010 and were followed up until 2016 or 2017. A polygenic risk score was calculated, and participants were classified as low (lowest quintile), intermediate (quintiles 2 to 4) or high (highest quintile) risk. Healthy lifestyle scores (no current smoking, regular physical activity, healthy diet and moderate alcohol consumption) were categorised into favourable, intermediate and unfavourable.

In addition to its role in preventing dementia physical activity may exert beneficial effects in people who have dementia or are at increased risk of developing dementia. Several studies have examined this issue with generally positive outcomes. One example is a RCT conducted in Perth, Western Australia between 2004 and 2007. This study involved 170 volunteers who reported memory problems but did not meet criteria for dementia. Participants were randomly allocated to an education and usual care group or to a six-month home-based programme of physical activity. The main outcome measure was change in the Alzheimer Disease Assessment Scale-Cognitive Subscale (ADAS-Cog) scores (possible range 0–70) over 18 months. Participants in the intervention group improved 0.26 points and those in the usual care group deteriorated 1.04 points on the ADAS-Cog at the end of the six-month intervention. After 18 months, participants in the intervention group improved 0.73 points compared with 0.04 points in the usual care group. The authors concluded that physical activity provoked a modest improvement in cognition in adults with subjective memory impairment (Lautenschlager et al. 2008). Another RCT conducted in the United States found that exercise training in combination with behavioural management improved physical health and depression in patients with Alzheimer disease (Teri et al. 2003). More recently the Finnish Alzheimer Disease Exercise Trial demonstrated a beneficial effect of a one-year exercise intervention programme on physical functioning – assessed by the Functional Independence Measure and the Short Physical Performance Battery (SPPB) – in 210 patients with Alzheimer disease. These benefits were achieved without increasing health-care costs or causing significant adverse effects (Pitkälä et al. 2013).

EXERCISE AND SURVIVAL

Evidence that high levels of physical activity and physical fitness lower the risk of premature mortality is discussed in Chapter 3 and this evidence will not be re-examined here, but several notable studies will be highlighted. One pertinent report comes from the Nurses' Health Study and examined the relationship between physical activity in midlife (mean age 60 years) and 'successful survival' in women aged 70 years or older. Successful survival was defined as no history of any of ten major chronic diseases or coronary artery bypass graft surgery and no cognitive impairment, physical impairment, or mental health limitations. The study involved 14 years of follow-up. After multivariate adjustment for covariates, higher physical activity levels at midlife, as measured by metabolic-equivalent tasks, were significantly associated with two-fold better odds of successful survival (Sun et al. 2010). More recently a report from the Oslo Study concluded that 30 minutes of physical activity, six days per week was associated with a 40% mortality risk reduction in elderly men (mean age 73 at baseline) and a five-year increase in life expectancy (Holme and Anderssen 2015).

An area of increasing interest in recent years is the extent to which physical capability levels can predict survival. The term physical capability is used to describe a person's ability to do the physical tasks of everyday living. These can be assessed by self-report or via objective tests of strength, speed, agility and balance. A systematic review and meta-analysis conducted by Cooper and colleagues (2010) concluded that objective measures of physical capability (grip strength, walking speed, chair rising and standing balance) predict all-cause mortality risk in older community dwelling populations and can be used as markers for current and future health. Cooper and colleagues (2010) suggest that these objective tests could serve as screening tools in the general population to identify people who may benefit from targeted intervention or among patient groups to assess response to treatment.

The ability of walking to predict survival has been the focus of many studies and a recent example is a report from the Women's Health Study involving 16,741 older women (mean age 72 years) followed for 4.3 years (Lee et al. 2019). Steps per day were measured over seven days in this cohort via accelerometers. Women who averaged approximately 4400 steps per day had significantly lower mortality rates during follow-up than women who took approximately 2700 steps per day. As more steps per day were accumulated, mortality rates progressively decreased before levelling at around 7500 steps per day. Stepping intensity was not clearly related to lower mortality rates after accounting for total steps per day. The investigators concluded that number of steps, rather than stepping intensity, was the metric most consistently related to lower mortality rates and suggested that these findings might serve as encouragement to sedentary individuals who find the commonly cited 10,000 steps per day goal unobtainable (Figure 12.14). Although walking volume is emphasised in the Women's

Figure 12.14 Dose–response association between mean steps per day and all-cause mortality in the Women's Health Study.

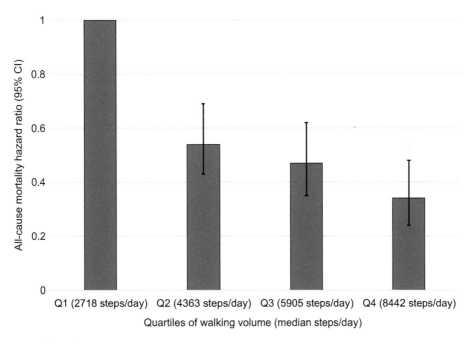

Note: n = 16,741 older women (mean age 72 years) followed for 4.3 years. Data are shown as hazard ratios with 95% CIs. Quartile 1 is the reference group. Values are adjusted for age; wear time; smoking status; alcohol use; intakes of saturated fat, fibre, fruits and vegetables; hormone therapy; parental history of myocardial infarction; family history of cancer; general health; history of cardiovascular disease; history of cancer; cancer screening, body mass index; history of hypertension, high cholesterol and diabetes.

Health Study (Lee et al. 2019) other studies have observed that slow walking speed is a predictor of cardiovascular and all-cause mortality (Dumurgier et al. 2009) and one study (Stanaway et al. 2011) recommends a minimum walking speed of 3 miles per hour (approximately 5 km per hour) for men aged 70 and above who wish to avoid the Grim Reaper!

A fascinating cohort study which sought to identify modifiable factors associated with longevity among adults aged 75 and older was conducted in the Swedish town of Kungsholmen, Stockholm (Rizzuto et al. 2012). This study involved 1810 adults aged 75 or older at baseline (1987) who were followed for 18 years (1987 to 2005) during which time 1661 (91.8%) participants died. Half of the participants lived longer than 90 years. Half of the current smokers died one year earlier than non-smokers. Of the leisure activities examined, physical activity was most strongly associated with survival; the median age at death of participants who regularly swam, walked, or did gymnastics was two years greater than those who did not. The median survival of people with a low-risk profile (healthy lifestyle behaviours, participation in at least one leisure activity, and a rich or moderate social network) was 5.4 years longer than those with a high-risk profile (unhealthy lifestyle behaviours, no participation in leisure activities, and a limited or poor social network). Even among the oldest old (85 years or older) and people with chronic conditions, the median age at death was four years higher for those with a low-risk profile than those with a high-risk profile. These findings suggest that even after age 75 lifestyle behaviours such as not smoking and physical activity are associated with longer survival. The low-risk profile was estimated to add five years to women's lives and six years to men's lives. These associations, although attenuated, were also present among the oldest old (≥85 years) and in people with chronic conditions (Figure 12.15). This cohort study cannot prove causality and a variety of limitations are acknowledged by the authors and other commentators (Glymour and Osypuk 2012). Nevertheless, the findings are thought provoking and provide further insight to the factors associated with healthy ageing and survival.

Can physical activity delay the ageing process? There is some evidence to support this idea, although it is observational and thus falls short of proving cause and effect. A report published in the *Archives of Internal Medicine* assessed the association between leisure-time physical activity and leukocyte telomere length in 2401 twin volunteers (2152 women and 249 men) from the UK Adult Twin Registry (Cherkas et al. 2008). Telomeres are pieces of DNA at the end of chromosomes. They protect the chromosomes from damage, but every time the cell divides telomeres shorten. Telomere length can therefore be used as an index of biological age – longer telomeres being suggestive of a lower biological age. Cherkas and colleagues (2008) found that higher levels of leisure-time physical activity were associated with longer telomeres, suggesting an anti-ageing effect of exercise (Figure 12.16). The study authors observed that inactive participants may be biologically older by ten years than more active participants. Genetic factors are a possible confounding factor in this study, but the researchers addressed this issue by comparing leukocyte telomere length in monozygotic and dizygotic twin pairs discordant for physical activity. The relationship between telomere length and physical activity remained significant in this analysis, suggesting that genetic factors are not responsible for the differences in telomere length between active and inactive individuals. These findings are supported by those of Werner and colleagues

Figure 12.15 Median age at death in four risk groups according to combinations of modifiable factors among entire population, men and women separately, older adults (75–84 years) and oldest old adults (≥85 years), and by status of chronic conditions.

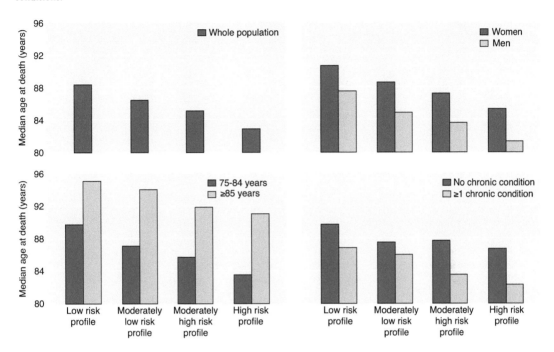

Source: Reproduced from the *British Medical Journal*, Rizzuto, D. et al., 345: e5568, copyright © 2012 with permission from BMJ Publishing Group Ltd.
Note: Findings are from a cohort study conducted in the Swedish town of Kungsholmen, Stockholm. n = 1810 adults aged 75 or older at baseline (1987) who were followed for 18 years (1987 to 2005) during which time 1661 (91.8%) participants died. Results are adjusted for multiple covariates. A low-risk profile was characterised by healthy lifestyle behaviours, participation in at least one leisure activity, and a rich or moderate social network. A high-risk profile was characterised by unhealthy lifestyle behaviours, no participation in leisure activities, and a limited or poor social network.

(2009) who observed that a three-week wheel running intervention upregulated telomerase activity in mice and that young and middle-aged human endurance athletes exhibit higher telomerase activity than their untrained counterparts. Telomerase is a reverse transcriptase enzyme involved in telomere elongation hence these findings suggest a telomere stabilising effect of exercise in mice and humans (Werner et al. 2009). Although these findings are exciting a recent review concluded that at least 50% of studies have failed to find an association between physical activity levels and telomere length (Chilton et al. 2017) and further work is required to explain this inconsistency.

Another potential mechanism by which physical activity may delay ageing and extend life is by facilitating an energy deficit and acting synergistically with calorie restriction. A six-month intervention trial reported that exercise in combination with calorie restriction was effective in reducing fasting insulin and body temperature (two biomarkers of longevity) in men and women who were overweight (body mass index

Figure 12.16 Association between mean leukocyte telomere length and leisure-time physical activity levels in middle-aged men and women.

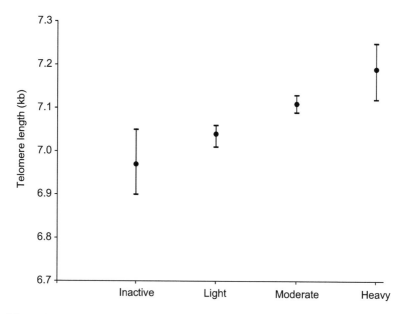

Source: Adapted from Cherkas et al. (2008).

Note: The subjects were 2401 white twins (2152 women and 249 men) from the UK Adult Twin Registry. The sample comprised 167 monozygotic twin pairs, 915 dizygotic twin pairs and 237 unpaired twins. Physical activity levels were assessed using questionnaires. kb, kilobases. Values are mean and SD.

25 to <30 kg m^{-2}) as well as reducing DNA damage. If such changes were maintained over the long term, they have the potential to attenuate the ageing process (Heilbronn et al. 2006). It should be emphasised that far more work is required to understand the significance of telomere length for ageing, the extent to which calorie restriction can delay ageing/extend life in humans and how exercise might contribute to this. At present these are merely possibilities. The evidence explored in this chapter leaves no doubt, however, that physical activity is one ingredient required for successful ageing.

SUMMARY

- Although people are living longer than ever before, ageing is associated with an increased risk of disability and chronic disease some of which is due to factors related to secondary ageing including a lack of physical activity.
- Physical capacities decline with age. Most noteworthy among these are $\dot{V}O_2$max and muscle strength. Flexibility, balance and general mobility also decline with age, and there are changes in body composition, most notably a decline in muscle mass.
- Loss of muscle mass is a major reason for the decline in muscle strength with age. It may also explain a large portion of the decline in $\dot{V}O_2$max.

- Some of the decline in physical function with age is due to inactivity rather than a genuine effect of ageing. Older adults who continue training and competing retain relatively high $\dot{V}O_2$max values and are capable of high levels of physical performance into their eighth decade of life and beyond.
- The body retains the ability to adapt to exercise training throughout life. Adaptations include increases in $\dot{V}O_2$max, skeletal muscle oxidative enzyme activity, skeletal muscle capillarisation, muscle mass, muscle fibre area and muscle strength.
- The decline in physical function associated with ageing eventually impairs strength, walking speed, general mobility and the ability to perform activities of daily living. This leads to a loss of independence and quality of life and is also predictive of disability, morbidity and mortality.
- Physical activity intervention programmes demonstrate multiple benefits for older adults, even the oldest old and in those who are institutionalised and hospitalised. These benefits include improvements in strength, endurance and mobility helping to counteract age-related declines in functional capacities and preserve independence.
- Along with declines in physical function, cognitive function also declines with age. Exercise may have benefits for reducing age-related cognitive decline and preserving brain volume and function although there is inconsistency in the evidence. Further research is required to ascertain whether physical activity has an independent role in counteracting age-related cognitive decline.
- Although the extent to which exercise can influence the risk of dementia is uncertain, physical activity is an important component of a package of healthy lifestyle behaviours which appear to be effective for reducing dementia risk. There is also evidence that exercise provides benefits for people suffering from or at increased risk of dementia although this is an under-researched area requiring further study.
- Evidence consistently demonstrates that regular physical activity is important for healthy ageing, compressed morbidity, longevity and survival even among the oldest old.

STUDY TASKS

1   Describe the major changes in physical function associated with ageing. What evidence is there to suggest that some of these changes are due to disuse rather than ageing?
2   Identify the range of $\dot{V}O_2$max values (ml kg^{-1} min^{-1}) you might expect to see in men and women in their 60s and 70s. Discuss the possible physiological mechanisms that might underlie a decline in $\dot{V}O_2$max with age and the extent to which regular exercise can influence these mechanisms.
3   Give examples of the different tests used to assess general mobility and physical capability in older adults. What is the relevance of these tests for health and how might they be used?
4   Identify and explain the methodology and findings of two RCTs which have demonstrated the benefits of physical activity/exercise for one or more aspects of physical function in older adults.

5 Discuss the strengths and limitations of the evidence linking physical activity with improved cognition and a reduced risk of dementia. Explain the mechanisms which could explain how physical activity preserves/improves brain volume and cognition in older adults.
6 Discuss the evidence that exercise can benefit health and longevity even in the oldest old.
7 What evidence is available to suggest that physical activity can slow the ageing process? How convincing is this evidence?

FURTHER READING

Booth, F.W., Laye, M.J. and Roberts, M.D. (2011) Lifetime sedentary living accelerates some aspects of secondary ageing. *Journal of Applied Physiology* 111: 1497–504.

Cartee, G.D., Hepple, R.T., Bamman, M.M. and Zierath, J.R. (2016) Exercise promotes healthy aging of skeletal muscle. *Cell Metabolism* 23: 1034–47.

Chilton, W., O'Brien, B. and Charchar, F. (2017) Telomeres, ageing and exercise: guilty by association? *International Journal of Molecular Sciences* 18: 2573. doi: 10.3390/ijms18122573.

Chin A Paw, M.J.M., van Uffelen, J.G.Z., Riphagen, I. and van Mechelen, W. (2008) The functional effects of physical exercise training in frail older people. A systematic review. *Sports Medicine* 38: 781–93.

Chodzko-Zajko, W.J., Proctor, D.N., Fiatarone Singh, M.A., Minson, C.T., Nigg, C.R., Salem, G.J. and Skinner, J.S. (2009) Exercise and physical activity for older adults: ACSM position stand. *Medicine and Science in Sports and Exercise* 41: 1510–30.

Erickson, K.I., Hillman, C., Stillman, C.M., Ballard, R.M., Bloodgood, B., Conroy, D.E. et al. for 2018 Physical Activity Guidelines Advisory Committee. (2019) Physical activity, cognition, and brain outcomes: a review of the 2018 physical activity guidelines. *Medicine and Science in Sports and Exercise* 51: 1242–51.

Harridge, S.D. and Lazarus, N.R. (2017) Physical activity, ageing, and physiological function. *Physiology* 32: 152–61.

Kusy, K. and Zielinski, J. (2015) Sprinters versus long-distance runners: how to grow old healthy. *Exercise and Sport Sciences Reviews* 43: 57–64.

Lazarus, N.R. and Harridge, S.D.R. (2017) Declining performance of master athletes: silhouettes of the trajectory of healthy human ageing? *Journal of Physiology* 595: 2941–8.

Lazarus, N.R. and Harridge, S.D.R. (2018) The inherent human aging process and the facilitating role of exercise. *Frontiers in Physiology* 9: 1135. doi: 10.3389/fphys.2018.01135.

Valenzuela, P.L., Castillo-García, A., Morales, J.S., de la Villa, P., Hampel, H., Emanuele, E. et al. (2020) Exercise benefits on Alzheimer's disease: state-of-the-science. *Ageing Research Review.* 62: 101108. doi: 10.1016/j.arr.2020.101108.

Voss, M.W., Nagamatsu, L.S., Liu-Ambrose, T. and Kramer, A.F. (2011) Exercise, brain, and cognition across the life span. *Journal of Applied Physiology* 111: 1505–13.

Wilkinson, D.J., Piasecki, M. and Atherton, P.J. (2018) The age-related loss of skeletal muscle mass and function: measurement and physiology of muscle fibre atrophy and muscle fibre loss in humans. *Ageing Research Reviews* 47: 123–32.

Young, A. and Dinan, S. (2005) Activity in later life. *British Medical Journal* 330: 189–91.

REFERENCES

Abbott, R.D., White, L.R., Ross, G.W., Masaki, K.H., Curb, J.D. and Petrovitch, H. (2004) Walking and dementia in physically capable elderly men. *Journal of the American Medical Association* 292: 1447–53.

Ades, P.A., Ballor, D.L., Ashikaga, T., Utton, J.L. and Nair, K.S. (1996) Weight training improves walking endurance in healthy elderly persons. *Annals of Internal Medicine* 124: 568–72.

American College of Sports Medicine. (2010) *ACSM's guidelines for exercise testing and prescription*. 8th edn, Philadelphia, PA: Wolters Kluwer Health/Lippincott Williams and Wilkins.

Baker, L.A., Frank, L.L., Foster-Schubert, K., Green, P.S., Wilkinson, C.W., McTiernan, A. et al. (2010) Effects of aerobic exercise on mild cognitive impairment: a controlled trial. *Archives of Neurology* 67: 71–9.

Broskey, N.T., Greggio, C., Boss, A., Boutant, M., Dwyer, A., Schlueter, L. et al. (2014) Skeletal muscle mitochondria in the elderly: effects of physical fitness and physical training. *Journal of Clinical Endocrinology and Metabolism* 99: 1852–61.

Cartee, G.D., Hepple, R.T., Bamman, M.M. and Zierath, J.R. (2016) Exercise promotes healthy aging of skeletal muscle. *Cell Metabolism* 23: 1034–47.

Chakravarty, E.F., Hubert, H.B., Lingala, V.B. and Fries, J.F. (2008) Reduced disability and mortality among aging runners: a 21-year longitudinal study. *Archives of Internal Medicine* 168: 1638–46.

Cherkas, L.F., Hankin, J.L., Kato, B.S., Richards, B., Gardner, J.P., Surdulescu, G.L. et al. (2008) The association between physical activity in leisure time and leukocyte telomere length. *Archives of Internal Medicine* 168: 154–8.

Chilton, W., O'Brien, B. and Charchar, F. (2017) Telomeres, ageing and exercise: guilty by association? *International Journal of Molecular Sciences* 18: 2573. doi: 10.3390/ijms18122573.

Chin A Paw, M.J.M., van Uffelen, J.G.Z., Riphagen, I. and van Mechelen, W. (2008) The functional effects of physical exercise training in frail older people: a systematic review. *Sports Medicine* 38: 781–93.

Chodzko-Zajko, W.J., Proctor, D.N., Fiatarone Singh, M.A., Minson, C.T., Nigg, C.R., Salem, G.J. and Skinner, J.S. (2009) Exercise and physical activity for older adults: ACSM position stand. *Medicine and Science in Sports and Exercise* 41: 1510–30.

Coggan, A.R., Spina, R.J., King, D.S., Rogers, M.A., Brown, M., Nemeth, P.M. and Holloszy, J.O. (1992) Skeletal muscle adaptations to endurance training in 60- to 70-yr-old men and women. *Journal of Applied Physiology* 72: 1780–6.

Coggan, A.R., Spina, R.J., Rogers, M.A., King, D.S., Brown, M., Nemeth, P.M. and Holloszy, J.O. (1990) Histochemical and enzymatic characteristics of skeletal muscle in masters athletes. *Journal of Applied Physiology* 68: 1896–901.

Cooper, R., Kuh, D. and Hardy, R.; Mortality Review Group on behalf of the FALCon and HALCyon study teams (2010) Objectively measured physical capability levels and mortality: systematic review and meta-analysis. *British Medical Journal* 341: c4467. doi: 10.1136/bmj.c4467.

Daley, M.J. and Spinks, W.L. (2000) Exercise, mobility and aging. *Sports Medicine* 29: 1–12.

de Souto Barreto, P., Rolland, Y., Vellas, B. and Maltais, M. (2019) Association of long-term exercise training with risk of falls, fractures, hospitalizations, and mortality in older adults: a systematic review and meta-analysis. *Journal of the American Medical Association Internal Medicine* 179: 394–405.

Dong, X., Milholland, B. and Vijg, J. (2016) Evidence for a limit to human lifespan. *Nature* 538: 257–9.

Dumurgier, J., Elbaz, A., Ducimetière, P., Tavernier, B., Alpérovitch, A. and Tzourio C. (2009) Slow walking speed and cardiovascular death in well functioning older adults: prospective cohort study. *British Medical Journal* 339: b4460. doi: 10.1136/bmj.b4460.

Elwood, P., Galante, J., Pickering, J., Palmer, S., Bayer, A., Ben-Shlomo, Y. et al. (2013) Healthy lifestyles reduce the incidence of chronic diseases and dementia: evidence from the Caerphilly cohort study. *PLoS One* 8: e81877. doi: 10.1371/journal.pone.0081877.

Erickson, K.I., Hillman, C., Stillman, C.M., Ballard, R.M., Bloodgood, B., Conroy, D.E. et al. for 2018 Physical Activity Guidelines Advisory Committee. (2019) Physical activity, cognition, and brain outcomes: a review of the 2018 physical activity guidelines. *Medicine and Science in Sports and Exercise* 51: 1242–51.

Erickson, K.I., Raji, C.A., Lopez, O.L., Becker, J.T., Rosano, C., Newman, A.B. et al. (2010) Physical activity predicts gray matter volume in late adulthood: The Cardiovascular Health Study. *Neurology* 75: 1415–22.

Erickson, K.I., Voss, M.W., Prakash, R.S., Basak, C., Szabo, A., Chaddock, L. et al. (2011) Exercise training increases size of hippocampus and improves memory. *Proceedings of the National Academy of Sciences* 108: 3017–22.

Etgen, T., Sander, D., Huntgeburth, U., Poppert, H., Förstl, H. and Bickel, H. (2010) Physical activity and incident cognitive impairment in elderly persons: the INVADE study. *Archives of Internal Medicine* 170: 186–93.

Fiatarone, M.A., O'Neill, E.F., Ryan, N.D., Clements, K.M., Solares, G.R., Nelson, M.E. et al. (1994) Exercise training and nutritional supplementation for physical frailty in very elderly people. *New England Journal of Medicine* 330: 1769–75.

Frontera, W.R., Hughes, V.A., Fielding, R.A., Fiatarone, M.A., Evans, W.J. and Roubenoff, R. (2000) Aging skeletal muscle: a 12-yr longitudinal study. *Journal of Applied Physiology* 88: 1321–6.

Frontera, W.R., Hughes, V.A., Lutz, K.J. and Evans, W.J. (1991) A cross-sectional study of muscle strength and mass in 45- to 78-year old men and women. *Journal of Applied Physiology* 71: 644–50.

Frontera, W.R., Meredith, C.N., O'Reilly, K.P., Knuttgen, H.G. and Evans, W.J. (1988) Strength conditioning in older men: skeletal muscle hypertrophy and improved function. *Journal of Applied Physiology* 64: 1038–44.

Glymour, M.M. and Osypuk, T.L. (2012) Promoting health and improving survival into very old age. *British Medical Journal* 345: e6452. doi: 10.1136/bmj.e6452.

Gries, K.J., Raue, U., Perkins, R.K., Lavin, K.M., Overstreet, B.S., D'Acquisto, L.J. et al. (2018) Cardiovascular and skeletal muscle health with lifelong exercise. *Journal of Applied Physiology* 125: 1636–45.

Guralnik, J.M., Ferrucci, L., Simonsick, E.M., Salive, M.E. and Wallace, R.B. (1995) Lower-extremity function in persons over the age of 70 years as a predictor of subsequent disability. *New England Journal of Medicine* 332: 556–61.

Hagberg, J.M., Graves, J.E., Limacher, M., Woods, D.R., Leggett, S.H., Cononie, C. et al. (1989) Cardiovascular responses of 70- to 79-yr-old men and women to exercise training. *Journal of Applied Physiology* 66: 2589–94.

Hawkins, S.A. and Wiswell, R.A. (2003) Rate and mechanism of maximal oxygen consumption decline with aging. *Sports Medicine* 33: 877–88.

Heath, G.W., Hagberg, J.M., Ehsani, A.A. and Holloszy, J.O. (1981) A physiological comparison of young and older endurance athletes. *Journal of Applied Physiology* 51: 634–40.

Heilbronn, L.K., de Jonge, L., Frisard, M.I., DeLany, J.P., Larson-Meyer, D.E., Rood, J. et al. for the Pennington CALERIE Team (2006) Effect of 6-month calorie restriction on biomarkers of longevity, metabolic adaptation, and oxidative stress in overweight individuals: a randomized trial. *Journal of the American Medical Association* 295: 1539–48.

Holme, I. and Anderssen, S.A. (2015) Increases in physical activity is as important as smoking cessation for reduction in total mortality in elderly men: 12 years of follow-up of the Oslo II study. *British Journal of Sports Medicine* 49: 743–8.

Ingram, D.K. (2000) Age-related decline in physical activity: generalization to nonhumans. *Medicine and Science in Sports and Exercise* 32: 1623–9.

Joyner, M.J. and Barnes, J.N. (2013) I am 80 going on 18: exercise and the fountain of youth. *Journal of Applied Physiology* 114: 1–2.

Kaminsky, L.A., Arena R. and Myers, J. (2015) Reference standards for cardiorespiratory fitness measured with cardiopulmonary exercise testing: data from the fitness registry and the importance of exercise national database. *Mayo Clinic Proceedings* 90: 1515–23.

Kivimäki, M., Singh-Manoux, A., Pentti, J., Sabia, S., Nyberg, S.T., Alfredsson, L. et al. on behalf of the IPD-Work consortium (2019) Physical inactivity, cardiometabolic disease, and risk of dementia: an individual-participant meta-analysis. *British Medical Journal* 365: l1495. doi: 10.1136/bmj.l1495.

Lautenschlager, N.T., Cox, K.L., Flicker, L., Foster, J.K., van Bockxmeer, F.M., Xiao, J. et al. (2008) Effect of physical activity on cognitive function in older adults at risk for Alzheimer disease: a randomized trial. *Journal of the American Medical Association* 300: 1027–37.

Lee, I.-M., Shiroma, E.J., Kamada, M., Bassett, D.R., Matthews, C.E. and Buring, J.E. (2019) Association of step volume and intensity with all-cause mortality in older women. *Journal of the American Medical Association Internal Medicine* 179: 1105–12.

Liu-Ambrose, T., Nagamatsu, L.S., Graf, P., Beattie, B.L., Ashe, M.C. and Handy, T.C. (2010) Resistance training and executive functions: a 12-month randomized controlled trial. *Archives of Internal Medicine* 170: 170–8.

Lourida, I., Hannon, E., Littlejohns, T.J., Langa, K.M., Hyppönen, E., Kuźma, E. and Llewellyn, D.J. (2019) Association of lifestyle and genetic risk with incidence of dementia. *Journal of the American Medical Association* 322: 430–7.

Mackey, R.H. (2008) Weighing benefits for older runners. *Archives of Internal Medicine* 168: 1948–9.

Malbut, K.E., Dinan, S. and Young, A. (2002) Aerobic training in the 'oldest old': the effect of 24 weeks of training. *Age and Ageing* 31: 255–60.

Martinez-Velilla, N., Casas-Herrero, A., Zambom-Ferraresi, F., Sáez de Asteasu, M.L., Lucia, A., Galbete, A. et al. (2019) Effect of exercise intervention on functional decline in very elderly patients during acute hospitalization: a randomized clinical trial. *Journal of the American Medical Association Internal Medicine* 179: 28–36.

McDermott, M.M., Guralnik, J.M., Criqui, M.H., Ferrucci, L., Liu, K., Spring, B. et al. (2015) Unsupervised exercise and mobility loss in peripheral artery disease: a randomized controlled trial. *Journal of the American Heart Association* 4: e001659. doi: 10.1161/JAHA.114.001659.

McGuire, D.K., Levine, B.D., Williamson, J.W., Snell, P.G., Blomqvist, G., Saltin, B. and Mitchell, J.H. (2001a) A 30-year follow-up of the Dallas bed rest and training study. I. Effect of age on the cardiovascular response to exercise *Circulation* 104: 1350–7.

McGuire, D.K., Levine, B.D., Williamson, J.W., Snell, P.G., Blomqvist, G., Saltin, B. and Mitchell, J.H. (2001b) A 30-year follow-up of the Dallas bed rest and training study. II. Effect of age on cardiovascular adaptation to exercise training. *Circulation* 104: 1358–66.

Middleton, L.A., Manini, T.M., Simonsick, E.M., Harris, T.B., Barnes, D.E., Tylavsky, F. et al. (2011) Activity energy expenditure and incident cognitive impairment in older adults. *Archives of Internal Medicine* 171: 1251–7.

Myers, J., Prakash, M., Froelicher, V., Do, D., Partington, S. and Atwood, J.E. (2002) Exercise capacity and mortality among men referred for exercise testing. *New England Journal of Medicine* 346: 793–801.

Nagamatsu, L.S., Flicker, L., Kramer, A.F., Voss, M.W., Erickson, K.I., Hsu, C.L. and Liu-Ambrose, T. (2014) Exercise is medicine, for the body and the brain. *British Journal of Sports Medicine* 48: 943–4.

Newman, A.B., Simonsick, E.M., Naydeck, B.L., Boudreau, R.M., Kritchevsky, S.B., Nevitt, M.C. et al. (2006) Association of long-distance corridor walk performance with mortality, cardiovascular disease, mobility limitation, and disability. *Journal of the American Medical Association* 295: 2018–26.

Pahor, M., Guralnik, J.M., Ambrosius, W.T., Blair, S., Bonds, D.E., Church, T.S. et al. (2014) Effect of structured physical activity on prevention of major mobility disability in older adults: the LIFE study randomized clinical trial. *Journal of the American Medical Association* 311: 2387–96.

Pitkälä, K.H., Pöysti, M.M., Laakkonen, M-L., Tilvis, R.S., Savikko, N., Kautiainen, H. and Strandberg, T.E. (2013) Effects of the Finnish Alzheimer disease exercise trial (FINALEX): a randomized controlled trial. *Journal of the American Medical Association Internal Medicine* 173: 894–901.

Rabin, J.S., Klein, H., Kirn, D.R., Schultz, A.P., Yang, H.-S., Hampton, O. et al. (2019) Associations of physical activity and β-amyloid with longitudinal cognition and neurodegeneration in clinically normal older adults. *Journal of the American Medical Association Neurology* 76: 1203–10.

Rasmussen, L.J.H., Caspi, A., Ambler, A., Broadbent, J.M., Cohen, H.J., d'Arbeloff, T. et al. (2019) Association of neurocognitive and physical function with gait speed in midlife. *Journal of the American Medical Association Network Open* 2: e191312. doi: 10.1001/jamanetworkopen.2019.13123.

Rizzuto, D., Orsini, N., Qiu, C., Wang, H.-X. and Fratiglioni, L. (2012) Lifestyle, social factors, and survival after age 75: population-based study. *British Medical Journal* 345: e5568. doi: 10.1136/bmj.e5568.

Rovio, S., Kåreholt, I., Helkala, E.-L., Viitanen, M., Winblad, B., Tuomilehto, J. et al. (2005) Leisure-time physical activity at midlife and the risk of dementia and Alzheimer's disease. *Lancet Neurology* 4: 705–11.

Sabia, S., Dugravot, A., Dartigues, J.F., Abell, J., Elbaz, A., Kivimäki, M. and Singh-Manoux, A. (2017) Physical activity, cognitive decline, and risk of dementia: 28-year follow-up of Whitehall II cohort study. *British Medical Journal* 357: j2709. doi: 10.1136/bmj.j2709.

Sabia, S., Fayosse, A., Dumurgier, J., Schnitzler, A., Empana, J.P., Ebmeier, K.P. et al. (2019) Association of ideal cardiovascular health at age 50 with incidence of dementia: 25 year follow-up of Whitehall II cohort study. *British Medical Journal* 366: l4414. doi: 10.1136/bmj.l4414.

Scarmeas, N., Luchsinger, J.A., Schupf, N., Brickman, A.M., Cosentino, S., Tang, M.X. and Stern, Y. (2009) Physical activity, diet and risk of Alzheimer disease. *Journal of the American Medical Association* 302: 627–37.

Shaaban, C.E., Aizenstein, H.J., Jorgensen, D.R., Mahbubani, R.L.M., Meckes, N.A., Erickson, K.I. et al. (2019) Physical activity and cerebral small vein integrity in older adults. *Medicine and Science in Sports and Exercise* 51: 1684–91.

Spartano, N.L., Davis-Plourde, K.L., Himali, J.J., Andersson, C., Pase, M.P., Maillard, P. et al. (2019) Association of accelerometer-measured light-intensity physical activity with brain volume: The Framingham Heart Study. *Journal of the American Medical Association Network Open* 2: e192745. doi: 10.1001/jamanetworkopen.2019.2745.

Spina, R.J., Ogawa, T., Kohrt, W.M., Martin, W.H., Holloszy, J.O. and Ehsani, A.A. (1993) Differences in cardiovascular adaptations to endurance exercise training between older men and women. *Journal of Applied Physiology* 75: 849–55.

Stanaway, F.F., Gnjidic, D., Blyth, F.M., Le Couteur, D.G. Naganathan, V., Waite, L. et al. (2011) How fast does the Grim Reaper walk? Receiver operating characteristics curve analysis in healthy men aged 70 and over. *British Medical Journal* 343: d7679. doi: 10.1136/bmj.d7679.

Sun, Q., Townsend, M.K., Okereke, O.I., Franco, O.H., Hu, F.B. and Grodstein, F. (2010) Physical activity at midlife in relation to successful survival in women at age 70 years or older. *Archives of Internal Medicine* 170: 194–201.

Tanaka, H. and Seals, D.R. (1997) Age and gender interactions in physiological functional capacity: insight from swimming performance. *Journal of Applied Physiology* 82: 846–51.

Ten Brinke, L.F., Bolandzadeh, N., Nagamatsu, L.S., Hsu, C.L., Davis, J.C., Miran-Khan, K., Liu-Ambrose, T. (2015) Aerobic exercise increases hippocampal volume in older women with probable mild cognitive impairment: a 6-month randomised controlled trial. *British Journal of Sports Medicine* 49: 248–54.

Teri, L., Gibbons, L.E. McCurry, S.M., Logsdon, R.G., Buchner, D.M., Barlow, W.E. et al. (2003) Exercise plus behavioural management in patients with Alzheimer disease: a randomized controlled trial. *Journal of the American Medical Association* 290: 2015–22.

Trappe, S., Hayes, E., Gaplin, A., Kaminsky, L., Jemiolo, B., Fink, W. et al. (2013) New records in aerobic power among octogenarian lifelong endurance athletes. *Journal of Applied Physiology* 114: 3–10.

Tricco, A.C., Thomas, S.M., Veroniki, A.A., Hamid, J.S., Cogo, E., Strifler, L. et al. (2017) Comparisons of interventions for preventing falls in older adults: a systematic review and meta-analysis. *Journal of the American Medical Association* 318: 1687–99.

Valenzuela, P.L., Castillo-García, A., Morales, J.S., de la Villa, P., Hampel, H., Emanuele, E. et al. (2020) Exercise benefits on Alzheimer's disease: state-of-the-science. *Ageing Research Review* 62: 101108. doi: 10.1016/j.arr.2020.101108.

Vercambre, M.-N., Grodstein, F., Manson, J.E., Stampfer, M.J. and Kang, J.H. (2011) Physical activity and cognition in women with vascular conditions. *Archives of Internal Medicine* 171: 1244–50.

Voss, M.W., Nagamatsu, L.S., Liu-Ambrose, T. and Kramer, A.F. (2011) Exercise, brain, and cognition across the life span. *Journal of Applied Physiology* 111: 1505–13.

Werner, C., Fürster, T., Widmann, T., Pöss, J., Roggia, C., Hanhoun, M. et al. (2009) Physical exercise prevents cellular senescence in circulating leukocytes and in the vessel wall. *Circulation* 120: 2438–47.

Westerterp, K.R. (2015) Daily physical activity as determined by age, body mass and energy balance. *European Journal of Applied Physiology* 115: 1177–84.

Weuve, J., Kang, J.H., Manson, J.E., Breteler, M.M.B., Ware, J.H. and Grodstein, F. (2004) Physical activity, including walking, and cognitive function in older women. *Journal of the American Medical Association* 292: 1454–61.

Wilkinson, D.J., Piasecki, M. and Atherton, P.J. (2018) The age-related loss of skeletal muscle mass and function: measurement and physiology of muscle fibre atrophy and muscle fibre loss in humans. *Ageing Research Reviews* 47: 123–32.

World Masters Athletics records [online], available at: https: //world-masters-athletics.com/ (accessed 8 August 2019).

Wroblewski, A.P., Amati, F., Smiley, M.A., Goodpaster, B. and Wright, V. (2011) Chronic exercise preserves lean muscle mass in masters athletes. *Physician and Sportsmedicine* 39: 172–8.

Young, J., Angevaren, M., Rusted, J. and Tabet, N. (2015) Aerobic exercise to improve cognitive function in older people without known cognitive impairment. *The Cochrane Database of Systematic Reviews* 4: CD005381. doi: 10.1002/14651858.CD005381.pub4.

Part IV
Physical activity – risks and opportunities

13 Hazards

Adrianne E. Hardman

INTRODUCTION

Physical activity can be hazardous as well as beneficial to health. For example, jogging, walking and cycling inevitably increase exposure to the risk of injury through falls or collisions with vehicles. Cycling is particularly hazardous because around one-third of serious injuries are to the head. Every year there are reports of deaths during swimming – mainly drowning and especially among children.

Sudden cardiac events during participation in sports invariably attract much publicity, particularly when they happen to young people in high-profile sports. These and other cardiac issues are discussed later in this chapter.

Prolonged exercise in the heat can lead to exertional heat stroke (rectal temperature >40°C), particularly if fluid intake is insufficient, and even to dangerously low levels of serum sodium (<135 mmol l^{-1}). Exercise-associated collapse can result from either of these potentially life-threatening pathologies but it is more often due to transient postural hypotension caused by pooling of blood in the lower extremities once the athlete stops running.

Hypothermia (rectal temperature <35⁰C) can be experienced by people engaging in water sports, hill-walking and even marathon running if the environmental temperature is low. Rhabdomyolysis (sporadic appearance in blood of abnormal levels of myoglobin) has been reported among endurance runners engaged in high-volume training and there may be an increased likelihood of osteoarthritis in people who engage over many years in sports involving a lot of high impacts and/or torsional loading of joints (see Chapter 9).

Exercise 'dependence' – a craving for activity that results in uncontrollable excessive exercise behaviour – has been identified as a potential problem for some individuals. Criteria to define 'how much exercise is too much' and the development of more objective measures are needed, however, before this research area yields secure findings.

Specific hazards are, of course, associated with physical activity for people with existing disease. Exercise can lead to hypoglycaemia in diabetics because it increases the rate of glucose uptake into muscle. Asthma may be precipitated by exercise – running in cold weather is a particularly potent trigger. Another problem for asthmatics is that, in urban environments, air contains small amounts of gases and particulates other than its normal constituents. The increased ventilation of the lungs during exercise increases exposure to this pollution and may exacerbate existing respiratory problems. Even in healthy people, ozone and sulphur dioxide can impair lung function.

Sports and recreation-related injuries are a common type of injury seen in emergency departments and some require in-patient care. Annually, across the European Union, nearly 6 million people need treatment in hospital due to sport-related injuries. The survey 'Physical Activity Netherlands', based on a representative sample of more than 85,000 citizens, reported that nearly one in five participants sustained a sports injury per year and that 50% of these had to be treated medically (Schmikli et al. 2009). In a representative sample of the Danish population 18% of adults and 19% of children aged 7–15 years reported having had an injury within the past 12 months (Bueno et al. 2018). Sports injuries are not a trivial problem and can have important consequences for the individual and for society. Their prevention is part of the research agenda of the US Centers for Disease Control and Prevention.

Thus, in some situations – and for some individuals – participation in exercise or sports can be hazardous. The best-documented hazards are: musculoskeletal injuries; adverse cardiac effects; the 'Female Athlete Triad' – also known as Relative Energy Deficiency in Sports – and impairment of aspects of immune function.

MUSCULOSKELETAL INJURIES

Musculoskeletal injuries fall into two categories, i.e. acute traumatic and overuse. Incidence rates for acute exercise-related (including sport-related) injuries are rather low in the general population but are higher, of course, among specific populations that are vigorously active; around 50% of people participating in team sports will sustain one or more injuries over a season and the annual rate of musculoskeletal injuries among military trainees is between 25% and 50%. The majority of sports injuries are to the lower limb, especially the knee and ankle (e.g. ligament sprains, meniscal tears) and two out of three occur during team sports. Soccer in particular gives rise to a high number of injuries, even when corrected for the number of people who play. As mentioned in Chapter 9, traumatic damage to joints is an important predisposing factor for osteoarthritis which is such a troublesome disease in later life. Cervical spine injuries are occasionally incurred in sports such as rugby, diving, trampolining, gymnastics and horse-riding and long-term adverse neurocognitive effects are a cause for concern in boxers. A heightened risk for early-onset dementia in soccer players, probably due to repeated heading of the ball in training as well as in competition, is also giving rise to increasing concern.

Running

Running carries a high risk of injury. Among recreational runners who are training steadily and participate in a long-distance run every now and then, the yearly incidence rate for injuries has been reported to be between 37% and 56%. In a large, representative study in the Netherlands, the incidence rate was 2.5 higher in novice runners than in experienced runners (Kemler et al. 2018). Competitive athletes typically incur between 2.5 and 5.8 injuries per 1,000 hour hours of running, depending on their speciality. Most injuries are to the lower limb, predominantly the knee, and the majority appear to be due to the constant repetition of the same movement and impact; that is, they are overuse injuries, often stress fractures. Common sites for stress fractures, together with notes on definition, symptoms and diagnosis are shown in Figure 13.1.

Many overuse injuries lead to a reduction in or cessation of training. Weekly distance run is the most important determinant of such injuries for both men and women and their incidence increases rapidly when average weekly distance run exceeds 40 miles (64 km). Other predisposing factors include previous injury (injury recurrence is common), lack of running experience, running to compete and a rapid increase in training distance or intensity. In women, the risk of bone stress injury increases markedly with the number of triad components present (Barrack et al. 2014; see discussion later in this chapter). Running on hard surfaces and running in poor shoes are implicated in

Figure 13.1 Common sites of stress fractures to lower limb.

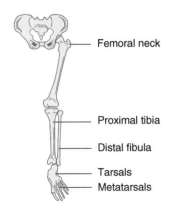

- Femoral neck
- Proximal tibia
- Distal fibula
- Tarsals
- Metatarsals

Stress fractures

- **Definition** – tiny cracks in bone, either through overuse or through normal use when bone has been weakened by a condition such as osteoporosis (see later section on athletic amenorrhoea)
- **Symptoms** – localised pain and swelling
- **Individuals at high risk** – athletes, military recruits, sedentary people who suddenly adopt an active lifestyle
- **Diagnosis** – may not be apparent on X-ray until several weeks after appearance of symptoms. Confirmation through various imaging techniques (magnetic resonance imaging, bone scans, computerised tomography)
- **Prevention** – avoid sudden changes to training regimen, alternate activities, appropriate footwear, ensure adequate calcium and other nutrients in diet.

about 5% of injuries. Age and sex do not appear to be important aetiological factors. That said, there is concern – at least in the US – that the incidence of running-related injuries in children and adolescents is increasing. One factor may be that the age of initiation of intense training in young athletes is coming down.

Moderate-intensity physical activity

Information about injury rates among people who engage in 'ordinary' amounts of moderate-intensity activity is limited as the risks have rarely been systematically evaluated. However, researchers have documented the prevalence and nature of injuries among participants in the Aerobics Center Longitudinal Study (Hootman et al. 2002). The subjects (5,028 men, 1,285 women), who were aged 20–85, provided information on their physical activity habits and injury experiences during one year immediately preceding a follow-up survey. A quarter of participants reported at least one musculo-skeletal injury and 83% of these were activity-related, two-thirds of them to the lower limb (Figure 13.2). Among both men and women, those participating in sports were the most likely to have an activity-related injury (27%), followed by runners (23–24%) and walkers (17–20%). However, 16% of subjects classified as inactive also reported

Figure 13.2 Distribution and percentage of activity-related musculoskeletal injuries among participants in the US Aerobics Center Longitudinal Study. 'Other' injuries, not depicted in the figure, comprised 1.9% and 5.7% of total injuries to men and women, respectively.

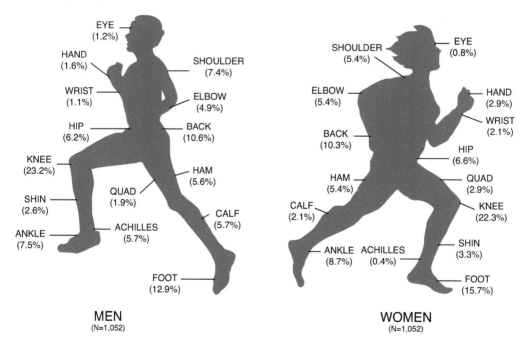

Source: Reprinted with permission from Wolters Kluwer Health, Inc.: Hootman, J.M. et al. (2002) 'Epidemiology of musculoskeletal injuries among sedentary and physically active adults', *Medicine and Science in Sports and Exercise*, 34: 838–44. Available at: https://doi.org/10.1097/00005768-200205000-00017.

activity-related injuries and so not all the injuries among the active groups could be attributed to physical activity purposefully taken for reasons of health benefit.

Few randomised intervention trials report data on injuries associated with adopting a habit of moderate activity. One is the Diabetes Prevention Program Group report (mentioned in Chapter 5). Their findings are broadly in line with those from the Aerobics Center Longitudinal Study. Among men and women at risk of type 2 diabetes whose goal was 'moderate exercise such as brisk walking for at least 150 minutes per week' the incidence rate of musculoskeletal injury was low (24.1 per 100 person-years) and about the same as that experienced by the placebo group (Knowler et al. 2002). In a later, multi-centre trial of more than 5000 patients with type 2 diabetes, participants in the intervention group (aim – at least 175 minutes of moderate exercise per week) did not experience more fractures likely to be exercise-related than those in the control group (Look AHEAD Research Group 2013).

Thus, moderate amounts and intensities of physical activity are not associated with a high risk of musculoskeletal injuries and walking carries a particularly low risk. In the Aerobics Center Longitudinal Study, men and women who walked for exercise experienced few 'excess' injuries; that is, above and beyond those reported in the inactive group. Increasing duration of walking per week was not associated with an increased risk of injury (Hootman et al. 2001). In an early study of 21 elderly men and women who trained by walking briskly for three sessions per week, increasing to 45 minutes per session, only one injury was sustained over 13 weeks (Pollock et al. 1991).

ADVERSE CARDIOVASCULAR EVENTS

Endurance exercise increases the physiological demands on the heart and, when undertaken regularly, leads to structural, functional and electrical cardiac adaptations. Collectively, these (together with effects on risk factor for cardiovascular disease (CVD)) probably explain the extensive epidemiological evidence suggesting that level of regular physical activity reduces the risk of CVD in a graded manner. Nevertheless, exercise can have both acute and, possibly chronic, adverse cardiac effects.

Acute cardiac events

Vigorous physical activity can acutely and transiently increase the risk of heart attack or even sudden cardiac death in susceptible individuals. Who is 'susceptible' and why? Just how risky is vigorous exercise for the heart? What factors modify that risk? Research has provided some of the answers to these questions.

First, people who experience an exercise-related cardiac event invariably have underlying heart disease. In young adults this is typically some sort of hereditary or congenital cardiovascular abnormality, the most common being hypertrophic cardiomyopathy or coronary artery abnormalities. Ventricular arrhythmias are the immediate cause of death in these conditions. By contrast, in middle-aged and older individuals who experience sudden cardiac death, atherosclerotic coronary artery disease is the most frequent pathological finding; autopsy reports commonly include evidence for acute disruption of an atherosclerotic plaque, with thrombotic occlusion of a coronary artery.

Can the increased risk of a cardiac event associated with vigorous exercise be quantified? In a classic study in Seattle, limited to previously asymptomatic individuals, the incidence of cardiac arrest during exercise was 25 times higher than at all other times (Siscovick et al. 1984). Findings from the later US Physicians' Health Study bolster these conclusions: among more than 12,000 men followed for 12 years, the risk of sudden cardiac death associated with an episode of vigorous exercise was 17 times higher than at all other times (Albert et al. 2000).

Besides the presence or absence of existing disease, the most important factor that modifies the increase in risk of a cardiac event during exercise is level of habitual exercise. In Germany (Willich et al. 1993) and in the United States (Mittleman et al. 1993), researchers interviewed patients soon after they were admitted to hospital with myocardial infarction. Vigorous exercise was clearly one trigger to myocardial infarction but a striking finding in both studies was that the increase in risk during or after vigorous exercise differed greatly according to patients' usual frequency of this level of exercise. In the American study the exercise-associated risk was 2.4 among those reporting regular vigorous exertion but it was 107 among inactive men, with clear evidence of a dose–response relationship (Figure 13.3). Thus the risk of a sudden cardiac

---

Figure 13.3 Relative risk of onset of myocardial infarction during a single session of heavy exertion, compared with all other times, according to the habitual frequency of heavy exertion at ≥6 METs.

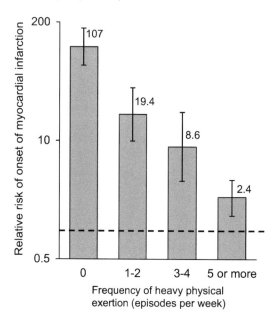

Source: From the *New England Journal of Medicine*, Mittleman, M.A. et al., 'Triggering of acute myocardial infarction by heavy physical exertion: protection against triggering by regular exertion', 329: 1677–83. Copyright © 1993 Massachusetts Medical Society. Reprinted with permission from Massachusetts Medical Society.

Note: The relative risk is shown on a logarithmic scale because the extremely high relative risk in habitually inactive people (107) was so different from that in people who reported that they regularly engaged in heavy exertion five or more times per week (2.4, $P < 0.001$). The horizontal line represents the baseline risk; that is, the risk during no exertion or during light exertion. Bars represent 95% confidence intervals.

event associated with a bout of vigorous exertion is much greater in habitually inactive men than in men accustomed to this level of exertion.

These findings are not inconsistent with extensive, robust evidence that regular, frequent exercise lowers the risk for cardiovascular events; acute bouts of exercise can clearly trigger cardiovascular events but regular exercisers exhibit a much smaller increase in risk during each bout of exercise and, most importantly, a lower overall risk in the long term (Figure 13.4).

At this point it is important to distinguish between the *relative* risk during exercise and the *absolute* risk. Although the *relative* risk is clearly increased during a session of exercise compared with other times, the *absolute* risk is extremely low in ostensibly healthy people. For example, the Physicians' Health Study reported just one death per 1.51 million episodes of exercise during a 12-year follow-up of nearly 21,500 men (Albert et al. 2000). Even in the marathon, the incidence rates for cardiac events are low, of the order of 1 to 1.75 per 100,000 runners for sudden cardiac arrest and around 0.6 per 100,000 runners for sudden cardiac death (Kim et al. 2012; Webner et al. 2012). The incidence of sudden cardiac death in young, apparently healthy, athletes during other competitive sports is even lower although such events invariably receive much publicity. Such high-profile incidents seldom involve women athletes as the incidence of sudden cardiac death in sports is ten times greater in men than in women (Colombo and Finocchiaro 2018).

As might be expected, the incidence of exercise-related deaths among high-risk adults is higher. Based on reports of medically supervised cardiac rehabilitation programmes, one may expect one cardiac arrest per 116,906 patient hours of rehabilitative exercise,

Figure 13.4 Schematic representation of risk for myocardial infarction in active and inactive people. The dashed line shows the large transient increase in risk associated with an isolated episode of vigorous exercise in inactive people. The solid line shows that people who are habitually active have a lower level of risk whilst at rest but also a much smaller transient increase in risk associated with each episode of exercise.

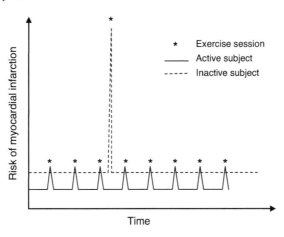

Source: Adapted with permission from Wolters Kluwer Health, Inc.: Mittleman, M.A. and Mostofsky, E. (2011) 'Physical, psychological and chemical triggers of acute cardiovascular events: preventive strategies', *Circulation*, 124: 346–54. Available at: https://doi.org/10.1161/CIRCULATIONAHA.110.968776.

one myocardial infarction per 219,970 patient hours and one fatality per 752,365 patient hours (Thompson et al. 2007).

Cardiac overuse injury – a hypothesis

The previous discussion focused on acute cardiac events but it can be argued that extreme levels of prolonged high-intensity endurance exercise over years may lead to cardiac maladaptations. Proponents of this 'extreme exercise hypothesis' speculate that the dose–response relationship between level of physical activity and benefits for cardiovascular health – long described as curvilinear – may in fact be U- or J-shaped (Eijsvogels et al. 2018) (Figure 13.5). Their argument is based on two main lines of evidence, i.e. epidemiological studies and observations in cohorts of endurance athletes.

There are reports in prospective studies that the disease/mortality risk in the most active group studied was smaller than that in groups with lower levels of activity. Examples include the classic study of Harvard alumni (Paffenbarger et al. 1986, see Chapter 4) as well as a later pooled analysis of the dose-response relationship (Arem et al. 2015). In the Copenhagen City Heart Study joggers as a group had a remarkable 44% lower risk for all-cause mortality than non-joggers over 35 years (Schnohr et al. 2013). However, when joggers were further categorised as light, moderate or strenuous

Figure 13.5 Conceptual overview of the extreme exercise hypothesis depicting a curvilinear relationship between volume of exercise and health benefits. Speculatively, there exists a volume of exercise training beyond which benefits may be partially lost. The schematic takes no account of exercise intensity.

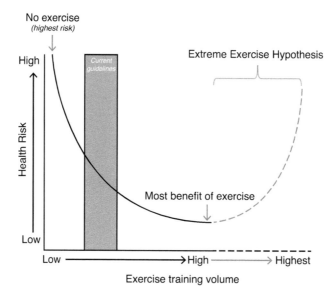

Source: Reprinted with no modifications from 'The "Extreme Exercise Hypothesis"; recent findings and cardiovascular health implications', Eijsvogels, T.M.H. et al., *Current Treatment Options in Cardiovascular Medicine*, 2018, 20: 84. Article distributed under the terms of the Creative Commons Attribution 4.0 International (CC BY) Licence (http://creativecommons.org/licenses/by/4.0/).

according to quantity, speed and frequency of jogging, the hazard ratio for mortality was lowest in light joggers, followed by moderate joggers and then strenuous joggers. Mortality among strenuous joggers was not significantly different from that in the sedentary group, suggesting a U-shaped association between mortality and 'dose' of jogging (Schnohr et al. 2015).

Such observations appear to challenge the notion that 'more is better' for the health benefits of activity. Epidemiological studies, however, seldom have the power to explore the top end of the dose–response relationship and have typically been concerned to identify the *minimum* effective dose of activity as this is the most important element of recommendations for public health.

What evidence is there for mechanisms that might explain potential adverse cardiac effects of extreme exercise? First, there are reports of a higher prevalence of cardiac fibrosis in lifelong endurance athletes than controls, as detected by magnetic resonance imaging (van de Schoor et al. 2016). An explanation might be that individual sessions of extreme endurance exercise cause acute volume overload of the chambers of the heart which leads to overstretching and micro-tears in the myocardium. Such damage leads to infiltration of collagen and subsequent cardiac fibrosis. Cardiac fibrosis is associated with myocardial stiffness and poor ventricular systolic function which is a common phenomenon in the late stages of diverse cardiac diseases. Not all endurance athletes demonstrate myocardial fibrosis, however, and the clinical implications in those who do are unknown.

Based on changes in cardiac biomarkers, a session of challenging endurance exercise certainly leads to cardiac stress. One such marker is troponin – a protein found in cardiac myocytes which is a standard marker in blood for diagnosis of myocardial infarction. Circulating troponin levels were increased in every runner studied during the 2011 Boston marathon (Eijsvogels et al. 2014) (Figure 13.6). Such elevations in cardiac

Figure 13.6 Increases in concentrations in cardiac troponin after running a marathon. Each bar represents one runner. All individuals demonstrated an increase in cardiac troponin

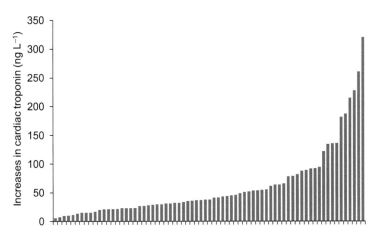

Source: Reprinted from *The American Journal of Cardiology*, 114: 624–8, Eijsvogels, T.M.H. et al., 'Impact of statin use on exercise-induced cardiac troponin elevations', page 626, copyright © 2014, with permission from Elsevier.

biomarkers appear to return to baseline within a week, however, so once more, their clinical implications are uncertain.

Coronary artery calcification, an excellent predictor of future cardiac events, has been reported to be more extensive in marathon runners (≥5 races) than in controls matched for age and Framingham score (a composite risk factor score) (Mohlenkamp et al. 2008). On the other hand, individuals who engage in mild to moderate levels of activity have typically been found to have lower coronary artery calcification scores than those of control groups. There is no consensus on the possibility of accelerated coronary atherosclerosis with extreme endurance exercise.

Research has much to clarify in these and related areas but there is already sufficient evidence to justify concern that, after years or decades of training for and competing in events such as marathons, ultramarathons or ironman triathlons, pathological changes may adversely affect cardiac function.

Atrial fibrillation

Atrial fibrillation refers to chaotic electrical activity that replaces normal sinus rhythm, impairing left ventricular filling and hence cardiac output. Its prevalence in the UK and the US ranges from 2% in under 65s to around 9% in people aged 65 and over. It is associated with a five-fold risk of stroke because of the blood stasis it creates in the atria.

Whilst low levels of physical activity appear to be associated with reduced prevalence of atrial fibrillation, maybe because of a blood pressure lowering effect (hypertension is an important risk factor for atrial fibrillation), long-term high levels of endurance exercise are rather consistently associated with *increased* prevalence (Wehrens et al. 2013). For example, in the US Physicians' Health Study, the risk for atrial fibrillation increased with the number of days per week of vigorous physical activity reported (Aizer et al. 2009). Even among athletes, prevalence seems to increase with the amount of intense endurance training undertaken and is raised in veteran athletes. Norwegian researchers evaluated veteran cross-country skiers who were followed up 28–30 years later. The final analysis included 78 skiers and the overall prevalence of atrial fibrillation in the group was 16.7% (Grimsmo et al. 2010).

Potential mechanisms which might explain the higher prevalence of atrial fibrillation in athletes include anatomic changes arising from long-standing volume and/or pressure overload, alterations to the autonomic nervous system, as demonstrated in an animal model (Guasch et al. 2013), exposure to sustained inflammatory responses and fluid shifts with associated challenges to electrolyte homeostasis.

Because of the links between atrial fibrillation and risk for stroke, clinicians recommend that athletes with this condition should always be investigated. It appears, however, that endurance athletes suffer fewer strokes *despite* their higher prevalence of atrial fibrillation. Researchers drew on comprehensive records of 203,000 participants in the World's largest ski-race, the Swedish Vasaloppet. Stroke rates among this physically active group were compared with those in a population drawn randomly from that country's Total Population Register and then matched with the skiers according to key variables; the stroke rate among skiers did not differ from that in the non-skiers, despite their higher prevalence of atrial fibrillation (Hållmarker et al. 2015).

In summary, evidence to support the extreme endurance hypothesis is essentially circumstantial at the time of writing – and based almost entirely on male athletes. The adverse adaptations described may be limited to susceptible individuals and further research is needed before a firm conclusion can be drawn in a potential safe upper limit to physical activity. In the meantime, case reports paint differing pictures. For example, the heart of a six-time ultramarathon winner who had accumulated more than 50,000 hours of training and competition over 35 years, averaging 25–30 hours per week was found at autopsy to be 'quite normal' (Araújo et al. 2014). On the other hand, when Micah True, an American who dropped out of modern civilisation to live and run daily distances of 25 to 100 miles with the Tarahumara Indians, dropped dead at the age of 58 whilst on a modest 12-mile training run his death was attributed to an unclassified cardiomyopathy which resulted in cardiac dysrhythmia (Hutchinson 2012).

Paradoxically then, exercise can be hazardous – as well as beneficial – for the heart. Does this diminish its role as part of a population-based preventive strategy against CHD? The answer to this question – crucial for public health – is clearly 'no'. There is no evidence that the risks of engaging in recommended amounts and intensities of physical activity outweigh the benefits for healthy people. Rather, the converse is true – benefits outweigh risks. Emerging evidence for potential cardiac harms with prodigious amounts of exercise has, though, stimulated debate concerning dose–response issues. The search for the lowest effective dose of activity for health will continue because levels of inactivity are typically so high but there is now good reason to question the assumption that more is always better. The issue of benefit versus risk for CHD at a population level is discussed more fully in Chapter 14 in the context of public health.

FEMALE ATHLETE TRIAD (RELATIVE ENERGY DEFICIENCY IN SPORT)

For most women, important health benefits accrue from leading a physically active lifestyle. On the other hand, extremely active girls and women may be at risk of developing a syndrome known as the 'female athlete triad'. This term was first adopted in the early 1990s by a group convened by the ACSM to describe the association of 'disordered eating, amenorrhea and osteoporosis' observed in some female athletes. These clinical endpoints were the diagnostic criteria initially adopted but it soon became clear that many female athletes with less severe manifestations of the triad components still faced important health issues.

Consequently, subsequent Position Stands of the American College of Sports Medicine (ACSM) and the International Olympic Committee (IOC) employed a wider definition of the triad as the pathological end of a spectrum of inter-related *sub*clinical conditions, i.e. low energy availability (with or without eating disorders), amenorrhea and osteoporosis which, singly or in combination, pose significant health risks (IOC Medical Commission Working Group Women in Sport 2005; Nattiv et al. 2007). Later, an international group of leading triad researchers went on to specify triad diagnostic components as: (i) low energy availability (with or without disordered eating), (ii) menstrual dysfunction and (iii) low bone mineral density (De Souza et al. 2014).

Whilst there is wide agreement that low energy availability is the defining feature of the triad, controversy is evident between different expert groups. The IOC consensus group proposed a new name – relative energy deficiency in sport (RED-S). Their model

Figure 13.7 Definition of the female athlete triad: athletes may present with one or more of the three inter-related components.

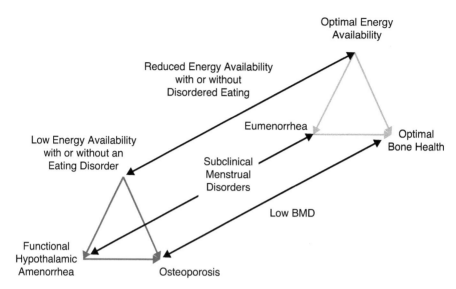

Source: Adapted with permission from Wolters Kluwer Health, Inc.: Nattiv, A. et al. (2007) 'American College of Sports Medicine position stand: The female athlete triad', *Medicine and Science in Sports and Exercise*, 39: 1867–82. Available at: https://doi.org/10.1249/mss.0b013e318149f111.

depicts energy deficiency as the 'central hub' from which a number of physiological sequelae besides menstrual dysfunction and bone health arise; it also includes male and 'para' athletes (Mountjoy et al. 2014, 2018). Other high-profile researchers in the field question the validity of the IOC group's postulation that energy deficiency exerts direct effects on systems such as immunological, cardiovascular and gastrointestinal health (De Souza et al. 2017). Until further evidence confirms the proposed links, the conservative approach is to retain the model depicted in the 2007 ACSM position stand on the female athlete triad and the 2014 female athlete triad coalition consensus statement (De Souza et al. 2014; Nattiv et al. 2007) (Figure 13.7). For review of the historical development of research in the area the reader is referred to Slater and colleagues (2017).

Energy availability

In exercise physiology, energy availability is defined as dietary energy intake minus exercise energy expenditure, i.e. the amount of dietary energy available for other bodily functions after exercise training. When this is too low, physiological mechanisms adapt by reducing the amount of energy used for cellular maintenance, thermoregulation, growth and reproduction. While this compensation tends to restore energy balance and promote survival, it impairs health.

The reader should note that energy *availability* is not the same as energy *balance*. The latter term is defined as dietary energy intake minus *total* energy expenditure, i.e. the amount of dietary energy added to or lost from the body's energy stores after the body's physiological systems have 'done their work for the day'. For further clarification of this important distinction see Loucks and colleagues (2011).

Four distinct origins of low energy availability can be identified in athletes. The first is obsessive disordered eating. Such behaviours can progress to clinical eating disorders such as anorexia nervosa or bulimia nervosa. The second is intentional efforts to reduce body size and fatness in order to succeed in events that require or prize leanness. The third is the *inadvertent* failure to increase energy intake to compensate for the energy expended in exercise: an athlete may be eating normally for a non-athlete but not realise that her energy intake is insufficient to meet her enhanced energy needs. This may be a particular problem among girls as their food intake must also cover the energy costs of growth. Fourthly, female athletes may also under-eat for reasons unrelated to sport, for perceived 'improvement of appearance', for instance. For elite athletes, the challenge of balancing strict training and travel schedules with mealtimes may also be a factor influencing energy availability.

So, what constitutes *low* energy availability? This question can be answered by ascertaining the level at which physiological processes are compromised. For example, careful laboratory studies have found that, when energy availability is less than 126 kJ (30 kcal) per kg fat-free mass per day, reproductive function is disrupted and bone health is impaired. This threshold, which roughly equates to the average resting metabolic rate, will be higher in growing adolescents. Measuring energy availability in free-living athletes is fraught with problems, however, and estimates are used in diagnosis and monitoring (Burke et al. 2018b).

When energy availability is low, the neuroendocrine functions of the hypothalamus are impaired and the ensuing absence of normal menses is termed *functional hypothalamic amenorrhoea*: oestrogen levels fall, compromising both bone mineralisation and the rate of bone protein synthesis. Low energy availability also suppresses type 1 immunity that mounts the body's defence against intracellular pathogens like viruses.

Menstrual dysfunction

Menarche has been reported to occur later in athletic girls – gymnasts and dancers, for example – than in those who are less active. This may be indicative of primary amenorrhoea (no menarche by age 16, despite normal secondary sexual characteristics) but is more likely accounted for by the self-selection of late-maturing girls into these activities. By contrast, the high prevalence of menstrual dysfunction among women athletes is clearly associated with their eating and exercise behaviours. This can take the form of secondary amenorrhoea (the absence of menstrual cycles for three or more months in women with previously normal menstruation) or oligomenorrhoea (menstrual cycles at intervals longer than 35 days). Luteal deficiency and anovulation, other important forms of dysfunction, have no perceptible symptoms.

The first systematic study of menstrual dysfunction in athletes found that between 6% and 43% of women runners participating in the 1977 US National Collegiate Cross-Country Championships had amenorrhoea and that its prevalence was linearly related to training distance (Feicht et al. 1978) (Figure 13.8). Training intensity was

Figure 13.8 Incidence of secondary amenorrhoea in women runners in relation to distance run during training.

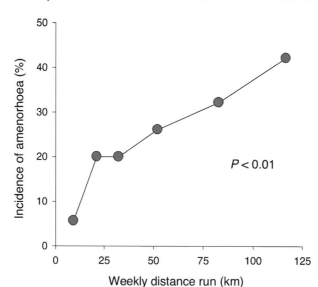

Source: Reprinted from *The Lancet*, 312: 1145–6, Feicht, C.B. et al., 'Secondary amenorrhoea in athletes', page 1145, copyright © 1978, with permission from Elsevier.

highest among the amenorrhoeic athletes and they were also better runners than those who were menstruating regularly.

In the ensuing decades a strong body of evidence supporting and extending this finding has been published. Reports of the prevalence of menstrual disorders in athletes vary widely but, in general, this is highest in sports where leanness influences performance or where weight categories define competition. Based on meta-analysis of the findings of 65 studies, clinical dysfunction (amenorrhoea/oligomenorrhoea) in adult female athletes ranges from 1% to 63% (Gibbs et al. 2013). Where valid comparisons have been made, prevalence is much higher than in non-athletic women of comparable age in the general population. Predisposing factors include youth (women who take up a sport as adults are less likely to become amenorrhoeic), a low level of body fatness and a high training intensity or volume. Intense training for non-sporting activity is also associated with amenorrhoea; for example, around 40% of ballet dancers are amenorrhoeic.

Menstrual disturbances can be induced when a habit of strenuous exercise is begun. In one prospective study, women began running 6.4 km (4 miles) per day, progressing to 16.1 km (10 miles) per day by the fifth week as well as engaging daily in moderate intensity sports (Bullen et al. 1985). Based on hormonal measurements, only four of 28 participants had a normal menstrual cycle whilst pursuing this training regimen. Within six months of the end of the study, all participants were again experiencing normal menstrual cycles, confirming the causal role of strenuous training in menstrual disorders.

Reproductive function is often impaired even in women who have a normal pattern of menstrual bleeding. Researchers have undertaken careful comparisons of the characteristics of menstrual cycles of recreational exercisers with those of inactive age- and weight-matched controls, using daily measurements of reproductive hormones over two to three months (De Souza et al. 2010). Exercising women had average values for $\dot{V}O_2$max and BMI of 44 ml kg^{-1} min^{-1} and 22.0 kg m^{-2}, respectively. They engaged in 'purposeful' exercise for an average of 7.5 hours per week. Among the inactive group, the prevalence of subtle menstrual disturbances was only 4%, with 96% of cycles defined as ovulatory. In stark contrast, amongst exercising women presenting with regular, repeatable cycles of about 28 days, 52% showed luteal phase defects or anovulation (Figure 13.9). These findings, and others, demonstrate that studies relying solely on self-report to document menstrual function are likely to underestimate the prevalence of disorders – probably one reason for the wide variation in reported prevalence.

Figure 13.9 Prevalence of subtle menstrual disturbances among (a) inactive (n = 20) and (b) exercising (n = 48) women. Compared with inactive women, a greater proportion of exercising women displayed anovulatory cycles ($P < 0.001$) and luteal phase defects ($P < 0.05$).

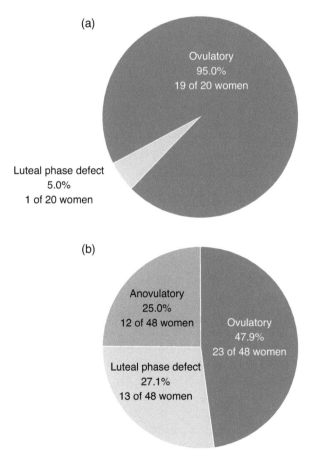

Source: M.J. De Souza, R.J. Toombs, J.L. Scheid et al. High prevalence of subtle and severe menstrual disturbances in exercising women: confirmation using daily hormone measures. *Human Reproduction* (2010) 25: 491–503, doi: 10.1093/humrep/dep411. Adapted with permission from Oxford University Press on behalf of the European Society of Human Reproduction and Embryology.

If low energy availability is indeed the important causal factor in the menstrual disorders of athletes, then these should be prevented or reversed by dietary intervention without any moderation of the exercise regimen. Disruption of the normal preovulatory surge in luteinising hormone[1] constitutes a marker for menstrual and ovarian dysfunction. Any combination of dietary restriction and exercise energy expenditure that reduces energy availability disrupts the pulsatile secretion of this hormone within days, in proportion to the magnitude of the energy deficit. These findings are consistent with an extensive literature showing that reproductive function in animals is dependent on energy availability. When women with a habit of exercise supplement their diet to compensate fully for their exercise energy expenditure, disruption of luteinising hormone pulsatility is prevented.

'Athletic amenorrhoea' can be reversed by modest weight gain and/or a reduced level of training which restore adequate energy availability. In a five-year retrospective study of 50 amenhorrhoeic/oligomenorrhoeic college athletes, those with a weight gain of 2.27 kg (5 lb) were twice as likely to resume menses as those with less weight gain (Arends et al. 2012). Thus amenorrhoea is not necessarily, in itself, a long-term hazard to reproductive health. Its most obvious short-term consequence is infertility; amenorrhoeic women are not developing egg cells that can be fertilised. Short luteal phases and low progesterone can also lead to infertility due to failures of implantation. Paradoxically, without contraception, irregularly menstruating athletes may be at increased risk for unwanted pregnancy because their day of ovulation is less predictable.

On the other hand, long episodes of amenorrhoea have important consequences for health beyond their impact on reproductive physiology. The best-documented consequence of low oestrogen states is skeletal demineralisation.

Low bone mineral density

Amenorrhoea can predispose athletes to low bone mineral density (BMD) and put them at higher risk of fragility fractures. Several reports in the early 1980s showed that women with exercise-associated amenorrhoea had lower spinal BMD than age-matched physically active or inactive eumenorrhoeic women. Retrospective analysis of the menstrual histories of nearly 100 runners found that spinal BMD correlated with the degree (severity and duration) of their amenorrhoea (Drinkwater et al. 1990) (Figure 13.10). Moreover, as newer techniques became available, it has become clear that bone loss in amenorrhoeic athletes is not restricted to the spine, but may be observed at multiple skeletal sites, suggesting that this is a generalised effect and that even sites subjected to impact loading during exercise may be affected. The problem of low BMD is not restricted to women with exercise-associated oligo/amenorrhoea. Physically active women with regular menstrual cycles but who are anovulatory and/or have short luteal phases also experience bone loss.

As would be expected when BMD is compromised, stress fractures are common among amenorrhoeic athletes (Duckham et al. 2012). A dose–response relationship is evident with respect to such injuries, for which the strongest predictors are low BMD, low BMI and 12 or more hours per week of purposeful exercise (Barrack et al. 2014). A high prevalence is also evident in other groups of vigorously exercising women. Among

Figure 13.10 Relationship between bone mineral density and menstrual history for 97 active women aged between 18 and 38.

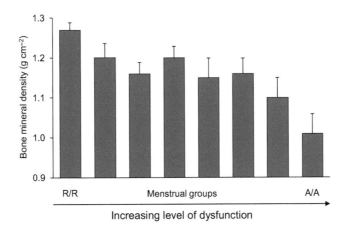

Source: Adapted from Drinkwater et al. (1990).
Note: Values are mean and standard error. Subjects were categorised according to both pattern of menstrual function at time of observation and previous menstrual history; R/R regular menstrual cycles at time of study and previously; A/A amenorrhoeic at the time of study and previously. Other groups had histories intermediate between these two.

female recruits in basic training for the US Marine Corps, amenorrhoeic women had an almost three-fold increase in the risk of a lower extremity stress fracture (Rauh et al. 2006). In another study, every one of a group of amenorrhoeic ballet dancers who practised for more than five hours per day had experienced a stress fracture (Kadel et al. 1992).

No large prospective trials are available to evaluate the long-term consequences for skeletal health in women who have experienced long episodes of oligo/amenorrhoea. Eight-year follow-up data have been reported for a group of 29 athletes; despite several years of normal menses or use of oral contraceptives, formerly oligomenorrhoeic athletes still had values for vertebral BMD that were 15% lower than those of the athletes who had regular menses throughout (Keen and Drinkwater 1997). Amenorrhoeic athletes are clearly at risk for a decrease in bone mass and this may be irreversible. It is not known whether or not these women are at risk for premature osteoporotic fractures as they age. Even if regular menstrual cycles are restored with pharmacological therapy – and evidence for this is mixed – the metabolic factors that impair bone health will not be normalised. It is widely accepted that, at least among postmenopausal women, lost bone cannot be restored.

The effect of menstrual dysfunction on BMD is of special concern for young athletes; BMD normally doubles during adolescence and anything that impairs bone mineral accrual during this stage of life may lead to low peak BMD in adulthood. A prospective study of 40 adolescent runners with a mean age of 15.9 years found that 90% of those with low bone mass for age at baseline failed to increase this to normal levels three years later, emphasising the importance of optimising bone mineral accrual during early to mid-adolescence (Barrack et al. 2011).

Disordered eating

Disordered eating includes a range of abnormal eating behaviours, including restrictive eating, fasting, frequently skipping meals, binge-eating and purging or even use of laxatives and diuretics. It leads to low energy availability and the consequences of this. Moreover, disordered eating can progress to clinical eating disorders that are often accompanied by other psychiatric illnesses.

The prevalence of disordered eating in adult athletes is high and, in general, exceeds rates found in non-athletic controls. For example, a controlled study of the entire population of Norwegian female elite athletes aged 15–39 (n = 572) found that 20% exhibited eating disorders, compared with 9% of controls (Sundgot-Borgen and Torstveit 2004). The prevalence of disorders was highest (42%) in athletes competing in 'aesthetic' sports such as figure skating, gymnastics and dancing where female athletes may feel under pressure to reduce weight in order to perform well. Disordered eating was also prevalent in sports that employ weight categories, for example judo and karate, where many athletes often want to compete in a class below their 'ordinary' weight. Disordered eating is also apparent in non-sporting groups. Dance students and professional ballerinas have been reported to consume less than 70% of the energy needed to meet body weight targets.

However, to put this into perspective, some studies have found that the prevalence of disordered eating is actually higher in controls than in athletes. For example, researchers made comparisons between 15–16-year-old pupils from elite sport high schools in Norway and age-matched controls (Martinsen et al. 2010). Amongst non-athletic girls, 71% of controls practised disordered eating, compared with 45% of athletes. In boys, this behaviour was also more prevalent in controls than in athletes (30% vs 13%). This same pattern was found in another robust study of high school pupils, this time in Germany (Rosendahl et al. 2009).

So, whilst disordered eating is clearly one reason for energy deficiency in athletes, other young females (and males) are also at risk of low energy availability – particularly during adolescence – because social success and attractiveness are often equated with thinness.

Prevalence

In athletes, the prevalence of disordered eating, menstrual dysfunction and low BMD varies widely. However, low energy availability – the defining feature of the triad – can be present even in the absence of disordered eating often because of compulsive exercise. The prevalence of the triad and its components is still poorly documented and the issue remains complicated by the different definitions employed.

Only a handful of studies have investigated the simultaneous occurrence of disordered eating, menstrual disorders and low BMD, identifying the latter by criteria appropriate to premenopausal women. One large survey was conducted in Norway, where all female elite athletes aged 13–39 (n = 938) from 66 diverse sports were invited to participate in a study, along with 900 controls in the same age group (Torstveit and Sundgot-Borgen 2005). Controls were randomly selected from the total female population. Eight athletes (4.3%) and five controls (3.4%) met all the authors' criteria for the triad (Figure 13.11). Other studies have found the entire triad in 2.7% of collegiate

Figure 13.11 Prevalence of the three components of the female athlete triad in elite Norwegian athletes and age-group-matched controls randomly selected from the Norwegian population. Data are given in numbers with percentages in brackets.

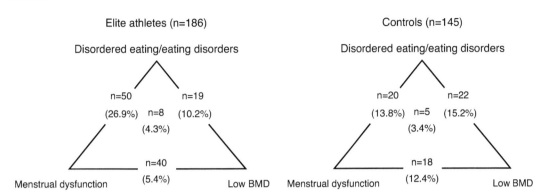

Source: Adapted with permission from Wolters Kluwer Health, Inc.: Torstveit, M.K. and Sundgot-Borgen, J., (2005) 'The female athlete triad exists in both elite athletes and controls', *Medicine and Science in Sports and Exercise*, 37: 1449–59. Available at: https://doi.org/10.1249/01.mss.0000177678.73041.38.

athletes (3/112) and in 1.2% of high school athletes (2/170) but the reported prevalence varies widely (Gibbs et al. 2013). Readers interested in the methodological challenges of research in this area are referred to Loucks (2006), Nattiv and colleagues (2007) and Williams and De Souza (2006).

What about male athletes?

The above discussion, like much of the literature in this area, has focused on women. Do male athletes exhibit features of the triad? A subset of male athletes, especially in those sports emphasising leanness, do exhibit similar features and the issue is now an active area of research, stimulated by the introduction of the concept RED-S (Mountjoy et al. 2014, 2018).

The risk of low energy availability is apparently heightened in male cyclists, rowers, athletes in combat sports, distance runners and jockeys. Disordered eating has been reported in male athletes but the prevalence is lower than in their female contemporaries, at around 4–8%. In particular, the need to make weight in some sports leads to cyclical management of body mass which is detrimental to both energy availability and maintenance of levels of micronutrients. Young male athletes typically report enhanced performance as a reason for dieting (Martinsen et al. 2010).

Reproductive hormone responses are probably depressed by regular exercise in men as well as in women but, without an overt sign such as absence of menses, are difficult to document. Male endurance runners have been reported to exhibit plasma testosterone concentrations that are around 15% lower than those of inactive men, but clinical reproductive dysfunction is rare.

Based on cross-sectional studies, male athletes in weight-bearing sports typically have higher BMD than non-athletes but there are reports of surprisingly low values in cyclists, particularly in the lumbar spine (Smathers et al. 2009). Whilst a representative prevalence of low BMD in male athletes is unknown, it has been suggested that groups most at risk for impaired bone health are those participating in endurance and weight-class sports (Burke et al. 2018a; Tenforde et al. 2016).

IMPAIRED IMMUNE FUNCTION

As explained in Chapter 8, moderate exercise benefits immune function. By contrast, prolonged, intense exercise or training may elicit effects that may be dramatic and similar to clinical stresses such as trauma, burns, surgery and sepsis.

The most common illnesses in athletes, accounting for up to one third of non-injury presentations at sports medicine clinics, are upper respiratory tract illnesses with symptoms which include a sore throat, headache, fatigue, runny nose and/or watery eyes. Observational reports suggest that, during periods of heightened training or after marathon-type events, athletes are at increased risk of such episodes. For example, their incidence was studied in a group of 2,300 marathon runners who had applied to enter the Los Angeles marathon (Nieman et al. 1990). After the race, runners reported information about their training habits and about upper respiratory tract symptoms before and for one week after the race. Nearly 13% of participants reported having an episode during the week after the race, compared with only 2.2% of similarly experienced runners who had applied but did not participate (for reasons other than sickness). Participants were six times more likely to report upper respiratory tract illness during the week after the race than the non-participating runners. Runners training more than 96 km (60 miles) per week were twice as likely as those running less than 32 km (20 miles) per week to have experienced symptoms during the two months leading up to the marathon.

In a group of French professional swimmers monitored over four years, researchers found that a 10% increase in training load was associated with a 10% increase in the risk of upper respiratory tract illness (Hellard et al. 2015). Similar links between increases in training load and illness have been found in elite rugby union players and in American college football players.

Despite this sort of observational evidence, uncertainties remain as to what proportion of upper respiratory tract symptoms reported by athletes are in fact caused by infection. Symptoms such as sore throat can also be attributable to allergic responses to inhaled allergens or inflammation caused by inhalation of cold, dry or polluted air as well as other factors such as psychological stress, lack of sleep, exposure to environmental extremes (for example, high temperature or high altitude). Another possibility was raised by a substantial study of runners in the Stockholm marathon where the increased risk of post-race upper respiratory tract illness was strongly related to *pre*-race illness, suggesting that participating in the race somehow reactivates an existing problem (Ekblom et al. 2006). The phenomenon known as viral reactivation may provide an explanation. Nevertheless, the weight of the evidence does support the idea that exercise-induced immune suppression increases susceptibility to symptoms of infection or inflammation.

A plethora of studies have investigated potential mechanisms that might explain increased susceptibility to upper respiratory tract infections in athletes. After prolonged, intensive exercise there are complex changes to the populations of cells that constitute a first line of defence against infection, i.e. macrophages, neutrophils and natural killer cells. (Macrophages have phagocytic and cytotoxic capacities; neutrophils, also phagocytic, are important in the non-specific killing of bacteria; natural killer cells seek out and destroy virus-infected cells.) Macrophage antiviral function, neutrophil function and natural killer cell activity are all impaired for several hours after a session of high-intensity exercise, particularly if this is prolonged. The function of T lymphocytes (important cells of the adaptive immune system) is also altered in these circumstances. These cells are pivotal for anti-viral responses and of particular relevance. In the light of these findings, it has been suggested that a prolonged session of high-intensity endurance exercise leads to transient, but clinically important, changes in immune function which give rise to an 'open window' of altered immunity (which may last 3–72 hours) during which viruses and bacteria may gain a foothold.

Impairment of mucosal immunity by prolonged, intense exercise may also contribute to increased susceptibility to upper respiratory tract symptoms. Secretion of immunoglobulins protects mucosal surfaces in the mouth and respiratory system, providing defence against pathogens present at mucosal surfaces. Functionally, the most important of these is immunoglobulin A (IgA), which is relatively easily measured in saliva. Very prolonged exercise and periods of intensified training can result in its decreased secretion in saliva and reduced levels are associated with increased risk of upper respiratory tract infections.

One weakness of evidence in this field is that investigators have yet to link most markers of immunosuppression after exercise with an actual increased incidence of infections or inflammation. It is difficult (and expensive) to confirm the cause of reported symptoms. There is no single marker of immune function to adopt as an outcome measure and the need to employ a large spectrum of parameters restricts research activity. Measurement of IgA in tear fluid may prove a useful, non-invasive biomarker suitable for use in the field (Walsh and Oliver 2016). Despite these limitations to our understanding of the mechanisms involved, there is a consensus that the majority of elite athletes do experience symptoms of upper respiratory tract illness more frequently during periods of high-intensity training or after a competition.

PREVENTION

Some of the hazards of exercise are preventable.

Protective equipment offers an obvious and effective strategy in some sports. Examples include helmets, mouth guards, shin pads and knee pads: the compulsory use of a face mask in ice hockey has virtually eliminated eye injuries in this sport. Safety is improved if cyclists display lights and wear reflective clothing. Helmets offer protection for the head for cyclists, although there are reports from Canada, Australia and the United States that the increasing wearing of these has not been associated with a reduction in fatalities. However, measures of incidence are difficult to obtain in the absence of robust data on exposure: how much cycling is being engaged in by the population at-risk? Runners can decrease their risk of injury through traffic accidents by wearing clothing that ensures that they can easily be seen, and selecting their routes carefully. For many activities the risk of injury is influenced by environmental factors. For example, for the most part, roads are not configured to separate vulnerable pedestrians and cyclists from vehicle traffic.

As physical activity levels increase in a population, so do the numbers of injuries, with the social and economic consequences of these. Moreover, when a habit of activity is interrupted by injury its health benefits (for the individual and society) are lost. Injury prevention is thus an active research area and qualitative methods now complement the quantitative approach so that the context in which injuries occur is understood (Bolling et al. 2018).

The identification of effective preventive measures is important but researchers are also concerned to understand the determinants of 'preventive behaviour' – not only in sportsmen and women but also in referees, physiotherapists and governing bodies of sports (Verhagen et al. 2010). Head injuries in soccer provide an example. Most head injuries in soccer are due to the illegal use of the elbow in tackling when a player is heading a ball. Instructions by FIFA to referees to implement the 'elbow rule' more strictly were associated with a decline in the number of head injuries from 25 in the 2002 World Cup to 13 in the 2006 event.

Community-based attempts to prevent injuries have been reported. Swedish researchers compared injury rates in a year-long injury prevention intervention population with those in a comparable control population (Timpka and Lindqvist 2001). The intervention comprised: an injury prevention course for physical education teachers; a programme for coaches and referees on discouraging foul play; compulsory use of shin pads in soccer; increased supervision of novices in all sports; and courses for coaches on proper physical preparation. In the intervention population the total morbidity rate for sports-related injuries decreased by 14%; the rate of moderately severe injuries halved and minor injuries increased, but there was no change in the rate of severe injuries. However, there was no tendency towards a decreased injury rate among the over 40s, probably because they do not participate as much in the traditional, mainly team, sports targeted by this particular intervention.

Physical activity is an important cause of injuries in children; in the US, for example, over one-third of school-aged children sustain an injury severe enough to be treated by a doctor or nurse. Systematic review and meta-analysis of 21 exercise-based injury prevention programmes found that participation in such a programme halved injury risk in children and adolescents (Butler et al. 2017). Preventive behaviour may be particularly important for injury risk in young people because parental influence is strong.

Prevention of running injuries may best be tackled through education about rehabilitation after injury, early recognition of symptoms of overuse and of training principles. This is an important area since injury is the main reason for discontinuation of a running programme. Education on gradual entry into any sort of conditioning programme may be particularly important for middle-aged and older people especially if – often after long periods of an inactive lifestyle – they intend to enter or re-enter the competitive arena. However, the effectiveness of 'pre-conditioning' programmes on preventing running-related injuries has yet to be demonstrated.

One obvious way to reduce the risk for adverse cardiovascular events is to recommend that previously inactive individuals begin exercising at a low/moderate level and progress only gradually to more vigorous exercise. Other strategies include: preparing fitness personnel and facilities to identify and deal with cardiovascular emergencies; increasing health-care professionals' knowledge of pathological conditions that may increase risk; and educating physically active adults to recognise symptoms that may be indicative of cardiac disease.

Arguably, pre-participation screening could reduce exercise-related cardiac events. Guidance from working groups of clinicians in the US and Europe is that individuals deemed to be at heightened risk (because they have two or more CVD risk factors or because they are diabetic) should be considered for exercise testing before beginning a vigorous exercise training programme (Corrado et al. 2011; Thompson et al. 2007). However, the appropriate methodology for evaluation of *asymptomatic* adults who are physically active or intend to become active remains controversial. There is concern that a requirement for pre-participation health screening may constitute an unnecessary barrier to adopting an exercise programme. Accordingly, an ACSM roundtable of experts has proposed a new, logical model for screening such that physically inactive but otherwise healthy asymptomatic individuals may begin light- to moderate-intensity exercise without medical clearance (Riebe et al. 2015).

For young athletes, pre-participation practices vary. The issue here is that exercise in young people with hidden (usually hereditary or congenital) coronary heart disease may increase both exercise-related and non-exercise-related sudden death. The European Society of Cardiology recommends routine ECGs for all athletes as part of a comprehensive pre-participation evaluation. On the other hand, the American Heart Association, while recommending pre-participation screening for high school and college athletes, does not advocate that ECG is routinely included. In the UK there are no recommendations for widespread screening.

Reasons for not instigating widespread screening for young athletes include: the low incidence of cardiac events in this group; cost–benefit issues; the low specificity (proportion of true negatives correctly identified) of ECG as a screening tool in an athletic population; and the problem of 'false positives' – results that indicate a problem where one does not exist. The efficacy of screening remains contentious, with conflicting findings from an observational study in Italy (Corrado et al. 2006) and a survey of cardiac arrest events in Israel where medical screening of all competitive athletes became mandatory in 1997 (Steinvil et al. 2011).

Noting that, at least in Europe, the sport in which sudden cardiac death occurs most often is soccer, FIFA adopted in 2005 a comprehensive pre-competition medical assessment (Higgins and Andino 2013). They have also made it mandatory for all stadiums to have appropriately trained medical personnel available, initiatives which probably contributed to the full recovery made by Fabrice Muamba who went into cardiac arrest during an English Premier League game in 2012.

Prevention of the female athlete triad must focus on discouraging athletes from restrictive eating and on increasing understanding among athletes, coaches and health-care professionals of nutritional principles. Very active women and men – and athletes in particular – need to take special care to maintain energy intake at a sufficient level to match their high levels of energy expenditure. Education, not only of athletes, but also of parents and coaches is the key for prevention and early intervention. For many athletes, nutrition counselling and monitoring are sufficient, but both the ACSM and the IOC recommend that athletes are assessed for the triad at any health-screening opportunity or whenever they present with any of the associated clinical conditions. For a full discussion of issues concerning prevention, diagnosis, management and treatment, readers are referred to Consensus Statements from the IOC (Mountjoy et al. 2018) and the Female Athlete Triad Expert Panel (De Souza et al. 2014).

Finally, a constellation in athletes of symptoms such as fatigue, performance decline and mood disturbances known as the overtraining syndrome (Meeusen et al. 2013) is now an active area of research. The IOC has convened expert groups to address the question 'How much is too much?' in sport. These groups developed the concept of load, defining it 'broadly to include rapid changes in training and competition load, competition calendar congestion, psychological load and travel'. The evidence for the relationships of load with health outcomes in sports has been examined and it is clear that poorly managed training loads, combined with a saturated competition calendar may damage the health of athletes, increasing the risk for both injury (Soligard et al. 2016) and illness (Schwellnus et al. 2016). Conversely, good load management configures training, competition and other aspects of load to maximise adaptation and performance whilst minimising the risk for injury and illness. Both IOC statements provide guidelines for athletes and their support staff to help the achievement of these aims. Fundamentals include the right balance between training and recovery (Kellmann et al. 2018) and nutritional support to ensure robust immune function (Gleeson 2016).

In practice, most of the hazards of exercise may be avoided by pursuing a habit of moderate exercise, rather than high-volume, intense training. As explained earlier, the transient risk of a cardiac event during exercise is much lower in people who are physically active on a regular basis than in those who rarely take exercise. Inactive individuals who begin low-intensity activity and progress gradually to more and more intense activity will minimise their cardiovascular and injury risk. Women (and men) who engage in moderate-intensity activity and allow the physiological mechanisms of hunger and satiety to govern their eating behaviour are not at high risk of reproductive dysfunction or its consequences. Similarly, recreational exercisers are unlikely to experience problems with immune function or overtraining syndrome. It is clear from the comprehensive literature published over a period of more than 50 years that substantial health benefits can be gained from regular physical activity. Recognition that some risks are associated with some types of activity – as described in this chapter – does not alter this conclusion.

SUMMARY

- Participation in vigorous exercise or sports can be hazardous but moderate amounts and intensities of exercise carry little risk.
- Exercise-related musculoskeletal injuries are common. The majority are to the lower limb and two out of three occur during team sports.

- Vigorous exertion acutely and transiently increases the risk of sudden cardiac death and heart attack in susceptible people. Risk is much higher among people unaccustomed to vigorous exercise than in people who are habitually active at this level.
- Extreme levels of prolonged high-intensity endurance exercise over years may lead to cardiac maladaptations, including an increased prevalence of atrial fibrillation.
- The female athlete triad (Relative Energy Deficiency in Sport) is a syndrome evident in some women who are very active, particularly in activities that emphasise leanness. It is characterised by three inter-related problems: low energy availability (with or without disordered eating), irregular or absent menses and low bone mineral density. There is concern that bone loss may be largely irreversible. Even when menstrual periods are regular, there may be abnormalities that reduce fertility.
- Male athletes in sports emphasising leanness or involving weight categories do exhibit features of the triad but the body of literature is not extensive. The alternative term 'low energy density in sport' has been coined partly because of the need to include men.
- Immune function may be compromised for some hours after prolonged vigorous exercise, providing a 'window of opportunity' for infection and/or inflammation to gain a foothold and give rise to symptoms of upper respiratory tract illness.
- Some hazards may be prevented through protective equipment. Those mainly associated with excessive exercise may be attenuated through avoidance of low energy availability and/or by moderation of the training regimen.

STUDY TASKS

1 What are the most common musculoskeletal injuries among runners? Discuss the factors that predispose to these and suggest preventive strategies.
2 The risk of a heart attack is greater during or shortly after a session of vigorous exercise than at other times. Describe the evidence justifying this statement, explaining why this increase in risk differs between different groups.
3 Explain the different reasons why energy availability may be low in female athletes training for endurance sports.
4 Distinguish between eumenorrhoea, oligomenorrhoea and amenorrhoea. Give examples of sports where women are at high risk of menstrual dysfunction and suggest reasons.
5 Describe one cross-sectional study that suggests that spinal bone mineral density in women athletes is related to their menstrual history. What are the limitations to this study?
6 The majority of elite athletes experience symptoms of upper respiratory tract infections at a rate similar to the general population. However, rather than following the usual seasonal pattern, the episodes of these symptoms among athletes tend to occur during or around competitions. Discuss possible reasons for this difference.
7 Do you think pre-participation screening of asymptomatic middle-aged people is justified? Explain your view as fully as possible.

NOTE

1 Luteinising hormone plays a critical role in the menstrual cycle: a surge in its secretion by the pituitary brings about ovulation.

FURTHER READING

De Souza, M.J., Koltun, K.J., Etter, C.V. and Southmayd, E.A. (2017) Current status of the Female Athlete Triad; update and future directions. *Current Osteoporosis Reports* 15: 577–87.

Gleeson, M., Bishop, N. and Walsh, N. (eds) (2013) *Exercise immunology*. London: Routledge.

Lancaster, G.I. and Febbraio, M.A. (2016) Exercise and the immune system; implications for elite athletes and the general population. *Immunology and Cell Biology* 94: Editorial page 115 and series of papers that follow.

Logue, D., Madigan, S.M., Delahunt, E., Heinen, M., McDonnell, S.-J., and Corish, C.A. (2018) Low energy availability in athletes: a review of prevalence, dietary patterns, physiological health, and sports performance. *Sports Medicine* 48: 73–96.

Mountjoy, M., Sundgot-Borgen, J., Burke, L., Ackerman, K.E., Blauwet, C., Constantini, N. et al. (2018) International Olympic Committee (IOC) Consensus statement on Relative Energy Deficiency in Sport (RED-S): 2018 update. *International Journal of Sport Nutrition and Energy Metabolism* 28: 316–31. doi: 10.1123/ijsnem.2018-0136.

Riebe, D., Franklin, B.A., Thompson, P.D., Garber, C.E., Whitfield, G.P., Magal, M. and Pescatello, L.S. (2015) Updating ACSM's recommendations for exercise preparticipation health screening. *Medicine and Science in Sports and Exercise* 47: 2473–9.

Tenforde, A.S., Barrack, M.T., Nattiv, N. and Fredericson, M. (2016) Parallels with the female athlete triad in male athletes. *Sports Medicine* 46: 171–82.

Thompson, P.D., Franklin, B.A., Balady, G.J., Blair, S.N., Corrado, D., Mark Estes, N.A. et al. (2007) Exercise and acute cardiovascular events placing the risks into perspective: a scientific statement from the American Heart Association Council on nutrition, physical activity, and metabolism and the Council on clinical cardiology, in collaboration with the American College of Sports Medicine. *Circulation* 115: 2358–68.

Verhagen, E.A.L.M., van Sluijs, E.M.F. and van Mechelen, W. (2012) Risks of physical activity, in C. Bouchard, S.N. Blair and W.L. Haskell (eds) *Physical activity and health*, 2nd edn, Champaign, IL: Human Kinetics.

REFERENCES

Aizer, A., Gaziano, J.M., Cook, N.R., Manson, J.E., Buring, J.E. and Albert, C.M. (2009) Relation of vigorous exercise to risk of atrial fibrillation. *American Journal of Cardiology* 103: 1572–7.

Albert, C.M., Mittleman, M.A., Chae, C.U., Lee, I.-M., Hennekens, C.H. and Manson, J.E. (2000) Triggering of sudden death from cardiac causes by vigorous exertion. *New England Journal of Medicine* 343: 1355–61.

Araújo, C.G.S., Belém, L. and Gottlieb, I. (2014) A six-time winner and a normal heart: a case report. *SAGE Open Medical Case Reports* 2: 2050313X14522439. doi: 10.1177/2050313X14522439.

Arem, H., Moore, S.C., Patel, A., Hartge, P., Berrington de Gonzalez, A., Visvanathan, J. et al. (2015) Leisure time physical activity and mortality: a detailed pooled analysis of the dose-response relationship. *Journal of the American Medical Association Internal Medicine* 175: 959–67.

Arends, J.C., Cheung, M.-Y.C., Barrack, M.T. and Nattiv, A. (2012) Restoration of menses with nonpharmacologic therapy in college athletes with menstrual disturbances. *International Journal of Sport Nutrition and Exercise Metabolism* 22: 98–108.

Barrack, M.T., Gibbs, J.C., De Souza, M.J., Williams, N.I., Nichols, J.F., Rauh, M.J. and Nattiv, A. (2014) Higher incidence of bone stress injuries with increasing Female Athlete Triad-related risk factors. A prospective multisite study of exercising girls and women. *American Journal of Sports Medicine* 42: 949–58.

Barrack, M.T. van Loan, M.D. Rauh, M.J. and Nichols J.F. (2011) Body mass, training, menses, and bone in adolescent runners: a 3-yr follow-up. *Medicine and Science in Sports and Exercise* 43: 959–66.

Bolling, C., van Mechelen, W., Pasman, H.R. and Verhagen, E. (2018) Context matters: revisiting the first step of the 'Sequence of Prevention' of sports injuries. *Sports Medicine* 48: 2227–34.

Bueno, A.M., Pilgaard, M., Hulme, A, Forsberg, P., Ramskov, D., Damsted, C. and Nielsen, R.O. (2018) Injury prevalence across sports: a descriptive analysis on a representative sample of the Danish population. *Injury Epidemiology* 5: 6. doi: 10.1186/s40621-018-0136-0.

Bullen, B.A., Skrinar, G.S., Beitins, I.Z., von Mering, G., Turnbull, B.A. and McArthur, J.W. (1985) Induction of menstrual disorders by strenuous exercise in untrained women. *New England Journal of Medicine* 312: 1349–53.

Burke, L.M., Glose, G., Lundy, B., Mooses, M., Morton, J.P. and Tenforde, A.S. (2018a) Relative energy deficiency in sport in male athletes: a commentary on its presentation among selected groups of male athletes. *International Journal of Sport Nutrition and Exercise Metabolism* 28: 364–74.

Burke, L.M., Lundy, B., Fahrenholtz, I.L. and Melin, A.K. (2018b) Pitfalls of conducting and interpreting estimates of energy availability in free-living athletes. *International Journal of Sport Nutrition and Exercise Metabolism* 28: 350–63.

Butler, P., Kamper, S.J. and Williams, C.M. (2017) Exercise-based programmes reduce sports injury in adolescents (PEDro synthesis). *British Journal of Sports Medicine* 52: 690–1.

Colombo, C.S.S.S. and Finocchiaro, G. (2018) The female athlete's heart: facts and fallacies. *Current Treatment Options in Cardiovascular Medicine* 20: 101. doi: 10.1007/s11936-018-0699-7.

Corrado, D., Basso, C., Pavei, A., Michieli, P., Schiavon, M., and Thiene, G. (2006) Trends in sudden cardiovascular death in young competitive athletes after implementation of a preparticipation screening program. *Journal of the American Medical Association* 296: 1593–601.

Corrado, D., Schmied, C., Basso, C., Borjesson, M., Schiavon, M., Pelliccia, A. et al. (2011) Risk of sports; do we need a pre-participation screening for competitive and leisure athletes? *European Heart Journal* 32: 934–44.

De Souza, M.J., Koltun, K.J., Etter, C.V. and Southmayd, E.A. (2017) Current status of the Female Athlete Triad; update and future directions. *Current Osteoporosis Reports* 15: 577–87.

De Souza, M.J., Nattiv, A., Joy, E., Misra, M., Williams, N.I., Mallinson, R.J. et al. (2014) 2014 Female Athlete Triad Coalition Consensus Statement on treatment and return to play of the Female Athlete Triad. *British Journal of Sports Medicine* 48: 289–309.

De Souza, M.J., Toombs, R.J., Scheid, J.L., O'Donnell, E., West, S.L. and Williams, N.I. (2010) High prevalence of subtle and severe menstrual disturbances in exercising women: confirmation using daily hormone measures. *Human Reproduction* 25: 491–503.

Drinkwater, B.L., Bruemner, B. and Chesnut, C.H. (1990) Menstrual history as a determinant of current bone density in young athletes. *Journal of the American Medical Association* 263: 545–8.

Duckham, R.L., Peirce, N., Meyer, C., Summers, G.D., Cameron, N. and Brooke-Wavell, K. (2012) Risk factors for stress fracture in female endurance athletes. *British Medical Journal Open* 2: e001920. doi: 10.1136/bmjopen-2012-001920.

Eijsvogels, T.M.H., Januzzi, J.L., Taylor, B.A., Isaacs, S.K., D'Hemecourt, P., Zaleski, A. et al. (2014) Impact of statin use on exercise-induced cardiac troponin elevations. *American Journal of Cardiology* 114: 624–8.

Eijsvogels, T.M.H., Thompson, P.D. and Franklin, B.A. (2018) The 'Extreme Exercise Hypothesis'; recent findings and cardiovascular health implications. *Current Treatment Options in Cardiovascular Medicine* 20: 84. doi: 10.1007/s11936-018-0674-3.

Ekblom, B., Ekblom, Ö. and Malm, C. (2006) Infectious episodes before and after a marathon race. *Scandinavian Journal of Medicine and Science in Sports* 16: 287–93.

Feicht, C.B., Johnson, T.S., Martin, B.J., Sparkes, K.E. and Wagner, W.W. (1978) Secondary amenorrhoea in athletes. *The Lancet* 312: 1145–6.

Gibbs, J.C., Williams, N.I. and De Souza, M.J. (2013) Prevalence of individual and combined components of the female athlete triad. *Medicine and Science in Sports and Exercise* 45: 985–6.

Gleeson, M. (2016) Immunological aspects of sport nutrition. *Immunology and Cell Biology* 94: 117–23.

Grimsmo, J., Grundvold, I., Maehlum, S. and Arnesen, H. (2010) High prevalence of atrial fibrillation in long-term endurance cross-country skiers; echocardiographic findings and possible predictors – a 28–30 years follow-up study. *European Journal of Cardiovascular Prevention and Rehabilitation* 17: 100–5.

Guasch, E., Benito, B., Qi, X., Cifelli, C., Naud, P., Shi, Y. et al. (2013) Atrial fibrillation promotion by endurance exercise; demonstration and mechanistic exploration in an animal model. *Journal of the American College of Cardiology* 62: 68–77.

Hållmarker, U., Åsberg, S., Michaëlsson, K., Ärnlöv, J., Hellberg, D., Lindbäck, J. et al. (2015) Risk of recurrent stroke and death after first stroke in long-distance ski race participants. *Journal of the American Heart Association* 4: e002469. doi: 10.1161/JAHA.115.002469.

Hellard, P., Avalos, M., Guimaraes, F., Toussaint, J.F. and Pyne, D.B. (2015) Training-related common illnesses in elite swimmers over a 4-yr period. *Medicine and Science in Sports and Exercise* 47: 698–707.

Higgins, J.P. and Andino, A. (2013) Soccer and sudden cardiac death in young competitive athletes: a review. *Journal of Sports Medicine* 2013: Article ID 967183. doi: 10.1155/2013/967183.

Hootman, J.M., Macera, C.A., Ainsworth, B.E., Addy, C.L., Martin, M. and Blair, S.N. (2002) Epidemiology of musculoskeletal injuries among sedentary and physically active adults. *Medicine and Science in Sports and Exercise* 34: 838–44. Erratum in *Medicine and Science in Sports and Exercise* 2003, 35: 183.

Hootman, J.M., Macera, C.A., Ainsworth, B.E., Martin, M., Addy, C.L. and Blair, S.N. (2001) Association among physical activity level, cardiorespiratory fitness, and risk of musculoskeletal injury. *American Journal of Epidemiology* 154: 251–8.

Hutchinson, A. (2012) Did running cause Micah True's death? *Runners World*, 13 May.

International Olympic Committee Medical Commission Working Group Women in Sport. (2005) Position stand on the female athlete triad [online], available at: https://www.olympic.org/news/ioc-consensus-statement-on-the-female-athlete-triad (accessed 18 February 2019).

Kadel, N.J., Teits, C.C. and Kronmal, R.A. (1992) Stress fractures in ballet dancers. *American Journal of Sports Medicine* 20: 445–9.

Keen, A.D. and Drinkwater, B.L. (1997) Irreversible bone loss in former amenorrheic athletes. *Osteoporosis International* 7: 311–15.

Kellman, M., Bertollo, M., Bosquet, L., Brink, M., Coutts, A.J., Duffield, R. et al. (2018) Recovery and performance in sport: consensus statement. *International Journal of Sports Physiology and Performance* 13: 240–5.

Kemler, E., Blokland, D., Backx, F. and Huissted, B. (2018) Differences in injury risk and characteristics of injuries between novice and experienced runners over a 4-year period. *Physician and Sports Medicine* 46: 485–91.

Kim, J.H., Malhotra, R., Chiampas, G., d'Hemecourt, P., Troyanos, C., Cianca, J. et al. for the Race Associated Cardiac Arrest Event Registry (RACER) Study Group. (2012) Cardiac arrest during long-distance running races. *New England Journal of Medicine* 366: 130–40.

Knowler, W.C., Barrett-Connor, E., Fowler, S.E., Hamman, R.F., Lachin, J.M., Walker, E.A. and Nathan, D.M. for the Diabetes Prevention Program Research Group (2002) Reduction in the incidence of type 2 diabetes with lifestyle intervention or Metformin. *New England Journal of Medicine* 346: 393–403.

Look AHEAD Research Group; Wing, R.R., Bolin, P., Brancati, F.L., Bray, G.A., Clark, J.M., Co-day, M. et al. (2013) Cardiovascular effects of intensive lifestyle intervention in type 2 diabetes. *New England Journal of Medicine* 369: 145–54.

Loucks, A.B. (2006) Methodological problems in studying the female athlete triad. *Medicine and Science in Sports and Exercise* 38: 1020. doi: 10.1249/01.mss.0000218146.91864.b5.

Loucks, A.B., Kiens, B. and Wright, H.H. (2011) Energy availability in athletes. *Journal of Sports Sciences* 29: S7–15.

Martinsen, M., Bratland-Sanda, S., Eriksson, E.K. and Sundgot-Borgen, J. (2010) Dieting to win or to be thin? A study of dieting and disordered eating among adolescent elite athletes and non-athlete controls. *British Journal of Sports Medicine* 44: 70–6.

Meeusen, R., Duclos, M., Foster, C., Fry, A., Gleeson, M., Nieman, D. et al. (2013) Prevention, diagnosis of the overtraining syndrome: joint consensus statement of the European College of Sport Science and the American College of Sports Medicine. *Medicine and Science in Sports and Exercise* 45: 186–205.

Mittleman, M.A., Maclure, M., Tofler, G.H., Sherwood, J.B., Goldberg, R.J. and Muller, J.E. for the Determinants of Myocardial Infarction Onset Study Investigators. (1993) Triggering of acute myocardial infarction by heavy physical exertion: protection against triggering by regular exertion. *New England Journal of Medicine* 329: 1677–83.

Mittleman, M.A. and Mostofsky, E. (2011) Physical, psychological and chemical triggers of acute cardiovascular events: preventive strategies. *Circulation* 124: 346–54. doi: 10.1161/CIRCULATIONAHA.110.968776.

Mohlenkamp, S., Lehmann, N., Breuckmann, F., Brocker-Preuss, M., Nassenstein, K., Halle, M. et al. (2008) Running: the risk of coronary events: prevalence and prognostic relevance of coronary atherosclerosis in marathon runners. *European Heart Journal* 29: 1903–10.

Mountjoy, M., Sundgot-Borgen, J., Burke, L., Ackerman, K.E., Blauwet, C., Constantini, N. et al. (2018) International Olympic Committee (IOC) Consensus statement on Relative Energy Deficiency in Sport (RED-S): 2018 update. *International Journal of Sport Nutrition and Energy Metabolism* 28: 316–31.

Mountjoy, M., Sundgot-Borgen, J., Burke, L., Carter, S., Constantini, N., Lebrun, C. et al. (2014) The IOC consensus statement: beyond the Female Athlete Triad – Relative Energy Deficiency in Sport (RED-S). *British Journal of Sports Medicine* 48: 491–7.

Nattiv, A., Loucks, A.B., Manore, M.M., Sanborn, C.F., Sundgot-Borgen, J. and Warren, M.P. (2007) Position stand of the American College of Sports Medicine: the female athlete triad. *Medicine and Science in Sports and Exercise* 39: 1867–82.

Nieman, D.C., Johansson, A.M., Lee, J.W. and Arabatzis, K. (1990) Infectious episodes in runners before and after the Los Angeles Marathon. *Journal of Sports Medicine and Physical Fitness* 30: 316–28.

Paffenbarger, R.S., Hyde, R.T., Wing, A.L. and Hsieh, C.C. (1986) Physical activity, all-cause mortality, and longevity of college alumni. *New England Journal of Medicine* 314: 605–13.

Pollock, M.L., Carroll, J.F., Graves, J.E., Leggett, S.H., Braith, R.W., Limacher, M. and Hagberg, J. (1991) Injuries and adherence to walk/jog and resistance training programs in the elderly. *Medicine and Science in Sports and Exercise* 23: 1194–200.

Rauh, M.J., Macera, C.A., Trone, D.W., Shaffer, R.A. and Brodine, S.K. (2006) Epidemiology of stress fracture and lower-extremity overuse injury in female recruits. *Medicine and Science in Sports and Exercise* 38: 1571–7.

Riebe, D., Franklin, B.A., Thompson, P.D., Garber, C.E., Whitfield, G.P., Magal, M. and Pescatello, L.S. (2015) Updating ACSM's recommendations for exercise preparticipation health screening. *Medicine and Science in Sports and Exercise* 47: 2473–9.

Rosendahl, J., Bormann, B., Aschenbrenner, K., Aschenbrenner, F. and Strauss, B. (2009) Dieting and disordered eating in German high school athletes and non-athletes. *Scandinavian Journal of Medicine and Science in Sports* 19: 731–9.

Schmikli, S.L., Backx, F.J.G., Kemler, H.J. and van Mechelen, W. (2009) National survey on sports injuries in the Netherlands: target populations for sports injury prevention programs. *Clinical Journal of Sports Medicine* 19: 101–6.

Schnohr, P., Marott, J.L., Lange, P. and Jensen, G.B. (2013) Longevity in male and female joggers: the Copenhagen City Heart Study. *American Journal of Epidemiology* 177: 683–9.

Schnohr, P., O'Keefe, J.H., Marott, J.L., Lange, P. and Jensen, G.B. (2015) Dose of jogging and long-term mortality: the Copenhagen City Heart Study. *Journal of the American College of Cardiology* 65: 411–19.

Schwellnus, M., Soligard, T., Alonso, J.-M., Bahr, R., Clarsen, B., Dijkstra, H.P. et al. (2016) How much is too much? (Part 2). International Olympic Committee consensus statement on load in sport and risk of illness. *British Journal of Sports Medicine* 50: 1043–52.

Siscovick, D.S., Weiss, N.S., Fletcher, R.H. and Lasky, T. (1984) The incidence of primary cardiac arrest during vigorous exercise. *New England Journal of Medicine* 311: 874–7.

Slater, J., Brown, R., McLay-Cooke, R. and Black, K. (2017) Low energy availability in exercising women: historical perspectives and future directions. *Sports Medicine* 47: 207–20. doi: 10.1007/s40279-016-0583-0.

Smathers, A.M., Bemben, M.G. and Bemben, D.A. (2009) Bone density comparisons in male competitive road cyclists and untrained controls. *Medicine and Science in Sports and Exercise* 41: 290–6.

Soligard, T., Schwellnus, M., Alonso, J.-M., Bahr, R., Clarsen, B., Dijkstra, H.P. et al. (2016) How much is too much? (Part 1) International Olympic Committee consensus statement on load in sport and risk of injury. *British Journal of Sports Medicine* 50: 1030–41.

Steinvil, A., Chundadze, R., Zeltser, D., Rogowski, O., Halkin, A., Galily, Y. et al. (2011) Mandatory electrocardiographic screening of athletes to reduce their risk for sudden death: proven fact or wishful thinking? *Journal of the American College of Cardiology* 57: 1291–6.

Sundgot-Borgen, J. and Torstveit, M.S. (2004) Prevalence of eating disorders in elite athletes is higher than in the general population. *Clinical Journal of Sports Medicine* 14: 25–32.

Tenforde, A.S., Barrack, M.T., Nattiv, N. and Fredericson, M. (2016) Parallels with the male athlete triad in male athletes. *Sports Medicine* 46: 171–82.

Thompson, P.D., Franklin, B.A., Balady, G.J., Blair, S.N., Corrado, D., Estes III, N.A.M. et al. (2007) Exercise and acute cardiovascular events placing the risks into perspective: a scientific statement from the American Heart Association Council on Nutrition, Physical Activity, and Metabolism and the Council on Clinical Cardiology in collaboration with the American College of Sports Medicine. *Circulation* 115: 2358–68.

Timpka, T. and Lindqvist, K. (2001) Evidence based prevention of acute injuries during physical exercise in a WHO safe community. *British Journal of Sports Medicine* 35: 20–7.

Torstveit, M.K. and Sundgot-Borgen, J. (2005) The female athlete triad exists in both elite athletes and controls. *Medicine and Science in Sports and Exercise* 37: 1449–59.

van de Schoor, F.R., Aegevaeren, V.L., Hopman, M.T.E., Oxborough, D.L., George, K.P., Thompson, P.D. and Eijsovogels, T.M.H. (2016) Myocardial fibrosis in athletes. *Mayo Clinic Proceedings* 91: 1617–31.

Verhagen, E.A.L.M., van Stralen, M.M. and van Mechelen, W. (2010) Behaviour, the key factor for sports injury prevention. *Sports Medicine* 40: 899–906.

Walsh, N.P. and Oliver, S.J. (2016) Exercise, immune function and respiratory infection: an update on the influence of training and environmental stress. *Immunology and Cell Biology* 94: 132–9.

Webner, D., Duprey, K.M., Drezner, J.A., Cronholm, P. and Roberts, W.O. (2012) Sudden cardiac arrest and death in United States marathons. *Medicine and Science in Sports and Exercise* 44: 1843–5.

Wehrens, X.H.T., Chang, D.Y. and Li, N. (2013) Chronic exercise – a contributing factor to atrial fibrillation? *Journal of the American College of Cardiology* 62: 78–80.

Williams, N.I. and De Souza, M.J. (2006) Female athlete triad errors and misunderstandings. *Medicine and Science in Sports and Exercise* 38: 1021. doi: 10.1249/01.mss.0000218189.10155.0a.

Willich, S.N., Lewis, M., Löwel, H., Arntz, H.-R., Schubert, F. and Schröder, R. (1993) Physical exertion as a trigger of acute myocardial infarction. *New England Journal of Medicine* 329: 1684–90.

14 Public health

Marie H. Murphy and Adrianne E. Hardman

INTRODUCTION

After the Second World War research in public health began to focus on the influence of individual behaviours on non-communicable diseases such as cardiovascular disease (CVD), cancer, chronic respiratory diseases and type 2 diabetes. The work of the late Professor Jeremy Morris (who wrote the Forewords to earlier editions of this book) on the role of exercise in protection against heart attack, alongside that of Doll and Hill on smoking and lung cancer, was instrumental in defining this new vision of public health.

Non-communicable diseases kill 41 million people each year and account for 71% of all deaths, worldwide (World Health Organization 2018). They share four common and preventable risk factors, i.e. lack of physical activity, tobacco use, an unhealthy diet and the harmful use of alcohol. Conservative estimates show that, worldwide, physical inactivity causes 6–10% of the burden of disease from coronary heart disease (CHD), type 2 diabetes and breast and colon cancers and 9% of premature mortality (Lee et al. 2012). Moreover, as discussed in earlier chapters, physical activity has beneficial effects on other diseases and health conditions – falls, hip fractures and depression, for example – making *in*activity a major public health burden.

How does physical inactivity compare with other risk factors for poor health? Figure 14.1 addresses this question by presenting data for inactivity alongside that for smoking. Globally, smoking and inactivity each contribute about 7.2 million of the 41 million deaths each year from non-communicable diseases (World Health Organization 2018). Although the *relative risk* for all-cause mortality of inactivity (defined as below the minimum recommended level) is lower than that of smoking, the *population-attributable risks* are similar because the prevalence of inactivity is greater than that of smoking. Consequently, inactive people are contributing a mortality 'burden' as large as tobacco smoking and even a 10% decrease in the prevalence of inactivity could potentially avoid more than 533,000 deaths, worldwide, each year (Lee et al. 2012).

What implications does this information have for public health strategies? Two approaches to primary prevention may be identified. In the context of physical activity, the first requires identification of the least active individuals followed by individually targeted interventions including guidance on physical activity and/or opportunities and encouragement to participate in an exercise programme. The second involves encouraging the whole population to become a little more active by targeting individual behaviour and its social, environmental and policy determinants. These approaches are not mutually exclusive of course. However, the priority for public health, as opposed to clinical medicine, is to reduce overall disease incidence and the most effective way to do this is probably to attempt to shift the whole distribution of risk (Rose 1981).

Figure 14.1 Comparison of the global burden of disease between smoking and physical inactivity.

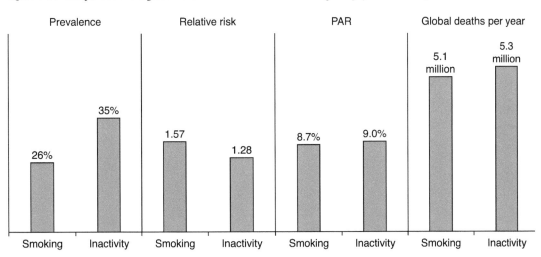

Source: Reprinted from *The Lancet*, 380: 192–3, Wen, C.P. and Wu, X., 'Stressing harms of physical inactivity to promote exercise', page 192, copyright © 2012, with permission from Elsevier.
Note: PAR, population-attributable risk.

Indeed, getting the least active to engage in a moderate amount of physical activity may bring the best return on investment. For inactivity, this requires a population-based strategy to increase physical activity across all sectors. Whilst this has now become a mainstream part of health policy, the gap between the size of the problem and the scale of the public health response remains large (Pratt et al. 2014).

Manifestos by governments and international bodies typically emphasise the role of physical activity as an important part of primary and secondary disease prevention. Public health agencies (governmental and non-governmental) work to develop strategies that are appropriate to particular settings, implement these and monitor their effectiveness. The scientific guidelines that underpin public health recommendations for physical activity are summarised in the next section, with introductory notes about the history of their development.

RECOMMENDATIONS FOR PHYSICAL ACTIVITY

Early in the twentieth century there was concern in the United Kingdom at the poor fitness of recruits to the armed services. As this impaired the country's capability to wage war, the government took action to improve the fitness of young people, introducing 'physical training' (PT as it was called) into schools. Nowadays, governments around the world instigate strategies to increase fitness and/or physical activity for a different reason – the benefits to personal and public health.

The development of recommendations on physical activity began in the middle of the twentieth century when scientific interest in the biological effects of exercise and training gathered momentum. By the 1970s this had generated a considerable literature about the type, intensity, frequency and duration of exercise needed to improve fitness – invariably interpreted as cardiorespiratory fitness, measured as maximum oxygen uptake ($\dot{V}O_2$max). The first formal document was from the American College of Sports Medicine (ACSM) in their 'Position statement on the recommended quantity and quality of exercise for developing and maintaining fitness in healthy adults' (American College of Sports Medicine 1978). The recommendation was for 'continuous aerobic activity', three to five days per week at an intensity of 50–85% of $\dot{V}O_2$max for 15–60 minutes per session. Both this position stand and the 1990 update (American College of Sports Medicine 1990) were soundly based in that if healthy adults followed their recommendations most would improve fitness. Many people assumed, probably correctly, that this regimen would also lead to health benefits but this was not the basis on which the recommendations were formulated.

The need to expand the 'exercise training-physical fitness' model to include a 'physical activity-health' model was addressed during the 1990s (Haskell 1994), leading to recommendations from several authorities, namely: the ACSM/US Centers for Disease Control and Prevention (Pate et al. 1995); the US National Institutes of Health Consensus Development Panel (1995); and the landmark US Surgeon General's Report (US Department of Health and Human Services 1996). These differed in several important respects from earlier recommendations by:

- recognising the benefit from moderate-intensity activity, including activities of daily living (if performed at an intensity corresponding to brisk walking);

- accepting that the *volume* of activity is the important determinant of health benefits so that shorter periods of vigorous-intensity exercise may be substituted for longer periods of moderate-intensity activity;
- asserting that multiple short episodes of activity during a day are one way to fulfil the recommendations;
- emphasising the need for frequent, preferably daily, activity.

These recommendations had a strong influence on public health strategies and statements in other developed countries, for example the UK Chief Medical Officer's Report in 2004 'At least five a week' and the 2005 National Physical Activity Guidelines for Adults, published by the Department of Health and Ageing in Australia.

In 2007, updated recommendations for adults aged 18–65 were published jointly by the ACSM and the American Heart Association (Haskell et al. 2007). These largely confirmed the guidance included in the 1996 Surgeon General's Report, while placing greater emphasis on the possibility to combine moderate and vigorous activities in bouts of at least ten minutes. They also specified that activities to maintain or increase muscular strength and endurance should be performed at least twice a week and stated that people would benefit from exceeding the recommended minimum amount of activity. These core recommendations underpin, for the most part, subsequent guidelines from various authoritative bodies in different countries. An important addition is that later guidelines such as the UK Chief Medical Officers' Guidelines (Department of Health 2011, 2019) invariably include the need to limit sedentary behaviour.

Specific guidance for adults aged 65 and over was published for the first time in 2007 by the ACSM and the American Heart Association and includes a recommendation for exercises to maintain or improve balance (Nelson et al. 2007). Improving 'neuromotor fitness' was also included in guidelines for Americans a few years later (American College of Sports Medicine 2011). Subsequent guidelines for older people from, for example, the UK, the US Department of Health and Human Services and the World Health Organization have adopted a similar approach.

Recognising the importance of lifelong physical activity, guidelines have been published specifically for children and young people and, in Canada, the US and the UK, for the under 5s. Several include a stipulation on minimising sitting time or 'screen time'. Particular importance has been attached to this issue by the Canadians who have published guidance on this for the 'early years' (0–4) and for children (5–17) (Canadian Society for Exercise Physiology 2020).

Evidence review from the US underscores the positive association between physical activity and the maintenance of healthy weight, stating that attenuation of weight gain is most pronounced when physical activity is *above* 150 minutes per week (Physical Activity Guidelines Advisory Committee 2018). Thus there is concern that minimal compliance with the recommendations summarised in Box 14.1 may be insufficient to prevent the gradual transition to overweight or obesity.

RATIONALE FOR RECOMMENDATIONS

Inactive people, who account for much of the public health burden, are the primary target population for public health recommendations. Thus, these are based on the

---

BOX 14.1 GUIDELINES FOR PHYSICAL ACTIVITY FOR HEALTH ACROSS THE LIFETIME*.

Pre-school-aged children (3 to 5 years)

- Should be physically active in play throughout the day.

Children and adolescents (6 to 17 years)

- Should engage in 60 minutes or more of physical activity daily.
  - *Most* of this should be moderate- or vigorous-intensity aerobic activity, with the vigorous intensity on at least three days per week.
  - *Part* of this should be muscle-strengthening activity on at least three days a week.
  - *Part* of this should be bone-strengthening activity on at least three days a week.

Adults (19 to 64 years)

- For some health benefits adults should sit less and move more. Any moderate-to-vigorous physical activity is better than none.
- For substantial health benefits they should, throughout the week:
  - do at least 150 to 300 minutes per week of moderate-intensity aerobic physical activity;
  - *or* at least 75 to 150 minutes per week of vigorous-intensity aerobic activity;
  - *or* an equivalent combination of moderate- and vigorous-intensity aerobic activity.
- In addition, adults should do muscle-strengthening activities that involve all major muscle groups on two or more days per week.

Older adults (65 years and older)

- Should follow the above guidelines for adults, within the limits of their individual functional capabilities and any chronic conditions.
- In addition, older adults should do activities to improve balance and flexibility on at least two days per week.

Source: Adapted from Physical Activity Guidelines for Americans (US Department of Health and Human Services 2018) which are based on the 2018 report of the Physical Activity Guidelines Advisory Committee (2018).
Note: The 2018 US guidelines are consistent with UK guidelines (Department of Health 2019). US guidelines also exist for pregnancy and the post-partum period as well as for adults with chronic conditions and disabilities (not shown).

---

minimally effective 'dose' of activity. Indeed, it has been suggested that the largest health gains *for the population* occur when inactive people undertake between 15 and 29 minutes of physical activity per day (Wen and Wu 2012). The following rationale should be read with this in mind and with the knowledge that guidelines invariably include the rider that physical activity above the recommended level will bring greater benefits.

The evidence upon which public health guidelines are based is drawn from two different research literatures; observational epidemiological studies and experimental exercise training studies, both of which are referred to in the following section.

Intensity – moderate to vigorous[1]

Intensity of exercise can be described in *absolute* terms or *relative* to the capacity of the individual. In absolute terms, it is the rate of energy expenditure demanded by an activity, invariably estimated from the associated oxygen uptake. In relative terms, intensity is this oxygen uptake expressed as a percentage of the individual's maximum. This distinction is important because it is the relative intensity of activity that determines not only many of the beneficial adaptations, but also some of the risks associated with physical activity. For practical reasons, large population studies have to measure and describe intensity in absolute terms. On the other hand, experimental studies invariably express intensity relative to each individual's capacity.

In many epidemiological studies moderate-intensity physical activity has been associated with beneficial health outcomes, for example a lower risk of all-cause or CVD mortality, type 2 diabetes and some cancers (Chapters 3, 5 and 8 provide further discussion and main references). For example, the amount of walking – moderate-intensity exercise for most middle-aged people – has been specifically linked to the risk of each of these disease endpoints. Moreover, lower rates of CHD are consistently reported for people categorised as moderately active or having moderate levels of fitness than for those in the least active or least fit categories (Chapter 4).

Complementing these epidemiological findings, exercise training studies have found that regular moderate-intensity activity will improve fitness in previously inactive people (see section below on walking) and benefit some health-related outcomes.

Two other considerations underpin the decision to recommend moderate-intensity physical activity for previously inactive people. First, experience worldwide with earlier recommendations and campaigns has shown how difficult it is to increase the proportion of people engaging in vigorous exercise (Biddle and Batterham 2015). Second, the hazards of physical activity appear to be associated more with its intensity than with its frequency or duration (Chapter 13).

The risks of vigorous exercise give rise to concern about an upsurge of interest in high-intensity training, high-intensity interval training or sprint interval training for individuals who have been inactive for many years. There is no doubt that a training regimen comprising very brief, maximal efforts – an approach which has its roots in the Wingate test – improves various metabolic and vascular risk factors, including insulin sensitivity (Kessler et al. 2012; Whyte et al. 2010). This sort of regimen has been advocated as a time-efficient strategy to achieve these and other health benefits. However, when essential warm-up and recovery time between the sprints are included, the total time commitment may be no different from 30 minutes of continuous activity. Whilst this sort of sprint training may be one activity option for individuals without pre-existing disease, particularly if they progress to it after an initial period of moderate-intensity activity, it is difficult to envisage that it is appropriate for widespread recommendation to the population at large.

Amount, volume of activity

Epidemiological studies typically describe the volume of activity in one of three ways: either duration within a specified intensity range; or in MET-h per week; or as energy expenditure in kcal per week (less often, MJ per week). The unit MET-h was explained in Chapter 2; in brief, it is the intensity in METs (multiples of resting metabolic rate) multiplied by the duration of activity in hours. When activity is reported in energy units these are typically based on estimates of rates of energy expenditure, with an assumption about body mass.

Recommendations for at least 150 minutes per week of moderate-intensity physical activity are based on evidence from large prospective cohort studies of diverse populations that this volume of activity is associated with lower rates of CVD and premature mortality. At an intensity of 3–5.9 METS (and for people with body mass 70–90 kg) it approximates to an energy expenditure of 1000 kcal (~4.2 MJ) per week or 10 MET-h per week. Ten MET-h can also be achieved with ≥20 min of vigorous intensity activity (≥6 METs) on three or more days per week or for a total of about 75 minutes per week.

Systematic review and meta-analysis of 22 cohort studies including 977,925 people found that 2.5 hours per week (equivalent to 30 minutes on five days each week) of moderate-intensity activity was associated with a 19% lower all-cause mortality risk, compared with no activity, justifying the recommendation for 'at least' 150 minutes of moderate-intensity activity each week (Woodcock et al. 2011).

Can longer periods of non-vigorous activity be substituted for shorter periods of vigorous activity – as stipulated in most recent guidelines? Several small experimental studies have compared the short-term effects on a health outcome of exercise sessions that differ in intensity but expend the same energy. Outcomes where similar benefits have been reported include insulin sensitivity and the plasma triglyceride response to a test meal. So, there is some evidence that intensity *can* be traded for duration but the number of outcomes studied is limited.

We can be fairly confident that intensity can be traded for duration with regard to weight control because reviews and meta-analyses have consistently found that it is the total energy expended in physical activity or exercise that determines its influence on body weight or fatness (see Chapter 7). An important caveat is, however, that the few epidemiological studies that have compared the benefits of different intensities of exercise whilst controlling for energy expenditure have consistently found greater benefits – at least in terms of protection against CHD – from vigorous, rather than moderate, exercise (Swain and Franklin 2006). This finding is congruent with the relationship observed between level of fitness and incidence of heart disease but evidence for other health outcomes is scant.

Patterning of activity, accumulation

Current recommendations advise that activity may be accumulated in shorter bouts undertaken over the course of the day. Support for this view comes from the fact that much of the activity reported in epidemiological studies and found to be associated with health benefits was probably not undertaken in sessions of long duration. Examples include walking, stair climbing, gardening and household chores. There are few data to confirm the (probably fairly safe) assumption that most such activities are performed intermittently, but one report from the Harvard Alumni study does provide some. Between 1988 and 1993 participants reported the frequency and average duration of each episode of activity; researchers found that longer sessions did not have a different effect on risk than shorter sessions, as long as the total energy expended was similar (Lee et al. 2000).

Experimental studies that have compared responses to contrasting patterns of activity of the same total duration are another source of data on the efficacy of accumulating activity. These include both training studies and studies of the acute, short-term effects of a single session of exercise.

In one classic training study, previously inactive middle-aged men did 30 minutes of jogging per day, five days per week for eight weeks (DeBusk et al. 1990). One group did this in a single, 30-minute session per day, while a second group did three ten-minute sessions per day (no control group). Increases in $\dot{V}O_2$max and loss of body weight were similar in both groups. Another study, this one randomly controlled, allocated middle-aged women to train for ten weeks by brisk walking in either one 30-minute session or three ten-minute sessions per day (Murphy and Hardman 1998). Fitness improvements were similar in each walking group (relative to controls who remained inactive) and three ten-minute sessions were at least as effective in decreasing body fatness as one long bout (Table 14.1). A subsequent study found that training by brisk walking for three ten-minute sessions per day increased high-density lipoprotein (HDL)-cholesterol and decreased total cholesterol and triglycerides to a similar extent as training by one 30-minute session daily (Murphy et al. 2002).

Recent systematic review and meta-analysis of data from 19 studies that compared interventions of continuous with accumulated exercise concluded that changes in fitness, blood pressure, blood lipids, insulin or glucose were independent of the pattern of exercise; there was limited evidence that beneficial changes in body mass and low-density lipoprotein cholesterol may be more marked with an accumulated approach (Murphy et al. 2019).

Several studies have compared the acute effects of several short sessions of brisk walking accumulated throughout the day with one longer session of equivalent total

Table 14.1 Changes with different patterns of brisk walking in previously inactive, middle-aged women.

	CONTROLS N = 10	THREE TEN-MINUTE SESSIONS, N = 12	ONE 30-MINUTE SESSION, N = 12
Body mass, kg	+0.6 (0.7)	−1.7 (1.7)*	−0.9 (2.0)
Sum 4 skinfold thicknesses, mm	+2.6 (2.8)	−3.3 (3.5)*	−2.8 (3.8)*
Waist circumference, cm	+0.6 (1.0)	−3.0 (2.4)*	−1.8 (2.4)
Systolic blood pressure, mm Hg	−2.0 (6.9)	−7.4 (7.3)	−4.6 (5.9)
$\dot{V}O_2$max, ml kg^{-1} min^{-1}	−0.5 (0.1)	+2.3 (0.1)*	+2.4 (0.1)*

Source: Reprinted with permission from Wolters Kluwer Health, Inc.: Murphy, M.H. and Hardman, A.E., (1998) 'Training effects of short and long bouts of brisk walking in sedentary women', *Medicine and Science in Sports and Exercise*, 30: 152–7. Available at: https://doi.org/10.1097/00005768-199801000-00021.

Note: * Values are mean (standard deviation). Change from baseline significantly different from change in controls, $P < 0.05$. Training was either one 30-minute session per day or three ten-minute sessions per day, five days per week for ten weeks. Comparisons are with controls who remained sedentary.

duration. For example, the effects on postprandial plasma triglycerides and blood pressure were compared in a group of healthy men, using a two-day protocol (Miyashita et al. 2008). On day one, participants either rested (control) or walked briskly for ten three-minute bouts or walked briskly for one 30-minute bout (gross energy expenditure 1.1 MJ, ~ 260 kcal); on day two, blood pressure and postprandial triglycerides were measured over a seven-hour period. Brisk walking in short bouts was just as effective in reducing postprandial triglycerides (16% lower, Figure 14.2) and resting systolic blood pressure (6–7% lower) as one continuous bout.

In another study, changes in ambulatory blood pressure after four ten-minute walks were compared with changes after one 40-minute walk in healthy but pre-hypertensive people (Park et al. 2006). Both systolic and diastolic pressures were reduced for longer after multiple short bouts of walking than after the single, longer bout, i.e. 11 hours and seven hours respectively. This finding was confirmed in a subsequent study where the blood-pressure lowering effect of three ten-minute bouts of walking spaced throughout the day persisted throughout the night and into the next morning (Bhammar et al. 2012).

Using an entirely different approach, the associations of short and longer bouts (≤10 minutes vs ≥10 minutes, measured using accelerometry) with several CVD risk factors were compared in a large, cross-sectional observational study of more than 2,000 participants in the Third Generation Framingham Heart Study. Both patterns of activity were significantly associated with lower circulating triglycerides, BMI, waist

Figure 14.2 Multiple short bouts of brisk walking reduce postprandial triglycerides to the same extent as one continuous bout of equivalent energy expenditure.

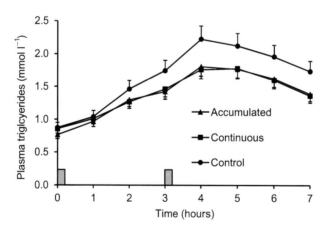

Source: Miyashita, M. et al., 'Accumulating short bouts of brisk walking reduces postprandial plasma triacylglycerol concentrations and resting blood pressure in healthy young men', *American Journal of Clinical Nutrition*, 2008, 88: 1225–31, by permission of Oxford University Press.
Notes: Fifteen healthy men each undertook three trials, each in a two-day protocol. On day one they either rested (Control) or walked briskly for 30 minutes in one continuous bout (Continuous) or walked briskly for 30 minutes in ten three-minute bouts (Accumulated). The following day, plasma triglycerides were measured over a seven-hour period, during which two high-fat test meals were consumed (blue rectangles). Values are mean and standard error. Both patterns of walking reduced the postprandial response by 16%, compared with Control ($P < 0.005$).

circumference and overall Framingham risk score and higher HDL-cholesterol (Glazer et al. 2013).

Given the prominence afforded in public health recommendations to the efficacy of accumulating physical activity throughout the day, research on this topic is still inadequate. However, the body of evidence is strengthening and it seems likely that it is not only long, continuous episodes of activity which result in health benefits – accumulating activity throughout the day is effective too. What about the distribution of bouts of activity throughout the *week*? Does this matter?

Particularly relevant for people who work a typical Monday–Friday pattern, a few studies have investigated the so-called 'weekend warrior' pattern whereby an individual meets the 150 minutes of moderate intensity physical activity in just two sessions per week rather than spread across most days of the week. One prospective cohort study found that this pattern of exercise was indeed associated with lower rates of premature mortality, compared with being sedentary, but only among men without major CVD risk factors (Lee et al. 2004) (Figure 14.3).

A recent study of British adults found that those who reported that they were regularly active three or more times per week in either ≥150 minutes per week of moderate intensity or in ≥75 minutes per week of vigorous intensity had similar reductions in risk of all-cause, cardiovascular and cancer mortality (O'Donovan et al. 2017).

Another pattern of activity has been known traditionally as interval training. This involves varying intensity within a single bout of exercise and is commonly used by athletes because it can increase the total volume of exercise the athlete can achieve in a

Figure 14.3 Relative risks of mortality according to physical activity pattern in the Harvard Alumni Study 1988–1997.

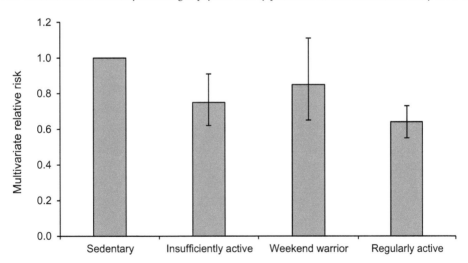

Source: Lee et al. (2004).
Notes: Mean and 95% confidence interval for multivariate-adjusted data. Referent group is described as 'sedentary'. Physical activity pattern defined as follows: sedentary (men expending <500 kcal week^{-1} in walking, climbing stairs and sports/recreation); insufficiently active (men expending 500–999 kcal week^{-1} in these same activities); weekend warrior (men expending ≥1,000 kcal week^{-1} by participation in sports/recreation once or twice a week); and regularly active (all other men expending ≥1,000 kcal week^{-1} in walking, climbing stairs and sports/recreation).

session. Short-term (≤3 months) interval training has been shown to result in similar or greater improvements in fitness and some cardio-metabolic markers, compared with single-intensity exercise.

Non-exercise physical activity

There is overlap here with topics discussed earlier as much of this type of activity is of light to moderate intensity and undertaken intermittently. It includes self-selected leisure, occupational or household activities or activities involved in 'getting about' engaged in as part of everyday life – but *excludes* intentional exercise. An alternative term is 'lifestyle physical activity'. This type of activity may be particularly important for people who dislike structured exercise for whom it may be better maintained than structured exercise programmes. It can increase energy expenditure by as much as regular aerobic exercise, making it an attractive approach for weight control.

Intervention studies conducted in the 1990s demonstrated that lifestyle activity can improve cardiovascular risk factors. For example, in a two-year randomised (but not controlled) trial, called Project Active, researchers compared the effects of increased lifestyle/non-exercise activities with those of a traditional structured exercise programme in 235 healthy, slightly overweight men and women aged 35–60 (Dunn et al. 1999). Energy expenditure increased by a similar amount in both groups. By 24 months, there was no significant difference between groups in the modest increases in $\dot{V}O_2$max but both groups experienced similar small decreases in body fatness and blood pressure. Interestingly, participants in the lifestyle group increased their physical activity mainly through increases in walking (mean of 19 additional mins per day). That study and others (several of overweight or obese individuals) provide support for the proposition that a generally active daily life benefits health.

This proposition is further supported by studies that have demonstrated inverse associations between time spent in non-exercise activity and CVD risk and all-cause mortality. One prospective cohort study conducted in Sweden followed more than 4,000 people for 12.5 years, reporting that a high level of non-exercise physical activity was associated with a lower risk of a first CVD event and lower mortality, regardless of regular intentional exercise (Ekblom-Bak et al. 2014).

Frequent, almost daily, activity – reversibility

Physical activity does not need to result in a training effect to elicit a health benefit – although benefits may be enhanced when it does. Some health-related changes are due largely to acute biological responses that persist for some time following each session. For example, blood pressure is lowered for up to 12 hours after an exercise session and plasma triglyceride concentrations are reduced for even longer. Of course, for such changes to decrease disease risk in the longer term, people need to be physically active on an almost daily basis. This is well illustrated by 'de-training' studies. At least two beneficial metabolic characteristics (low postprandial triglycerides, good insulin sensitivity) have been shown to deteriorate rapidly when a habit of exercise is interrupted (Figure 14.4).

Figure 14.4 (a) Changes in fasting and postprandial plasma concentrations of triglyceride in ten endurance-trained athletes during a 6.5-day interruption to training (mean and standard error); and (b) changes in insulin sensitivity in nine moderately-trained men and women during a seven-day interruption to training (mean and standard deviation).

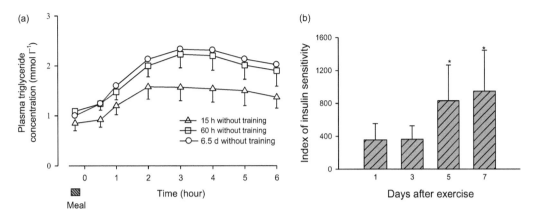

Sources: (a) Hardman et al. (1998); and (b) reproduced from the *Journal of Applied Physiology*, King, D.S. et al., 78: 17–22, copyright © 1995 with permission from the American Physiological Society.
Notes: (a) A high-fat mixed meal was completed at time 0 h. The area under the plasma triglyceride x time curve was 45% lower after 15 h without training than after 60 h without training ($P < 0.05$). (b) Insulin sensitivity measured as the product of insulin and glucose areas under concentration versus time curves (low values indicate good sensitivity).
* Significantly different from one and three days after interruption to training.

Acute responses to bouts of exercise are likely to be augmented when a person's fitness improves because the absolute intensity of exercise that can be sustained is increased. This will be the case for any benefit determined by the magnitude of the energy expended during an exercise session. Thus there is an important interaction between acute and chronic (training) effects in this regard.

Sedentary behaviour

Sedentary behaviour has been a topic of much research interest in the last decade, as discussed in Chapter 3. Sitting (the archetypal sedentary behaviour) for over eight to nine hours per day has been associated with elevated risk for all-cause and cardiovascular mortality (Patterson et al. 2018) and sedentary time is strongly and consistently associated with the risk for diabetes (Wilmot et al. 2012). Its potential for harm is thus an important public health issue.

Biomarkers such as blood glucose, insulin and lipoproteins have been reported to be worse with high levels of self-reported sedentary behaviour (Staiano et al. 2014). The venous stasis associated with uninterrupted sitting heightens thrombotic risk and, furthermore, prolonged sitting has been implicated in endothelial cell dysfunction. Thus metabolic and/or pro-coagulant mechanisms may plausibly explain these detrimental effects of prolonged uninterrupted sitting. Links to intervention data on longer-term health outcomes are, however, lacking.

An interesting practical suggestion is that people should take short activity breaks from sitting. Interrupting long periods of sitting with two-minute bouts of gentle walking has been reported to avoid some potent negative metabolic and pro-coagulant effects (Howard et al. 2013). However breaking up prolonged sitting with standing – rather than walking – did not influence markers of metabolic health, suggesting that the walking may be key rather than the interruption to sitting *per se* (Yates et al. 2020).

An important theme in this area is the idea, widely promulgated by the media, that sedentary behaviour may be detrimental to health even among people who are active at the recommended level (see Chapter 3). One synthesis of early studies concluded that high levels of sitting time and TV viewing time (over eight to nine hours per day) are both associated with greater risk for several major chronic disease outcomes *independent* of physical activity (Patterson et al. 2018). On the other hand, meta-analysis of data on sitting time (also self-reported) and premature mortality found that 60–75 mins per day of self-reported moderate intensity activity seem to eliminate the increased risk associated with high sitting time (Ekelund et al. 2016). A subsequent meta-analysis of (presumably more objective) accelerometry studies found that *both* higher levels of total physical activity, at any intensity, *and* less time spent sedentary were both associated with premature mortality in a dose–response manner (Ekelund et al. 2019). In the context of this ongoing debate, the reader is reminded just how difficult it is fully to control for factors associated with sedentary behaviours which may themselves confer an increased risk of disease (see Chapter 2). Reverse causation – illness or over-fatness causing people to become sedentary – is an issue, as is effect modification because time spent in physical activity reduces the time available for sitting.

It remains possible that sitting is mostly the inverse of physical activity, as pointed out in a thoughtful review by Stamatakis and colleagues (2019). They argue that the evidence base to include quantitative recommendations on sitting in public health guidance, e.g. reducing work time sitting by up to four hours per day (Buckley et al. 2015), is insecure and incomplete. This dialogue is not just about semantics since, once guidelines are established, they are difficult to modify without confusing the public. Stamatakis and colleagues (2019) are of the opinion that available data seem to support a message to 'move more (at any intensity)' rather than 'sit less'. The reader must arrive at his or her own opinion.

Muscular strength and endurance

Activities that increase muscular strength and endurance promote musculoskeletal and other health benefits (for discussion see Williams et al. 2007). In particular, mechanical loading by resistance exercise stimulates an increase in bone formation in young adults and slows bone loss in middle-age. Bone strength is increased in the bones stressed by the exercise. These effects are expected to lower risk of osteoporosis and bone fracture in the later years (see Chapter 9).

Activities that increase muscular strength also promote the development of a large metabolically active muscle mass, helping to maintain insulin sensitivity. This may be one reason why higher levels of muscular strength have been associated with better cardio-metabolic risk profiles, lower risk of all-cause mortality, fewer cardiovascular events and a lower risk of developing functional limitations. Muscle-strengthening activities can slow the age-related decline in muscle mass helping older individuals to continue to live independently and, alongside balance exercises, decrease the risk for falls (see Chapters 9 and 12).

Overall evaluation of evidence underpinning recommendations

The process of refining evidence-based recommendations is ongoing. Meta-analysis has quantified the dose–response relationship of non-vigorous activity and all-cause mortality (Woodcock et al. 2011), although these relationships remain poorly described for many health outcomes. The health dangers of sedentariness are a topic of active research as is the role of activity (structured/intentional and other) in individuals with existing disease.

Public health recommendations can never reflect the complexities of the relationships between physical activity, sedentary living and health. Consequently, individuals (or those who counsel them) will always have to interpret recommendations in relation to personal needs, priorities and physical capabilities. Comprehensive guidance on the prescription of individualised exercise is available in the ACSM's guidance for prescribing exercise (Garber et al. 2011).

As the Canadian HERITAGE Family Study has shown, individual responses to a given amount and/or type of activity are heterogeneous. People will get different 'rewards' for their investment in activity. Changes in fitness, HDL-cholesterol and blood pressure all varied greatly among the 700 study participants, despite a carefully standardised 20-week training programme. This variation clustered in families and so must reflect a degree of genetic predisposition and/or gene–environment interactions. For further discussion of this topic the reader is referred to Rankinen and colleagues (2010) and Pérusse and colleagues (2013).

However, the evidence that physical activity benefits health for people of all ages is irrefutable and more than sufficient to underpin public health policies and programmes that aim to improve population levels of physical activity. Concerns about the inadequacy of information in some areas should be viewed in the context of this certainty.

The relative importance of physical *activity* versus physical *fitness* for health benefits has been widely debated. As the level and intensity of activity is one determinant of fitness and the indices used to measure these parameters have different attributes, this is not always helpful. However, the emphasis on moderate-intensity exercise in current recommendations has sometimes been interpreted to mean that physical activity at this intensity is the only goal. However, fitness *does* matter because it enables an individual to sustain a higher rate of energy expenditure without becoming fatigued. This, in turn, helps weight regulation, enhances the acute biological responses to each session of activity and opens up a wide choice of leisure-time pursuits. A given task (e.g. shovelling snow, playing football with the children) demands a lower proportion of $\dot{V}O_2max$ for a fit person, so they can do it with something in reserve. Finally, the process of developing fitness – regular participation in at least moderately vigorous exercise – attenuates the cardiovascular risk associated with each session (Chapter 13).

Steps per day – a different approach

Physical activity guidelines have been 'translated' into related indices based on pedometer readings of steps per day that approximate the associated energy expenditure. This approach enshrines the principle that accumulating activity is one way to achieve the recommended level of activity. It has its origins in the Japanese walking clubs of more than 30 years ago and is popular with the media because of the simplicity of the concept. For apparently healthy adults, a target of 10,000 steps per day has been widely adopted as a reasonable estimate of an appropriate level of daily activity. This target is, however, not appropriate for individuals starting from a base of low physical activity and probably not sustainable for older adults or those whose capacities are constrained by chronic disease.

Studies are emerging that document the health benefits of attaining numbers of steps per day that approximate this target (reviewed in Tudor-Locke et al. 2011) and step-count data are being converted into minutes of active time in line with public health guidelines. Targets are being refined for children, older adults and those living with disability and/or chronic illness. Canadian researchers have reported that 12,000 steps per day is equivalent to the guideline 60 minutes per day of moderate- to vigorous-intensity activity for 6 to 19 year-olds (Colley et al. 2012) and that pre-school children (3–5 years) meet the guideline of 180 minutes of any physical activity with a step count of 6,000 per day (Gabel et al. 2013).

Besides simplicity and ease of measurement, the 'steps per day' approach has the potential for objective assessment of the volume of activity. It may be utilised to motivate individuals and as a tool for surveillance of population physical activity levels. Suggested cut-off points for classifying levels of activity according to recorded steps per day may provide a framework for translating physical activity guidelines. Figure 14.5 attempts, schematically, to link steps per day to guidelines expressed as time spent in moderate-to-vigorous physical activity.

WALKING – THE NEAREST TO PERFECT EXERCISE

Epidemiological evidence shows that the biggest difference in risk for all-cause mortality is between inactive people and those who, whilst reporting some activity, are insufficiently active to meet current recommendations for moderate-intensity activity (Figure 14.6 and Figure 14.7). The greatest rewards in public health terms are, therefore, likely to be achieved if the most inactive people become just a little more active. Walking is the obvious starting point. It is safe, inexpensive, popular and sociable[2] and can take place in all sorts of environments. Not surprisingly therefore it is the most popular physical activity reported by adults in most physical activity surveys. It has the potential to improve fitness in most middle-aged and older adults (Kelly et al. 2011) and its health benefits are clear from a plethora of epidemiological studies.

Figure 14.5 'Translation' of public health guidelines for moderate-to-vigorous physical activity into steps per day for different groups within the population.

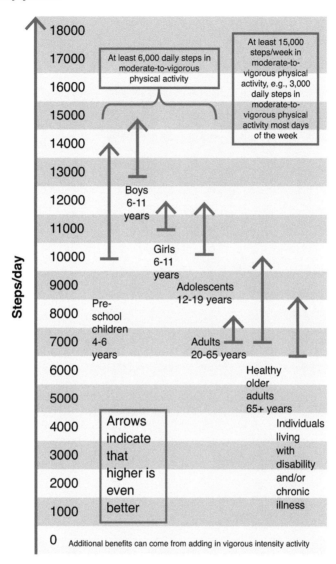

Source: Reprinted with no modifications from 'How many steps/day are enough? For older adults and special populations', Tudor-Locke, C. et al., *International Journal of Behavioral Nutrition and Physical Activity*, 2011, 8: 80. Article distributed under the terms of the Creative Commons Attribution 4.0 International (CC BY) Licence (http://creativecommons.org/licenses/by/4.0/).

Walking and fitness

At a 'normal/ordinary' pace, say 4.8 km h^{-1} (3 mile h^{-1}) on level ground, walking increases the metabolic rate more than three-fold, demanding about 3.5 METs. At a 'brisk' pace of around 5.6 km h^{-1} (3.5 mile h^{-1}) this rises to 3.8 METs. Such brisk

Figure 14.6 Relative risk of mortality (all-cause, cardiovascular disease and cancer) in people categorised according to whether or not they met recommendations for moderate and/or vigorous activity. Bars represent 95% confidence intervals.

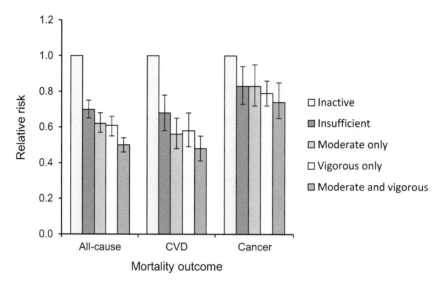

Source: Leitzmann et al. (2007).

Notes: Moderate activity – at least 30 minutes on most days of the week. Vigorous activity – at least 20 minutes, three times per week.

Figure 14.7 Association between (MET-h week^{-1}) of non-vigorous physical activity and the relative risk for all-cause mortality.

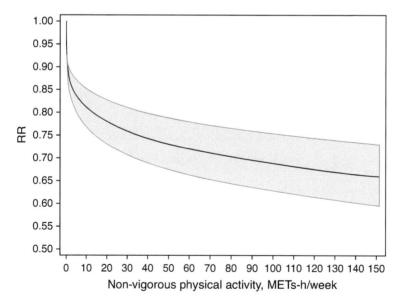

Source: Woodcock, J. et al., 'Non-vigorous physical activity and all-cause mortality: systematic review and meta-analysis of cohort studies', *International Journal of Epidemiology*, 2011, 40: 121–38, by permission of Oxford University Press.

Notes: Shaded area represents 95% confidence intervals. Based on 29 estimates from 22 studies.

Figure 14.8 Differences in the relative intensity of exercise (expressed as both %$\dot{V}O_2$max and as %$\dot{V}O_2$max reserve) for individuals with a range of $\dot{V}O_2$max values when walking at a 'brisk' pace, utilising 3.8 METs.

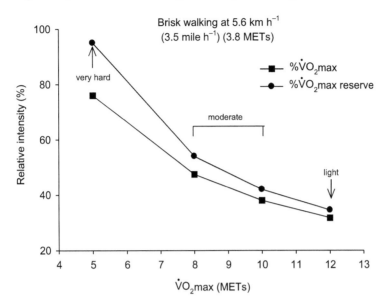

Source: Adapted from Howley (2001).

walking constitutes light activity for the average young person, but moderate or even vigorous activity for those with lower functional capacities (Figure 14.8). Notice that this figure expresses the intensity of exercise relative to $\dot{V}O_2$max reserve, i.e. capacity above the resting metabolic rate of 1 MET (see Chapter 2), as well as to $\dot{V}O_2$max. For people with very low $\dot{V}O_2$max values, such as patients with cardiac or respiratory problems, this distinction is important as there is little capability to increase oxygen uptake above the resting level. For such individuals brisk – or even normal-paced – walking constitutes vigorous exercise.

When asked to walk 'briskly', inactive middle-aged men and women typically select a pace that elicits nearly 60% $\dot{V}O_2$max. It is therefore not surprising that regular brisk or fast walking has been found to improve fitness in controlled trials in both men and women in this age group. Based on meta-analysis of intervention studies with a mean length of 35 weeks, the average increase is typically 9% for people with initial $\dot{V}O_2$max values around 30 ml kg^{-1} min^{-1} (Murphy et al. 2007). Such increases, although modest, are consistent with meaningful reductions to the risk of CVD morbidity and mortality (see Chapter 4).

Walking and health outcomes

Walking (amount and/or usual pace) has been specifically studied in observational and prospective epidemiological studies and shown to be independently associated with a lower risk of all-cause mortality, CHD/CVD, ischaemic stroke, type 2 diabetes, cognitive decline and weight gain. On average, the risk of CHD/CVD is around 20–30% lower for individuals who walk briskly for at least half an hour per day, compared with inactive individuals. Meta-analysis revealed a dose–response relationship between measures of walking and the risk of CHD, with a 19% reduction associated with a weekly walking increment of 8 MET-h (Zheng et al. 2009). Intervention studies provide complementary evidence that regular walking leads to improvements in risk markers for CHD such as blood lipids and blood pressure (Murtagh et al. 2010).

Comprehensive analyses of walking behaviour, for example, the Women's Health Initiative Observational Study (Manson et al. 2002), found that both amount and pace of walking were strongly related in a dose–response manner to the risk of a cardiovascular event (Figure 14.9).

However, according to meta-analysis, the effects on total and CVD mortality may be stronger for walking pace than for volume of walking (Hamer and Chida 2008b). In a 40-year follow-up of the prospective Whitehall Study, disease-specific mortality was reported in relation to self-rated walking pace in more than 19,000 male civil servants; walking pace was inversely related to mortality from all causes, CHD and all cancer (Figure 14.10). An analysis of pooled data from 50,225 walkers from 11 British population cohorts suggests that increasing walking pace could reduce risk for all-cause and CVD mortality (Stamatakis et al. 2018).

Walking has been related specifically to the risk of breast cancer: among postmenopausal women who reported walking as their only recreational physical activity,

Figure 14.9 Effect of volume (a) and pace (b) of walking on the relative risk of cardiovascular disease among postmenopausal women in the US Women's Health Initiative Observational Study.

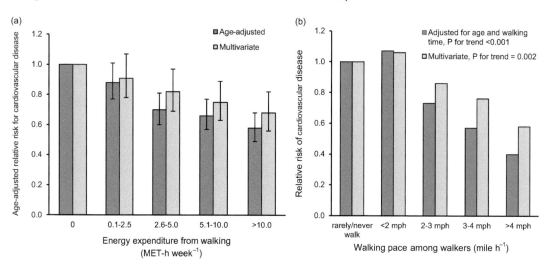

Source: From the *New England Journal of Medicine*, Manson, J.E. et al., 'Walking compared with vigorous exercise for the prevention of cardiovascular events in women', 347: 716–25. Copyright © 2002 Massachusetts Medical Society. Reprinted with permission from Massachusetts Medical Society.

Notes: 10 MET-h is equivalent to walking for 3 h 20 mins at an 'ordinary' pace of 4.8 km h^{-1} (3 mile h^{-1}). Mean and 95% confidence intervals for analysis of volume of walking. No confidence intervals reported for analysis by pace.

Figure 14.10 Relationships between self-rated walking pace and mortality outcomes in male civil servants: 40-year follow-up data from the Whitehall study.

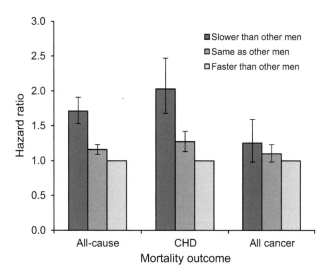

Source: Batty et al. (2010).

Notes: Hazard ratios (mean with 95% confidence intervals) are fully adjusted for known confounders. Men rated their usual speed of walking. The question asked was: 'Compared with other men of your age, do you tend to walk slower, faster or about the same pace?'

risk was 14% lower for those who reported ≥ 7 h week^{-1} than for those who reported ≤ 3 h week^{-1} (Hildebrand et al. 2013).

The increasing age of the population, one of the important modern trends identified in Chapter 1, makes research on the risk factors for diminished cognitive function essential. Cohort studies of people in their 70s have reported that regular walking is associated with better cognitive function and less cognitive decline in women (Weuve et al. 2004) and with a lower risk of developing dementia in men (Abbott et al. 2004).

In a number of observational studies, regular walking has been associated with a lower risk of hip fracture in women. Potential explanations include an osteogenic effect and/or improvements in strength and balance that reduce the risk of falling. While walking does not elicit an *optimal* osteogenic response, if brisk or fast, it can stimulate activity in the lower limb skeleton through alterations to the direction and rate of loading that increase ground and hip reaction forces. Effects are less likely at the lumbar spine. However, even a small difference in bone mineral density (BMD) can reduce the propensity to fracture. Moreover, older women enjoy walking and compliance can be excellent. For example, one trial ($n = 78$) reported 91% adherence among women aged 60–70 during the first year of the intervention and 94% during the follow-up year (Brooke-Wavell et al. 2001).

Regular walking has been specifically associated with prevention of weight gain in prospective studies. For example, after an eight-year follow-up, premenopausal women who walked for more than 30 minutes per day were 30% less likely to gain weight than those who walked for less than ten minutes daily (Mekary et al. 2009). This is

---

BOX 14.2 WALKING AND PUBLIC HEALTH – IMPLICATIONS FOR PREVENTION.

- A 17% decrease in colon cancer would be expected if three hours of walking per week were to be added to the physical activity of all participants in the US Health Professionals Follow-up Study (18,000 fewer deaths) (Colditz et al. 1997).
- In the Honolulu Heart Study of Japanese men aged 61–81, for every five men who walked at least 2 miles daily, one fewer died over 12 years, compared with those who walked less than 1 mile per day (Hakim et al. 1998). A walking group that includes 60 men in this age group may therefore be expected to save one life each year.
- In a prospective study of nearly 3,000 diabetics in the US, walking half an hour per day was associated with a 50% lower risk of cardiovascular and total mortality. Researchers estimated that '1 death per year may be preventable for every 61 people who could be persuaded to walk at least 2 h per week' (Gregg et al. 2003).
- Meta-analysis of studies of dose–response of walking in reducing CHD risk found that about 30 minutes of normal walking a day for five days a week was associated with a 19% reduction in risk (Zheng et al. 2009).

---

consistent with findings from intervention studies that regular walking for exercise decreases body weight and/or adiposity (or avoids increases seen in controls) (see, for example, data in Table 14.1).

Even when employed as planned exercise with the goal to improve fitness, walking is very injury-free. This is important because fear of sustaining an injury and stopping activity because of an injury have both been associated with failure to start or to maintain a physically active lifestyle. Furthermore, because walking constitutes moderate-intensity activity for so many people, it carries little risk for sudden cardiovascular events. Examples of potential benefits for public health if levels of walking could be increased within a population are presented in Box 14.2.

ACTIVE TRAVEL, COMMUTING

One reason that walking and cycling for personal transportation can be health-enhancing is because these activities are regular and performed on a near-daily basis. According to a UK survey, more than two-thirds of people who reported any active transport got sufficient activity to meet government guidelines by this means alone (Adams 2010).

Commuting to work by walking and cycling has been specifically studied. The first large-scale prospective study found that commuting by bicycle reduced the risk of premature mortality by approximately one-third (Andersen et al. 2000). Meta-analytic review of eight prospective cohort and case-control studies of physically active commuting concluded that this behaviour was associated with an 11% reduction in cardiovascular risk (Hamer and Chida 2008a). Other health-related outcomes reported to be associated with a lower risk in people with a habit of active commuting include certain cancers and all-cause mortality (Matthews et al. 2005, 2007). In the CARDIA cross-sectional study, men who used active commuting to work were fitter, less likely to be obese and exhibited lower CVD risk than other men (Gordon-Larsen et al. 2009). Even if commuting distances are too great to rely solely on walking and cycling, using public transport rather than a car increases the amount of walking (to and from bus and train stops) and so the promotion of public transport can have public health benefits.

Walking or cycling to school is a valuable source of activity for children and does not appear to displace time spent in active leisure pursuits. Children who travel to school by these means have higher daily step counts than those who are transported in vehicles (Murtagh and Murphy 2011). It has also been suggested that the ability to concentrate in the classroom is greater in children who walk or cycle to school than in those who travel in other ways; however, a recent meta-analysis of 12 studies found that there is insufficient evidence to support this association (Ruiz-Hermosa et al. 2019).

There are enormous differences in active travel to school between countries. Around three quarters of Dutch children walk or cycle to school, compared with about half in the UK and about 15% in Canada and the US. In many countries, the potential to increase walking and cycling for short commuting journeys – and/or to incorporate these activities into car journeys – is therefore considerable.

CHANGING PHYSICAL ACTIVITY BEHAVIOURS

Worldwide, many researchers have addressed the question: 'What works to increase physical activity levels?' A more recent, but just as relevant, question is: 'What works to decrease sedentary behaviours?' The answers are as yet far from clear.

A wide range of different interventions have been undertaken, including community-based, informational, behavioural, social, policy and environmental approaches. Nevertheless, more information is needed concerning their uptake, sustainability and cost-effectiveness as well as their applicability in different countries. A 'one-size fits all' approach is never likely to succeed – interventions need to be adapted to different cultures and to embrace the complexity of the entire system (Heath et al. 2012). One popular framework for health behaviour change is the COM-B system which suggests that interventions to increase physical activity should address an individual's capability, opportunity and motivation (Michie et al. 2011). Given the high levels of inactivity in the population, some have suggested that physical activity promotion should espouse a fresh approach. Invoking a parallel with tobacco control, it might be more effective to emphasise the *harms* of *in*activity than to continue solely to disseminate the message that exercise brings health benefits (Wen and Wu 2012).

Monitoring change is a prerequisite for evaluating effectiveness and developing policies to enhance physical activity. Comprehensive and systematic surveillance systems could, in future, use measurement tools such as accelerometers and inclinometers that capture all components of activity – and inactivity – as an adjunct to self-reported data. At a national level, these systems need routinely to sample diverse segments of the population in order to ensure representativeness.

Whole of community interventions

Early examples of effective interventions of this nature are the North Karelia project in Finland and the Stanford Five City project in the US which were implemented in the 1970s and 1980s. More recently effective community-based interventions have used a range of complementary, high-visibility strategies to encourage people to be more physically active. These include: social marketing to raise awareness and provide information; individual counselling by health professionals; working with voluntary and non-governmental organisations, including sporting clubs; working in specific settings such as schools, workplaces and shopping malls; and environmental change strategies such as provision of cycle lanes (Mummery and Brown 2009). Whilst there is a sound theoretical case for such interventions – and numerous studies have been undertaken – the body of evidence in support of their long-term effectiveness remains unconvincing.

Behavioural and social approaches

Interventions that are targeted at individuals or groups incorporate a range of behaviour change techniques such as goal-setting, social support and behavioural reinforcement. They can be delivered by email, internet, SMS messages, social media or telephone – separately or in combination. Targeted groups of the population may be, for example, the elderly, schoolchildren or patient groups. For individuals, an assessment of current physical activity levels and readiness to change form the basis of a tailored activity plan.

Nearly 50 trials have examined the effectiveness of interventions to promote walking. These include advice to individuals, group-based and community-level approaches, as well as a number based on walking as a means of transport (Ogilvie et al. 2007). There is clear evidence that people can be encouraged to walk more by interventions that are tailored to their needs, targeted at the most sedentary and/or at those most motivated to change and delivered either at the level of the individual, household or group. The most successful have been reported to increase walking by some 30–60 minutes per week. The availability of inexpensive pedometers means that individuals can monitor their levels of walking and use feedback to reinforce this behaviour change.

'Buddy' systems and support groups have been particularly successful at generating and sustaining walking behaviour. These usually organise walking partners or groups, provide initial training about walking and then facilitate the activity by providing maps. Regular telephone prompts reinforce behaviours and help to prevent relapse.

In the UK, an initiative called the 'Green Gym' brings together people who want to help the environment and, at the same time, increase their level of activity. Since its inception in the 1990s, more than 60 groups have been established, country-wide. It is run by a charity, with central government support. Volunteers meet once a week and do up to four hours of practical conservation or gardening work, with a refreshment break and a chance to socialise. Regular participants show improvements in cardiovascular fitness and strength and report that the activity is good for their mental health and wellbeing (Bowler et al. 2010).

Another grassroots initiative is parkrun, which began in Teddington, London in 2004. Events are organised by volunteers and are free. Groups of all ages meet on a Saturday morning for a timed walk, jog or run 5k in an open space. Participants register online and receive an email with their time. The scheme expanded rapidly and is now established in more than 21 countries, worldwide. Technology has facilitated another successful scheme, the nine-week running plan 'Couch to 5k', targeted at absolute beginners. Started by an American, Josh Clark, in the late 1990s the programme has been adopted by the National Health Service in the UK and is available to download as a smartphone app (over one million downloads in 2018).

Settings for interventions can be worksites, community centres or recreational facilities with practical sessions delivered by personal trainers or community coaches. Structured programmes often involve attendance at an exercise facility such as a gymnasium over several weeks or months. Sessions are generally supervised and this may help previously inactive people to avoid injury or other adverse events. It may also help them to appreciate the need to start gently, progress gradually and to incorporate different modes of activity – stretching, aerobic activity and muscle strengthening – into an exercise regimen.

Adherence to structured interventions has been reported to be good, with at least 80% of participants completing a typical programme. As well as improving fitness, such programmes appear to motivate people to be more active outside the structured activity; for example, they may do more walking, even on the days they attend an exercise class. On the other hand, their effectiveness at a population level is limited by the fact that only a small proportion of the inactive population enrol and they are less cost-effective than alternative population-level approaches. Moreover such facility- and personnel-dependent interventions may increase health inequalities.

The potential for primary care physicians to counsel inactive, apparently healthy, people to increase physical activity is increasingly recognised. A variety of interventions, including exercise referral schemes, motivational interviewing and introducing such patients to more active 'peer mentors' can all be effective, particularly among people initially classed as minimally active. Several randomised controlled trials (advice from a physician versus no advice) have found that counselling is effective, at least over 6–12 months. Physicians are more likely to offer such counselling if they are active themselves – as is the case with smoking behaviour. They can give advice, offer educational materials delivered by an ever-increasing range of media and/or refer patients to exercise specialists. The efficacy of these (probably complementary) approaches is a topic of continuing research interest, although there is still little information about longer-term effects on patients' physical activity levels. The cost-effectiveness of primary care interventions remains to be determined but, based on randomised controlled trials, researchers estimated that the number needed to 'treat' with an intervention for one additional inactive adult to meet recommended levels of activity at 12 months was 12 (Orrow et al. 2012).

The initiative 'Exercise is Medicine' was launched in 2007 by the American College of Sports Medicine and the American Medical Association in an attempt to make physical activity a standard component of disease prevention. The specific goal is to encourage all physicians 'to assess, to advocate for, and to review every patient's physical activity program (sic) during every comprehensive visit'. A website provides physicians, health and fitness professionals, policy makers, the media and the public with every kind of educational and practical resource to support the initiative (Exercise is

Medicine 2007). Physicians are encouraged to sign up to this policy and the public are encouraged to put pressure on their physicians to do so. The range of supporting organisations is vast and bodes well for the success of this initiative.

Physical activity is important in the management of patients suffering from a variety of conditions and may be best delivered if clinical and community resources are co-ordinated. However, a detailed discussion of this topic is beyond the scope of this book and the interested reader is referred to Pedersen and Saltin (2015).

School-based interventions targeted at children and adolescents are an attractive way to increase activity levels before sedentary behaviours become entrenched. Successful schemes are invariably multi-component and largely education-based, with classes about diet and physical activity as well as additional physical education sessions and opportunities to be active during the school day, at break times and after school. To reach their full potential, such interventions need actively to involve parents and families and to be linked to community initiatives.

Interventions to reduce sedentary behaviour in children and adolescents have been a focus of recent research. These have been delivered through a variety of settings and involved different components – educational, behavioural, environmental and social support. A 'review of reviews' found that interventions have a 'small but statistically significant effect' (Biddle et al. 2014). A supportive family environment was important for success. Interventions with children under six years old tended to be more effective, probably because parents have more control over behaviours at this age.

Policy and environmental approaches

Everyday physical activity is strongly influenced by the built environment (Sallis et al. 2012). For instance, the more attractive and 'walkable' streets and parks are, the higher the levels of walking – and the more likely residents are to meet physical activity guidelines. On the other hand, if they live in less 'walkable' areas, people are more likely to be overweight or obese.

Land use and transport policies and practice can therefore help to generate and sustain increases in physical activity at a population level. Arguably, this approach can benefit *all* community members, in contrast to targeted behaviour change programmes that focus on individuals who are motivated to take part. Changes to the built environment can influence physical activity levels, even in people who have no conscious intention to become more active. This approach is timely and attractive, complementing policies on air quality, noise pollution, climate change, 'liveability' of neighbourhoods, children's independent mobility, traffic congestion and sustainability. In the UK about 20% of all car journeys during the weekday morning rush hour are undertaken by parents taking children to school. Creating environments that support safe local walking and cycling is a prerequisite if more children (and parents) are to make frequent, short journeys without the use of a car.

Influences on walking include land use/mix and transportation infrastructure. People are more likely to walk if shops, bus stops and offices are nearby. More and better pavements (sidewalks) encourage walking, as do high street connectivity and improved street lighting. Safe bicycle paths and lanes encourage commuting by bicycle but bad weather, hills and fear of crime remain barriers.

Examples of initiatives to promote active travel

In 1976 the Danish government introduced legislation requiring that every child has a safe route to school. If there is no such route, free bus transport must be provided, giving authorities a financial incentive to invest in safe routes. More than 70% of Danish children now walk or cycle to school and this has been achieved alongside a reduction in the child accident rate. 'Safe routes to school' programmes are now in place throughout Europe and in Australia, New Zealand, Canada and the US. The cycling culture in Denmark is reinforced by other legislation. Cyclists are liable to a substantial fine if, for example, they: cycle on the road when a cycle path is available; fail to use hand signals to indicate turns; jump a red light; ride without lights; or use a hand-held telephone whilst cycling.

In the Netherlands, motorised traffic entering 6,500 residential zones (called Woonerf) is restricted to a speed of 'walking pace'. These areas typically combine shared walking/cycling/driving surfaces and use trees, planters and children's play areas to create a street space so unlike a traditional street that vehicle speeds are markedly reduced by instinctive, behavioural change in drivers. Under the unique Dutch legal system, motorists must yield to cyclists unless there are special road markings; they are held automatically to be responsible in collisions with cyclists, regardless of the circumstances of an accident. Cycling accounts for up to a third of journeys in Dutch and Danish cities – in sharp contrast to many other European countries and to the US where cycling comprises only 1–2% of trips.

With the aim of making Paris a quieter place, with less pollution and where people 'take up more of the space', this city has vigorously encouraged cycling through a variety of schemes. It now boasts some 370 km of bicycle paths, and bicycle use increased by nearly 50% between 2001 and 2007. Accident rates from cycling remained stable despite this big increase. It seems that, with more cyclists on the road, they are more visible to other road users. On Sundays and Bank Holidays the initiative 'Paris Breathes' permits pedestrians, cyclists and people on roller blades to benefit from the closure of many roads to cars. ('Ciclovía' initiatives have a similar approach and are rapidly spreading throughout the Americas and the Caribbean.) Many cities now have free or low-cost rental bicycles (as in the 'Rando Vélo' scheme in Paris) and allow users to pick up a bicycle from any station, returning it to any other. Most allow users to cycle for the first 30 minutes without charge.

Cities such as Berlin, Barcelona and Bogotá, where initiatives have included constructing bicycle facilities and bicycle-sharing systems, have seen a doubling of the share of trips undertaken by bicycle. These sorts of strategies are probably most effective when combined with promotional campaigns targeted, for example, at schools and workplaces. Actions by businesses and organisations can also promote active living. For example, in one intervention, installing locker rooms led to an increase in the number of employees walking or cycling to work. Simple changes within buildings, such as clear signing of staircases, can increase daily activity.

Policies or interventions to encourage active travel do not necessarily target walking and cycling *per se* but instead have an indirect effect by *dis*couraging travel by vehicle. Examples include road and parking pricing or improving public transport. London, for example, has seen a near doubling of levels of cycling since the introduction of a congestion charge for vehicles – but also significant investment in cycling infrastructure.

BENEFITS VERSUS RISKS

As discussed in Chapter 13, physical activity can be hazardous as well as beneficial to health. The risk–benefit ratio of exercise is therefore an important concern for public health, as well as for the individual, for whom it will be modified by pre-existing medical conditions.

Cardiovascular events

Some risk–benefit analysis is available for cardiac events. As discussed in Chapter 13, vigorous exercise is associated with a transient increase in the risk of a cardiovascular event during or soon after exertion.[3] Nevertheless, there is no evidence to suggest that the cardiovascular risks of physical activity outweigh the benefits for healthy people. Indeed, the converse is true: epidemiological, scientific and clinical evidence shows that habitual activity decreases overall risk (Goodman et al. 2011; Thompson et al. 2007).

The reader will recall that the increase in risk associated with exertion varies greatly according to level of habitual activity so that a disproportionate number of cardiac events occur in people performing vigorous activity to which they are unaccustomed. Thus, one of the most important defences against exercise-related cardiac events is to acquire and maintain physical fitness through regular physical activity. Whilst public health initiatives must encourage a high level of physical activity in the population they should also emphasise the need for inactive people to begin with low/moderate-intensity activity, progressing only gradually to longer-duration, high-intensity activity if they seek greater benefits.

A simple screening tool such as the well-established Canadian PAR-Q (physical activity readiness questionnaire) can identify individuals at high risk. If individuals answer 'no' to seven simple questions about their health, they are deemed to be at low risk and can exercise at low to moderate intensities with minimal or no supervision. The new PAR-Q+ incorporates seven 'evidence-based' questions, with further questions on specific chronic medical conditions to either clear the respondent for activity or refer them for further assessment in a risk stratification process (Bredin et al. 2013).

Injuries

Walking for exercise, gardening or yard work, bicycling or exercise cycling, dancing, swimming and golf are activities with the lowest injury rates (Physical Activity Guidelines Advisory Committee 2018) but risk–benefit analysis is not available. This is a cause for concern because injury prevalence will increase if the population becomes more active. It is particularly important for older adults, for whom the consequences of a fall can be catastrophic.

What is known is that rates of pedestrian and cyclist road traffic injuries are in fact reduced as walking and cycling become more commonplace (Jacobsen et al. 2009). The overall risk–benefit implications of a shift from private car use to bicycle use have been modelled by researchers in the Netherlands who estimated the effect on all-cause mortality if 500,000 people made the transition from car to bicycle for short trips on a daily basis. The benefit to the individual in terms of increased mortality (3–14 months gained) was substantially greater than the decrease through greater exposure to air pollution and the increase in traffic accidents (0.8–40 days lost) (de Hartog 2010).

Pharmacological interventions carry risks too

Finally, physical activity is not the only intervention aiming to benefit health that carries risks. Drugs have side effects too, ranging from the discomforting to the life-threatening. Their packaging therefore carries instructions on how to optimise effectiveness and minimise risks – rather like physical activity recommendations. For example, the Diabetes Prevention Program Group trial compared physical activity with metformin (a drug that improves insulin sensitivity) as means to prevent the development of type 2 diabetes in people with impaired glucose tolerance (Diabetes Prevention Program Research Group 2002). Subjects allocated to the drug therapy group were more likely not only to develop type 2 diabetes but also to experience a higher incidence of gastrointestinal disturbances (a side effect of the drug) than those in the lifestyle intervention group.

PHYSICAL ACTIVITY: A 'BEST BUY' IN PUBLIC HEALTH?

Promoting physical activity can be viewed as a health-care intervention. Professor Archie Cochrane, a pioneering clinical epidemiologist, introduced a hierarchy of evidence required before any health-care intervention can be applied to real-life situations. Three simple questions have to be answered satisfactorily (Table 14.2): *Can* it work (efficacy)? *Does* it work (effectiveness)? And *is* it worth it (cost-effectiveness)?

For pharmacological interventions that prevent disease, this scheme can be applied in a rather straightforward way because a drug is invariably targeted at a single health outcome. Physical activity interventions have multiple, often inter-related outcomes so the situation is vastly more complex. Nevertheless, it is clear that – for many important health outcomes – physical activity *is* efficacious (shown by intervention trials) and *is* effective in 'real world' settings (epidemiological evidence).

Table 14.2 Cochrane's scheme for hierarchy of evidence: criteria to be met before a health intervention is acceptable.

TYPE OF EVIDENCE	QUESTION	DESCRIPTION
Efficacy	Can it work?	The extent to which an intervention does more good than harm under ideal circumstances.
Effectiveness	Does it work in practice?	Whether an intervention does more good than harm when provided under usual circumstances.
Cost effectiveness	Is it worth it?	The effect of the intervention in relation to the resources it consumes

Source: Reproduced from the *British Medical Journal*, Järvinen, T.L.N. et al., 342: d2175, copyright © 2011 with permission from BMJ Publishing Group Ltd.

One issue that research has largely failed to address is the comparative effectiveness of exercise and drug interventions in reducing mortality. However, in a unique meta-epidemiological study, researchers compared mortality outcomes from four conditions (secondary prevention of CHD, rehabilitation of stroke, treatment of heart failure and prevention of diabetes) using data from meta-analyses (four exercise and 12 drug) of randomised controlled trials. Based on the limited evidence available, it was concluded that exercise and many drug interventions are often potentially similar in terms of their mortality benefits. Indeed, physical activity interventions were found to be *more* effective than drug treatments among patients with stroke (Naci and Ioannidis 2013).

Data are becoming available to quantify the economic burden of physical inactivity and examples for three countries are presented in Box 14.3. Estimates of the direct economic costs[4] attributable to inactivity range from 1.2% to 2.5% of total health-care expenditures in highly developed countries (Katzmarzyk 2011). The few available estimates for low- and middle-income countries are of the same order (Pratt et al. 2014). Few studies have estimated the indirect[4] costs of physical inactivity – because this involves more assumptions – but these likely markedly exceed direct medical costs, as has been estimated for Canada (Katzmarzyk and Janssen (2004).

So, what about the last question in Cochrane's hierarchy of evidence, on cost-effectiveness? Based on analyses extrapolated from epidemiological findings, substantial economic benefit may be expected if the prevalence of physical inactivity can be decreased (Box 14.4). One Australian study focused specifically on walking as a means of decreasing the health-care costs of CHD (Zheng et al. 2010). Prevention of CHD among the one-third of adults who engaged in 'sufficient walking' (defined as 30 minutes on five to seven days per week) at the start of the study in 2004 was estimated to save AU$126 million. Health-care cost savings were then estimated for three different plausible scenarios, i.e. a 1% increase in the prevalence of 'sufficient' walking among the Australian population, a 5% increase, a 10% increase and, more speculatively, a situation where the entire sedentary adult population achieved this goal. The corresponding potential net direct cost savings[5] are shown in Figure 14.11. Given the low injury risk and high adherence rate, walking was described as a 'key population-based primary intervention strategy for CHD prevention and health-care cost reduction' (Zheng et al. 2010).

BOX 14.3 THE ECONOMIC BURDEN OF PHYSICAL INACTIVITY; ESTIMATES FROM HIGHLY DEVELOPED COUNTRIES.

- In 2009, the direct and indirect health-care costs of physical inactivity in Canada were estimated as CAN$2.4 billion (£1.52 billion) and CAN$4.3 billion (£2.73 billion), respectively (Janssen 2012).
- Based on 2006–7 data, physical inactivity costs the UK National Health Service £0.9 billion (US$1.37 billion) annually (Scarborough et al. 2011).
- In 2008 in the Czech Republic, the financial cost of physical inactivity to public health insurance companies was almost 700 million CZ Koruna (£23.1 million or US$34.9 million) (Maresova 2014).

BOX 14.4 POTENTIAL ECONOMIC BENEFITS FROM INCREASING LEVELS OF PHYSICAL ACTIVITY.

- Increased urban walking and cycling in England and Wales could, over 20 years, lead to savings of roughly £17 million (US$25.8) (in 2010 prices) to the UK National Health Service through reductions in the prevalence of seven diseases (Jarrett et al. 2012). Assumed increases in average daily distances travelled were 1 mile (1.6 km) for walking and 2.1 miles (3.4 km) for cycling.
- In Australia, the potential net direct annual health-care savings[4] (2004 prices) from a 5–10% increased participation in sufficient walking (30 mins, 5–7 days a week) to prevent CHD were estimated as AU$145–164 million (US$143.8–162.7 million or £94.2–106.6 million) (Figure 14.11) (Zheng et al. 2010).
- In Australia, a 10% reduction in physical inactivity in would provide gains in working days (114,000) and gains in days of home-based production (180,000) (Cadilhac et al. 2011).

Figure 14.11 Estimates of the net direct health-care cost[4] savings in preventing CHD from increased participation in 'sufficient' walking (millions of Australian dollars). First group of bars represent savings from participation in 'sufficient' walking by Australian adults in 2004 at the time of the study (about one-third of the population); remaining bars show projected savings if 1%, 5% and 10% more Australians – or even the entire inactive population – were to engage in 'sufficient' walking.

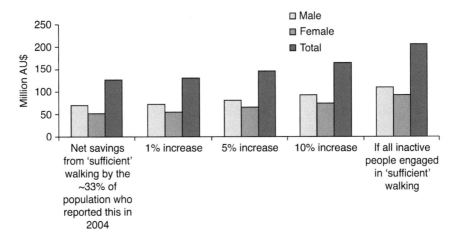

Source: Adapted by permission from Springer Nature Customer Service Centre GmbH: Springer Nature, *International Journal of Health Care Finance and Economics*, 'Economic evaluation of the direct healthcare cost savings resulting from the use of walking interventions to prevent coronary heart disease in Australia', Zheng, H. et al., copyright © 2010.
Notes: 'Sufficient' walking defined as 30 mins of normal walking a day on five to seven days per week. Estimates are for 2004. (1 Australian dollar is about £0.63; Australian and US dollars almost the same.)

Only actual cost-effectiveness trials of exercise interventions can fulfil with external validity the requirement of Cochrane's third criterion, 'Is it worth it?' One such trial has confirmed the cost-effectiveness of an exercise programme in preventing falls of older adults (Robertson et al. 2001) but more data are sorely needed. Interestingly, the scenario is no different for preventive drugs such as statins, anti-hypertensives and bisphosphonates where it has been asserted that there is 'a virtual absence of empirical cost-effective data' (Järvinen et al. 2011).

Of course, the whole economic picture associated with physical in/activity can probably never be modelled satisfactorily. As healthy life expectancy increases, people may work longer and pay more into the public purse through taxes; equally they may, in old age, draw more heavily on health services. Despite the many uncertainties and assumptions involved, available data on health economics are compelling and coherent with Professor Morris's memorable description of exercise as the 'best buy in public health' (Morris 1994).

However, as a justification for the promotion of physical activity economic benefits are neither necessary nor sufficient. Low fitness and physical inactivity are a waste of human potential, at the population level as well as at a personal level. For this reason alone, promotion of physical activity should be a priority for public health.

SUMMARY

- Non-communicable diseases are a major and increasing public health burden, in developing countries as well as in those with established market economies. Increasing physical activity levels would have an important impact on the incidence of these diseases.
- Adults need moderate-intensity aerobic activity for a minimum of 30 minutes on at least five days each week, or vigorous-intensity aerobic activity for a minimum of 20 minutes on three days each week or a combination of both. Children need more activity, of the order of 60 minutes at a moderate-to-vigorous intensity, most days of the week. Activity should be performed in bouts of at least ten minutes duration.
- Older adults should be as physically active as their abilities and conditions allow. They should also do exercises to maintain muscle mass, improve balance and prevent falls.
- All adults and children – even those whose activity levels meet recommendations – should minimise the time spent in sedentary behaviours and avoid prolonged uninterrupted periods of sitting.
- Walking is the obvious starting point for inactive people and regular walking has been associated, in a dose-dependent manner, with a number of health outcomes. Brisk or fast walking will improve fitness in most middle-aged and older men and in almost all adult women.
- Interventions, including community-wide campaigns, behavioural and social approaches as well as policy and environmental approaches, are active research areas. Multi-component interventions are the most likely to succeed but demand co-operation of different agencies and stakeholders.
- Physical activity has some adverse side effects, but these are mainly avoided if the intensity of activity is moderate. For the overwhelming majority of individuals, benefits clearly outweigh risks.
- Physical inactivity is a considerable economic burden and reduced levels would be expected lead to economic benefits.

STUDY TASKS

1 Name the major chronic non-communicable diseases and briefly describe their most important preventable risk factors.
2 Write an 'executive summary' of widely accepted recommendations for physical activity levels in adults.
3 'For most health outcomes, additional benefits occur as the amount of physical activity increases.' Explain the basis of this statement.
4 Is the pattern of exercise an important determinant of its health benefits and risks? Provide a reasoned argument for your view.
5 Explain why walking can be light or vigorous activity for different individuals, giving illustrative examples.
6 Identify and discuss different types of intervention that aim to increase levels of activity in a population.

NOTES

1 Moderate intensity: 3–5.9 METs or 40–60% $\dot{V}O_2$max: vigorous intensity $\geq$6 METs or >60% $\dot{V}O_2$max.
2 Dogs are good companions as well as people – in one Australian study around a quarter of all walking was dog walking (Bauman and Russell 2001)! Dog owners are much more likely than non-owners to be sufficiently active.
3 The media appreciate the relative risk (e.g. five-fold, 56-fold) but, in reporting sudden exercise-related deaths, do not explain to their readership that the absolute risk of a cardiac event during exercise is very low (Chapter 13).
4 Direct costs are those incurred in treatment, care and rehabilitation of injury or illness, in this instance CHD. (They do not include, for instance, the considerable costs to the economy of absence from work due to ill health.) Net direct costs are the gross costs less the costs of the intervention – deemed in this instance to be costs of walking shoes and medical care for injuries incurred during walking.
5 Net direct cost savings were estimated by subtracting the direct costs associated with walking (shoes and treatment of injuries incurred) from the direct medical cost savings to the health system attributable to Australians who participated in sufficient walking.

FURTHER READING

Biddle, S.J. and Batterham, A.M. (2015) High-intensity interval exercise training for public health: a big HIT or shall we HIT it on the head? *International Journal of Behavioral Nutrition and Physical Activity* 12: 95. doi: 10.1186/s12966-015-0254-9.
DiPietro, L., Buchner, D.M., Marquez, D.X., Pate, R.R., Pescatello, L.S. and Whitt-Glover, M.C. (2019) New scientific basis for the 2018 U.S. Physical Activity Guidelines. *Journal of Sport and Health Science* 8: 197–200.
Murphy, M.H., Lahart, I., Carlin, A. and Murtagh, E. (2019) The effects of continuous compared to accumulated exercise on health: a meta-analytic review. *Sports Medicine* 45: 1285–91.
O'Donovan, G., Lee, I.-M., Hamer, M. and Stamatakis, E. (2017) Association of 'weekend warrior' and other leisure time physical activity patterns with risks for all-cause, cardiovascular disease, and cancer mortality. *JAMA Internal Medicine* 177: 335–42.

Physical Activity Guidelines Advisory Committee. (2018) *2018 Physical activity guidelines advisory committee scientific report*. Washington, DC: U.S. Department of Health and Human Services.

Pratt, M., Norris, J., Lobelo, F., Roux, L. and Wang, G. (2014) The cost of physical inactivity: moving into the 21st century. *British Journal of Sports Medicine* 48: 171–3.

Reis, S.R., Salvo, D., Ogilvie, D., Lambert, E.V., Goenka, S., Brownson, R.C. and Lancet Physical Activity Series 2 Executive Committee. (2016) Scaling up physical activity interventions across the globe: stepping up to larger and smarter approaches to get people moving. *The Lancet* 388: 1337–48.

Stamatakis, E., Ekelund, U., Ding, D., Hamer, M., Bauman, A.E. and Lee, I.-M. (2019) Is the time right for quantitative public health guidelines on sitting? A narrative review of sedentary behaviour research paradigms and findings. *British Journal of Sports Medicine* 53: 377–82.

REFERENCES

Abbott, R.D., White, L.R., Ross, G.W., Masaki, K.H., Curb, J.D. and Petrovitch, H. (2004) Walking and dementia in physically capable elderly men. *Journal of the American Medical Association* 292: 1447–53.

Adams, J. (2010) Prevalence and sociodemographic correlates of 'active transport' in the UK: analysis of the UK time use survey 2005. *Preventive Medicine* 50: 199–203.

American College of Sports Medicine. (1978) The recommended quantity and quality of exercise for developing and maintaining fitness in healthy adults. *Medicine and Science in Sports* 10: vii–ix.

American College of Sports Medicine. (1990) Position Stand. The recommended quantity and quality of exercise for developing and maintaining cardiorespiratory and muscular fitness in healthy adults. *Medicine and Science in Sports and Exercise* 22: 265–74.

American College of Sports Medicine. (2011) Position Stand. Quantity and quality of exercise for developing and maintaining cardiorespiratory, musculoskeletal, and neuromotor fitness in apparently healthy adults: guidance for prescribing exercise. *Medicine and Science in Sports and Exercise* 43: 1334–59.

Andersen, L.B., Schnohr, P., Schroll, M. and Hein, H.O. (2000) All-cause mortality associated with physical activity during leisure time, work, sports and cycling to work. *Archives of Internal Medicine* 160: 1621–8.

Batty, G.D., Shipley, M.J., Kivimaki, M., Marmot, M. and Davey-Smith, G. (2010) Walking pace, leisure time physical activity, and resting heart rate in relation to disease-specific mortality in London: 40 years follow-up of the original Whitehall study. An update of our work with Professor Jerry N. Morris 1910–2009. *Annals of Epidemiology* 20: 661–9.

Bauman, A.E. and Russell, S.J. (2001) The epidemiology of dog walking in Australia: an underutilised population strategy for increasing physical activity levels. *Medicine and Science in Sports and Exercise* 33: S238.

Bhammar, D.M., Angadi, S.S. and Gaesser, G.A. (2012) Effects of fractionized and continuous exercise on 24-h ambulatory blood pressure. *Medicine and Science in Sports and Exercise* 44: 2270–6.

Biddle, S.J. and Batterham, A.M. (2015) High-intensity interval exercise training for public health: a big HIT or shall we HIT it on the head? *International Journal of Behavioral Nutrition and Physical Activity* 12: 95. doi: 10.1186/s12966-015-0254-9.

Biddle, S.J.H., Petrolini, I. and Pearson, N. (2014) Interventions designed to reduce sedentary behaviours in young people: a review of reviews. *British Journal of Sports Medicine* 48: 182–6.

Bowler, D.E., Buyung-Ali, L.M., Knight, T.M. and Pullin, A.S. (2010) A systematic review of evidence for the added benefits to health of exposure to natural environments. *BMC Public Health* 10: 456. doi: 10.1186/1471-2458-10-456.

Bredin, S.S.D., Gledhill, N., Jamnick, V.K. and Warburton, D.E.R. (2013) PAR-Q+ and ePARmed-X+: new risk stratification and physical activity clearance strategy for physicians and patients alike. *Canadian Family Physician* 59: 273–7.

Brooke-Wavell, K.S.F., Jones, P.R.M., Hardman, A.E., Tsuritani, I. and Yamada, Y. (2001) Commencing, continuing and stopping brisk walking: effects on bone mineral density, quantitative ultrasound of bone and markers of bone metabolism in postmenopausal women. *Osteoporosis International* 12: 581–7.

Buckley, J.P., Hedge, A., Yates, T., Copeland, R.J., Loosemore, M., Hamer, M. et al. (2015) The sedentary office: an expert statement on the growing case for change towards better health and productivity. *British Journal of Sports Medicine* 49: 1357–62.

Cadilhac, D.A., Cumming, T.B., Sheppard, L., Pearce, D.C., Carter, R. and Magnus, A. (2011) The economic benefits of reducing physical inactivity: an Australian example. *International Journal of Behavioral Nutrition and Physical Activity* 8: 99. doi: 10.1186/1479-5868-8-99.

Canadian Society for Exercise Physiology. (2020) Canadian 24-hour movement guidelines [online], available at: https://csepguidelines.ca/ (accessed 12 May 2020).

Colditz, G.A., Cannuscio, C.C. and Frazier, A.L. (1997) Physical activity and reduced risk of colon cancer: implications for prevention. *Cancer Causes and Control* 8: 649–67.

Colley, R.C., Janssen, I. and Tremblay, M.S. (2012) Daily step target to measure adherence to physical activity guidelines in children. *Medicine and Science in Sports and Exercise* 44: 977–82.

DeBusk, R.F., Stenestrand, U., Sheehan, M. and Haskell, W.L. (1990) Training effects of long versus short bouts of exercise in healthy subjects. *American Journal of Cardiology* 65: 1010–13.

De Hartog, J.J., Boogaard, H., Nijland, H. and Hoek, G. (2010) Do the health benefits of cycling outweigh the risks? *Environmental Health Perspectives* 118: 1109–16.

Department of Health. (2011) Start active, stay active. A report from the Four Home Countries' Chief Medical Officers [online], available at: https://assets.publishing.service.gov.uk/government/uploads/system/uploads/attachment_data/file/216370/dh_128210.pdf (accessed 30 July 2019).

Department of Health. (2019) UK Medical Officers' physical activity guidelines [online], available at: https://assets.publishing.service.gov.uk/government/uploads/system/uploads/attachment_data/file/832868/uk-chief-medical-officers-physical-activity-guidelines.pdf (accessed 7 May 2020).

Diabetes Prevention Program Research Group. (2002) Reduction in the incidence of type 2 diabetes with lifestyle intervention or metformin. *New England Journal of Medicine* 346: 393–403.

Dunn, A.L., Marcus, B.H., Kampert, J.B., Garcia, M.E., Kohl, H.W. and Blair, S.N. (1999) Comparison of lifestyle and structured interventions to increase physical activity and cardiorespiratory fitness. *Journal of the American Medical Association* 281: 327–34.

Ekblom-Bak, E., Ekblom, B, Vikström, M., de Faire, U. and Hellénius, M.-L. (2014) The importance of non-exercise physical activity for cardiovascular health and longevity. *British Journal of Sports Medicine* 48: 233–8.

Ekelund, U., Steene-Johanssessen, J., Brown, W.J., Fagerland, M.W., Owen, N., Powell et al. for the Lancet Physical Activity Series 2 Executive Committee and the Lancet Sedentary Behaviour Working Group. (2016) Does physical activity attenuate, or even eliminate, the detrimental association of sitting time with mortality? A harmonised meta-analysis of data from more than 1 million men and women. *The Lancet* 388: 1302–10.

Ekelund, U., Tarp, J., Steene-Johannessen, J., Hansen, B.H., Jefferis, B., Fagerland, M.W. et al. (2019) Dose-response associations between accelerometry measured physical activity and sedentary time and all-cause mortality: systematic review and harmonised meta-analysis. *British Medical Journal* 366: l4570. doi: 10.1136/bmj.l4570.

Exercise is Medicine. (2007) A programme launched by the American College of Sports Medicine and the American Heart Association [online], available at: https://exerciseismedicine.org/ (accessed 30 July 2019).

Gabel, L., Proudfoot, N.A., Obeid, J., Macdonald, M.J., Bray, S.R., Cairney, J. and Timmons, B.W. (2013) Count targets corresponding to new physical activity guidelines for the early years. *Medicine and Science in Sports and Exercise* 45: 314–18.

Garber, C.E., Blissmer, B., Deschenes, M.R., Franklin, B.A., Lamonte, M.J., Lee, I.-M. et al. (2011) American College of Sports Medicine Position Stand: quantity and quality of exercise for developing and maintaining cardiorespiratory, musculoskeletal, and neuromotor fitness in apparently healthy adults: guidance for prescribing exercise. *Medicine and Science in Sports and Exercise* 43: 1334–59.

Glazer, N.L., Lyass, A., Esliger, D.W., Blease, S.J., Freedson, P.S., Massaro, J.M. et al. (2013) Sustained and shorter bouts of physical activity are related to cardiovascular health. *Medicine and Science in Sports and Exercise* 45: 109–15.

Goodman, J.M., Thomas, S.G. and Burr, J. (2011) Evidence-based risk assessment and recommendations for exercise testing and physical activity clearance in apparently healthy individuals. *Applied Physiology, Nutrition and Metabolism* 36: S14–32.

Gordon-Larsen, P., Boone-Heinonen, J.E., Sidney, S., Sternfeld, B., Jacobs, D.R. and Lewis, C.E. (2009) Active commuting and cardiovascular risk: the CARDIA study. *Archives of Internal Medicine* 169: 1216–23.

Gregg, E.W., Cauley, J.A., Stone, K., Thompson, T.J., Bauer, D.C., Cummings, S.R. and Ensrud, K.E. (2003) Relationship of changes in physical activity and mortality among older women. *Journal of the American Medical Association* 289: 2379–86.

Hakim, A.A., Petrovitch, H., Burchfiel, C.M., Ross, G.W., Rodriguez, B.L., White, L.R. et al. (1998) Effects of walking on mortality among non-smoking retired men. *New England Journal of Medicine* 338: 94–9.

Hamer, M. and Chida, Y. (2008a) Active commuting and cardiovascular risk: a meta-analytic review. *Preventive Medicine* 46: 9–13.

Hamer, M. and Chida, Y. (2008b) Walking and primary prevention: a meta-analysis of prospective cohort studies. *British Journal of Sports Medicine* 42: 238–43.

Hardman, A.E., Lawrence, J.E.M. and Herd, S.L. (1998) Postprandial lipaemia in endurance-trained people during a short interruption to training. *Journal of Applied Physiology* 84: 1895–901.

Haskell, W.L. (1994) Health consequences of physical activity: understanding and challenges regarding dose-response. *Medicine and Science in Sports and Exercise* 26: 649–60.

Haskell, W.L., Lee, I.-M., Pate, R.R., Powell, K.E., Blair, S.N., Franklin, B.A. et al. (2007) Physical activity and public health: updated recommendation for adults from the American College of Sports Medicine and the American Heart Association. *Medicine and Science in Sports and Exercise* 39: 1423–34.

Heath, G.W., Parra, D.C., Sarmiento, O.L., Andersen, L.B., Owen, N., Goenka, S. et al. for the Lancet Physical Activity Series Working Group. (2012) Evidence-based intervention in physical activity: lessons from around the world. *Lancet* 380: 272–81.

Hildebrand, J.S., Gapstur, S.M., Campbell, P.T., Gaudet, M.M. and Patel, A.V. (2013) Recreational activity and leisure-time sitting in relation to postmenopausal breast cancer risk. *Cancer Epidemiology, Biomarkers and Prevention* 22: 1906–12.

Howard, B.J., Fraser, S.F., Sethi, P., Cerin, E., Hamilton, M.T., Owen, N. et al. (2013) Impact on hemostatic parameters of interrupting sitting with intermittent activity. *Medicine and Science in Sports and Exercise* 45: 1285–91.

Howley, E.T. (2001) Type of activity: resistance, aerobic and leisure versus occupational physical activity. *Medicine and Science in Sports and Exercise* 33: S364–9.

Jacobsen, P.L., Racioppi, F. and Rutter, H. (2009) Who owns the roads? How motorised traffic discourages walking and bicycling. *Injury Prevention* 15: 369–73.

Janssen, I. (2012) Health care costs of physical inactivity in Canadian adults. *Applied Physiology, Nutrition and Metabolism* 37: 803–6.

Jarrett, J., Woodcock, J., Griffiths, U.K., Chalabi, Z., Edwards, P., Roberts, I. and Haines, A. (2012) Effect of increasing active travel in urban England and Wales on costs to the National Health Service. *The Lancet* 379: 2198–205.

Järvinen, T.L.N., Sievänen, H., Kannus, P., Jokihaara, J. and Kahn, K.M. (2011) The true cost of pharmacological disease prevention. *British Medical Journal* 342: d2175. doi: 10.1136/bmj.d2175.

Katzmarzyk, P.T. (2011) Cost-effectiveness of exercise is medicine. *Current Sports Medicine Reports* 10: 217–23.

Katzmarzyk, P.T. and Janssen, I. (2004) The economic costs associated with physical inactivity and obesity in Canada: an update. *Canadian Journal of Applied Physiology* 29: 90–115.

Kelly, P., Murphy, M., Oja, P., Murtagh, E.M. and Foster, C. (2011) Estimates of the number of people in England who attain or exceed vigorous intensity exercise by walking at 3mph. *Journal of Sports Science* 29: 1629–34.

Kessler, H.S., Sisson, S.B. and Short, K.R. (2012) The potential for high intensity interval training to reduce cardiometabolic disease risk. *Sports Medicine* 42: 489–509.

King, D.S., Baldus, R.J., Sharp, R.L., Kesl, L.D., Feltmeyer, T.L. and Riddle, M.S. (1995) Time course for exercise-induced alterations in insulin action and glucose tolerance in middle-aged people. *Journal of Applied Physiology* 78: 17–22.

Lee, I.-M., Sesso, H.D., Oguma, Y. and Paffenbarger, R.S. (2004) The 'weekend warrior' and risk of mortality. *American Journal of Epidemiology* 160: 636–41.

Lee, I.-M., Sesso, H.D. and Paffenbarger, R.S. (2000) Physical activity and coronary heart disease risk in men: does the duration of episodes predict risk? *Circulation* 102: 981–6.

Lee, I.-M., Shiroma, E.J., Lobelo, F., Puska, P., Blair, S.N. and Katzmarzyk, P.T. for the Lancet Physical Activity Series Working Group. (2012) Effect of physical inactivity on major non-communicable diseases world-wide: an analysis of burden of disease and life expectancy. *Lancet* 380: 219–29.

Leitzmann, M.F., Park, Y., Blair, A., Ballard-Barbash, R., Mouw, T., Hollenbeck, A.R. and Schatzkin, A. (2007) Physical activity recommendations and decreased risk of mortality. *Archives of Internal Medicine* 167: 2453–60.

Manson, J.E., Greenland, P., LaCroix, A.Z., Stefanik, M.L., Mouton, C.P., Oberman, A. et al. (2002) Walking compared with vigorous exercise for the prevention of cardiovascular events in women. *New England Journal of Medicine* 347: 716–25.

Maresova, K. (2014) The costs of physical inactivity in the Czech Republic in 2008. *Journal of Physical Activity and Health* 11: 489–94.

Matthews, C.E., Jurj, A.L., Shu, X.O., Li, H.L., Yang, G., Li, Q. et al. (2007) Influence of exercise, walking, cycling and overall nonexercise physical activity on mortality in Chinese women. *American Journal of Epidemiology* 165: 1343–50.

Matthews, C.E., Xu, W.H., Zheng, W., Gao, Y.T., Ruan, Z.X., Cheng, J.R. et al. (2005) Physical activity and risk of endometrial cancer: a report from the Shanghai endometrial cancer study. *Cancer Epidemiology, Biomarkers and Prevention* 14: 779–85.

Mekary, R.A., Feskanich, D., Malspeis, S., Hu, F.B., Willett, W.C. and Field, A.E. (2009) Physical activity patterns and prevention of weight gain in premenopausal women. *International Journal of Obesity* 33: 1039–47.

Michie, S., Van Stralen, M.M. and West, R. (2011) The behaviour change wheel: a new method for characterising and designing behaviour change interventions. *Implementation Science* 6: 42. doi: 10.1186/1748-5908-6-42.

Miyashita, M., Burns, S.F. and Stensel, D.J. (2008) Accumulating short bouts of brisk walking reduces postprandial plasma triacylglycerol concentrations and resting blood pressure in healthy young men. *American Journal of Clinical Nutrition* 88: 1225–31.

Morris, J.N. (1994) Exercise in the prevention of coronary heart disease; today's best buy in public health. *Medicine and Science in Sports and Exercise* 26: 807–14.

Mummery, W.K. and Brown, W.J. (2009) Whole of community physical activity interventions: easier said than done. *British Journal of Sports Medicine* 43: 39–43.

Murphy, M.H. and Hardman, A.E. (1998) Training effects of short and long bouts of brisk walking in sedentary women. *Medicine and Science in Sports and Exercise* 30: 152–7.

Murphy, M.H., Lahart, I., Carlin, A. and Murtagh, E. (2019) The effects of continuous compared to accumulated exercise on health: a meta-analytic review. *Sports Medicine* 45: 1285–91.

Murphy, M.H., Nevill, A.M., Murtagh, E.M. and Holder, R.L. (2007) The effect of walking on fitness, fatness and resting blood pressure: a meta-analysis of randomised, controlled trials. *Preventive Medicine* 44: 377–85.

Murphy, M.H., Nevill, A.M., Neville, C., Biddle, S.J.H. and Hardman, A.E. (2002) Accumulating brisk walking for fitness, cardiovascular risk, and psychological health. *Medicine and Science in Sports and Exercise* 34: 1468–74.

Murtagh, E.M. and Murphy, M.H. (2011) Active travel to school and physical activity levels of Irish primary schoolchildren. *Pediatric Exercise Science* 23: 230–6.

Murtagh, E.M., Murphy, M.H. and Boone-Heinonen, J. (2010) Walking – the first steps in cardiovascular disease prevention. *Current Opinion in Cardiology* 25: 490–6.

Naci, H. and Ioannidis, J.P.A. (2013) Comparative effectiveness of exercise and drug interventions on mortality outcomes: metaepidemiological study. *British Medical Journal* 347: f5577. doi: 10.1136/bmj.f5577.

Nelson, M.E., Rejeski, J.W., Blair, S.N., Duncan, P.W., Judge, J.O., King, A.C. et al. (2007) Physical activity and public health in older adults: recommendation from the American College of Sports Medicine and the American Heart Association. *Medicine and Science in Sports and Exercise* 39: 1435–45.

O'Donovan, G., Lee, I.-M., Hamer, M. and Stamatakis, E. (2017) Association of 'weekend warrior' and other leisure time physical activity patterns with risks for all-cause, cardiovascular disease, and cancer mortality. *JAMA Internal Medicine* 177: 335–42.

Ogilvie, D., Foster, C.E., Rothnie, H., Cavill, N., Hamilton, V., Fitzsimons, C.F. and Mutrie, N. (2007) Interventions to promote walking: systematic review. *British Medical Journal* 334: 1204–14.

Orrow, G., Kinmonth, A.-L., Sanderson, S. and Sutton, S. (2012) Effectiveness of physical activity promotion based in primary care: systematic review and meta-analysis of randomised controlled trials. *British Medical Journal* 344: e1389. doi: 10.1136/bmj.e1389.

Park, S., Rink, L.D. and Wallace, J.P. (2006) Accumulation of physical activity leads to a greater blood pressure reduction than a single continuous session, in prehypertension. *Journal of Hypertension* 24: 1761–70.

Pate, R.R., Pratt, M., Blair, S.N., Haskell, W.L., Macera, C.A., Bouchard, C. et al. (1995) Physical activity and public health: a recommendation from the Centers for Disease Control and

Prevention and the American College of Sports Medicine. *Journal of the American Medical Association* 273: 402–7.

Patterson, R., McNamara, E., Tainio, M., Hérick de Sá, T., Smith, A.D., Sharp, S.J. et al. (2018) Sedentary behaviour and risk of all-cause, cardiovascular and cancer mortality, and incident type 2 diabetes: a systematic review and dose response meta-analysis. *European Journal of Epidemiology* 33: 811–29.

Pedersen, B.K. and Saltin, B. (2015) Exercise as medicine – evidence for prescribing exercise in 26 different chronic diseases. *Scandinavian Journal of Medicine and Science in Sports* 25 (Supplement 3): 1–72.

Pérusse, L., Rankinen, T., Hagberg, J.M., Loos, R.J.F., Roth, S.M., Sarzynski, M.A. et al. (2013) Advances in exercise, fitness, and performance genomics in 2012. *Medicine and Science in Sports and Exercise* 45: 824–31.

Physical Activity Guidelines Advisory Committee (2018) *2018 Physical activity guidelines advisory committee scientific report.* Washington, DC: U.S. Department of Health and Human Services.

Pratt, M., Norris, J., Lobelo, F., Roux, L. and Wang, G. (2014) The cost of physical inactivity: moving into the 21st century. *British Journal of Sports Medicine* 48: 171–3.

Rankinen, T., Roth, S.M., Bray, M.S., Loos, R., Pérusse, L., Wolfarth, B. et al. (2010) *Advances in exercise, fitness and performance genomics.* 42: 835–46.

Robertson, M.C., Gardner, M.M., Devlin, N., McGee, R. and Campbell, A.J. (2001) Effectiveness and economic evaluation of a nurse delivered home exercise programme to prevent falls. Part 2. Controlled trial in multiple centres. *British Medical Journal* 322: 701–4.

Rose, G. (1981) Strategy of prevention: lessons from cardiovascular disease. *British Medical Journal* 282: 1847–51.

Ruiz-Hermosa, A., Álvarez-Bueno, C., Cavero-Redondo, I., Martínez-Vizcaíno, V., Redondo-Tébar, A. and Sánchez-López, M. (2019) Active commuting to and from school, cognitive performance, and academic achievement in children and adolescents: a systematic review and meta-analysis of observational studies. *International Journal of Environmental Research and Public Health* 16: 1839–61.

Sallis, J.F., Floyd, M.F., Rodríguez, D.A., and Saelens, B.E. (2012) Role of built environments in physical activity, obesity, and cardiovascular disease. *Circulation* 125: 729–37.

Scarborough, P., Bhatnagar, P., Wickramasinghe, K.K., Allender, S., Foster, C. and Rayner, M. (2011) The economic burden of ill health due to diet, physical inactivity, smoking, alcohol and obesity in the UK: an update to 2006–07 NHS costs. *Journal of Public Health* 33: 527–35.

Staiano, A.E., Harrington, D.M., Barreira, T.V. and Katzmarzyk, P.T. (2014) Sitting time and cardiometabolic risk in US adults: associations by sex, race, socioeconomic status and activity level. *British Journal of Sports Medicine* 48: 213–19.

Stamatakis, E., Ekelund, U., Ding, D., Hamer, M., Bauman, A.E. and Lee, I.-M. (2019) Is the time right for quantitative public health guidelines on sitting? A narrative review of sedentary behaviour research paradigms and findings. *British Journal of Sports Medicine* 53: 377–82.

Stamatakis, E., Kelly, P., Strain, T., Murtagh, E.M., Ding, D. and Murphy, M.H. (2018) Self-rated walking pace and all-cause, cardiovascular disease and cancer mortality: individual participant pooled analysis of 50 225 walkers from 11 population British cohorts. *British Journal of Sports Medicine* 52: 761–8.

Swain, D.P. and Franklin, B.A. (2006) Comparison of cardioprotective benefits of vigorous versus moderate intensity aerobic exercise. *American Journal of Cardiology* 97: 141–7.

Thompson, P.D., Franklin, B.A., Balady, G.J., Blair, S.N., Corrado, D., Estes III, N.A. et al. (2007) Exercise and acute cardiovascular events placing the risks into perspective: a scientific statement from the American Heart Association Council on Nutrition, Physical Activity, and Metabolism and the Council on Clinical Cardiology. *Circulation* 115: 2358–68.

Tudor-Locke, C., Craig, C.L., Aoyagi, Y., Bell, R.C., Croteau, K.A., de Bourdeaudhuij, I. et al. (2011) How many steps/day are enough? For older adults and special populations. *International Journal of Behavioral Nutrition and Physical Activity* 8: 80–99.

US Department of Health and Human Services. (1996) *Physical Activity and Health: A Report of the Surgeon General*. Atlanta, GA: Centers for Disease Control and Prevention.

US Department of Health and Human Services. (2018) *2018 Physical Activity Guidelines for Americans 2nd Edition* [online], available at: https://health.gov/paguidelines/second-edition/pdf/ Physical_Activity_Guidelines_2nd_edition.pdf (accessed 31 July 2019).

US National Institutes of Health Consensus Development Panel. (1995) Physical activity and cardiovascular health: NIH consensus statement [online], December 18–20; 13(3): 1–33, available at: http://consensus.nih.gov/1995/1995ActivityCardivascularHealth101html.htm (accessed 17 May 2013).

Wen C.P. and Wu, X. (2012) Stressing harms of physical inactivity to promote exercise. *The Lancet* 380: 192–3.

Weuve, J., Kang, J.H., Manson, J.E., Breteler, M.M., Ware, J.H. and Grodstein, F (2004) Physical activity, including walking, and cognitive function in older women. *Journal of the American Medical Association* 292: 1454–61.

Whyte, L.J., Gill, J.M.R. and Cathcart, A.J. (2010) Effect of 2 weeks of sprint interval training on health-related outcomes in sedentary overweight/obese men. *Metabolism* 59: 1421–8.

Williams, M.A., Haskell, W.L., Ades, P.A., Amsterdam, E.A., Bittner, V., Franklin, B.A. et al. (2007) Resistance exercise in individuals with and without cardiovascular disease: 2007 update: a scientific statement from the American Heart Association Council on Clinical Cardiology and Council on Nutrition, Physical Activity, and Metabolism. *Circulation* 116: 572–84.

Wilmot, E.G., Edwardson, C.L., Achana, F.A., Davies, M.J., Gorely, T., Gray, L.J. et al. (2012) Sedentary time in adults and the association with diabetes, cardiovascular disease and death: systematic review and meta-analysis. *Diabetologia* 55: 2895–905.

Woodcock, J., Franco, O.H., Orsini, N. and Roberts, I. (2011) Non-vigorous physical activity and all-cause mortality: systematic review and meta-analysis of cohort studies. *International Journal of Epidemiology* 40: 121–38.

World Health Organization. (2018) Noncommunicable diseases factsheet [online], available at: https://www.who.int/news-room/fact-sheets/detail/noncommunicable-diseases (accessed 30 July 2019).

Yates, T., Edwardson, C.L., Celis-Morales, C., Biddle, S.J.H., Bodicoat, D., Esliger, D. et al. (2020) Metabolic effects of breaking up prolonged sitting with standing or light walking in older South Asians and white Europeans: a randomized acute study. *Journals of Gerontology. Series A, Biological Sciences and Medical Sciences* 75: 139–46.

Zheng, H., Ehrlich, F. and Amin, J. (2010) Economic evaluation of the direct healthcare cost savings resulting from the use of walking interventions to prevent coronary heart disease in Australia. *International Journal of Health Care Finance and Economics* 10: 187–201.

Zheng, H., Orsini, N., Amin, J., Wolk, A., Nguyen, V.T.T. and Ehrlich, F. (2009) Quantifying the dose–response of walking in reducing coronary heart disease risk: meta-analysis. *European Journal of Epidemiology* 24: 181–92.

Epilogue

Since the authors started writing this book the world has faced a major pandemic which has necessitated major societal change. COVID-19 is a respiratory infection caused by a newly discovered virus, severe acute respiratory syndrome coronavirus 2 (SARS-CoV-2). The outbreak began in Wuhan, China, in December 2019 (World Health Organization (WHO) 2021). Whilst most infected people recover without needing hospital treatment, about 15% become seriously ill and develop difficulty breathing (WHO 2020). The most common symptoms are fever, dry cough, tiredness and loss of taste and/or smell. As of 24 April 2021 (16 months after the disease emerged) it has been estimated that, worldwide, there have been more than 145 million COVID-19 cases and more than 3 million attributable deaths (Johns Hopkins University 2021).

The rapid spread of the disease is explained by its virulence and the fact that it can be spread by asymptomatic individuals. These characteristics caused governments in many countries to respond by placing populations into lockdown to decrease social interactions and hence transmission. A huge research effort began to identify the characteristics of those most severely affected by the virus. It quickly became clear that, although anyone can become infected with SARS-CoV-2, older adults and those with underlying health conditions are most likely to be severely incapacitated. Reports from the United States (Stokes et al. 2020) and from the UK (Docherty et al. 2020) noted a particularly high incidence of the disease in people who were in their seventies and eighties. Those with cardiovascular disease, diabetes, chronic lung disease and (in the UK study) chronic kidney disease were more likely to be admitted to hospital or to die than those without pre-existing disease. Men were more likely to be severely ill than women and people from ethnic minority groups were disproportionately affected. Once these important aspects of the risk of severe disease were established, older people and others who are particularly vulnerable were advised to shield in their homes.

Aside from advanced age and chronic disease, another major factor influencing the severity of COVID-19 is obesity. Epidemiological data have consistently identified obesity as a risk factor for a variety of outcomes related to COVID-19, in some cases as a very potent risk factor. One French study, for example, reported a seven-fold higher risk of invasive mechanical ventilation due to COVID-19 in patients with a BMI >35 kg m^{-2} compared with those with a BMI <25 kg m^{-2}, independent of age, diabetes and hypertension (Simonnet et al. 2020). A systematic review and meta-analysis involving 75 studies found that individuals with obesity had a greater risk of testing positive for COVID-19 (odds ratio 1.46). They also had a greater risk of hospitalisation (odds ratio 2.13), intensive care unit admission (odds ratio 1.74) and death (odds ratio 1.48) (Popkin et al. 2020).

Explanations for this enhanced risk include that obesity is associated with a chronic pro-inflammatory state, elevated oxidative stress and impaired immunity (Caci et al. 2020). Such a state may dysregulate innate and adaptive immune functions, leading to an aggressive inflammatory response and the 'cytokine storm' associated with COVID-19 fatalities (Hinchliffe et al. 2020). Excess ectopic fat deposition with obesity may be a 'unifying risk factor' for severe COVID-19 infection as detailed by Sattar and colleagues (2020). It is also associated with adverse effects on lung function, diminishing forced expiratory volume and forced vital capacity which, in turn, may contribute to a poor response to mechanical ventilation (Caci et al. 2020; Sattar et al. 2020).

So, what of the implications of this pandemic – and the consequences of enforced changes in behaviour – for physical activity? One might expect that the lockdowns enforced around the world would lead to reductions in levels of activity, and preliminary evidence suggests this to be the case. Tison and colleagues (2020) used data collected via a smartphone app to compare physical activity levels before and after the WHO declared COVID-19 to be a pandemic on 11 March 2020. They estimated that, based on findings in 187 countries, there was a 5.5% decrease in mean steps per day (287 steps) within ten days of the declaration and a 27.3% decrease (1,432 steps) within 30 days. Reductions in step counts were greater in countries which implemented more severe lockdowns; for example, there was a 48.7% maximal decrease in step counts in Italy compared with a 6.9% decrease in Sweden.

Whilst these data provide evidence for a global and worrying decrease in daily physical activity, the picture is far from simple and step counts alone do not describe the complexity of the behaviour changes occasioned by the pandemic. Many opportunities to be physically active were suspended when lockdowns closed essential infrastructure such as gyms, leisure centres, pools, sports pitches/courts and even public parks, shutting down most structured exercise and sport.

The impact on physical activity levels of children and adolescents is of particular concern. School closures removed what is for many their main daily opportunity to be active. Sport England surveyed physical activity behaviours in children at weekly, then monthly, intervals from the beginning of April (Sport England 2020). Whilst most children under 16 continued to do something to stay active during lockdown, the amount they did fell markedly – only about 20% were meeting national guidelines and a worrying 7% were doing nothing. Barriers to being active included lack of access to usual clubs and facilities (36%), local spaces/pitches (24%) and concerns about the virus (14%). An adverse impact of the COVID-19 outbreak on physical activity levels has also been documented among Canadian children and young people (Moore et al. 2020); based on a national sample of parents, only 4.8% of children (aged 5–11 years) and 0.6% of young people (aged 12–17 years) were found to be meeting recommendations.

At the other end of the lifespan, decreased opportunities for physical activity have profound consequences for older people because deconditioning quickly diminishes functional reserves, increasing the risk of failing to attain thresholds for independent living. As the epidemic took hold, older people and those with chronic health conditions were advised to 'shield' (UK) or 'shelter in place' (USA). Decline in function due directly to inactivity is likely to have been exaggerated by reduced access to rehabilitation services as well as sub-optimal management of chronic conditions. Data from Japan describe reductions in physical activity among older people during the pandemic. Yamada and colleagues (2020) reported that total physical activity time decreased by a median 65 minutes per week (26.5%) between January and April 2020. In earlier years, measures of physical activity were typically higher in April than in January, suggesting that the effect of the pandemic might be even more pronounced than these data show.

The Sport England survey referred to above reported changes in physical activity after lockdown among adults as well as children. In the early weeks, between 34% and 41% of adults reported doing less activity than pre-lockdown and this figure remained in this range through to mid-July (Sport England 2020). By contrast, initially 31%, rising to 35% reported doing *more* physical activity than pre-lockdown. Clearly, contrasting changes in exercise behaviour were occurring. One factor appears to have been that, in countries such as the UK and Australia, governments specified that going out to exercise was one of only four permitted reasons to leave the house – the others being to shop for food, for medical needs or for work if essential. As a general practitioner and vice-chairman of the Royal College of General Practitioners is reported to have said, 'The fact that people are limited to going out just for exercise is making them do it' (in Chandler-Wilde and Mintz 2020). Another factor is surely that infection risk is markedly lower outside than indoors so going out, say, walking meant that limited socialising (at a distance) was possible.

One activity that increased considerably during lockdown is cycling. Vivacity Labs recorded the number of cyclists on the roads of several cities across England; on 5 April 2020, for instance, bicycle traffic was around 250% higher than normal (Chandler-Wilde and Mintz 2020). In May, Cycling Scotland reported an increase in cycling of more than 300%, compared with 2019 (Bol 2020). A record-breaking number of people hired the so-called 'Boris bikes' during lockdown. According to Transport for London, more than two million were rented out in May and June 2020 (Morrison 2020). Collectively, these data show a surge in cycling in the UK, both for recreation and for personal transport. Contributory factors include quieter roads, the perceived need for exercise, more discretionary time, increased health awareness – and probably the warm weather. These factors may also explain the clear increase in the number of people reporting walking for exercise. Around 60% of adults in England reported walking for exercise throughout lockdown and continued to do so as lockdown began to be eased (Sport England 2020). Anecdotally, many more families are choosing to walk for exercise. Following 'unprecedented levels of cycling and walking' across the UK during the pandemic', UK government initiatives to encourage walking and cycling included protecting road space for cyclists and walkers and even issuing vouchers to help pay for repairs to old bicycles. Such policies aim to reduce pressure on public transport (Department of Transport 2020) – and thus diminish the risk of community infection.

The requirement 'to stay at home' focused attention on online/digital exercise regimens. Popular freely available classes have included Pilates, yoga and all-round body conditioning – all of which help people to remain active without leaving the house. As many as 43% of adults reported engaging in such activities during lockdown

(Sport England 2020). Practical guidelines on how to remain active, including through home-based activities, have been made available by bodies such as the American College of Sports Medicine, the Centres for Disease Control, the British Association for Sport and Exercise Medicine, the WHO and the Canadian Society for Exercise Physiology. Print media have also been a productive source of information on accessible home-based exercise programmes as health journalists took up the challenge.

An innovative Australian study used Google Trends data to assess physical activity-related social and lifestyle changes associated with the pandemic (Ding et al. 2020). Community interest was explored before and during COVID-19 outbreaks in Australia, the UK and the USA. The use of search terms related to exercise, such as 'workouts' and 'fitness training', was assessed between May 2019 and May 2020 (to take account of seasonal variation) and contrasted with those for 'television show', a common sedentary activity. Interest in exercise-related topics surged immediately after the lockdown, then declined but remained at a higher level than before the lockdown. Interest in 'television show' remained an overall more searched topic but the surge in interest in 'exercise' was so large that it surpassed 'television show' for the two weeks after the lockdown in Australia and in the UK. In another study, data from Garmin fitness trackers suggested that, despite step-count decreases during COVID-19, exercise, particularly indoor exercise, increased substantially (Stables 2020), in line with the Sport England Survey finding that 31% of adults questioned actually reported more physical activity than pre-lockdown (Sport England).

So, is COVID-19 going to exacerbate an existing 'pandemic' of inactivity (Hall et al. 2020) or 'nudge' people to be more active (Ding et al. 2020)? If the former then, bearing in mind the many and varied links between physical activity and health highlighted in this book, lasting decreases in physical activity levels provide a significant challenge to the maintenance of metabolic health (King et al. 2020) – and maybe in the years to come if such a trend continues. If the latter, public health initiatives should capitalise on the increased awareness of and interest in physical activity to promote active lifestyles post COVID-19 (Ding et al. 2020). Of course, these effects are not mutually exclusive, and the pandemic may polarise changes in physical activity behaviours in different sections of society.

A different and important question is, 'Might a high habitual level of physical activity pre-infection limit the severity of illness due to COVID-19?' A definitive answer will require further research but emerging evidence from the UK Biobank study suggests that physical inactivity is a risk factor for hospitalisation due to COVID-19 (Hamer et al. 2020). In this study physical inactivity was associated with a 32% higher risk (relative risk 1.32) while the co-existence of multiple unhealthy factors (physical inactivity, smoking, obesity and heavy alcohol consumption) was associated with a 441% higher risk (relative risk 4.41). These findings are preliminary and observational but they raise the possibility that being physically active might lessen disease severity in those who become infected with SARS-CoV-2, possibly due to amelioration of the chronic low-grade inflammation often seen in those who are physically active (Hamer et al. 2020).

Another issue requiring clarification is the prescription of exercise/physical activity for individuals who have been infected with SARS-CoV-2. When can they start exercising again? Does physical activity facilitate recovery and/or rehabilitation from the disease? Should recovering patients be encouraged to exercise and, if so, how much should they do? The answer to these questions will depend on disease severity and the existence of other health conditions. Of crucial importance is the finding that COVID-19 can have adverse effects on the heart including acute myocardial injury, myocarditis and cardiac arrhythmias (Driggin et al. 2020). Exercise during the acute phase of COVID-19 could accelerate viral replication and increase inflammation, exacerbating these adverse effects (Phelan et al. 2020). Cardiac damage may be detectable and cardiac function may be impaired even in patients who have recovered from COVID-19 (Puntmann et al. 2020). Further research is required to answer these questions and many others including whether regular exercise will improve the immune response to a COVID-19 vaccine. Such questions are the tip of the iceberg and the call by Sallis and colleagues (2020) for an international physical activity and public health research agenda to inform COVID-19 policies and practices is pertinent and timely.

It should be clear from this brief Epilogue that the contents of this book are of fundamental importance and relevance to the current pandemic. So much could be said about COVID-19 in relation to every chapter in this book and to do so comprehensively would require another book! The relationship between chronic diseases (including cardiovascular disease, diabetes and obesity) and the severity of COVID-19 reinforces the importance of physical activity as preventative behaviour for these conditions and as a means of maintaining cardio-metabolic health. Likewise, the role of physical activity in children's health and healthy ageing takes on added significance, as does the potential of physical activity to alleviate the mental health challenges created by COVID-19. Consideration is required of the potential adverse consequences of physical activity for those infected with or recovering from COVID-19 but most importantly the current pandemic emphatically reinforces the potential health benefits that may be gained by the implementation of public health policies to promote and enhance physical activity levels worldwide.

REFERENCES

Bol, D. (2020) Coronavirus in Scotland: huge rise in cycling to escape lockdown blues. *The Herald*, 13 April. Available at: https://www.heraldscotland.com/news/18377069.coronavirus-scotland-huge-rise-cycling-escape-lockdown-blues/ (accessed 18 September 2020).

Caci, G., Albini, A., Malerba, M., Noonan, D.M., Pochetti, P. and Polosa, R. (2020) COVID-19 and obesity: dangerous liaisons. *Journal of Clinical Medicine* 9: 2511. doi.org/10.3390/jcm9082511.

Chandler-Wilde, H. and Mintz, L. (2020). The surprising health benefits of the coronavirus lockdown. *The Telegraph*, 18 May. Available at: https://www.telegraph.co.uk/health-fitness/body/surprising-health-benefits-coronavirus-lockdown/ (accessed 18 September 2020).

Department of Transport (2020) Two billion package to create new era for cycling and walking. Available at: https://www.gov.uk/government/news/2-billion-package-to-create-new-era-for-cycling-and-walking (accessed 18 September 2020).

Ding, D., del Pozo, B., Green, M.A. and Bauman, A.E. (2020) Is the COVID-19 lockdown nudging people to be more active: a big data analysis. *British Journal of Sports Medicine* Epub ahead of print: doi: 10.1136/bjsports-2020-102575.

Docherty, A.B., Harrison, E.M., Green, C.A., Hardwick, H.E., Pius, R., Norman, L. et al. on behalf of the ISARIC4C investigators. (2020) Features of 20,133 UK patients in hospital with covid-19 using the ISARIC WHO Clinical Characterisation Protocol: prospective observational cohort study *British Medical Journal* 369: doi: 10.1136/bmj.m1985.

Driggin, E., Madhavan, M.V., Bikdeli, B., Chuich, T., Laracy, J., Biondi-Zoccai, G. et al. (2020) Cardiovascular considerations for patients, health care workers, and health systems during the COVID-19 pandemic. *Journal of the American College of Cardiology* 75: 2352–71.

Hall, G., Laddu, D.R., Phillips, S.A, Lavie, C.J. and Arena, R. (2020) A tale of two pandemics: how will COVID-19 and global trends in physical inactivity and sedentary behaviour affect one another? *Progress in Cardiovascular Diseases* 64: 108–10. doi:10.1016/jcad.2020.04.005.

Hamer, M., Kivimäki, M., Gale, C.R. and Batty, G.D. (2020) Lifestyle risk factors, inflammatory mechanisms and COVID-19 hospitalisation: a community-based cohort study of 387,109 adults in the UK. (2020) *Brain, Behavior and Immunity* 87: 184–7. doi:10.1016/j.bbi.2020.05.059.

Hinchliffe, N., Bullen, V., Haslam, D. and Feenie, J. (2020) COVID-19 and obesity. *Practical Diabetes* 37: 149–51.

Johns Hopkins University (2021) Coronavirus Resource Centre. Available at: https://coronavirus.jhu.edu/map.html (accessed 24 April 2021).

King, A.J., Burke, L.M., Halson, S.L. and Hawley, J.A. (2020) The challenge of maintaining metabolic health during a global pandemic. *Sports Medicine* 50: 1233–41.

Moore, S.A., Faulkner, G., Rhodes, R.E., Brussoni, M., Chulak-Bozzer, T., Ferguson, L.J. et al. (2020) Impact of the COVID-19 virus outbreak on movement and play behaviours of Canadian children and youth: a national survey. *International Journal of Behavioral Nutrition and Physical Activity* 17: 85.

Morrison, S. (2020) Coronavirus crisis sparks huge surge in London cycle hire as 2 million people pick up 'Boris Bikes'. *Evening Standard*, 29 July. Available at: https://www.standard.co.uk/news/transport/cycle-hire-london-boris-bikes-spike-coronavirus-crisis-a4512006.html (accessed 18 September 2020).

Phelan, D., Kim, J.H. and Chung, E.H. (2020) A game plan for the resumption of sport and exercise after coronavirus disease 2019 (COVID-19) infection. *Journal of the American Medical Association Cardiology*: doi: 10.1001/jamacardio.2020.2136.

Popkin, B.A., Du, S., Green, W.D., Beck, M.A., Algaith, T., Herbst, C.H. et al. (2020) Individuals with obesity and COVID-19: a global perspective on the epidemiology and biological relationships. *Obesity Reviews* 21: e13128. doi: 10.1111/obr.13128.

Puntmann, V.O., Carerj, L., Wieters, I., Fahim, M., Arendt, C., Hoffmann, J. et al. (2020) Outcomes of cardiovascular magnetic resonance imaging in patients recently recovered from coronavirus disease 2019 (COVID-19) *Journal of the American Medical Association Cardiology* 5: 1265–73. doi: 10.1001/jamacardio.2020.3557.

Sallis, J.F., Adlakha, D., Oyeyemi, A. and Salvo, D. (2020) An international physical activity and public health research agenda to inform coronavirus disease-19 policies and practices. *Journal of Sport and Health Science* 9: 328–34.

Sattar, N., McInnes, I.B. and McMurray, J.J.V. (2020) Obesity a risk factor for severe COVID-19 infection: multiple potential mechanisms. *Circulation* 142: 4–6.

Simonnet, A., Chetboun, M., Poissy, J., Raverdy, V., Noulette, J., Duhamel, A. et al. on behalf of the LICORN and the Lille COVID-19 and Obesity study group. (2020) High prevalence of obesity in severe acute respiratory syndrome coronavirus-2 (SARS-CoV-2) requiring invasive mechanical ventilation. *Obesity* 28: 1195–9.

Sport England (2020) COVID-19 Briefing: exploring attitudes and behaviours in England during the COVID-19 pandemic. Available at: https://indd.adobe.com/view/793b48d5-bbcd-4de3-a50f-11d241a506b3 (accessed 18 September 2020).

Stables, J. (2020) Garmin data reveals how the world is working out during the lockdown. Wareable, 11 April. Available at: https://www.wareable.com/garmin/garmin-data-lockdown-7940 (accessed 18 September 2020).

Stokes, E.K., Zambrano, L.D., Anderson, K.N., Marder, E.P., Raz, K.M., Felix, S.E.B. et al. (2020) Coronavirus disease 2019 case surveillance – United States, January 22–May 30, 2020. *Morbidity and Mortality Weekly Report* 69: 759–65.

Tison, G.H., Avram, R., Kuhar, P., Abreau, S., Marcus, G.M., Pletcher, M.J. and Olgin, J.E. (2020) Worldwide effect of COVID-19 on physical activity: a descriptive study. *Annals of Internal Medicine*. doi: 10.7326/M20-2665.

World Health Organization (2020) Coronavirus disease (COVID-19) What happens to people who get COVID-19? Available at: https://www.who.int/news-room/q-a-detail/coronavirus-disease-covid-19 (accessed 21 May 2021).

World Health Organization (2021) Q and A on coronaviruses (COVID-19). Available at: https://www.who.int/emergencies/diseases/novel-coronavirus-2019/question-and-answers-hub/q-a-detail/q-a-coronaviruses (accessed 4 March 2021).

Yamada, M., Kimura, Y., Ishiyaa, D., Otobe, Y., Suzuki, M., Koyama, S. et al. (2020) Effect of the COVID-19 epidemic on physical activity in community-dwelling older adults in Japan: a cross-sectional online survey. *Journal Nutrition and Health in Aging* 24: 948–50. doi: 10.1007/s12603-020-1423-2.

GLOSSARY

Abdominal fat Fat on the trunk of the body between the waist and the diaphragm.

Accelerometer A device that senses motion in one or more planes. It yields a count of movements in arbitrary units.

Accuracy The extent to which measured values reflect the true values.

Acute biological response Physiological or metabolic changes arising from a single session of exercise.

Adiponectin A hormone and adipokine which helps to regulate glucose and fat breakdown and which has anti-atherogenic and anti-inflammatory properties.

Adventitia External layer of an artery or vein.

All-cause mortality Death from any cause.

Amenorrhoea Absence of menses. Primary amenorrhoea – normal menses never established; secondary amenorrhoea – cessation of menses after these were established.

Angina Severe but temporary attack of cardiac pain.

Angiogenesis Development of new blood vessels.

Anorexia nervosa A common psychological illness. There is minimal food intake, leading to loss of weight and sometimes death from starvation.

Anxiety Feelings of apprehension, worry or fear accompanied by somatic symptoms (e.g. increased respiration, muscle tension) and behavioural responses (e.g. avoidance, pacing).

Anxiety disorder A category of mental disorders in which anxiety is the predominant feature including generalised anxiety disorder, agoraphobia, panic disorder, social anxiety disorder and specific phobias.

Apoptosis Active ('programmed') cell death.

Arteriovenous difference for oxygen The difference between the oxygen content of arterial and mixed venous blood. This indicates how much oxygen has been extracted from arterial blood and utilised (predominantly) by muscle. Often written as $(a - \bar{v})$ O_2 diff.

Asthma Episodic obstruction of airway resulting from inflammation and characterised by cough, wheeze and breathlessness.

Atherosclerosis A progressive disease that leads to hardening and thickening of the walls of arteries and to narrowing of these vessels.

Atrial fibrillation An abnormal heart rhythm resulting from disorganised electrical impulses in the atria.

β-hydroxyacyl-CoA dehydrogenase   The rate-limiting enzyme in the mitochondrial β-oxidation pathway.

Bias   Error that produces results that differ in a systematic manner from the true values.

Body mass index   Body mass (in kilograms) divided by height (in metres) squared, i.e. body mass (kg)/height (m)^2. Used as a measure of obesity.

Bone mineral density (BMD)   The mass of bone mineral per unit area of volume.

Bronchitis   A lung disease characterised by excessive mucus production in the bronchial tree, causing coughing to get rid of sputum. Small airways become inflamed and narrowed and mucus may occlude small bronchi.

Bulimia nervosa   Self-induced vomiting after meals.

Calcification   The deposit of calcium salts within a tissue.

Cancer   A set of diseases characterised by unregulated cell growth leading to invasion of surrounding tissues and spread to other parts of the body.

Carcinogen   Agent capable of causing cancer.

Carcinogenesis   Processes involved in the development of a cancer.

Cardiomyopathy   Disorder of the heart muscle of unknown aetiology.

Case-control study   A study comparing the occurrence of a possible cause/risk factor between cases (people with a disease or other outcome variable) and suitable controls (unaffected by the disease or outcome variable).

Case-report or case-series   A study describing the characteristics of a patient or number of patients with a specific disease or attribute.

Cerebrovascular disease   Stroke.

Cholesterol   A steroid molecule necessary for the synthesis of steroid hormones and bile salts and an integral component of cell membranes.

Cholesterol esters   Cholesterol in combination with long chain fatty acids, i.e. esterified.

Chronic obstructive pulmonary disease (COPD)   Progressive, sometimes partially reversible, airflow obstruction that does not vary over a long period. Predominantly caused by cigarette smoking that results in emphysema, chronic bronchitis and small airways disease.

Chylomicron   A lipoprotein, its main function is the transport of dietary fat (triglyceride) to adipose tissue and muscle.

Citrate synthase   An enzyme involved in oxidative metabolism within the mitochondria. One of the enzymes in Kreb's cycle.

Claudication   The primary symptom of peripheral vascular disease which is defined as walking-induced pain in one or both legs (primarily the calves).

Clustering   Co-exist more commonly than would be expected by chance.

Cohort study   A study in which a group of people (a cohort), free of disease, are followed up to see how the development of new cases of the disease (or other outcome) differs between subgroups of the cohort classified according to their exposure to a potential cause/risk factor.

Confounding   A factor associated both with an exposure (for example, physical activity) and the outcome being studied which, if unequally distributed between the exposure subgroups, may confuse the findings. This distorts the estimated exposure effect.

Coronary angioplasty   A procedure to open up a blocked artery using a catheter.

Coronary artery bypass graft   A procedure to bypass a blocked coronary artery using a healthy artery or vein.

Coronary collaterals   Additional blood vessels that may grow in the heart, enhancing coronary blood flow.

Correlational study   A study describing relationships between potential risk factors and a disease (or other outcome). Populations or groups are the units of analysis, rather than individuals.

Cortical bone   Dense, strong bone that forms the outer covering of bone, and shaft of long bones.

C-reactive protein   A protein made in the liver and released into the bloodstream in response to inflammation.

Cytotoxic   Toxic to cells.

Depressive disorder   A mood disorder characterised by low mood and/or loss of interest along with associated symptoms such as appetite or weight changes, fatigue, sleep or psychomotor changes, feelings of worthlessness or guilt, cognitive problems, suicidal thoughts.

Diabetes insipidus   A disease caused by a low secretion of vasopressin (antidiuretic hormone, ADH) from the pituitary gland and hence a low rate of reabsorption of water in the kidneys.

Diabetes mellitus   A disease characterised by either an inability of the pancreas to secrete insulin (type 1 diabetes) or an inability of the cells to respond to insulin (type 2 diabetes).

Diabetic foot   An informal term for the damage caused by microvascular disease of the extremities. Tissue damage leads to pain and, in severe cases, can lead to the need for amputation.

Diaphysis (plural diaphyses)   Shaft of long bones.

Disability   Restriction or lack of ability to perform an activity in a manner or within the range considered normal for a human being.

Dyslipidaemia   Abnormal concentrations in the blood of plasma lipoprotein lipids.

Dyspnoea   Uncomfortable sensation of breathlessness, difficulty in breathing or laboured breathing.

Dose–response   The relationship between level of exposure to a factor such as physical activity and the response to this in terms of health (or disease) outcome.

Dual energy X-ray absorptiometry (DXA)   An X-ray-based technique that provides 2-D scans for measuring body composition and areal bone mineral density.

Effect modification   The magnitude or direction of the association under study differs according to the level of another factor.

Effect size   A statistic used to determine whether a difference between two means (different groups or same group in different conditions) is sufficiently large to be considered meaningful.

Emphysema   A lung disease characterised by enlargement of air spaces distal to the terminal bronchiole, with destruction of their walls. Parts of the capillary bed are destroyed.

Endosteum   The inner lining of bone that faces the bone marrow.

Endothelial function Ability of the endothelium to invoke vasodilation or vasoconstriction by interacting with vascular smooth muscle.

Epidemiology The study of the distribution and determinants of health-related states or events in specified populations, and the application of this study to control of health problems.

Euglycaemic clamp technique Also known as the 'hyperinsulinaemic euglycaemic clamp' or the 'glucose clamp'. A technique used to determine insulin sensitivity by measuring how much glucose the body can dispose of (via oxidation and storage) in response to a fixed insulin concentration.

Eumenorrhoea Normal menses, 10–13 cycles per year.

Excess post-exercise oxygen consumption (EPOC) The elevation in oxygen consumption above resting levels which occurs after an acute bout of exercise.

Exercise snacking The completion of multiple smaller bouts of exercise throughout the day rather than a single larger bout of exercise.

Experimental study A study in which researchers attempt to change a variable in one or more groups. Also called an intervention study.

Exposure A measure of an individual's experience or 'dose' of a specified risk factor. (Exposure has two dimensions, level and duration; for physical activity it depends not only on the level of activity but also on number of years during which an individual has engaged in physical activity.)

Fat-free mass Total body mass minus fat mass.

Fibrillation Rapid uncoordinated contraction or twitching of cardiac muscle.

Fibrinogen A plasma protein, the precursor of fibrin.

Fibrinolysis The breakdown of fibrin in blood clots.

Flow-mediated dilation (FMD) Vasodilation in response to the increased shear stress on the endothelium when blood flow is increased.

Free radical A highly chemically reactive molecule or molecular fragment that can damage cellular components such as DNA and lipid-rich membranes.

Generalisability The extent to which results are applicable to different populations.

Gluconeogenesis The synthesis of glucose from non-carbohydrate sources including pyruvate, lactate, glycerol and amino acids.

Glucose tolerance The ability of the body to respond to the ingestion of glucose. Usually determined using the blood glucose concentration measured at the 2-h point in an oral glucose tolerance test.

GLUT4 An insulin-sensitive receptor located on membranes of cells in muscle and adipose tissue, which aids in the transport of glucose across the membrane into the cell.

Glycated haemoglobin (HbA1c) Haemoglobin which is chemically linked to glucose and provides a measure of average blood glucose levels over the previous three months.

Glycosuria The presence of excessive amounts of glucose in the urine.

Gonadotrophins Hormones that control the endocrine functions of the gonads (ovaries in women, testes in men).

Haemorrhagic Due to a haemorrhage (bleed).

HbA1c See glycated haemoglobin.

Health status Disease-specific quality of life (a concept), usually measured with questionnaires.

Heart failure   The inability of the heart to pump blood at a sufficient rate to meet the metabolic demands of the body.

High-density lipoproteins   Species of lipoproteins that, amongst other functions, promote the removal of excess cholesterol from cells in a process termed reverse cholesterol transport.

Hyperglycaemia   Abnormally high concentration of glucose in the blood.

Hyperinsulinaemia   Abnormally high concentration of insulin in the blood.

Homocysteine   A sulphur-containing amino acid, high plasma concentrations of which may be associated with an increased risk of cardiovascular disease.

Hypertension   Abnormally high arterial blood pressure.

Hypertrophic cardiomyopathy   A familial cardiac disease characterised morphologically by an enlarged and non-dilated left ventricle.

Hypotension   Abnormally low arterial blood pressure.

Hypothermia   Abnormally low deep body temperature.

Incidence   The number of new events/cases that develop in a defined population during a specified time interval.

Infarction   Death of a section of tissue because the blood supply has been cut off, as in myocardial infarction (heart attack).

Insulin-dependent diabetes mellitus   Alternative name for type 1 diabetes.

Insulin resistance   A loss of sensitivity to the effects of insulin.

Insulin sensitivity   A measure of how effectively the cells remove glucose from the blood in response to insulin.

Intima   Internal layer of a blood vessel.

Intima media thickness (IMT)   Measurement of the thickness of the intima and media layers of the arterial wall most commonly assessed using ultrasound. Carotid IMT is used as a surrogate indicator of subclinical atherosclerosis in the carotid artery.

Ischaemic   Impaired blood flow.

Isokinetic   Movement at a constant speed or angular velocity.

Ketoacidosis   A life-threatening situation in which an excess of ketone bodies leads to an increase in the acidity (reduction in pH) of the blood.

Ketogenesis   The formation of ketone bodies.

Kyphosis   Excessive flexion of the spine.

Leukocytes   White blood cells that help defend the body against pathogens and remove toxins, waste and damaged cells at sites of infection or injury.

Lipolytic   Chemical breakdown of fat by enzymes.

Lipoproteins   Macromolecular complexes composed of lipid and protein, responsible for transporting triglycerides and cholesterol in the blood.

Low-density lipoprotein   The main carrier of cholesterol in the blood, responsible for delivering cholesterol to the cells.

Lumen   The central space within an artery through which blood flows.

Lymphoma   Tumour of lymphatic tissue.

Macrophages   Cells that scavenge foreign bodies and cell debris.

Magnetic resonance imaging (MRI)   A non-invasive imaging technology which can produce three-dimensional anatomical images.

Maximal oxygen uptake   The highest rate of oxygen uptake reached when there is little or no further increase (plateau) in oxygen uptake despite an increase in exercise intensity during a maximal exercise test. Expressed either in absolute terms (units $l\ min^{-1}$) or relative to body mass (ml $kg^{-1}\ min^{-1}$). Sometimes predicted from heart rate and oxygen uptake during submaximal exercise. Used as a marker for aerobic/endurance fitness.

Media   Middle layer of a blood vessel.

Mental disorder   A psychiatric illness involving changes in mood, thinking or behaviour and impairment of personal or occupational functioning.

Mental health   A state of psychological wellbeing that involves realising potential, coping with normal life stressors, working productively and contributing to community.

MET   Metabolic equivalent of task. A multiple of the resting metabolic rate. One MET is defined as the energy requirement at rest, designated as an oxygen uptake of 3.5 ml $kg^{-1}\ min^{-1}$.

Meta-analysis   The statistical analysis of a collection of analytic results for the purpose of integrating the findings.

Metastasis   Process by which cancers escape to other parts of the body.

Metformin   A drug used in the treatment of type 2 diabetes.

Microalbuminuria   A measure of the urinary protein albumin which is recognised as an early sign of vascular damage in the heart and kidneys.

Mutation   A heritable change in DNA.

Myocardial perfusion   The extent to which blood suffuses the muscle of the heart.

Nitric oxide   A gas released by endothelial cells which acts as a vasodilator.

Non-enzymatic glycation   A process whereby glucose molecules are bound to proteins to form glycoproteins.

Non-esterified fatty acids   Fatty acids not combined with glycerol in triglyceride.

Non-insulin-dependent diabetes mellitus   Alternative term for type 2 diabetes. An imprecise term since insulin is required by some individuals with type 2 diabetes.

Odds ratio   The ratio of the odds (likelihood) of exposure to the variable of interest in one group to the odds of exposure to this variable in another group.

Oligomenorrhoea   Infrequent menstruation, cycle prolonged beyond 35 days.

Oncogenes   A gene whose protein product contributes to carcinogenesis.

Osteoarthritis   A condition characterised by joint pain and deterioration that becomes more prevalent with age.

Osteoblasts   Cells that produce bone matrix to build new bone.

Osteoclasts   Cells responsible for bone resorption, removing old bone.

Osteocytes   Mature bone cells which may be involved in activation of bone turnover and regulation of extracellular calcium.

Osteomalacia   Demineralisation of the mature skeleton, with softening of the bone and bone pain.

Osteopenia   Lower than average bone mineral density.

Osteoporosis   A condition characterised by low bone mineral density and generalised skeletal fragility, leading to fractures with minimal trauma.

Pandemic   An epidemic of disease that has spread across a large region, such as multiple continents, affecting a substantial number of people.

Pathophysiology   The deranged physiological processes associated with disease.

Peak oxygen uptake   The highest rate of oxygen uptake recorded during an exercise test to volitional exhaustion. This term is often used instead of 'maximal oxygen uptake' as a marker for aerobic/endurance fitness when a plateau in oxygen uptake is not attained or cannot be verified at voluntary exhaustion. Expressed either in absolute terms (units $l\ min^{-1}$) or relative to body mass ($ml\ kg^{-1}\ min^{-1}$).

Peripheral vascular disease A disease caused by narrowing of peripheral arteries which compromises blood flow.

Plaques Complicated atheromatous lesions that are raised and obstruct blood flow.

Plasminogen A zymogen or proenzyme, the inactive precursor of plasmin.

Plasminogen activator inhibitor-1 Plasma constituent that inhibits fibrinolysis by opposing the conversion of plasminogen to plasmin.

Platelets Cell fragments in the blood that contain enzymes and other substances important for clotting.

Platelet aggregation The tendency for blood platelets to stick together.

Population-attributable risk The incidence of a disease or characteristic in a population that is associated with an exposure to a risk factor. Describes the relative importance of an exposure for that population.

Postprandial After a meal.

Precision The extent to which the same measurements, when repeated, yield the same values. Also called repeatability.

Prevalence The number of cases in a defined population at a specified point in time.

Primary care First level contact with the health-care system (in UK, with general practitioners).

Primary prevention Prevention of the development of disease in healthy people.

Procoagulant Leading to formation of a blood clot.

Quantitative computed tomography (QCT) An X-ray-based technique that images slices of bone, allowing a 3D representative and measurement of volumetric bone mineral density.

Relative risk The ratio of occurrence of a disease (or other outcome) among exposed people to that among the unexposed.

Repeated measures An experimental design where measurements are repeated on the same individuals in different conditions.

Resistant hypertension Hypertension that is poorly responsive to treatment and requires the use of multiple medications to achieve acceptable blood pressure ranges.

Resorption The breaking down of bone into soluble constituents.

Resting metabolic rate The energy expenditure at rest after an overnight fast and eight hours of sleep.

Rhabdomyolysis Sporadic appearance in blood of abnormal levels of myoglobin, indicative of muscle damage.

Rheumatic heart disease Damage to the myocardium due to rheumatic fever.

Rickets A disorder of calcium and phosphate metabolism, associated with deficiency of vitamin D, and beginning most often in infancy and early childhood. It leads to softening and bending of the long weight-bearing bones.

Risk difference The (absolute) difference in rates of occurrence between exposed and unexposed groups.

Sarcoma Cancer of connective tissues.

Secondary prevention Decrease in the risk of mortality and further morbidity in patients with existing disease.

Sedentary behaviour   Any waking behaviour characterised by an energy expenditure ≤ 1.5 metabolic equivalents (METs), while in a sitting, reclining or lying posture.

Sensitivity (of clinical tests)   The proportion of true positives that are correctly identified by the test.

Shear stress   The force exerted on the endothelium by blood flow.

Specificity (of clinical tests)   The proportion of true negatives that are correctly identified by the test.

Stenoses   Narrowing, for example of coronary vessels due to atherosclerosis.

Statistical power   The ability of a study to detect a specified (often 'clinically important') difference, i.e. the probability of rejecting the null hypothesis when this is in fact false and should be rejected. It depends on sample size, and on the level of significance chosen.

Stoichiometry   Calculation of quantitative relationships between the reactants and products in a chemical reaction. The mathematics of chemistry.

Strain   Deformation of a material, measured as the change in dimension produced by force, divided by the original dimension. One unit of 'strain' is thus equivalent to a one percent change.

Subcutaneous abdominal fat   Abdominal fat stored under the skin.

Succinate dehydrogenase   An enzyme involved in oxidative metabolism within the mitochondria. One of the enzymes in Kreb's cycle.

Syndrome   A group of symptoms which, occurring together, produce a pattern typical of a particular disease.

Thermic effect   Increase in energy expenditure. For example, the thermic effect of food is the increase in energy expenditure due to digestion, absorption and storage of food; the thermic effect of activity is the increase in energy expenditure due to physical activity.

Thromboembolytic   Due to the formation of a thrombus (blood clot) that has blocked a blood vessel.

Thrombosis   Formation of a blood clot.

Thrombus   A blood clot.

Trabeculae   Curved plates and rods organised to withstand the particular forces to which each part of a bone is normally subjected. They confer bone's essential property of 'strength with lightness'.

Trabecular bone   Spongy bone made up of a three-dimensional lattice-work of trabeculae (always enclosed in a hard outer crust of cortical bone). It has more surface area and a more active metabolism than cortical bone.

Training effect   An adaptive response to training, not merely a short-term biological response to a single session of exercise.

Triglyceride   A lipid molecule composed of glycerol and three fatty acids that is the storage form of fat in the body. From a biochemical perspective, it is correctly called triacylglycerol but the term triglyceride is still widely used, particularly in the clinical literature.

Tumour   A swelling or growth, i.e. a mass of tissue which fulfils no useful purpose and which grows at the expense of the body. It can be benign or cancerous.

Type I (alpha) error   Rejecting the null hypothesis when this is true, i.e. finding an effect when there is none (a 'false positive').

Type II (beta) error   Accepting the null hypothesis when this is false, i.e. failing to find an effect when one is there (a 'false negative').

Validity   The extent to which a study measures what it purports to measure.

Vascular conductance   The ease with which blood flows through a circulation (or vascular bed) at a given pressure difference (the reciprocal of resistance).

Vascular resistance   The hindrance to blood flow in a circulation (or a vascular bed) at a given pressure difference (the reciprocal of conductance).

Visceral fat   Fat stored within the abdominal cavity.

Waist circumference   The preferred surrogate marker for abdominal obesity.

Waist-hip ratio   The ratio of waist circumference to hip circumference, used as a surrogate marker for abdominal obesity.

INDEX